STEDMAN'S

RADIOLOGY & ONCOLOGY WORDS

SECOND EDITION

Edited by
Catherine S. Baxter, CMT

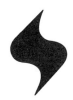

Stedman's

RADIOLOGY & ONCOLOGY
WORDS

SECOND EDITION

Including:
HIV-AIDS
Hematology

Williams & Wilkins

BALTIMORE • PHILADELPHIA • HONG KONG
LONDON • MUNICH • SYDNEY • TOKYO

A WAVERLY COMPANY

Series Editor: Elizabeth B. Randolph
Associate Managing Editor: Maureen Barlow Pugh
Editor: Catherine S. Baxter, CMT
Illustration Planner: Ray Lowman
Production Coordinator: Barbara J. Felton
Cover Design: Reuter & Associates

Copyright © 1995
Williams & Wilkins
351 W. Camden St
Baltimore, Maryland 21201-2436, USA

Printed in the United States of America

First Editions 1993

Library of Congress Cataloging-in-Publication Data

Stedman's radiology & oncology words: including HIV-AIDS, hematology/ edited by Catherine S. Baxter.—2nd ed.
  p. cm.—(Stedman's word book series)
  Developed from the database of Stedman's medical dictionary and supplemented by terminology found in current medical literature.
  Includes bibliographical references.
  ISBN 0-683-07966-2
1. Radiology—Terminology. 2. Radiography, Medical—Terminology. 3. Diagnosis, Radioscopic—
Terminology. 4. Oncology—Terminology. I. Baxter, Catherine S. II. Stedman, Thomas Lathrop, 1853-1938.
Medical dictionary. III. Series. IV. Series: Stedman's word books.
  [DNLM: 1. Radiology—terminology. 2. Medical Oncology—terminology. 3. Hematology—terminology.
4. HIV Infections—terminology. WN 15 S8115 1995].
RC78.A3S74 1995
616.07'57'014—dc20
DNLM/DLC
for Library of Congress   95-24138
                                                                                                                  CIP

97 98 99
3 4 5 6 7 8 9 10

Contents

PREFACE TO THE SECOND EDITION vii

ACKNOWLEDGMENTS ix

EXPLANATORY NOTES xi

A-Z WORD LIST 1

APPENDICES A1

   1. Radiographic Anatomy and Positioning A2

   2. Contrast Media A14

   3. AIDS Laboratory Tests A18

   4. AIDS-Related Drugs A20

   5. Chemotherapy Protocols A22

   6. Cancer Classification/Grading/Staging Systems A49

   7. National Cancer Institute (NCI)-designated
      Comprehensive Cancer Centers A52

Preface to the Second Edition

The question is inevitable. "Why did you put radiology and oncology words together in one book?" What at first glance seems like an odd couple really is the perfect match.

Although most patients undergoing radiologic procedures have relatively straightforward diagnostic imaging requirements, oncology patients receive comprehensive diagnosis, treatment, and followup care for a prolonged period of time. The depth of their evaluations can be measured by the width and weight of their charts, literally. Much of the volume of a cancer patient's chart comprises imaging reports that serially follow the course of the patient's treatment.

From the start, most cancer patients do not have all "normal" diagnostic imaging reports. One "abnormal" report leads to a multitude of additional diagnostic procedures ranging from the basic flat plate of the abdomen to radioisotope scanning to locate an occult metastasis. In addition, complex oncologic therapy protocols require frequent imaging studies for documentation of the patient's response to treatment. Rarely is an oncology report of any type dictated without mention of at least one diagnostic imaging report.

Have I answered the original question, "Why radiology and oncology?" I think they go hand-in-hand to provide a comprehensive one-stop guide to radiology and oncology terminology.

Each specialty was researched and compiled separately as if for an expanded second edition of its respective first edition Stedman's Word Book. Then, the terms from both specialties were blended into one A-Z format to serve the needs of radiology and oncology transcriptionists and other healthcare professionals.

This allowed us to provide more information for less money. More for less . . . what a refreshing concept! Since most of us work with our reference books adjacent to our PCs, the goal was to provide coverage of two specialties that could be accessed with one hand and at one economical price.

Williams & Wilkins has proven time and time again that it is dedicated to educating and assisting those professionals in a variety of healthcare-related professions, whose income is derived from the language of medicine. We really do have an industry supporter in Williams & Wilkins.

Many thanks go to the editors, contributors, and support personnel from Williams & Wilkins who once again combined forces to prepare *Stedman's Radiology & Oncology Words, Second Edition.*

In addition, I would like to dedicate this book to the memory of Robert Love, whose love of and respect for the profession of medical transcription was an inspiration to me. His warmth, concern, commitment, and guidance will be missed by all and forgotten by none.

Catherine S. Baxter, CMT

Acknowledgments

An important part of our editorial process is the involvement of medical transcriptionists—as advisors, reviewers and/or editors.

A special thank you goes to Catherine Baxter CMT, who in her usual style dedicated herself to the job of proofing the first edition of *Stedman's Oncology Words*, editing the new manuscript, and compiling the appendices for this second edition. Thanks also to Connie Davis who proofread the first edition of *Stedman's Radiology Words* and reviewed the new radiology terms we added to this second edition. Judy Johnson, CMT did an excellent job of editing the list of all the new oncology terms for this edition and reviewing the appendices.

Thanks also go to our *Stedman's Radiology & Oncology Words* MT Editorial Advisory Board, consisting of Darla Haberer CMT, Janet Christie Pugh CMT, Beth Tribelhorn CMT, and Janet Kelly. These medical transcriptionists served as editors and advisors, and spent hours perusing texts, journals, and manufacturer's information to compile the latest terms in interventional and diagnostic radiology, oncology, AIDS, and hematology.

Other important contributors to this revised edition include: Janice Deal RN, BSN, Marilyn Grebin, Deloris Hedge CMT, Theresa Lamberson CMT, Helen Littrell CMT, Averill Ring CMT, Linda Stewart, Donna Taylor, and Robin McRae Wasley, all of whom gathered new words and/or provided invaluable suggestions. Once again, Barb Ferretti did a terrific job updating the database.

As with all our Stedman's word references, we have benefited from the suggestions and expertise of our many contacts in the medical transcriptionist community. Thanks to all our advisory board participants, reviewers and editors, AAMT meeting attendees, and others who have written in with requests and comments—keep talking, and we'll keep listening.

Explanatory Notes

Users of the first editions of *Stedman's Radiology Words* and *Stedman's Oncology Words* will notice the merging of these two word books for this second edition. In this "combined" word book, we have edited, updated, and expanded the radiology and oncology content from the first editions. *Stedman's Radiology & Oncology Words, Second Edition*, offers an authoritative assurance of quality and exactness to the wordsmiths of the health care professions—medical transcriptionists, medical editors and copy editors, health information management personnel, court reporters, and the many other users and producers of medical documentation.

Stedman's Radiology & Oncology Words, Second Edition, can be used to validate both the spelling and the accuracy of terminology specific to radiology, oncology, HIV and AIDS, and hematology. The user will find the following radiology-specific topics: diagnostic and interventional radiology terms, radiographic anatomy, and the modalities of radiology—plain film/x-ray, nuclear medicine, computed tomography (CT), magnetic resonance imaging (MRI), and ultrasound radiology. Radiographic findings and radiopharmaceuticals are also covered.

Oncology-related topics include: chemotherapy, radiation oncology, surgical therapy, molecular cell biology, gynecologic oncology, tumors, and anticancer drug names. In addition, the user will find listed thousands of drugs, protocols, diagnostic and therapeutic procedures, new techniques and maneuvers, and lab tests, as well as equipment, instrument, and device names. Abbreviations and acronyms are also included. For quick reference, lists of contrast media, AIDS laboratory tests, AIDS-related drugs, chemotherapy protocols, and cancer classification/grading/staging systems appear in appendices at the back of the book.

Because our goal has been to provide a comprehensive yet streamlined reference tool, we have omitted terminology that is not specific to these specialties. Thus, some terms (such as anatomy and physiology terms) that are often dictated in these specialties are not included in this text, as they can be found in general medical dictionaries.

This compilation of over 54,500 entries, fully cross-indexed for quick access, was built from a base vocabulary of over 32,800 medical words, phrases, abbreviations, and acronyms. The extensive A-Z list was developed from the database of *Stedman's Medical Dictionary* and supplemented by terminology found in current medical literature (please see list of References on page xv).

Medical transcription is an art as well as a science. Both are needed to correctly interpret a physician's dictation, whose language is a product of education, training, and experience. This variety in medical language means that there are several acceptable ways to express certain terms, including jargon. This second edition of *Stedman's Radiology & Oncology Words* provides variant spellings and phrasings for many terms. This, in addition to complete cross-indexing, makes *Stedman's Radiology & Oncology Words, Second Edition,* a valuable resource for determining the validity of terms as they are encountered.

Alphabetical Organization

Alphabetization of entries is letter by letter as spelled, ignoring punctuation, spaces, prefixed numbers, Greek letters, or other characters. For example:

acid-fast staining methods
acid formaldehyde hematin
α-acid glycoprotein
acid hematin

In subentries, the abbreviated singular form or the spelled-out plural form of the noun main entry word is ignored in alphabetization.

Format and Style

All main entries are in **boldface** to speed up location of a sought-after entry, to enhance distinction between main entries and subentries, and to relieve the textual density of the pages.

Irregular plurals and variant spellings are shown on the same line as the singular or preferred form of the word. For example:

alveolus, pl. **alveoli**

disk, disc

Possessives
Possessive forms have been dropped in this reference for the sake of consistency and to conform to the guidelines outlined by the American Association for Medical Transcription (AAMT) and other groups. It should be noted, however, that retaining the possessive is a question of style, not of accuracy, and thus is a matter of choice. To form the possessive of a word, simply add the apostrophe or apostrophe "s" to the end of the word.

Cross-indexing
The word list is in an index-like main entry-subentry format that contains two combined alphabetical listings:

(1) A *noun* main entry-subentry organization typical of the A-Z section of medical dictionaries like **Stedman's:**

catheter
  Broviac c.
  central venous c.
  femoral arterial c.
  Foley c.
  Groshong c.

lymphadenopathy
  angioblastic l.
  angioimmunoblastic l.
  axillary l.
  benign l.
  dermatopathic l.

(2) An *adjective* main entry-subentry organization, which lists words and phrases as you hear them. The main entries are the adjectives or modifiers in a multi-word term. The subentries are the nouns around which the terms are constructed and to which the adjectives or modifiers pertain:

percutaneous
  p. aspiration
  p. biopsy
  p. cholecystostomy
  p. enterostomy

diffuse
  d. abdominal calcification
  d. air space disease
  d. alveolar hemorrhage
  d. bacterial nephritis

This format provides the user with more than one way to locate and identify a multi-word term. For example:

cyst
    bone c.

bone
b. cyst

pattern
    band p.
    bull's-eye p.
    centrum semiovale p.

bull's-eye
b.-e. analysis
b.-e. lesion
b.-e. pattern

It also allows the user to see together all terms that contain a particular descriptor as well as all types, kinds, or variations of a noun entity. For example:

leukemia
    chronic neutrophilic l.
    l. cutis
    embryonal l.
    feline l.
    l. inhibitory factor

Wherever possible, abbreviations are separately defined and cross-referenced. For example.

PID
    pelvic inflammatory disease

pelvic
    p. inflammatory disease (PID)

disease
    pelvic inflammatory d. (PID)

References

In addition to the manufacturers' literature we gather at various medical meetings, scientific reports from hospitals, and our MT Editorial Advisory Board members' word lists (from their daily work transcription), we used the following sources for new words for *Stedman's Radiology & Oncology Words, Second Edition:*

Ang K. Radiotherapy for head and neck cancers: indications and techniques. Baltimore: Williams & Wilkins, 1994.

Bartlett JG. The Johns Hopkins Hospital guide to medical care of patients HIV infection. 3rd ed. Baltimore: Williams & Wilkins, 1994.

Broder S. Textbook of AIDS medicine. Baltimore: Williams & Wilkins, 1994.

Callen PW. Ultrasonography in obstetrics & gynecology 3ed. Philadelphia: WB Saunders, 1993.

Cope C. Current techniques in interventional radiology. Philadelphia: Current Medicine, 1993.

Dahnert W. Radiology review manual. 2nd ed. Baltimore: Williams & Wilkins, 1993.

De Lorenzo B. Oncologic word book. Springhouse, PA: Springhouse Corporation, 1992.

Dorland's Hematology/Oncology speller. Philadelphia: WB Saunders, 1993.

Khaw BA. Monoclonal antibodies in cardiovascular diseases. Baltimore: Williams & Wilkins, 1993.

Littrell H. Immunologic and AIDS word book. Springhouse, PA: Springhouse Corporation, 1992.

Littrell H. The oncology word book. Philadelphia: FA Davis, 1993.

Evaluation and management of early HIV infection. Leverett, MA: Rector Pr., Ltd., 1994.

Pizzo P. Pediatric Aids: the challenge of HIV infection in infants, children, and adolescents 2nd ed. Baltimore: Williams & Wilkins, 1994.

Pugh J. The radiology transcriptionist's quick reference guide. Columbus, GA, 1991.

Rao K. MRI and CT of the spine. Baltimore: Williams & Wilkins, 1993.

Sartoris. Principles of shoulder imaging, 1994.

Stedman's medical dictionary. 26th ed. Baltimore: Williams & Wilkins, 1995.

Stedman's oncology words. Baltimore: Williams & Wilkins, 1993.

Stedman's radiology words. Baltimore: Williams & Wilkins, 1993.

Tollison CD. Handbook of pain management. 2nd ed. Baltimore: Williams & Wilkins, 1994.

Clinical practice guideline #9: management of cancer pain. Rockville, MD: US Department of Health and Human Services, 1994.

Journals

American Journal of Neuroradiology. Oakbrook, IL: American Society of Neuroradiology, 1994.

Cancer. Philadelphia: J.B. Lippincott Company, 1992–1995.

Contemporary Oncology. Montvale, NJ: Medical Economics, 1992–1994.

Emergency Radiology: A Journal of Practical Imaging. Baltimore: Williams & Wilkins, 1994.

Journal of Contemporary Oncology. Philadelphia: WB Saunders Company, 1992–1995.

Magnetic Resonance in Medicine. Baltimore: Williams & Wilkins, 1994.

Radiation Therapist. Albuquerque: American Society of Radiologic Technologists, 1994.

The Radiologist. Baltimore: Williams & Wilkins, 1994.

Your Medical Word Resource Publisher

We strive to provide you with the most up-to-date and accurate word references available. Your use of this word book will prompt new editions, which will be published as often as justified by updates and revisions. We welcome your suggestions for improvements, changes, corrections, and additions—whatever will make this *Stedman's* product more useful to you. Please use the postpaid card at the back of this book and send your recommendations to the Reference Division at Williams & Wilkins.

A

A 1 segment
A 2 segment

63178A

GR 63178A

A$_2$

hemoglobin A$_2$

AACR

American Association for Cancer Research

AAS

atomic absorption spectrophotometry

Abbe-Zeiss counting cell
Abbokinase catheter
ABC

avidin-biotin complex

ABCD

amphotericin B colloidal dispersion

abdomen

acute a.
gasless a.
scaphoid a.

abdominal

a. abscess
a. abscess drainage catheter
a. adenopathy
a. adhesion
a. air collection
a. aneurysm
a. angina
a. aorta
a. aortic aneurysm
a. aortography
a. biopsy
a. cavity
a. diffuse calcification
a. distention
a. fibromatosis
a. great vessel
a. hemorrhage
a. hysterectomy
a. irradiation
a. lymph node biopsy
a. mass
a. pain
a. plain film
a. roentgenography
a. sonography

a. space
a. strip radiotherapy
a. trauma
a. vascular calcification
a. wall calcification
a. wall defect
a. wall desmoid tumor
a. wall hernia

abdominis

rectus a.
rectus a. musculocutaneous flap
rectus a. myocutaneous flap

abdominopelvic

a. cavity
a. mass

abdominoperineal resection
abdominosacral resection
abducent nerve
abduction
abduction-external rotation fracture
abductor

a. muscle

Abelson murine leukemia virus
Abernethy sarcoma
aberrant

a. intrahepatic bile duct
a. right subclavian artery
a. subclavian artery

ABH

Ativan, Benadryl, Haldol
ABH blood group carbohydrate antigen

ABH/Lewis-related antigen
ABH(O) cell surface antigen
ABI

ankle-brachial index

ability

tumor-targeting a.

ABL

acute basophilic leukemia

abl

abl oncogene
abl proto-oncogene

ablation

adrenal a.
androgen a.
ethanol a.
marrow a.
organ a.

ablation *(continued)*
  ovarian a.
  parathyroid tumor a.
  percutaneous ethanol a.
  percutaneous tumor a.
  renal cyst a.
  a. therapy
  thyroid nodule a.
  tumor a.
ablative neurosurgery
ABMR
  autologous bone marrow rescue
ABMS
  autologous bone marrow support
ABMT
  allogeneic bone marrow
    transplant
  autologous bone marrow
    transplant
abnormal
  a. fetal urogenital tract
  a. staining
abnormality
  arterial blood gas a.
  bladder congenital a.
  breast a.
  caliceal a.
  cardiopulmonary a.
  chromosomal a.
  congenital a.
  diverticulation a.
  endocrine a.
  extremity a.
  facial a.
  figure-of-eight a.
  focal limb a.
  growth a.
  histopathologic a.
  immune function a.
  intracranial vascular a.
  labeling a.
  limb a.
  limb reduction a.
  nonpalpable a.
  nuclear a.
  nuclear membrane a.
  osseous a.
  protein-binding a.
  rostrocaudal extent signal a.
  snowman a.
  spinal cord injury without
    radiographic a.
    (SCIWORA)

  taste a.
  urachal a.
  vascular a.
  vertebral border a.
  vertebral endplate a.
abnormally
  a. contracting regions
  a. thin skull
ABO
  ABO blood group
  ABO incompatibility
abortion
  inevitable a.
  missed a.
  spontaneous a.
  threatened a.
abortive
  a. calyx
  a. neurofibromatosis
abortive neurofibromatosis
abortus
above-knee amputation
ABOV protocol
ABPA
  acute bronchopulmonary asthma
ABPAP
  avidin-biotin-peroxidase-
    antiperoxidase
Abrams biopsy needle
abrasion
  cortical a.
  subperiosteal cortical a.
A/B ratio
  apnea/bradycardia ratio
Abrodil
abruptio
  placenta a.
  a. placentae
abruption
  placental a.
abscess
  abdominal a.
  amebic a.
  anchovy paste a.
  annular a.
  aortic annulus a.
  appendiceal a.
  brain a.
  breast a.
  Brodie a.
  candidal a.
  chocolate sauce a.
  chronic breast a.

diverticular a.
a. drainage
epidural a.
frontal a.
granulomatous a.
hepatic a.
iliac fossa a.
intraperitoneal a.
intrascrotal a.
liver a.
lung a.
mediastinal a.
orbital a.
ovarian a.
pancreatic a.
parapharyngeal a.
paraspinal a.
parotid a.
pelvic a.
pericholecystic a.
perinephric a.
perirenal a.
pharyngeal a.
premasseteric space a.
pyogenic a.
renal a.
retropharyngeal a.
scrotal a.
soft tissue a.
space of Retzius a.
spinal epidural a.
splenic a.
sternal a.
subdiaphragmatic a.
subhepatic a.
subphrenic a.
testicular a.
thyroid a.

tuboovarian a.
ventral epidural a.
abscission needle
absent kidney
absolute
a. blood flow
a. curative resection
a. dose intensity (ADI)
a. ethanol
a. linearity
a. noncurative resection
absorbed dose
absorber
Hollister wound exudate a.
absorptiometry
dual-energy x-ray a. (DXA)
dual-photon a. (DPA)
single photon a.
absorption
a. coefficient
drug a.
electromagnetic a.
laser energy a.
photoelectric a.
radiofrequency a.
abuse
intravenous drug a. (IVDA)
ABV
Adriamycin, bleomycin,
vinblastine
ABVD
Adriamycin, bleomycin,
vinblastine, dacarbazine
AC
Adriamycin, cyclophosphamide
Acacia
Skiodan A.

NOTES

acalculia
acalculous cholecystitis
acantholytic dermatosis
acanthosis
    glycogen a.
    a. nigricans
acardia
ACBE
    air contrast barium enema
accelerated
    a. fractionation
    a. phase
    a. phase gain
acceleration
    fetal growth a.
    fetal heart rate a.
    growth a.
accelerator
    dual-energy linear a.
    a. factor
    high-energy a.
    linear a. (LINAC)
    particle a.
accentuation
    paramagnetic
      enhancement a.
access
    central venous a.
    hemodialysis a.
    translumbar a.
    vascular a.
    venous a.
accessioning
accessory
    a. adhesion molecule
    a. fissure
    a. hemidiaphragm
    a. hepatic vein
    a. lobe
    a. middle cerebral artery
    a. muscle
    a. nerve
    a. ossicle
    a. ossification center
    a. spleen
accident
    cerebrovascular a. (CVA)
accordion
    a. catheter
    a. vertebra
accreta
    placenta a.
accrual plan

Accucore II biopsy needle
accumulative phase
AccuProbe
Accutane
ACE
    Adriamycin, cyclophosphamide,
      etoposide
    angiotensin-converting enzyme
    ACE inhibitor
acemannin
    lyophilized a.
acervuloma
acetabula (*pl. of* acetabulum)
acetabular
    a. cavity
    a. fossa
    a. fracture
    a. posterior wall fracture
    a. protrusion
    a. residual dysplasia
    a. rim fracture
    a. roof
acetabuli
    protrusio a.
acetabulum, pl. acetabula
    Y-shaped a.
acetaminophen
acetanilide
acetate
    cellulose a.
    cortisone a.
    cyproterone a.
    depo-medroxyprogesterone a.
      (DMPA)
    goserelin a.
    leuprolide a. (LA)
    leuprorelin a.
    manganese a.
    medroxyprogesterone a.
      (MPA)
    megestrol a.
    methylprednisolone a.
acetazolamide
acetic
acetone
acetorphine
acetrizoate
acetrizoic acid
N-acetylaspartate (NAA)
acetylation
    histone a.
acetylator
acetylcholine

acetylsalicylic acid
acetyltransferase
    chloramphenicol a. (CAT)
achalasia
    cricopharyngeal a.
achievable
    as low as reasonably a.
    (ALARA)
Achilles
    A. tendon
    A. tendon reflex test
achlorhydria
    watery diarrhea,
    hypokalemia, a. (WDHA)
achondrogenesis
achondroplasia
    heterozygous a.
    homozygous a.
    hyperplastic a.
achondroplastic dwarfism
achoresis
achrestic anemia
achromic erythrocyte
achylic anemia
acid
    acetrizoic a.
    acetylsalicylic a.
    all-trans-retinoic a. (ATRA)
    amidotrizoic a.
    aminocaproic a.
    ε-aminocaproic a.
    arachidonic a.
    benzoic a.
    bile a.
    chenodeoxycholic a.
    cis-retinoic a.
    13-cis-retinoic a. (13-CRA)
    conjugated lineoleic a.
    cyclohexenediaminete-
      traacetic a. (CDTA)
    deoxyribonucleic a. (DNA)
    diatrizoic a.
    diethylenetriamine
      pentaacetic a. (DTPA)
    dihydroxybenzohydrox-
      amic a. (DIDOX)

    diisopropyliminodiacetic a.
      (DISIDA)
    dimercaptosuccinic a.
      (DMSA)
    dimethyl iminodiacetic a.
    eicosapentaenoic a.
    epsilon-aminocaproic a.
      (EACA)
    erucic a.
    ethacrynic a.
    ethylenediaminetetraacetic a.
      (EDTA)
    flavone acetic a. (FAA)
    flufenamic a.
    fluoro-6-thia-heptadecanoic a.
    folic a.
    folinic a.
    gadolinium
      cyclohexanediaminete-
      traacetic a. (Gd-CDTA)
    gadolinium-diethylenetriamine
      pentaacetic a. (Gd-DTPA)
    gadolinium
      ethylenediaminete-
      traacetic a. (Gd-EDTA)
    gadolinium
      tetraazacyclododecanete-
      traacetic a. (Gd-DOTA)
    gadopentetic a.
    glutaric a.
    glycyrrhetinic a.
    hepatic 2,6-
      dimethyliminodiacetic a.
      (HIDA)
    hippuric a.
    homocholic a.
    homocysteic a.
    hyaluronic a.
    4-
      hydroperoxy-
      cyclophosphamide a.
    hydroperoxyeicosatetrae-
      noic a. (HPETE)
    5-hydroxyindoleacetic a. (5-
      HIAA)
    iminodiacetic a. (IDA)
    iobenzamic a.

NOTES

5

acid *(continued)*
    iobutoic a.
    iocarmic a.
    iodamic a.
    iodoalphionic a.
    iodoxamic a.
    ioglicic a.
    ioglycamic a.
    iopanoic a.
    iophenoic a.
    iophenoxic a.
    ioprocemic a.
    iopronic a.
    iosefamic a.
    ioseric a.
    iosumetic a.
    ioteric a.
    iothalamic a.
    iotroxic a.
    ioxaglic a.
    ioxithalamic a.
    iozomic a.
    ipodic a.
    lipid-associated sialic a.
    long-chain fatty a.
    meclofenamic a.
    mefenamic a.
    metrizoic a.
    nitriloacetic a.
    nucleic a.
    okadaic a.
    oleic a.
    p-aminobenzoic a.
    a. phosphatase
    phosphonoformic a.
    pleural-fluid hyaluronic a.
    polylactic a.
    propanoldiaminotetraacetic a.
      (PDTA)
    prostanoic a.
    retinoic a.
    ribonucleic a. (RNA)
    serum methylmalonic a.
    sialic a.
    technetium-99m
      dimercaptosuccinic a.
    a. test
    tetraazacyclododecanete-
      traacetic a. (DOTA)
    thromboanoic a.
    tranexamic a.
    trans-retinoic a. (TRA)
    trichloracetic a.
    triiodobenzoic a.
    tyropanoic a.
    uric a.
    ursodeoxycholic a.
    valproic a.
    vanillylmandelic a. (VMA)

acid-base disorder

acidemia
    isovaleric a.
    methylmalonic a.

acid-fast
    a.-f. bacillus
    a.-f. stain

acidophilic adenoma

acidosis
    lactic a.
    metabolic a.
    renal tubular a.

acid-Schiff
    periodic a.-S. (PAS)
    a.-S. stain

acinar
    a. adenocarcinoma
    a. carcinoma
    a. cell carcinoma
    a. pattern
    a. sarcoidosis

acinarization

Acinetobacter lwoffi

acinic
    a. cell adenocarcinoma
    a. cell carcinoma
    a. cell tumor

acinus, pl. **acini**

acivicin

Ackermann needle

aclacinomycin A

aclarubicin

aclasis
    diaphyseal a.
    tarsoepiphyseal a.

acne
    propionibacterium a.

ACNU
    nimustine

acoustic
    a. canal
    a. enhancement
    a. gel
    a. imaging
    a. impedance
    a. lens
    a. meatus

a. nerve
a. nerve sheath tumor
a. neurinoma
a. neuroma
a. noise
a. pressure
a. pressure amplitude
a. response technology (ART)
a. schwannoma
a. shadow
a. velocity
a. wave
acoustical shadowing
acquired
a. agammaglobulinemia
a. drug resistance
a. hemolytic anemia
a. hepatocerebral degeneration
a. ichthyosis
a. immunity
a. immunodeficiency syndrome (AIDS)
a. renal cystic disease
a. spinal stenosis
acquisition
continuous volumetric a.
gradient a.
interleaved a.
a. matrix
multiple gated a. (MUGA)
spoiled gradient-recalled a.
a. time
a. window
acral
a. erythema
a. lentiginous melanoma
acrania
acridine orange
acridinyl anisidide
acrocephalosyndactyly
acrodermatitis enteropathica
acrokeratosis
paraneoplastic a.
acrolein
acromegaly

acromelia
acromelic
a. dwarfism
a. dysplasia
acromicria
acromioclavicular
a. joint
a. joint separation
a. space
acromion
hooked a.
a. process
acromioplasty
acroosteolysis
familial a.
idiopathic a.
acropachy
thyroid a.
acrylic microsphere
ACS
American Cancer Society
Act
CARE A.
Comprehensive AIDS Resources Emergency Act
Comprehensive AIDS Resources Emergency A. (CARE Act)
Ryan White CARE A.
ACT-D
actinomycin D
ACTII
adrenocorticotropic hormone
ACTH-producing adenoma
Actimmune
actin
muscle a.
muscle-specific a. (MSA)
a. protein
smooth muscle a. (SMA)
actinic
a. granuloma
a. keratosis
a. reticuloid
actinomycin D (ACT-D)
actinomycosis

NOTES

action
    drug a.
activated partial thromboplastin time (APTT)
activation
    a. associated antigen
    cell a.
    a. factor
    functional a.
    intracellular a.
    lyl-1 oncogene a.
    lyt-10 oncogene a.
    oncogene a.
    T-lymphocyte a.
activator
    lymphocyte a.
    tissue plasminogen a.
    urokinase-type
      plasminogen a.
active
    a. immunity
    a. immunization
    a. nonspecific
      immunotherapy
    a. shield
    a. shimming
    a. specific immunotherapy
activities of daily living (ADL)
activity
    antiviral a.
    blood pool a.
    bone morphogenetic a.
    burst-promoting a.
    downsloping a.
    endogenous biotin a.
    endogenous peroxidase a.
    erythroid a.
    immunoradiometric assay of
     antigen a.
    intrinsic tyrosine kinase a.
    lymphotoxin antitumor a.
    mast cell-enhancing a.
    peristaltic a.
    rotamase a.
    sexual a.
    veto a.
actuarial survival
acuity
acuminata
    condylomata a.
acuminatum
    condyloma a.
    papilloma a.

Acuson linear array transducer
acuta
    pityriasis lichenoides et
      varioliformis a. (PLEVA)
acute
    a. abdomen
    a. allergic extrinsic alveolitis
    a. anaphylaxis
    a. basophilic leukemia
      (ABL)
    a. bronchopulmonary asthma
      (ABPA)
    a. cholecystitis
    a. diffuse bacterial nephritis
    a. disseminated
      encephalomyelitis
    a. diverticulitis
    a. eosinophilic leukemia
    a. erythroblastic leukemia
    a. flank pain
    a. focal bacterial nephritis
    a. fracture
    a. granulocytic leukemia
    a. hepatitis
    a. interstitial nephritis
    a. lethal carditis
    a. leukemia
    a. lymphoblastic leukemia
      (ALL)
    a. lymphoblastic lymphoma
    a. lymphocytic leukemia
      (ALL)
    a. lymphoid leukemia
    a. megakaryoblastic
      leukemia
    a. megakaryocytic leukemia
    a. mixed lineage leukemia
    a. monoblastic leukemia
    a. monocytic leukemia
    a. myeloblastic leukemia
    a. myelocytic leukemia
      (AML)
    a. myelofibrosis
    a. myelogenous leukemia
      (AML)
    a. myeloid leukemia (AML)
    a. myelomonocytic leukemia
    a. myocardial infarction
    a. neuropathy
    a. nonlymphoblastic
      leukemia (ANLL)
    a. nonlymphocytic leukemia
      (ANLL)

a. nonlymphoid leukemia
a. nonsuppurative ascending cholangitis
a. pancreatitis
a. progranulocytic leukemia
a. promyelocytic leukemia (APL)
a. respiratory distress syndrome (ARDS)
a. retroviral syndrome
a. splenic tumor
a. suppurative ascending cholangitis
a. suppurative sialadenitis
a. suppurative thyroiditis
a. testicular torsion
a. traumatic aortic injury (ATAI)
a. tubular necrosis
acyanotic heart disease
acyclic metal chelate complex
acyclovir
a. sodium
acylated SK-plasminogen complex
acyl hypofluorite
AD
doxorubicin, dacarbazine
ADA
adenosine deaminase
Adagen
adamantinoma
Adamkiewicz
arteries of A.
A. artery
Adams-Stokes syndrome
Adam syndrome
Adapin
adaptation
adapted standard mammography unit
adapter
Christmas tree a.
Luer-Lok a.
Rutner nephroscopy a.
SafeTrak epidural catheter a.
Tuohy-Borst a.

adaptive correction
adaptogen
ADC
AIDS dementia complex
analog-to-digital converter
ADCC
antibody-dependent cell cytotoxicity
addictive androgen
Addis count
Addison
A. disease
A. syndrome
Addison-Biermer anemia
additive
Hemo-Dial dialysate a.
additivity
mode I a.
mode II a.
adduction
adductor
a. brevis
a. canal
a. hallucis
a. longus
a. magnus
a. pollicis
a. tubercle
adductus
metatarsus a.
adenectomy
adenine
a. arabinoside
a. phosphoribosyl transferase
adenitis
mesenteric a.
sclerosing a.
adenoacanthoma
adenoassociated virus
endometrial a.
adenocarcinoma
acinar a.
acinic cell a.
ampullary a.
bronchiolar a.
cervical a.
ciliated cell a.

NOTES

adenocarcinoma *(continued)*
    Clara cell a.
    clear cell a.
    cystic a.
    duct cell a.
    endometrial secretory a.
    gastrointestinal tract a.
    hepatoid a.
    intraluminal a.
    kidney a.
    Klatskin biliary a.
    Lucké a.
    mesonephric a.
    metastatic a.
    a. of Moll
    mucin-producing a.
    mucoid a.
    pancreatic a.
    papillary a.
    renal a.
    secretory a.
    serous a.
    a. in situ
    stomach a.
    a. of uterus
    vulvar adenoid cystic a.
    a. with squamous
      differentiation
adenofibroma
adenofibromyoma
adenoid
    a. cystic carcinoma
    a. squamous cell carcinoma
    a. tumor
adenoleiomyofibroma
adenolipoma
adenoma
    acidophilic a.
    ACTH-producing a.
    adnexal a.
    adrenal a.
    adrenal cortex a.
    adrenocortical a.
    aldosterone-producing a.
      (APA)
    apocrine a.
    autonomous a.
    basal cell a.
    basophilic a.
    a. of breast
    bronchial a.
    bronchoalveolar cell a.

carcinoma ex
    pleomorphic a.
carotid sheath a.
chromophilic a.
chromophobe a.
colloid a.
colorectal a.
corticotrophic a.
cystic a.
cystic pituitary a.
ductal a.
ectopic a.
ectopic parathyroid a.
embryonal a.
eosinophilic a.
fetal a.
fibroid a.
a. fibrosum
follicular a.
Fuchs a.
growth hormone-
    producing a.
hepatic a.
hepatocellular a.
Hürthle cell a.
islet cell a.
kidney a.
lactating a.
Leydig cell a.
liver cell a.
macrocystic a.
macrofollicular a.
a. malignum
mediastinal a.
microcystic a.
microfollicular a.
monomorphic a.
nephrogenic a.
a. of nipple
null cell a.
ovarian tubular a.
oxyphilic a.
papillary cystic a.
parathyroid a.
Pick tubular a.
pituitary a.
pleomorphic a.
polypoid a.
prolactin-producing a.
prostatic a.
proximal tubular a.
renal cortical a.
retrotracheal a.

sebaceous a.
a. sebaceum
somatotrophic a.
sweat duct a.
testicular tubular a.
thyroid a.
thyrotropin-producing a.
tubular a.
tubulovillous a.
undifferentiated cell a.
villotubular a.
villous a.
adenomatoid
a. hyperplasia
a. odontogenic tumor
a. tumor
adenomatous
a. colonic polyp
a. goiter
a. hyperplasia
a. polyp
a. polyposis syndrome
adenomyoma
adenomyomatosis
adenomyosarcoma
adenomyosis
a. in uterine enlargement
adenopathy
abdominal a.
axillary a.
cervical a.
hilar a.
mediastinal a.
mesenteric a.
metastatic a.
paratracheal a.
postinflammatory a.
pulmonary a.
retroperitoneal a.
secondary axillary a.
thoracic a.
tuberculous mediastinal a.
adenosarcoma
müllerian a.
adenosine
a. analog
a. arabinoside

a. deaminase (ADA)
a. deaminase deficiency
a. diphosphate
a. 5'-diphosphate (ADP)
a. monophosphate
a. triphosphate (ATP)
adenosis
microglandular a.
sclerosing a.
adenosyltransferase
cobalamin a.
adenoviral
adenovirus
a. colitis
a. infection
a. pneumonia
adenylate kinase (AK)
ADH
antidiuretic hormone
adherence
immune a.
adhesion
abdominal a.
a. molecule
pleuropericardial a.
adhesive
a. arachnoiditis
a. atelectasis
a. capsulitis
a. platelet
polymerizing tissue a.
tissue a.
ADI
absolute dose intensity
adiabatic
a. fast passage (AFP)
a. fast scanning
adipiodone
adipocyte
adipose
a. tissue
a. tumor
aditus ad antrum
adjuvant
a. analgesic
a. analgesic drug
a. chemotherapy

NOTES

adjuvant *(continued)*
   a. chronotherapy
   complete Freund a. (CFA)
   Freund a.
   Freund complete a. (FCA)
   a. immunotherapy
   incomplete Freund a. (IFA)
   a. irradiation
   a. therapy
adjuvanticity
ADL
   activities of daily living
administration
   contrast a.
   drug a.
   Food and Drug A. (FDA)
   intralymphatic
    radioactivity a.
   intraperitoneal drug a.
   intraspinal a.
   vasodilator a.
admixture lesion
adnexa
   lymphoma of ocular a.
   ocular a.
   transposed a.
adnexal
   a. adenoma
   a. carcinoma
   a. cyst
   a. embryo
   a. mass
   a. metastasis
adnexectomy
AD-OAP
   Adriamycin, Oncovin, ara-C,
    prednisone
AdoHcy
   S-adenosylhomocysteine
AdoHcyase
   S-adenosylhomocysteine
   hydrolase
Adolescent
   A. and Pediatric Pain Tool
    Scale
adolescent
   a. breast
   a. nulliparous patient
AdoMet
   S-adenosylmethionine
adoptive
   a. immunity
   a. immunotherapy

adozelesin
ADP
   adenosine 5'-diphosphate
ADR
   Adriamycin
   adverse drug reaction
ADR-529
adrenal
   a. ablation
   a. adenoma
   a. artery
   a. calcification
   a. carcinoma
   a. cortex
   a. cortex adenoma
   a. cyst
   a. cystic mass
   a. failure
   a. feminizing syndrome
   a. gland
   a. gland biopsy
   a. gland cancer
   a. hemorrhage
   a. hyperplasia
   a. insufficiency
   a. mass
   a. medullary disease
   a. metastasis
   a. myelolipoma
   a. rest
   a. scintigraphy
   a. tumor
   a. vein
   a. virilizing syndrome
adrenalectomy
adrenergic
   a. blocker
   a. receptor
β-adrenergic receptor
adrenoceptor
adrenocortical
   a. adenoma
   a. carcinoma
   a. disease
   a. macrocyst
   a. neoplasm
   a. rest cell tumor
   a. secretion
adrenocortical adenoma
adrenocorticoid
adrenocorticotropic hormone
   (ACTH)
adrenogenital syndrome

adrenoleukodystrophy
adrenoleukodystrophy-
  adrenomyeloneuropathy (ALD-
  AMN)
adrenomyeloneuropathy
Adriamycin (ADR)
Adriamycin, bleomycin, vinblastine
  (ABV)
Adriamycin, bleomycin, vinblastine
  (ABV)
Adriamycin, bleomycin, vinblastine,
  dacarbazine (ABVD)
Adriamycin, cyclophosphamide
  (AC)
Adriamycin, cyclophosphamide,
  etoposide (ACE)
Adriamycin (doxorubicin),
  bleomycin, vinblastine,
  dacarbazine
Adriamycin, 5-fluorouracil,
  methotrexate (AFM)
Adriamycin, Oncovin, ara-C,
  prednisone (AD-OAP)
Adriamycin PFS
Adriamycin RDF
Adrucil
Adson maneuver
Adson-Murphy needle
adult
  a. breast
  a. polycystic kidney disease
  a. progeria
  a. respiratory distress
    syndrome (ARDS)
  a. T-cell leukemia (ATL)
  a. T-cell lymphoma
advance directive
advanced multiple-beam
  equalization radiography
adventitia
  tunica a.
adventitial
  a. cell
  a. fibroplasia
adverse drug reaction (ADR)
advice
  against medical a. (AMA)

advocate
  patient a.
adynamic ileus
Aebi-Etter-Coscia fixation dens
  fracture
AEC
  3-amino-9-ethylcarbazole
AEGIS sonography management
  system
aegyptius
  Haemophilus a.
aequorin photoprotein
aeration
aerobe
aerobic gram-negative rod
AeroChamber
aerodigestive cancer
aerogenes
  Enterobacter a.
Aeroseb-Dex
aerosolized
  a. pentamidine
aeruginosa
  Pseudomonas a.
AFB
  aortofemoral bypass
  aspirated foreign body
afferent loop syndrome
afibrinogenemia
AFIP
  Armed Forces Institute of
    Pathology
AFM
  Adriamycin, 5-fluorouracil,
    methotrexate
AFP
  adiabatic fast passage
  alpha-fetoprotein
  AFP tumor marker
African
  A. Burkitt lymphoma
  A. Kaposi sarcoma
afterglow
afterload
afterloading
  a. catheter

NOTES

afterloading *(continued)*
    a. tandem and ovoids
    a. technique
afterretention catheter
Ag, ag
    antigen
against
    a. medical advice (AMA)
    militate a.
agammaglobulinemia
    acquired a.
    Bruton sex-linked a.
    common variable a.
    congenital a.
    Swiss-type a.
    X-linked a.
aganglionic
    a. megacolon
    a. segment
aganglionosis
agar
    a. gel electrophoresis
    Geliperm a.
    MacConkey a.
    Middlebrook a.
    Mycosel a.
    Schaedler blood a.
age
    bone a.
    fetal a.
    gestational a.
    large-for-gestational a. (LGA)
    menstrual a.
agenesis
    corpus callosum a.
    liver a.
    lumbosacral a.
    pulmonary a.
    renal a.
    sacral a.
    thymic a.
    unilateral pulmonary a.
    uterine a.
    vaginal a.
    vermian a.
agenetic fracture
agent
    alkylating a.
    antibacterial a.
    antidiarrheal a.
    antiemetic a.
    antifolic a.
    antifungal a.

    anti-inflammatory a.
    antimicrobial a.
    antimicrotubule a.
    antineoplastic a.
    antiparasitic a.
    antiplatelet a.
    antiproliferative a.
    antiviral a.
    bubble a.
    cardioprotective a.
    chelating a.
    chemotherapeutic a.
    contrast a.
    cycle-nonspecific a.
    cycle-specific a.
    cytotoxic a.
    dispersing a.
    Eaton a.
    fluid embolic a.
    fluid vascular-occluding a.
    glutathione-depleting a.
    hepatobiliary contrast a.
    high-osmolar contrast a.
    (HOCA)
    hormonal a.
    hypoxic cell cytotoxic a.
    intercalating a.
    intravascular a.
    ligand a.
    lighter-than-bile contrast a.
    neuroloptic a.
    nonalkylating a.
    nonmyelosuppressive a.
    Norwalk a.
    oncogenic a.
    oral bile desaturating a.
    oxazaphosphorine
    alkylating a.
    paramagnetic contrast a.
    Pittsburgh pneumonia a.
    platinating a.
    PRE a.
    progestational a.
    sclerosing a.
    superparamagnetic
    contrast a.
    targeting a.
    teratogenicity of contrast a.
    vasodilating a.
    ventilation a.
agger nasi air cells
agglomerans
    Enterobacter a.

agglutination
  a. assay
  chick-cell a.
  latex a.
  lectin a.
  platelet a.
agglutinin
  cold a.
  helix pomatia a. (HPA)
  immune a.
  Rh a.
  soybean a. (SBA)
  wheat germ a.
aggregate
  fibrinoplatelet a.
aggregation
  a. antibody-antigen complex
  platelet a.
aggregometer
aggressive
  a. fibromatosis
  a. infantile fibromatosis
Agnew tattooing needle
agnocobalamin
agnogenic myeloid metaplasia
agonist
  GNRH a.
  gonadotropin-releasing
    hormone a.
  LH-RF a.
  luteinizing hormone-
    releasing a.
  opioid a.
agonist-antagonist
  mixed opioid a.-a.
agranulocytosis
Agrelin
agretope
agyria
ahaustral
AICD
  automatic implantable
    cardioverter-defibrillator
aid
  pharmacologic a.

AIDS
  acquired immunodeficiency
    syndrome
    AIDS dementia complex
      (ADC)
    AIDS enteropathy
    feline AIDS (FAIDS)
    hemophilia-associated AIDS
    AIDS psychosis
    seronegative AIDS
    simian AIDS (SAIDS)
    transfusion-related AIDS
      (TRAIDS)
    AIDS wasting
AIDS-related
  AIDS-r. complex (ARC)
  AIDS-r. lymphoma
  AIDS-r. lymphomatous
    meningitis
AIHA
  autoimmune hemolytic anemia
AIL
  angiocentric
    immunoproliferative lesion
AILD
  angioimmunoblastic
    lymphadenopathy with
    dysproteinemia
AIN
  anal intraepithelial neoplasia
alnium disease
air
  a. bronchogram
  a. collection
  a. contrast barium enema
    (ACBE)
  a. contrast view
  a. encephalography
  a. esophagram
  a. exchange
  a. filtration system
  free a.
  a. gap
  high-efficiency, particulate a.
    (HEPA)
  intraperitoneal a.
  a. space disease

NOTES

air *(continued)*
    a. space enlargement
    a. trapping
air/bone/tissue boundary
airborne transmission
air-crescent sign
air-filled lung
air-fluid
    a.-f. level
    a.-f. line
air-gap
    a.-g. radiography
    a.-g. technique
airspace
airspace-filling pattern
air-swallowing
air-trapping
airway
    a. obstruction
    a. pattern
AITP
    autoimmune thrombocytopenic
      purpura
AJCC
    American Joint Committee on
      Cancer
AK
    adenylate kinase
akathisia
akinesis
AL
    anterolateral
ala, *pl.* **alae**
    sacral a.
alanine aminotransferase (ALT)
ALARA
    as low as reasonably achievable
albendazole
Albers-Schönberg disease
albicans
    Candida a.
Albright
    A. hereditary osteodystrophy
    A. syndrome
albuginea
    tunica a.
albumin
    human serum a.
    iodine-131 serum a.
    macroaggregated a. (MAA)
    neogalactosyl a.
    technetium-99m a.

    technetium-99m
      macroaggregated a., ^{99m}Tc
      macroaggregated a. (MAA)
Albuminar
albuminemia
Albumotope I-131
Albunex
albus
    Staphylococcus a.
alcaptonuria
Alcian blue
ALCL
    anaplastic large cell lymphoma
alcohol
    a. block
    polyvinyl a.
alcoholic
    a. cardiomyopathy
    a. cirrhosis
    a. gastritis
ALD-AMN
    adrenoleukodystrophy-
      adrenomyeloneuropathy
    ALD-AMN complex
aldehyde dehydrogenase
Alderson anthropomorphic
  phantoms
aldesleukin
aldophosphamide
aldosterone
    a. level
    a. secretion rate (ASR)
aldosterone-producing adenoma
  (APA)
aldosteronism
aldosteronoma
Aldrich syndrome
alendronate
aleukemic
    a. leukemia
    a. presentation
aleukocythemic leukemia
aleukocytosis
Alexander
    A. disease
    A. view
alfa
    epoetin a.
    interferon a.
alfa-2a
    interferon a., interferon-α-2a,
      Roferon-A

alfa-2b
> interferon a., interferon-α-2b, Intron A

alfa-n1
> interferon a.-n., Wellferon

alfa-n3
> interferon a.-n.

alfentanil
Alferon LDO
Alferon N
algorithm
> bone a.
> radix-two a.

aliasing artifact
alignment
> bony a.
> restoration of normal anatomic a.

alimentary
> a. tract
> a. tract calcification

alimentation
> intravenous a.

Alkaban-AQ
Alkaban-AW
alkaline
> a. burn
> a. phosphatase
> a. phosphatase-anti-alkaline phosphatase
> a. phosphatase-anti-alkaline phosphatase technique
> a. phosphatase isoenzyme tumor marker
> a. phosphatase-positive cell

alkalinity
> Engel a.

alkaloid
> periwinkle a.
> plant a.
> pyrrolizidine a.
> vinca a.

alkaptonuria
Alken-Marberger nephroscope
Alkeran
alkylating agent

alkylation
> busulfan a.
> a. resistance

alkylator
alkyl-lysophospholipid
alkyl transferase
ALL
> acute lymphoblastic leukemia
> acute lymphocytic leukemia

allantoic
> a. duct cyst

Alledronate
allele
allelic
> a. deletion
> a. exclusion
> a. gene

allelotype
Allen
> A. test
> A. treatment

allergen
allergic
> a. bronchopulmonary aspergillosis
> a. contact dermatitis
> a. disease
> a. granulomatosis
> a. granulomatous angiitis
> a. lung disorder
> a. reaction

allergy
> iodine a.

Allevyn hydrophilic polyurethane dressing
alligator forceps
alligator-jaw instrument
alloantibody
alloantigen
alloantin-D antibody
allocation
> fresh tissue a.
> a. of treatment

allogeneic
> a. antigen
> a. bone marrow cell

NOTES

allogeneic *(continued)*
    a. bone marrow transplant
      (ABMT)
    a. disease
    a. peripheral cell transplant
    a. stem cell
allogenic donor
allograft
    bone-chip a.
    pancreatic a.
    renal a.
allograft-mediated
    renal a.-m. hypertension
alloimmune
    a. disease
alloimmunization
    PNH prep a.
allopathic medicine
allophycocyanin
allopurinol
allosensitization
allotoxin
allotransplant recipient
allotype
alloxan-Schiff reaction
alloy
    Ostalloy 202 a.
all-trans-retinoic acid (ATRA)
alobar holoprosencephaly
alopecia
    drug-induced a.
    a. mucinosa
alpha
    a. 1 antitripsin
    a. antitrypsin deficiency
    a. chain thalassemia
    a. error
    a. heavy-chain disease
    interferon a.
    a. interferon
    a. interferon-2A
    a. interferon-2B
    a. interferon-N1
    a. interferon-N3
    a. islet cell neoplasm
    a. particle
    a. 1 proteinase inhibitor
    a. radiation
    recombinant interferon a.
      (rIFN-A)
    a. tocopherol
    transforming growth factor-
      a. 4 (TGF-alpha)

alpha-actinin protein
alpha-adrenergic blocker
alpha-fetoprotein (AFP)
    maternal serum a.-f.
      (MSAFP)
alpha-naphthyl
    a.-n. acetate esterase
    a.-n. butyrate esterase
alpha-tocopheral antioxidant
Alphavirus
ALP isoenzyme RNase
Alport syndrome
alprazolam
ALPSA
    anterior labroligamentous
    periosteal sleeve avulsion
ALT
    alanine aminotransferase
alta
    patella a.
altanserin
alteplase
alteration
    platelet aggregation a.
Alternaria
alternative
    a. donor
    a. medicine
alternator
ALT-RCC
    autolymphocyte-based treatment
    for renal cell carcinoma
altretamine
Altrigen
alumina
aluminum pneumoconiosis
alum-precipitated antigen
alvei
    Hafnia a.
alveolar
    a. cell carcinoma
    diffuse a. hemorrhage
    diffuse pulmonary a.
      hemorrhage
    a. disease
    a. duct
    a. echinococcosis
    a. epithelial hyperplasia
    a. foramina
    a. hemorrhage
    a. hypersensitivity
    a. infiltrate
    a. macrophage

a. microlithiasis
a. mucosal carcinoma
a. pattern
a. pneumonia
a. process
a. proteinosis
a. pulmonary edema
a. ridge
a. sac
a. sarcoidosis
a. soft part sarcoma
alveolaris
    Echinococcus a.
alveolarization
alveoli (*pl. of* alveolus)
alveolitis
    acute allergic extrinsic a.
    chronic diffuse sclerosing a.
    chronic extrinsic a.
    chronic fibrosing a.
    desquamative fibrosing a.
    diffuse sclerosing a.
    extrinsic a.
    extrinsic allergic a.
    fibrosing a.
    mural fibrosing a.
alveologram
alveolus, pl. alveoli
alvircept sudotox
alymphocytosis
Alzheimer disease
AMA
    against medical advice
    autoregressive moving average
amantadine
amastia
Amato body
amaurosis fugax
amazia
Ambazone
ambient
    a. cistern
    a. wing of the
      quadrigeminal cistern
ambiguous
ambiguus
    situs a.

AmBisome
amboceptor
AMBRI
    atraumatic, multidirectional,
      bilateral instability
    AMBRI syndrome
ambulette
amebiasis
amebic
    a. abscess
    a. dysentery
    a. granuloma
    a. infection
amebic granuloma
ameboma
amelanotic melanoma
amelia
ameloblast
ameloblastic
    a. adenomatoid tumor
    a. fibroma
    a. fibrosarcoma
    a. sarcoma
ameloblastoma
amenorrhea
    hypothalamic a.
    primary a.
American
    A. Association for Cancer
      Research (AACR)
    A. Cancer Society (ACS)
    A. College of Nuclear
      Physicians
    A. Foundation for AIDS
      Research (AmFAR)
    A. Joint Committee for
      Cancer Staging and End
      Results Reporting
    A. Joint Committee on
      Cancer (AJCC)
    A. Roentgen Ray Society
    A. Rolland
    A. Society of
      Neuroradiology
    A. Society of Preventive
      Oncology (ASPO)
    A. Society for Therapeutic

NOTES

American *(continued)*
Radiology and Oncology (ASTRO)
A. Stop Smoking Intervention Study for Cancer Prevention (ASSIST)
Ames test
amethopterin *(var. of* methotrexate)
AMeX method
AmFAR
American Foundation for AIDS Research
Amicar
amide
desacetyl vinblastine a. (DAVA)
amidotrizoic acid
Amifostine
amikacin
amine
a. precursor uptake
a. precursor uptake and decarboxylation (APUD)
sympathomimetic a.
amino acid sequence
9-aminocamptothecin
aminocaproate esterase
aminocaproic acid
ε-aminocaproic acid
6-aminochrysine-liposome
3-amino-9-ethylcarbazole (AEC)
aminoglutethimide
aminoglycoside
aminoguanidine
2-amino-6-mercaptopurine
4-amino-*N*-(a-aminophenyl) benzyamide
aminopeptidase
leucine a.
aminopeptidase N
aminopterin syndrome
aminothiadiazole (A-TDA)
aminotransferase
alanine a. (ALT)
aspartate a.
amiodarone
Amipaque
amitriptyline
AML
acute myelocytic leukemia
acute myelogenous leukemia
acute myeloid leukemia
amniocentesis
amniography
a. in hydatidiform mole
amnioinfusion
amnion
a. rupture
a. rupture sequence
amnionicity
amniotic, amnionic
a. band syndrome
a. cavity
a. fluid
a. fluid embolism
a. fluid index
a. fluid volume
a. membrane
a. sac
amobarbital
amonafide
amorphous
a. calcification
a. extracellular material
Amosite
AMPA
Amphethinile
amphipathic
amphotericin
a. B colloidal dispersion (ABCD)
a. B lipid complex
Amplatz
A. angiography needle
A. dilator set
A. double-J stent
A. dual-stiffness Malecot (Stamey) catheter
A. long tapered Teflon dilator
A. mechanical thrombolysis catheter
A. radiolucent handle
A. renal dilator
A. stiffening wire
A. tapered pyeloureteral stent
A. tapered-tip coaxial dilator
A. through-and-through basket
A. TLA needle
A. wire

Amplatz-Lund retrievable filter
amplification
    gene a.
amplifier
    image a.
    linear a.
    log a.
    Servox a.
    a. T-lymphocyte
amplitude
    acoustic pressure a.
    gradient a.
    a. mode
    a. modulation
    pressure a.
ampulla
    phrenic a.
    a. of Vater
    a. of Vater cyst
ampullary, ampullar
    a. adenocarcinoma
    a. carcinoma
    a. stenosis
amputated-foot view
amputation
    above-knee a.
    congenital a.
    Lisfranc a.
AMSA
    amsacrine
amsacrine (AMSA, mAMSA,
   m- AMSA)
Amsidyl
Amsler needle
Amsterdam dwarfism
Amussat operation
amylacea
    corpora a.
amylase
    a. level
amyl nitrite
amyloid
    a. arthropathy
    a. deposit
    a. oral cavity disease
    a. tumor
amyloidoma

amyloidosis
    a. of multiple myeloma
    primary systemic a.
    renal a.
    secondary a.
Amytal
Anadrol-50
anaerobe
anaerobic infection
anagen effluvium
anagrelide
anakinra
anal
    a. canal
    a. cancer
    a. condylomata
    a. copulation
    a. endosonography
    a. eroticism
    a. fisting
    a. herpes
    a. intraepithelial neoplasia
    (AIN)
    a. margin
    a. pterygoid
    a. region cancer
    a. rimming
    a. sadism
    a. sphincter
    a. triangle
analgesia
    epidural a.
    patient-controlled a. (PCA)
analgesic
    adjuvant a.
    a. nephropathy
    nonopioid a.
    opioid a.
    a. syndrome
analog, analogue
    adenosine a.
    butyrate a.
    camptothecin a.
    cisplatin a.
    echinocandin a.
    GnRH a.
    LHRH a.

NOTES

analog *(continued)*
    nucleoside a.
    purine a.
    rhodamine a.
    a. scan converter
    somatostatin a.
analog-to-digital converter (ADC)
analysis
    bayesian a.
    bivariant a.
    5-bromodeoxyuridine a.
    bull's-eye a.
    cell block a.
    cell cycle kinetics a.
    checkerboard a.
    chromosome a.
    cost-to-benefit a.
    Cox life-table regression a.
    cytogenetic a.
    data a.
    decision a.
    direct
      immunofluorescence a.
    DNA content a.
    dose intensity a.
    dot blot a.
    fetal blood a.
    five L a.
    flow cytometric a.
    Fourier a.
    heteroduplex a.
    histologic a.
    image a.
    image display and a. (IDA)
    immunocytochemical a.
    immunofluorescence a.
    immunogenotypic a.
    immunohistochemical a.
    immunophenotypic a.
    isobologram a.
    Kaplan-Meier univariant a.
    karyometric a.
    linkage a.
    molecular genetic a.
    multicolor data a.
    multivariant a.
    multivariant regressional a.
    neutron activation a.
    nonlinear least squares
      regression a.
    Northern blot a.
    Probit a.
    sensitivity a.

    slot-blot hybridization a.
    Southern blot a.
    Southern transfer a.
    S-phase a.
    univariant a.
    Western blot a.
    x-ray diffraction a.
analyte
analytic reconstruction
analyzer
    Dow hollow fiber a.
    pulse height a.
anamnestic response
Anandron
anaphylactic reaction
anaphylactoid reaction
anaphylaxis
    acute a.
anaplastic
    a. astrocytoma
    a. carcinoma
    cerebellar a.
    a. large cell Ki-1-positive
      lymphoma
    a. large cell lymphoma
      (ALCL)
    a. plasmacytoma
    a. thyroid carcinoma
Anaprox
anastomosis, pl. anastomoses
    arterial a.
    arteriovenous a.
    biliary-enteric a.
    Billroth I a.
    Billroth II a.
    colorectal a.
    end-to-end a.
    end-to-side a.
    Glenn a.
    graft a.
    hepatojejunal a.
    leptomeningeal a.
    percutaneous portocaval a.
    portopulmonary venous a.
    portosystemic a.
    side-to-side a.
    stenotic esophagogastric a.
    ureteroureteral a.
anastomotic
    a. aneurysm
    a. arterial circle
    a. stenosis
    a. stricture

anatomic
  a. barrier
  a. fracture
  a. snuffbox
anatomical variant
anatomy
  coronary vessel a.
  immune system a.
  Lowsley lobar a.
  normal planar MR a.
  plantar compartmental a.
  zonal a.
anaxirone
ANCA
  assay neutrophil cytoplasmic
  antibody
Ancef
anchovy paste abscess
anconeus muscle
ancrod
Anderson-Carr-Randall theory
Anderson disease
Anderson-Hutchins tibial fracture
androblastoma
androgen
  a. ablation
  addictive a.
  a. deprivation therapy
  a. receptor
androgen-independent prostate
  cancer
Android-F
android pelvis
androstenedione
anechoic
  a. thrombus
anembryonic pregnancy
Anemet
anemia
  achrestic a.
  achylic a.
  acquired hemolytic a.
  Addison-Biermer a.
  aplastic a.
  aregenerative a.
  autoimmune hemolytic a.
  (AIHA)

Bagdad Spring a.
Bartonella a.
Biermer a.
Biermer-Ehrlich a.
Blackfan-Diamond a.
cameloid a.
cancer-associated a.
chlorotic a.
Chvostek a.
congenital
  dyserythropoietic a.
congenital hypoplastic a.
Cooley a.
crescent cell a.
cytogenic a.
dimorphic a.
drepanocytic a.
Dresbach a.
drug-induced immune
  hemolytic a.
dyserythropoietic a.
Edelmann a.
elliptocytotic a.
erythronormoblastic a.
Estren-Damashek a.
Faber a.
Fanconi a.
globe cell a.
ground itch a.
Heinz body hemolytic a.
hemolytic a.
Herrick a.
hookworm a.
hypersplenic a.
hypochromic a.
iatrogenic a.
idiopathic a.
idiopathic hypochromic a.
immune hemolytic a.
iron deficiency a.
Jaksch anemia (*var. of* Von
  Jaksch a.)
Lederer a.
leukoerythroblastic a.
macrocytic a.
Mediterranean a.
megaloblastic a.

NOTES

23

anemia *(continued)*
    microangiopathic a.
    miner's a.
    mountain a.
    myelopathic a.
    myelophthisic a.
    normochromic a.
    normocytic a.
    nosocomial a.
    paraneoplastic a.
    pernicious a.
    phenylhydrazine a.
    polar a.
    pyridoxine-responsive a.
    refractory a.
    Runeberg a.
    scorbutic a.
    sickle cell a.
    sideroblastic a.
    simple achlorhydric a.
    spur cell a.
    thrombopenic a.
    tropical macrocytic a.
    Von Jaksch a., Jaksch
      anemia
anencephaly
anergy
    a. test
aneriosus
    ductus a.
anesthesia
    epidural a.
    general a.
    halothane a.
    local a.
    regional a.
    saddle block a.
anesthetic
    epidural a.
    eutectic mixture of
      local a.'s (EMLA)
    general a.
    local a.
    regional a.
    topical a.
aneuploid
    a. cell line
    a. NBX tumor
    a. tumor
aneuploidy
    DNA a.
    tumor a.

aneurysm
    abdominal a.
    abdominal aortic a.
    anastomotic a.
    aortic a.
    arterial a.
    arteriovenous a.
    bacterial a.
    berry a.
    bifurcation a.
    brain a.
    carotid a.
    carotid artery a.
    carotid-ophthalmic a.
    cavernous a.
    cavernous sinus a.
    celiac artery a.
    cerebral a.
    cirsoid a.
    communicating artery a.
    congenital left ventricular a.
    congenital renal a.
    coronary artery a.
    dissecting a.
    dissecting basilar artery a.
    false a.
    fusiform a.
    giant a.
    hepatic artery a.
    iliac artery a.
    inflammatory a.
    inflammatory aortic a.
    intracavernous carotid a.
    intracranial a.
    intracranial arterial a.
    left ventricular a.
    lower basilar a.
    mycotic a.
    mycotic aortic a.
    popliteal artery a.
    portal vein a.
    posterior communicating
      artery a.
    posterior-inferior cerebellar
      artery a.
    pulmonary arteriovenous a.
    pulmonary artery a.
    Rasmussen a.
    renal artery a.
    ruptured a.
    saccular a.
    sacral a.
    serpentine a.

sinus of Valsalva a.
splanchnic a.
supraclinoid carotid a.
suprarenal aortic a.
thoracic aorta a.
thrombosed giant vertebral
  artery a.
true a.
true ventricular a.
vein of Galen a.
ventricular a.
aneurysmal
  a. bone cyst
  a. clip
  a. dilatation
  a. proportions
aneurysmectomy
aneurysmogram
aneurysmograph
Anger camera
angiitis, angitis
  allergic granulomatous a.
  granulomatous a.
  necrotizing a.
angiitis-granulomatosis disorder
angina
  abdominal a.
  intestinal a.
  a. pectoris
  Prinzmetal a.
  unstable a.
angioblastic lymphadenopathy
angioblastoma
angiocardiography
  exercise radionuclide a.
  gated radionuclide a.
  radionuclide a.
Angiocath
angiocentric
  a. immunoproliferative
    disorder
  a. immunoproliferative
    lesion (AIL)
  a. lymphoproliferative lesion
  a. T-cell lymphoma
Angioconray
angiodynagraphy

angiodysgenetic
angiodysplasia
angioedema
angioendotheliomatosis
  malignant a.
  neoplastic proliferating a.
  reactive proliferating a.
angioendotheliosis
angiofibroma
  juvenile a.
angiofollicular
  a. hyperplasia
  a. lymph node hyperplasia
  a. and plasmacytic
    polyadenopathy
angiogenesis
  tumor a.
angiogenic cell
Angiografin
angiograph
  black blood a.
angiographic
  a. guidewire
  a. occlusion
  a. Teflon dilator
  a. two-wire snare
angiography
  aortic arch a.
  axial a.
  balloon occlusion
    pulmonary a.
  basilar a.
  biplane a.
  bronchial a.
  carotid a.
  a. catheter
  celiac a.
  cerebral a.
  contrast a.
  coronary a.
  2DFT time-of-flight MR a.
  digital celiac trunk a.
  digital subtraction a. (DSA)
  femoral runoff a.
  femorocerebral catheter a.
  hepatic a.
  interventional a.

NOTES

angiography *(continued)*
  intraarterial digital
    subtraction a.
  intracranial MR a.
  intraoperative a.
  intravenous digital
    subtraction a.
  magnetic resonance a.
    (MRA)
  magnification a.
  MR a.
  nuclear a.
  phase contrast a.
  pulmonary a.
  radionuclide a.
  renal a.
  scintigraphic a.
  selective arterial magnetic
    resonance a.
  selective venous magnetic
    resonance a.
  thoracic a.
  time-of-flight a.
  vertebral a.
angioimmunoblastic
  a. lymphadenopathy
  a. lymphadenopathy-like T-
    cell lymphoma
  a. lymphadenopathy with
    dysproteinemia (AILD)
  a. lymphadenopathy with
    dysproteinemia-like T-cell
    lymphoma
angioinfarction
angioleiomyoma
angiolipofibroma
angiolipoma
  epidural a.
  spinal epidural a.
angiolithic sarcoma
angiolymphoid hyperplasia
angioma
  arterial a.
  capillary a.
  cavernous a.
  cherry a.
  encephalic a.
  extracerebral cavernous a.
  a. lymphaticum
  pulmonary a.
  a. serpiginosum
  spider a.

  superficial a.
  telangiectatic a.
  a. venosum racemosum
  venous a.
angiomatoid
  a. malignant fibrous
    histiocytoma
  a. tumor
angiomatosis
  bacillary a.
  cystic a.
  encephalotrigeminal a.
  epithelioid a.
  retinal a.
  retinocerebellar a.
angiomatous
  a. disease
  a. lymphoid hamartoma
angiomyofibroma
angiomyolipoma
  renal a.
angiomyoma
angiomyosarcoma
angiomyxoma
angioneuromyoma
angioosteohypertrophy syndrome
angiopathy
  cerebral amyloid a.
angioplasty
  aortoiliac a.
  balloon a.
  a. balloon
  a. balloon catheter
  balloon dilation a. (BDA)
  coronary artery a.
  coronary balloon a.
  infrapopliteal a.
  infrapopliteal transluminal a.
  kissing-balloon a.
  laser-assisted balloon a.
  low-speed rotational a.
  patch a.
  percutaneous low-stress a.
  percutaneous transluminal a.
    (PTA)
  percutaneous transluminal
    coronary a. (PTCA)
  peripheral balloon a.
  renal a.
  tibioperoneal trunk a.
  transluminal a.
angioreticuloma

angiosarcoma
  hepatic a.
  uterine a.
angioscopic guidance
angioscopy
Angio-Seal
Angiostat
angiotensin-converting
  a.-c. enzyme (ACE)
  a.-c. hormone
angiotensin-II
angiotomosynthesis
angiotropic large cell lymphoma
angitis (*var. of* angiitis)
angle
  anterior angulation a.
  basal a.
  Boehler a.
  cardiophrenic a.
  carinal a.
  carpal a.
  cerebellopontine a.
  costophrenic a.
  Djian Annonier a.
  Doppler a.
  Ernst a.
  Ferguson a.
  flip a.
  gastroesophageal a.
  hepatic a
  Louis a.
  magic a.
  magnetization precession a.
  medial a.
  a. of orientation
  phase a.
  posterior urethrovesical a.
  precession a.
  pulse flip a.
  radiocarpal a.
  sphenoid a.
  splenic a.
  sternal a.
  subcarinal a.
  talocalcaneal a.
  tip a.
  tracheal bifurcation a.

  unsharpness of the
    costophrenic a.'s
angle-closure glaucoma
angular
  a. artery
  a. cheilitis
  a. frequency
  a. momentum
  a. velocity
angularis
  incisura a.
angulated fracture
angulation
  a. at the fracture site
  caudal a.
  coronal a.
  palmar a.
  volar a.
angustifolia
  Echinacea a.
anhydramnios
anicteric bile duct
anilingus
animal study
anion
  a. gap
aniridia
anisakiasis
anisidide
  acridinyl a.
anisocytosis
anisoleukocytosis
anisopoikilocytosis
anisotropic
  a. diffusion
  a. 3D imaging
  a. resolution
  a. rotation
  a. tissue
anisotropically-rotational
  a.-r. diffusion (ARD)
  a.-r. diffusion imaging
anisotropy
  chemical shift a.
  magnetic a.
ankle
  a. fracture

NOTES

27

ankle *(continued)*
 a. joint
 a. mortise
 a. mortise fracture
ankle-arm index
ankle-brachial
 a.-b. index (ABI)
 a.-b. pressure measurement
ankylosing
 a. hyperostosis
 a. spondylitis
ankylosis
 bony a.
ANLL
 acute nonlymphoblastic
 leukemia
 acute nonlymphocytic leukemia
Ann
 A. Arbor classification of
 Hodgkin disease staging
 A. Arbor staging system I-
 IV
anneal
annealing
annexin-V
annihilation photons
annotation
annular
 a. abscess
 a. array
 a. calcification
 a. constricting lesion
 a. disk bulge
 a. fiber
 a. fibrosis
 a. pancreas
 a. phased array
 hyperthermia
annulare
 granuloma a.
annuloaortic ectasia
annulus, anulus, pl. **annuli**
 bulging a.
 a. fibrosus
anode
 rotating a.
anomalous
 a. antigen expression
 a. branching
 a. innominate artery
 compression syndrome
 a. left coronary artery
 a. origin

 a. pulmonary venous return
 a. serum chemistry
anomaly
 anorectal a.
 atrioventricular junction a.
 congenital a.
 conjoined nerve-root a.
 craniofacial a.
 double-inlet ventricle a.
 duplication a.
 Ebstein a.
 fetal a.
 fetal cardiac a.
 fetal chest a.
 fetal gastrointestinal a.
 genitourinary a.
 heart a.
 jugular bulb a.
 kidney a.
 limb reduction a.
 May-Hegglin a.
 Michel a.
 Mondini a.
 müllerian duct a.
 numerary renal a.
 occipitoatlantoaxial a.
 Pelger-Huet a.
 presacral a.
 segmentation a.
 structural a.
 targeted imaging for
 fetal a.'s
 Undritz a.
 urinary tract a.
 uterine a.
 vascular a.
 vena cava a.
anopia
anorchia
anorectal
 a. anomaly
 a. atresia
 a. herpes
 a. malformation
 a. melanoma
 a. tuberculosis
anorectum
 cloacogenic carcinoma of
 the a.
anorexia
 a. nervosa
 paraneoplastic a.

anoxia
    cerebral a.
    perinatal a.
anoxic encephalopathy
ansamycin
Ansbacher unit
anserinus
    pes a.
antagonist
    calcium a.
    folate a.
    folic acid a.
    opioid a.
    pyrimidine a.
    RG 12915 serotonin a.
    serotonin a.
antalgic gait
antecolic
antecubital
    a. approach
    a. fossa
    a. vein
anteflexed uterus
antegrade
    a. catheterization
    a. flow
    ipsilateral a. arteriography
    a. puncture
    a. pyelogram
    a. venography
antenna
antepartum hemorrhage
anterior
    a. angulation angle
    a. cerebral artery
    a. choroidal artery
    a. clear space
    a. column fracture
    a. commissure
    a. communicating artery
    a. condylar canal
    a. condyloid foramen
    a. cruciate ligament
    a. exenteration
    a. horn cell disease
    a. iliac crest
    a. junction line

    a. labroligamentous
    periosteal sleeve avulsion
    (ALPSA)
    a. mediastinal mass
    a. osteophyte
    a. palatine foramen
    a. sacral foramen
    a. sagittal diameter (ASD)
    scalenus a.
    a. scalloping of vertebrae
    serratus a.
    a. spinal artery
    a. spinal artery syndrome
    a. spinal ligament
    calcification
    a. tibial bowing
    tibialis a.
    a. tibial tendon
    a. tracking of pML
anterior-posterior repair
anterior-to-posterior
    superior labrum, a.-t.-p.
    (SLAP)
anterolateral (AL)
    a. abdominal wall
    a. compression fracture
    a. system
anteroposterior (AP)
    a. projection
anteverted uterus
antherpetic
Anthophyllite
anthracenedione
anthracosilicosis
    conglomerate a.
anthracosis
anthracotic material
anthracycline
    morpholino a.
anthracycline-induced
  cardiomyopathy
anthrapyrazole
anthraquinone compound
anthrax
Anthron heparinized catheter
anti-ABO antibody
antiandrogen

NOTES

29

antianemia
 a. factor
 a. principle
antiangiogenesis factor
antiantibody formation
antiantitoxin
antiarrhythmic
anti-B4 blocked ricin
antibacterial agent
antibasement membrane antibody
anti-B cell antibody
antibiotic
 antitumor a.
 prophylactic a.
 a. prophylaxis
 a. therapy
antibiotic-resistant bacteria
antibioticus
 Streptomyces a.
antibody, pl. antibodies
 alloantin-D a.
 anti-ABO a.
 antibasement membrane a.
 anti-B cell a.
 anti-CALLA hybridoma a.
 anti-CD monoclonal a.
 anticentromere a.
 anti-CNA a.
 anticytokeratin a.
 anti-DNA a.
 anti-EBV a.
 anti-ETER a.
 antifibrin a.
 antifibronectin a.
 anti-GFAP a.
 antiglomerular basement
  membrane a.
 antigranulocyte a.
 anti-HIV a.
 anti-HLA a.
 anti-idiotype a.
 anti-immunocytokeratin a.
 anti-La a.
 antimitochondrial a.
 anti-MY9 monoclonal a.
 antimyosin a.
 antineuronal a.
 antinuclear a.
 antioxazolone a.
 antiphospholipid a.
 antiphospholipid a.
 anti-Ro a.
 anti-TAC a.

antithyroglobulin a.
anti-T12 monoclonal a.
assay neutrophil
 cytoplasmic a. (ANCA)
auto-anti-idiotypic a.
autologous a.
bifunctional a.
biotin-labeled a.
blocking a.
Campath-monoclonal a.
CD3 monoclonal a.
cell-bound a.
cell-fixed a.
cell-mediated a.
chelated a.
chimeric a.
cold a.
combining-site a.
complement-fixing a. (CFA)
cryptosporidiosis a.
CSLEX1 monoclonal a.
cytophilic a.
cytotoxic a.
DAB389 a.
a. deposition
direct fluorescent a. (DFA)
Donath-Landsteiner a.
duck virus hepatitis yolk a.
Duffy a.
erythrocyte and a. (EA)
F_2 a.
fluorescent a.
Forssman a.
GBM a.
heterogenetic a.
heterophil a.
high-affinity a.
HMB-45 a.
human antimouse a.
 (HAMA)
human antimouse a.
 (HAMA)
human immunodeficiency
 virus a. (HIV-AB)
humanized a.
humoral a.
hybridoma a.
idiotype a.
IgA a.
IgY a.
I-labeled B-cell-specific anti-
 CD20 monoclonal a.
 (BIMAb)

immune a.
immunofluorescence a. (IFA)
isophil a.
Kell a.
Ki-67 a.
Kidd a.
kidney-fixing a.
Ki-67 monoclonal a.
a. labeling
Leu monoclonal a.
Lewis a.
a. linkage method
Lutheran a.
Lym-1 monoclonal a.
lymphotoxic a.
M344 a.
mitochondrial a.
monoclonal a. (MAb)
monoclonal a. (MAb)
murine monoclonal a.
natural a.
OKB7 monoclonal a.
OKT3 anti-CD3
  monoclonal a.
opsonizing a.
Orthoclone OKT3
  monoclonal a.
Ortho-mune a.
osteosarcoma antigen-
  associated monoclonal a.
pan-B a.
pan-cytokeratin a.
a. panel
pan T-cell a.
PM-81 monoclonal a.
polyclonal a.
polyclonal CD3 a.
polyreactive a.
Prausnitz-Kustner a.
prophylactic a.
radiolabeled a.
a. reaction site
reaginic a.
resistance to a.
a. response
Rh a.
ricin-blocked a.

toxoplasma IgG a.
TSH-displacing a.
warm-reactive a.
antibody-absorbent
antibody-antigen complex
antibody-based detection system
antibody-dependent
  a.-d. cell cytotoxicity
    (ADCC)
  a.-d. cell-mediated
    cytotoxicity
  a.-d. enhancement
antibody-positive
  HLTV-I a.-p.
anti-CALLA hybridoma antibody
anticancer drug
anti-CD3, muromonab-CD3
anti-CD monoclonal antibody
anticentromere antibody
anticholinergic drug
anticipatory vomiting
anti-CNA antibody
anticoagulant
anticoagulation
anticodon
anticomplementary factor
anticonvulsant
anticrotalus serum
anti-cryptosporidium
  bovine a.-c.
anticytokeratin
  a. antibody
  monoclonal a. (MAK-6)
antidepressant
antidiarrheal agent
antidiuretic hormone (ADH)
anti-DNA antibody
antidote
  Hall a.
anti-EBV antibody
anti-EGFR
  anti-epidermal growth factor
  receptor
antiembolism stockings
antiemetic agent
anti-epidermal growth factor
  receptor (anti-EGFR)

NOTES

antiestrogen
anti-ETER antibody
antiferritin
    a. antibody linked to I-131
    yttrium-90-labeled a.
antifibrin
    a. antibody
antifibrinolysin
antifibronectin antibody
antifolate
antifolic agent
antifungal
    a. agent
    a. therapy
antigen (Ag, ag)
    ABH blood group
      carbohydrate a.
    ABH/Lewis-related a.
    ABH(O) cell surface a.
    activation associated a.
    allogeneic a.
    alum-precipitated a.
    Australian a.
    B1 a.
    B4 a.
    B5 a.
    B-cell lineage a.
    BE1 a.
    BE2 a.
    beef heart a.
    a. binding site
    blood group a.
    B-ly-7 a.
    Boivin a.
    CA 125 a.
    cancer a. (CA)
    cancer-associated serum a.
      (CASA)
    a. capture assay
    carbohydrate a.
    carcinoembryonic a. (CEA)
    carcinoid embryonic a.
    CD a.
    CD18 a.
    CD21 a.
    CD33 a.
    cell-bound a.
    cell membrane a.
    cell surface a.
    Chido-Rogers a.
    common acute leukemia a.
    common acute lymphoblastic
      leukemia a. (CALLA)

    common leukocyte a.
    conjugated a.
    cutaneous lymphocyte a.
    cytokeratin membrane a.
    cytoplasmic CD3 a.
    cytoskeletal a.
    a. deficiency
    delta a.
    a. determinant
    DF3 a.
    differentiation a.
    diphtheria a.
    Duffy a.
    E a.
    early a.
    endogenous a.
    endothelial localization of a.
    epithelial membrane a.
    exogenous a.
    a. expression
    extractable nuclear a.
    factor IX a.
    factor VII a. (VII:Ag)
    factor VIII-related a.
    factor X a. (X:Ag)
    fecal carcinoembryonic a.
    Forssman a.
    Frei a.
    Fy a.
    Gm a.
    Gross cell surface a.
    H a.
    H-2 a.
    Hangar-Rose skin test a.
    Helmes 3 a.
    hepatitis-associated a. (HAA)
    hepatitis B surface a.
      (HBsAg)
    heterogeneic a.
    heterologous a.
    heterophil a.
    histocompatibility a.
    HIV p24 a.
    HLA a.
    HLA-A1 a.
    HLA-B a.
    HLA-C a.
    HLA-D a.
    HLA-DR a.
    HLA-DR 1 a.
    HLA-DR 5 a.
    HLA-L a.
    homologous a.

human leukocyte a. (HLA)
human leukocyte Cw5 a.
HUTCH-1 a.
H-Y a.
Ia a.
idiotypic a.
intracellular a.
Inv group a.
isogeneic a.
isophil a.
K a.
Ki-1 a.
Ki-67 nuclear a.
Km a.
Kveim a.
L26 a.
large granular lymphocyte a.
late a.
LD a.
Le blood group a.
Leu-8 a.
leukocyte common a.
Lewis A a.
Lewis blood group a.
lineage-associated a.
Ly a.
Lyb a.
lymphocyte function a.
lymphogranuloma
  venereum a.
Lyt a.
M a.
M344 a.
Mac-1 a.
macrophage lineage a.
major histocompatibility a.'s
major histocompatibility
  complex a.
mammary serum a. (MSA)
melanoma-associated a.'s
Mitsuda a.
MO1 a.
monoclonal antibody-
  defined a.
monocyte lineage a.
mumps skin test a.
myeloid associated a.

myeloid lineage a.
myelomonocytic a.
natural killer cell a.
NR a.
nuclear a.
nuclear proliferation a.
O a.
oncofetal a.
organ-specific a.
Oz a.
p24 a.
pan B-cell a.
pancreatic oncofetal a.
panhematopoietic cell a.
pan T-cell a.
PC-1 a.
PC10 a.
PCA a.
PCA-1 a.
phytohemagglutinin a.
plasma cell a.
pollen a.
polysaccharide a.
Pr a.
preferential B-cell
  panhematopoietic a.
preferential T-cell
  panhematopoietic a.
a. presentation
private a.
progenitor cell a.
proliferating cell nuclear a.
proliferation a.
proliferation-associated a.
prostate-specific a. (PSA)
public a.
QA a.
radiolabeled a.
RD1 a.
a. receptor
a. receptor gene
red blood cell a.
red cell a.
a. restriction
Rh factor a.
SD a.
sequestered a.

NOTES

33

antigen *(continued)*
  serodefined a.
  serum hepatitis a.
  serum tissue polypeptide a.
    (S-TPA)
  SH a.
  sialyl Lewis
    necroinflammation-
    associated carbohydrate a.
  sialyl Lex a.
  sialyl Tn a. (STN)
  skin-specific
    histocompatibility a.
  Sm a.
  species-specific a.
  SR-1 a.
  SS-A a.
  SS-B a.
  surface a.
  surface membrane a.
  T a.
  T11 a.
  Tac a.
  T-cell lineage a.
  tetanus a.
  Thy 1 a.
  thymic lymphocyte a.
  thymus-dependent a.
  thymus-independent a.
  tissue polypeptide a. (TPA)
  tissue-specific a.
  a. titer
  a. tolerance
  transplantation a.
  tumor a.
  tumor-associated a. (TAA)
  tumor-associated
    glycoprotein-72 a.
  tumor-associated
    transplantation a. (TATA)
  tumor-specific a.
  tumor-specific
    transplantation a. (TSTA)
  a. unmasking
  very late a.
  Vi a.
  viral capsid a. (VCA)
  xenogeneic a.
  ZEBRA a.
antigen-antibody complex
antigenemia
antigenic
  a. determinant

  a. drift
  a. modulation
  a. paralysis
  a. target
antigenicity
  lowered tumor a.
  tumor a.
antigenotherapy
antigen-sensitive cell
anti-GFAP antibody
antiglomerular basement membrane
  antibody
antigonadotropin
antigranulocyte antibody
anti-G suit
antihelminthic drug
antihemagglutinin
antihemolytic
antihemophilic factor
antihemorrhagic
  a. factor
anti-hepatitis C virus-positive
  cirrhosis
antiherpetic
anti-HIV
  a.-HIV antibody
  a.-HIV immune serum
    globulin (HIVIG)
anti-HLA antibody
antihuman globulin
anti-icteric
anti-idiotype antibody
anti-idiotypic
  a.-i. affinity chromatography
  a.-i. immunoglobulin
    response
anti-immunocytokeratin antibody
anti-immunoglobulin
  biotin-labeled a.-i.
anti-inflammatory agent
anti-inhibitor coagulant complex
anti-La antibody
antilymphocyte
antimacrophage
antimetabolic
  10-Edam a.
antimetabolite
  purine a.
antimicrobial agent
antimicrotubule agent
antimitochondrial antibody
antimonium tungstate (HPA-23)
antimouse lymphocyte serum

anti-MY9 monoclonal antibody
antimycotic therapy
antimyosin
    a. antibody
    a. Fab-DTPA
    a. uptake
antineoplastic
    a. agent
    a. drug
    a. therapy
antineoplaston
antineuronal antibody
antinuclear
    a. antibody
    a. factor
antioncogene
antioxazolone antibody
antioxidant
    alpha-tocopheral a.
antiparasitic agent
antiphospholipid
    a. antibody
    a. syndrome
antiplasmin
    Stachrom a.
α_2-antiplasmin
antiplatelet
    a. agent
    a. therapy
antipneumocystis
antipolycythemic
antiproliferative agent
antireceptor
antiretroviral
    a. drug
    a. therapy
anti-Ro antibody
antisense
    a. oligonucleotide
    a. RNA
    a. technology
anti-shared idiotype
antisheep red blood cell
antishock suit
antistreptolysin O (ASO)
anti-T12 monoclonal antibody

anti-TAC antibody
antithrombin III (AT III)
antithymocyte globulin (ATG)
antithyroglobulin antibody
antitoxin
antitripsin
    alpha 1 a.
antitrypanosomal
α_1-antitrypsin
antitrypsin deficiency
antitumor
    a. antibiotic
    a. drug
antivenom
antiviral
    a. activity
    a. agent
    a. immunity
    a. therapy
antra (*pl. of* antrum)
antral
    a. beaking
    a. lavage
    a. mucosal diaphragm
    a. mucosal thickening
    a. padding
    a. polyp
    a. stricture
    a. ulcer
    a. web
Antril
antrochoanal polyp
antroduodenal motility
antrogen blockade
antropyloric canal
antrum, pl. antra
    aditus ad a.
    gastric a.
    maxillary a.
    pyloric a.
    retained gastric a.
anulus (*var. of* annulus)
    a. fibrosus tear
anuria
anus
    ectopic a.
    imperforate a.

NOTES

35

anxiolysis
anxiolytic
aorta
    abdominal a.
    ascending a.
    descending a.
    double-barrel a.
    native a.
    overriding a.
    tulip bulb a.
aortic
    a. aneurysm
    a. annulus abscess
    a. aperture
    a. arch
    a. arch angiography
    a. arch atresia
    a. atresia
    a. balloon pump
    a. bifurcation
    a. bifurcation prosthesis
    a. body tumor
    a. coarctation
    a. dissection
    a. flow volume
    a. foramen
    a. graft
    a. injury
    a. insufficiency
    a. isthmus
    a. kinking
    a. knob
    a. lymph node
    a. motion artifact
    a. nipple
    a. node metastasis
    a. opening
    a. regurgitation
    a. root
    a. rupture
    a. stenosis
    a. thrombosis
    tortuous a. arch
    a. transection
    a. valve
    a. valve atresia
    a. valve echocardiography
    a. valve lesion
    a. valvular disease
    a. window
aorticopulmonary
    a. window
    a. window shunt

aorticorenal graft
aortic-pulmonic window
aortitis
    bacterial a.
    giant cell a.
    luetic a.
    syphilitic a.
aortobifemoral bypass
aortoenteric fistula
aortofemoral
    a. bypass (AFB)
    a. bypass graft
    a. graft
aortography
    abdominal a.
    ascending a.
    retrograde a.
    translumbar a. (TLA)
aortoiliac
    a. angioplasty
    a. bypass graft
    a. disease
    a. inflow system
aortoplasty
aortovisceral bypass
AP
    anteroposterior
    AP projection
    AP repair
APA
    aldosterone-producing adenoma
APAAP technique
apallic syndrome
apatite deposition disease
APD
    bisphosphonate APD
aperta
    spina bifida a.
Apert syndrome
aperture
    aortic a.
    a. diaphragm
apeu virus
apex, pl. apices
    a. of the heart
    lung apices
    petrous a.
Aphanizomenon flos-aquae
aphasia
    stroke-like syndrome of a.
apheresis
    single-donor a.
    subclavian a.

aphidicolin
    a. glycinate
aphrophilus
    Haemophilus a.
aphtha, pl. aphthae
aphthous
    a. stomatitis
    a. ulcer
Aphthovirus
apical
    a. cap sign
    a. granuloma
    a. lordotic projection
    a. lordotic view
    a. notch
    a. petrositis
    a. pleural thickening
apices (*pl. of* apex)
APL
    acute promyelocytic leukemia
aplasia
    bone marrow a.
    a. cutis
    dens a.
    germinal a.
    idiopathic megakaryocytic a.
    pulmonary a.
    pure red cell a.
    radial a.
    red cell a.
    uterine a.
aplastic anemia
apnea
    sleep a.
apnea/bradycardia ratio (A/B ratio)
apocrine
    a. adenoma
    a. carcinoma
    a. cyst
apodization
Apogee RX400
apolipoprotein
aponeurotic fibroma
apophyseal
    a. fracture
    a. injury

apophysis
    ring a.
apoplexy
    pituitary a.
apoptosis
apoptotic cell death
apparatus
    Barcroft a.
    Golgi a.
    Hilal embolization a.
    Tiselius a.
    Warburg a.
apparent
    a. diffusion coefficient
    a. paramagnetism
appearance
    apple core a.
    apple peel a.
    apple sauce a.
    ball-in-hand a.
    beaded a.
    beaked a.
    beaten brass a.
    bolus-of-worms a.
    bone-within-bone a.
    bubble-like a.
    candle drippings a.
    candy cane a.
    cat's-eye a.
    cobblestone a.
    coffee bean a.
    coiled-spring a.
    comma a.
    corkscrew a.
    cotton ball a.
    cotton-wool a.
    cracked walnut a.
    cushingoid a.
    cystic a.
    double-bulb a.
    drumstick a.
    frayed string a.
    ground glass a.
    hair-standing-on-end a.
    hammered brass a.
    hammered silver a.
    harlequin a.

NOTES

appearance *(continued)*
    hole-within-hole a.
    honeycombed a.
    hot-cross-bun a.
    inverse comma a.
    inverted-T a.
    jail-bars a.
    jelly belly a.
    kernel of popcorn a.
    lace-like a.
    leafless tree a.
    light bulb a.
    lollipop tree a.
    moth-eaten a.
    mottled a.
    mushroom a.
    onion skin a.
    pancake a.
    panda a.
    peau d'orange a.
    picket fence a.
    picture frame a.
    popcornlike a.
    pruned-tree a.
    punched-out a.
    railroad track a.
    rugger jersey a.
    saber-shin a.
    sandwich a.
    scottie dog a.
    serrated a.
    shell-of-bone a.
    sign of the burnuous a.
    snake's head a.
    soap bubble a.
    spade-like a.
    stacked-coin a.
    stepladder a.
    stippled a.
    string-of-beads a.
    string-of-pearls a.
    sunburst a.
    Swiss Alps a.
    tam-o-shanter a.
    teardrop a.
    tree-in-winter a.
    trefoil a.
    walking-stick a.
    waterfall a.
    weblike a.
    windsock a.
    wineglass a.
    wormy a.

appendage
    atrial a.
appendectomy
appendiceal
    a. abscess
    a. cancer
appendicitis
    perforated a.
appendicolith
appendicular skeleton
appendix
    hot a.
    a. mucocele
    retrocecal a.
    vermiform a.
apple
    a. core appearance
    a. core carcinoma
    a. core lesion
    a. peel appearance
    a. sauce appearance
apposition
approach
    antecubital a.
    brachial artery a.
    femoral artery a.
    genetic a.
    molecular a.
    neurosurgical a.
    PEACH a.
    psychological a.
    retrograde endoscopic a.
    supine oblique a.
    therapeutic a.
    transcubital a.
    transgluteal a.
    transvaginal a.
APTT
    activated partial thromboplastin time
APUD
    amine precursor uptake and decarboxylation
apudoma
    a. tumor
Aquaplast mask
aqueduct
    cerebral a.
    cochlear a.
    sylvian a.
    a. of Sylvius
    vestibular a.

aqueductal
a. obstruction
a. stenosis
aqueous solution
AR-121
ara-A
ara-AC
arabinogalactan
arabinoside
adenine a.
adenosine a.
behenoylcytosine a.
cytosine a. (ara-C, ARA-C)
high-dose cytosine a.
(HI-DAC)
iodoazomycin a.
arabinoside-liposome
cytosine a.-l.
arabinosylcytosine
arabinosyl cytosine
Arabitin
ara-C, ARA-C
cytarabine
cytosine arabinoside
high-dose ara-C (HDARA-C)
ara-C 5'-triphosphate
(ara-CTP)
arachidonic
a. acid
a. acid metabolism
arachnodactyly, arachnodactilia
arachnoid
a. cyst
a. granulation calcification
a. retrocerebellar pouch
a. space
a. villi
a. villi obstruction
arachnoiditis
adhesive a.
cystic a.
neoplastic a.
ara-CTP
ara-C 5'-triphosphate
arborescens
lipoma a.
arbovirus

ARC
AIDS-related complex
arch
aortic a.
bovine a.
chimney-shaped high
aortic a.
circumflex retroesophageal a.
coracoacromial a.
double aortic a.
ductus a.
a. fracture
hypochordal a.
neural a.
osseocartilaginous a.
osseoligamentous a.
plantar a.
pubic a.
retroesophageal a.
tortuous aortic a.
zygomatic a.
architectural
a. disturbance
a. effacement
architecture
histologic a.
arcuate
a. artery
a. ligament
arcuatus
uterus a.
ARD
anisotropically-rotational
diffusion
ARD imaging
ARDS
acute respiratory distress
syndrome
adult respiratory distress
syndrome
area, pl. areae
Broca a.
cells per unit a.
echo-free a.
fat-density a.
a. gastrica
a. hepatica fibrosa

NOTES

area *(continued)*
    infraclavicular a.
    infrahilar a.
    motor a.
    parietooccipital a.
    peak a.
    perianal a.
    proliferation a.
    punched-out a.
    radiodensity a.
    retrocardiac a.
    scrotal a.
    skip a.
    speech a.
    a. under the curve (AUC)
    water density a.
    watershed areas
    Wernicke a.
areal density
Aredia
5a-reductase
aregenerative anemia
Arenavirus
Arensin
argentaffin
Argentinian hemorrhagic fever
arginine-glycine-aspartic acid moiety
argininemia
arginine vasopressin
argininosuccinicacidemia
argon laser
Argyle
    A. catheter
    A. feeding tube
    A. Ingram trocar catheter
Argyll-Robertson pupil
argyrophilic cell
arhinencephaly
Arimidex
Aristizabal
Arizona Cancer Center multiple myeloma staging system
armamentarium
armed
    A. Forces Institute of Pathology (AFIP)
    a. macrophage
Armidex
Arneth count
Arnoff external fixation device
Arnold body

Arnold-Chiari
    A.-C. deformity
    A.-C. malformation
    A.-C. syndrome
aromatase inhibitor
arotinoid
arousal
    sexual a.
array
    annular a.
    a. coil
    convex a.
    linear a.
    phased a.
    a. processor
    silicon diode a.
arrest
    maturation a.
arrhenoblastoma
arrhythmia
    cardiac a.
    fetal a.
arsenic poisoning
arsenism
    chronic a.
ART
    acoustic response technology
    ART transducer
artefact *(var. of* artifact*)*
arterial
    a. anastomosis
    a. aneurysm
    a. angioma
    a. blood
    a. blood gas abnormality
    a. bypass graft
    a. calcification
    a. disease
    a. dissection
    a. hypertension
    a. hypotension
    intraabdominal a. hemorrhage
    a. linear density
    a. occlusion
    a. oxygen saturation (SaO_2)
    a. phase
    a. pulsatility
    a. sheath
    a. spasm
    a. stenosis
    a. supply

transcatheter a.
  chemoembolization (TACE)
  a. wall
  a. wall dissection
  a. waveform
arterial-arterial fistula
arterial-portal fistula
arteria lusoria
arteries of Adamkiewicz
arteriobiliary fistula
arteriogenic impotence
arteriogram
  documentary a.
  pelvic a.
arteriography
  bilateral carotid a.
  bronchial a.
  carotid cerebral a.
  digital a.
  digital subtraction a. (DSA)
  femoral runoff a.
  intraoperative a.
  ipsilateral antegrade a.
  pulmonary a.
  renal a.
  splenic a.
arteriolar narrowing
arteriole
arteriomyomatosis
arteriopathy
  plexogenic pulmonary a.
arterioportal venous shunting
arterioportobiliary
  a. fistula
arteriosclerosis
arteriosclerotic
  a. occlusive disease
  a. renal disease
arteriosinusoidal
  a. fistula
  a. penile fistula
arteriosum
  ligamentum a.
arteriosus
  calcified ductus a.
  ductus a.
  patent ductus a. (PDA)

persistent truncus a.
pseudotruncus a.
railroad track ductus a.
truncus a.
arteriovascular calcification
arteriovenous (AV, A-V)
  a. anastomosis
  a. aneurysm
  a. fistula (AVF)
  a. hemangioma
  a. malformation (AVM)
  a. shunt
arteritis
  carotid artery a.
  cranial granulomatous a.
  giant cell a.
  granulomatous a.
  Takayasu a.
  temporal granulomatous a.
artery
  aberrant right subclavian a.
  aberrant subclavian a.
  accessory middle cerebral a.
  Adamkiewicz a.
  adrenal a.
  angular a.
  anomalous left coronary a.
  anterior cerebral a.
  anterior choroidal a.
  anterior communicating a.
  anterior spinal a.
  arcuate a.
  ascending pharyngeal a.
  atrial circumflex a.
  auricular a.
  axillary a.
  azygos anterior cerebral a.
  basal cerebral a.
  basilar a.
  brachial a.
  brachiocephalic a.
  bronchial a.
  bulbourethral a.
  callosomarginal a.
  candelabra a.
  caroticotympanic a.
  carotid a.

NOTES

41

artery *(continued)*
cavernous a.
cavernous internal
  carotid a.
celiac a.
central a.
cerebellar a.
cerebellolabyrinthine a.
cerebral a.
cervical a.
choroidal a.
circumflex a.
colic a.
common carotid a.
common femoral a.
common hepatic a.
common iliac a.
communicating a.
complete transposition of
  great a.'s
congenital absence of
  pulmonary a.
congenital aneurysm of
  pulmonary a.
coronary a.
corrected transposition of
  great a.'s
cortical a.
cremasteric a.
cystic a.
deferential a.
digital a.
dominant a.
dorsal a.
a. of Drummond
duodenal a.
ectatic carotid a.
ethmoidal a.
external carotid a.
external iliac a.
facial a.
falx a.
femoral a.
frontal a.
frontopolar a.
gastric a.
gastroduodenal a.
gonadal a.
helicine a.
hemorrhoidal a.
hepatic a.
hyaloid a.
hypogastric a.

ileocolic a.
iliac a.
iliofemoral a.
inferior mesenteric a.
innominate a.
intercostal a.
interlobar a.
internal carotid a. (ICA)
internal mammary a.
invisible main pulmonary a.
lacrimal a.
left anterior descending a.
left atrioventricular
  groove a.
left circumflex a.
left common carotid a.
left coronary a.
left pulmonary a.
lenticulostriate a.'s
lingual a.
lumbar a.
main pulmonary a.
mammary a.
maxillary a.
medullary a.
meningeal a.
meningohypophyseal a.
mesenteric a.
middle cerebral a.
nutrient a.
occipital a.
operculofrontal a.
ophthalmic a.
origin of the renal a.
ovarian a.
pancreaticoduodenal a.
pelvic a.
penile a.
pericallosal a.
periosteal a.
peroneal a.
persistent primitive
  trigeminal a.
pharyngeal a.
phrenic a.
popliteal a.
popliteal a. trifurcation
posterior cerebral a.
posterior communicating a.
posterior descending a.
posterior inferior
  cerebellar a.

posterior-inferior
   communicating a. (PICA)
posterior tibial a.
precentral a.
prefrontal a.
premammillary a.
primitive acoustic (otic) a.
primitive hypoglossal a.
profunda femoris a.
pterygoid a.
pulmonary a.
radial a.
radicular a.
ramus intermedius a.
renal a.
right coronary a.
Riolan a.
rolandic a.
segmental a.
single umbilical a.
spermatic a.
spinal a.
splenic a.
stapedial a.
subclavian a.
superficial femoral a. (SFA)
superficial temporal a.
superior mesenteric a.
   (SMA)
supernormal a.
supraorbital a.
supratrochlear a.
telencephalic
   ventriculofugal a.
temporal a.
temporooccipital a.
testicular a.
thalamoperforating a.
thoracoacromial a.
tibial a.
transposition of great a.'s
ulnar a.
umbilical a.
uterine a.
ventriculofugal a.
vertebral a.
vertebrobasilar a.

vidian a.
visceral a.
arthritis, pl. arthritides
   coccidioidomycosis a.
   degenerative a.
   facet joint a.
   gouty a.
   juvenile rheumatoid a.
   Kellgren a.
   Lyme a.
   metatarsophalangeal joint a.
   mixed rheumatoid and
      degenerative a.
   psoriatic a.
   rheumatoid a.
   septic a.
   a. syphilitica deformans
      (ASD)
   tuberculous a.
arthrography
arthrogryposis
   a. multiplex congenita
Arthropan
arthropathy
   amyloid a.
   Charcot a.
   cuff a.
   facet a.
   gouty a.
   hemodialysis a.
   hemophiliac a.
   Jaccoud a.
   neuropathic a.
   rotator cuff a.
arthroplasty
   Girdlestone a.
arthropneumoradiography
arthroscopic
arthroscopy
arthrotomography
Arthus reaction
articular
   a. cartilage
   a. disorder
   a. facet
   a. mass separation fracture
   a. pillar fracture

NOTES

articular *(continued)*
    a. process
    a. surface
articulation
    humeroradial a.
    triquetropisiform a.
artifact, artefact
    aliasing a.
    aortic motion a.
    barium a.
    beam-hardening a.
    "black comets" a.
    black spot a.
    bone hardening a.
    bowel gas a.
    braces a.
    broadband noise detection
      error a.
    calibration failure a.
    center line a.
    chemical shift a.
    chemical shift
      misregistration a. (CSMA)
    coin a.
    computer-generated a.
    construction a.
    corduroy a.
    crescent a.
    crinkle a.
    cross-talk effect a.
    crown a.
    crush a.
    data-clipping a.
    data-clipping detection
      error a.
    data spike detection
      error a.
    DC offset a.
    deodorant a.
    detector a.
    developer a.
    double-exposure drift a.
    double exposure drift a.
    eddy current a.
    eddy ringing a.
    edge a.
    equipment a.
    faulty radiofrequency
      shielding a.
    ferromagnetic a.
    flow a.
    flow effect a.
    flow-related enhancement a.

    fog a.
    foreign material a.
    geophagia a.
    ghost a.
    Gibbs phenomenon a.
    glass eye a.
    half-moon a.
    image postprocessing
      error a.
    imbalance of phase or
      gain a.
    intensifying screen a.
    kink a.
    kissing a.
    large clothing a.
    lettering a.
    "magic angle" a.
    magnetic susceptibility a.
    main magnetic field
      inhomogeneity a.
    mercury a.
    metallic a.
    mirror-image a.
    misregistration a.
    mitral regurgitation a.
    motion a.
    movement a.
    noise spike a.
    nuclear bubbling a.
    out-of-slice a.
    paramagnetic a.
    pellet a.
    phase cancellation
      intensity a.
    phase discontinuity a.
    phase-encoding a.
    phase shift a.
    pica a.
    propagation speed a.
    pseudofracture a.
    quadrature phase detector a.
    radiofrequency spatial
      distribution a.
    reconstruction a.
    reverberation a.
    screen craze a.
    side lobe a.
    signal drop-out a.
    simulated-echo a.
    skin fold a.
    skin lesion a.
    slice profile a.
    spatial misregistration a.

spatial offset image a.
split image a.
star a.
stimulated echo a.
stimulated-echo a.
subcutaneous injection of
  contrast a.
summation shadow a.
superimposition a.
susceptibility a.
swamp-static a.
temporal instability a.
tree a.
truncation a.
truncation band a.
view insufficiency a.
wheelchair a.
wraparound a.
wraparound ghost a.
wrinkle a.
zebra a.
zebra stripe a.
zipper a.
artifactual black boundary
Artma Virtual Patient
aryepiglottic
  a. cyst
  a. fold
  a. fold neurofibroma
arylsulfatase A deficiency
arytenoid
  a. cartilage
asbestos
  a. fibers
asbestosis
  pulmonary a.
asbestos-related
  a.-r. mesothelioma
  a.-r. pleural disease
ascariasis
  binary a.
Ascaris
ascending
  a. aorta
  a. aortography
  a. colon

a. medullary vein
  thrombosis
a. pharyngeal artery
Aschoff
  A. body
  A. cell
ascites
  chylous a.
  fetal a.
  gelatinous a.
  neonatal a.
  pancreatic a.
ascitic fluid
ascorbate
ASD
  anterior sagittal diameter
  arthritis syphilitica deformans
  atrial septal defect
aseptic
  a. meningitis
  a. necrosis
Asherman syndrome
**Ashhurst-Bromer classification of
  ankle fractures**
ash leaf patch
asialoglycoprotein
  a. receptor
Askin tumor
Ask-Upmark kidney
**as low as reasonably achievable
  (ALARA)**
ASN-ase
  asparaginase
    E. coli ASN-ase
    Erwinia ASN-ase
    polyethylene glycol-modified
      E. coli ASN-ase
ASO
  antistreptolysin O
  ASO titer
asoma
ASP
  asparaginase
L-ASP
  L-asparaginase

NOTES

L-ASP
    L-asparaginase
asparaginase (ASN-ase, ASP)
L-asparaginase (L-ASP)
    E. coli L-a.
    Erwinia L-a.
    native L-a.
    polyethylene glycol-
      conjugated L-a. (PEG-L-
      ASP)
L-asparaginase (L-ASP)
L-asparagine
aspartate aminotransferase
aspartic proteinase
aspect
    dorsal a.
    plantar a.
    psychosocial a.
aspergilloma
aspergillosis
    allergic bronchopulmonary a.
    bronchopulmonary a.
    cutaneous a.
    invasive pulmonary a.
    noninvasive a.
    pleural a.
    primary a.
    semi-invasive a.
Aspergillus
    A. flavus
    A. fumigatus
    A. niger
    A. torreus
asphyxia
    birth a.
    fetal a.
    perinatal a.
asphyxiating thoracic dysplasia
aspirated foreign body (AFB)
aspiration
    a. biopsy
    bone marrow a.
    breast cyst a.
    CT-guided needle a.
    cyst a.
    a. cytology
    fine-needle a. (FNA)
    guided fine-needle a.
    meconium a.
    mineral oil a.
    a. needle
    percutaneous fine-needle a.
      (PFNA)

    pleural fluid a.
    a. pneumonia
    ultrasound-guided needle a.
aspirator
    Vabra a.
aspirin
asplenia
    functional a.
    a. syndrome
ASPO
    American Society of Preventive
      Oncology
ASR
    aldosterone secretion rate
    atrial septal resection
assay
    agglutination a.
    antigen capture a.
    binding a.
    Boyden chamber a.
    CAM 125 antigen a.
    CEA-Roche a.
    clinical a.
    clonogenic a.
    Clorox bleach a.
    Coamate antithrombin a.
    colony-forming a. (CFA)
    complement a.
    DNA transfection a.
    dye exclusion a.
    EAC rosette a.
    enzyme-linked
      immunoabsorbent assay
      (ELISA)
    enzyme-linked
      immunoelectrodiffusion a.
      (ELIEDA)
    E rosette a.
    excision a.
    fluorescent cytoprint a.
    four-point a.
    gel-shift a.
    gene transfer
      transcription a.
    Guthrie bacterial
      inhibition a.
    hemolytic complement a.
    hemolytic plaque a.
    hormonal a.
    immunocytochemical a.
      (ICA)

immunofluorescence
antibody a.
immunoradiometric a.
(IRMA)
Jerne plaque a.
lymphoblast mutation a.
lymphocyte proliferation a.
a. methodology
microculture tetrazolium
dye a.
microcytotoxicity a.
microencapsulation a.
microhemagglutination assay-
Treponema pallidum a.
(MHA-TPA)
mobility shift a.
a. neutrophil cytoplasmic
antibody (ANCA)
a. normalization
Oncotech a.
Pace a.
pan-T antigen a.
p24 antigen capture a.
polymerase chain reaction a.
Promega Cell Titer 96 cell
proliferation a.
radioligand a.
radioreceptor a.
Raji cell a.
RAST inhibition a.
renin vein a.
runon transcription a.
sandwich a.
in situ a.
spleen colony a.
TARAP a.
a. target
a. technique
tetrazolium-based
colorimetric a.
Tietze cyclic reduction a.
in vitro antibody
production a. (IVAP)
in vitro transcription a.
Assera
A. AT III
A. vWF

Asserachrom
A. ATM
A. D-Di
A. D-Di ELISA
A. fibronectin
A. FPA
A. IX:Ag
A. PAI-1
A. PF4
A. protein C
A. β-TG
A. thrombospondin
A. VII:Ag
A. X:Ag
Assera-Plate
A.-P. AT III
A.-P. C4b-BP
A.-P. IX:Ag
A.-P. protein C
A.-P. protein S
A.-P. vWF
Assera protein
A. p. S
assessment
cell viability a.
Diagnostic and Therapeutic
Technology A. (DATTA)
Doppler a.
myocardial function a.
neurologic a.
nutritional a.
pretreatment a.
quantitative risk a.
sonographic a.
vascular a.
in vivo stereologic a.
weight estimation and a.
WHO toxicity a.
assignment
gender a.
sex a.
ASSIST
American Stop Smoking
Intervention Study for Cancer
Prevention
association
a. fiber

NOTES

association *(continued)*
    noncausal a.
    a. tract
    VATER a.
asterisk sign
asterixis
asteroid body
asteroides
        Nocardia a.
asthma
    acute bronchopulmonary a.
        (ABPA)
    atopic a.
    bronchial a.
    extrinsic a.
    intrinsic a.
    refractory a.
asthmatic bronchitis
Astler-Coller
    A.-C. modification of Dukes
        classification
    A.-C. staging system
astragalocalcanean
astragaloscaphoid
astragalotibial
Astragalus
ASTRO
    American Society for
        Therapeutic Radiology and
        Oncology
astroblastoma
astrocytic hamartoma
astrocytoma
    anaplastic a.
    cerebellar a.
    cerebral a.
    cystic a.
    fibrillary a.
    gemistocytic a.
    giant cell a.
    grade I-IV a.
    juvenile pilocytic a.
    macrocystic pilocytic
        cerebellar a.
    microcystic pilocytic
        cerebellar a.
    multifocal anaplastic a.
    pilocystic a.
    piloid a.
    protoplasmic a.
    subependymal giant cell a.
    supratentorial a.
Astrup blood gas value

asymmetric
    a. bile duct
    a. data sampling
    a. echo
    a. septal hypertrophy
asymmetry
asymptomatic
asynchrony
asynergy
AT90 regulated BRE3
Atabrine
ATAI
    acute traumatic aortic injury
atavaquone
ataxia
    a. telangiectasia
ataxia-hemiparesis syndrome
ataxia-telangiectasia
A-TDA
    aminothiadiazole
atelectasis
    adhesive a.
    cicatrizing a.
    compressive a.
    discoid a.
    passive a.
    plate-like a.
    resorptive a.
    round a.
    segmental a.
    subsegmental a.
atelectatic asbestos pseudotumor
atelosteogenesis
atevirdine mesylate
ATG
    antithymocyte globulin
Atgam
atherectomy
    a. device
    directional a.
    percutaneous a.
    Simpson a.
atherocath
    Simpson a.
atheroembolic renal disease
atherogenesis
atherolysis
    ultrasonic a.
atherolytic
    a. reperfusion wire
    a. reperfusion wire device
atheroma
atheromatous plaque

atherosclerosis
 a. obliterans
atherosclerotic
 a. change
 a. disease
 a. lesion
 a. plaque
 a. ulcer
Athrombin-K
AT-II-induced intraarterial
 chemotherapy
Ativan
Ativan, Benadryl, Haldol (ABH)
Atkin epiphyseal fracture
ATL
 adult T-cell leukemia
atlantoaxial
 a. joint
 a. subluxation
atlantodental
atlantooccipital dislocation
atlas fracture
ATM
 Asserachrom ATM
atomic
 a. absorption
  spectrophotometry (AAS)
 a. mass
atonic urinary bladder
atony, atonia
 gastric a.
atopic
 a. asthma
 a. dermatitis
atopy
atovaquone
ATP
 adenosine triphosphate
ATPase locus
ATRA
 all-trans-retinoic acid
atransferrinemia
atraumatic, multidirectional,
 bilateral instability (AMBRI)
atraumatic needle
atresia
 anorectal a.

 aortic a.
 aortic arch a.
 aortic valve a.
 biliary a.
 bronchial a.
 congenital biliary a.
 congenital intestinal a.
 duodenal a.
 esophageal a.
 ileal a.
 inner ear a.
 intestinal a.
 pulmonary a.
 small bowel a.
 tricuspid a.
atretic segment
atria (*pl. of* atrium)
atrial
 a. appendage
 a. circumflex artery
 a. fibrillation
 a. flutter
 a. mesenchymoma
 a. myxoma
 a. natriuretic factor receptor
 a. natriuretic peptide
 a. septal defect (ASD)
 a. septal resection (ASR)
 a. septostomy
 a. septum
 a. situs
 a. thrombosis
atrioventricular (AV, A-V)
 a. block
 a. bundle
 a. canal
 a. connection
 a. discordance
 a. junction
 a. junction anomaly
 a. node
 a. septal defect
 a. valve
atrium, pl. atria
 common a.

NOTES

atrophic
- a. fracture
- a. pyelonephritis

atrophy
- cerebellar a.
- cerebral a.
- cortical a.
- disuse a.
- focal a.
- hippocampal a.
- olivopontocerebellar a.
- postinflammatory renal a.
- postmenopausal uterine a.
- postobstructive renal a.
- renal a.
- spinal muscular a.
- Sudeck a.

atropine

attachment
- biopsy-guided a.
- meniscocapsular a.
- metal biopsy guidance a.

attack
- postmicturitional adrenergic a.
- transient hemispheric a.
- transient ischemic a.

attenuation
- beam a.
- broadband a.
- a. coefficient
- a. compensation
- a. correction
- digital beam a.
- a. level
- signal a.
- ultrasonic a.
- a. valve

attenuator

Atvogen

atypical
- a. cell of undetermined significance
- a. epithelium
- a. lymphoproliferative disorder
- a. measles pneumonia
- a. regenerative hyperplasia
- a. tuberculosis
- a. vessel colposcopic pattern

A770U
- BW A.

^{198}Au
- gold-198

Auberger blood group

AUC
- area under the curve

auditory
- a. canal
- a. tube

Auer
- A. body
- A. rods

Auger
- A. effect
- A. electron

augmentation
- bladder a.
- breast a.
- a. mammoplasty
- reverse a.
- thiol a.

augmented breast

aureus
- *Staphylococcus a.*

auricle

auricular artery

aurotherapy

auscultation

Austin
- A. Flint murmur
- A. Moore hip prosthesis

Australian antigen

Autenrieth and Funk method

Auth rotablation rotational atherectomy catheter

autoamputation

autoantibody
- platelet-derived a.
- vitiligo a.

autoantigen

auto-anti-idiotypic antibody

autochthonous tumor

autocrine
- a. effect
- a. growth factor
- a. mechanism
- a. motility factor receptor

autofluorescence

autogenous vein bypass graft

autograft
- a. cryopreservation
- double a.
- stem cell a.

autografting
peripheral blood stem
cell a.
autohemotherapy
autoimmune
a. disorder
a. hemolytic anemia (AIHA)
a. leukopenia
a. phenomenon
a. polyendocrine-candidiasis
syndrome
a. response
a. sialadenitis
a. thrombocytopenic purpura
(AITP)
autoimmunization
autointegration
autologous
a. antibody
a. blood
a. blood clot
a. blood stem cell
transplantation
a. bone marrow cell
a. bone marrow rescue
(ABMR)
a. bone marrow support
(ABMS)
a. bone marrow transplant
(ABMT)
a. donor
a. fat
a. graft
a. hematopoietic cell
a. material
a. muscle
a. red blood cell
a. red cell salvage
a. stem cell
a. vein graft
**autolymphocyte-based treatment for
renal cell carcinoma (ALT-RCC)**
autolysin
automated large-core breast biopsy
**automatic implantable cardioverter-
defibrillator (AICD)**
automation

automotility factor
autonephrectomy
autonomic nerve block
autonomous adenoma
autoradiography
**autoregressive moving average
(AMA)**
autoreinfusion
autosomal
a. dominant
a. dominant polycystic
kidney disease
a. gene
a. recessive
a. recessive polycystic
kidney disease
a. recessive SCID
autostapler
Autosyringe pump
autotoxic
autotransfusion
autotransplantation
autovaccination
AV, A-V
arteriovenous
atrioventricular
AV fistula
AV node
Avacryl
avascular necrosis
average
autoregressive moving a.
(AMA)
a. gradient number
a. radiation dose
signal a.
spatial average-pulse a.
(SAPA)
spatial average-temporal a.
(SATA)
spatial peak-temporal a.
(SPTA)
averaging
motional a.
volume a.
AVF
arteriovenous fistula

NOTES

avian
- a. E26 virus
- a. leukemia-sarcoma complex
- a. leukosis-sarcoma complex
- a. leukosis-sarcoma virus
- a. sarcoma virus

avidin

avidin-biotin
- a.-b. binding technique
- a.-b. complex (ABC)

avidin-biotin-peroxidase-antiperoxidase (ABPAP)
- a. b.-p.-a.-p. technique

avidin-biotin-peroxidase complex

Avitene

avium
- Mycobacterium a.

avium-intracellulare
- Mycobacterium a.-i.

Aviva mammography system

AVM
- arteriovenous malformation

avulsed fragment

avulsion
- anterior labroligamentous periosteal sleeve a. (ALPSA)
- a. fracture
- lumbar root a.
- peroneus longus muscle a.
- a. stress fracture
- testicular artery a.

avulsive cortical irregularity

axes (*pl. of* axis)

axetil
- cefuroxime a.

axial
- a. angiography
- a. cineangiography
- a. hernia
- a. image
- a. plane
- a. radiograph
- a. resolution
- a. section
- a. skeleton
- a. view

axilla, pl. axillae

axillary
- a. adenopathy
- a. artery
- a. dissection
- a. hematoma
- a. lymphadenopathy
- a. lymph node
- a. node involvement
- a. node metastasis
- a. region
- a. sheath
- a. skin lesion
- a. tail
- a. vein
- a. vessel
- a. view

axillobifemoral bypass graft

axillosubclavian vein thrombosis

axis, pl. axes
- celiac a.
- a. fracture
- hypothalamic-pituitary-adrenal a. (HPA)
- hypothalamic-pituitary-gonadal a.
- renal a.

axoplasmic flow

Ayerza disease

Ayurvedic medicine

azacitidine

5-azacitidine

5-aza-2'-deoxycytidine

8-azaguanine

azathioprine

azdu

azidothymidine (AZT)

azidouridine

Azimexon

azimuthal resolution

aziridinylbenzoquinone (AZQ)

azithromycin

azlocillin

azoospermia

azotemia

AZQ
- aziridinylbenzoquinone

AZT
- azidothymidine

Aztec

azurophilia

azurophilic granule

azygoesophageal
- a. line
- a. recess

azygos
- a. anterior cerebral artery
- a. continuation

a. fissure
a. lobe
a. lymph node

a. vein
a. vein enlargement
Azzopardi tumor

NOTES

B4
> B4 antigen
> B4 blocked ricin

B5
> B5 antigen
> B5 fixative

B7
> B-cell surface antigen B7
> B7 transfected melanoma cell vaccine

B23
> NSABT protocol B23

B72.3
> monoclonal antibody B72.3

2b
> IFN-alpha 2b

B1 antigen
B6 bronchus sign
Babesia microti
babesiosis
BAC
> BCNU, ara-C, cyclophosphamide

bacillary
> b. angiomatosis
> b. dysentery
> b. peliosis hepatis

bacille
Bacille Calmette-Guérin (BCG)
bacillus, pl. bacilli
> acid-fast b.
> Calmette-Guérin b.
> Friedländer b.

Bacillus anthracis **pneumonia**
backfire fracture
backflow
> pyelolymphatic b.
> pyelorenal b.
> pyelotubular b.
> pyelovenous b.

background equivalent radiation time
backprojection
back projection
backscatter
backwash ileitis
baclofen
BACOP
> bleomycin, Adriamycin, cyclophosphamide, Oncovin, prednisone

BACT
> BCNU, ara-C, cyclophosphamide, 6- thioguanine

Bactec
bacteremia
> catheter-associated b.
> venous access device-related b.

bacteria (*pl. of* bacterium)
> antibiotic-resistant b.
> endogenous b.
> Gram-negative b.
> Gram-positive b.

bacterial
> b. aneurysm
> b. aortitis
> b. endocarditis
> b. ependymitis
> b. epiglottitis
> b. infection
> b. meningitis
> b. nephritis
> b. osteomyelitis
> b. pneumonitis
> b. septicemia
> b. sinusitis
> b. toxin
> b. vaginosis
> b. vasculitis

bactericidal
bacteriobilia
bacteriolytic
bacteriophage
bacterium, pl. bacteria
bacteriuria
bacterohemolysin
Bacteroides
BactoAgar
Bactoshield antibacterial soap
Bactrim
> B. DS

baculovirus
badge
> ring b.

Bafverstedt syndrome
bagassosis
Bagdad Spring anemia

bag-of-bones effect
bag-of-worms effect
baileyi
 Cryptosporidium b.
baja
 patella b.
Baker cyst
BAL
 bronchoalveolar lavage
Balb/C sarcoma virus
ball
 fungus b.
 keratin b.
 renal fungus b.
 sludge b.
 b. thrombus
ball-and-socket
 b.-a.-s. epiphysis
 b.-a.-s. joint
 b.-a.-s. prosthesis
ball-in-hand appearance
ballistic material
balloon
 b. angioplasty
 angioplasty b.
 b. atrial septostomy (BAS)
 Balt b.
 Bardex b.
 Becton Dickinson b.
 Blue Max high-pressure b.
 b. bronchoplasty
 b. catheter
 b. catheter technique
 b. cell
 corset b.
 b. counterpulsation
 Debrun b.
 detachable b.
 b. dilation
 b. dilation angioplasty
  (BDA)
 b. dilation valvuloplasty
  (BDV)
 b. dilator
 b. embolotherapy
 b. epiphysis
 E-Z-EM b. enema
 Gianturco-Roubin b.
 Hieshima b.
 Hunter-Sessions b.
 laser b.
 latex b.
 low-profile angioplasty b.

 Moser b.
 b. occlusion
 b. occlusion pulmonary
  angiography
 Schwarten Microglide LP b.
 Spears laser b.
 Stealth catheter b.
 b. tamponade
 TEGwire b.
 b. test occlusion
 thermal b.
 transurethral b. dilatation
 ultrasmall-shafted b.
 ultrathin b.
balloon-cell melanoma
balloon-expandable
 b.-e. stent
 b.-e. tantalum stent
balloon-occluded arterial infusion
balloon-on-a-wire
Baltaxe-Mitty-Pollack needle
Balt balloon
bamboo spine
banana
 b. catheter
 b. fracture
 b. sign
bancrofti
 Wucheria b.
band
 b. cell
 crow's feet b.'s
 dense metaphyseal b.'s
 b. form
 germline b.
 HIV b.'s
 iliotibial b.
 intratesticular b.
 Ladd b.'s
 Mach b.
 metaphyseal b.'s
 monoclonal b.
 b. pattern
 Z b.
banded chromosome
bandemia
banding
 chromosome b.
band-pass filter
bandwidth (BW)
 gradient b.
 low b.
 receiver b.

bank
    cell b.
    gene b.
    tissue b.
Bankart
    B. fracture
    B. lesion
    B. procedure
banking
    cryopreserved tissue b.
Bannayan syndrome
Banti disease
bar
    coracoclavicular b.
    cricopharyngeal b.
    physeal b.
barber pole sign
barbiturate
Barcroft apparatus
Bard
    B. absorption dressing
    B. rotary atherectomy
      system (BRAS)
Bardex
    B. balloon
    B. catheter
bare
    b. fiber
    b. lymphocyte syndrome
bare-area sign
Bareggi reaction
Bargen streptococcus
baritosis
barium
    b. artifact
    b. bolus
    b. enema
    b. enema with air contrast
    b. examination
    holdup in flow of b.
    b. meal
    b. mixture
    b. pneumoconiosis
    pocketing of b.
    reflux of b.
    retained b.
    b. study

    b. sulfate
    b. suspension
    b. swallow
barium-filled colon
barium-water esophagram
Barlow
    B. syndrome
    B. test
baroreceptor
barotrauma
barrel-shaped lesion
Barrett
    B. epithelium
    B. esophagus
barrier
    anatomic b.
    blood-air b.
    blood-aqueous b.
    blood-brain b. (BBB)
    blood-cerebrospinal fluid b.
    blood-thymus b.
    cerebrospinal fluid-brain b.
    endothelial b.
    integumentary b.
    mucosal b.
Bart hemoglobin
Bartholin
    B. duct
    B. gland carcinoma
Bartonella anemia
bartonellosis
Barton fracture
Barton-Smith fracture
Bartter syndrome
BAS
    balloon atrial septostomy
basal
    b. angle
    b. cell adenoma
    b. cell carcinoma
    b. cell nevus syndrome
    b. cell papilloma
    b. cerebral artery
    b. cistern
    b. descent
    b. ganglia
    b. ganglia calcification

NOTES

basal *(continued)*
  b. ganglia hematoma
  b. ganglia infarct
  b. lamella
  b. neck fracture
  b. nucleus
  b. vein of Rosenthal
basalis layer
basaloid
  b. carcinoma
  b. nonkeratinizing carcinoma
  b. squamous cell carcinoma
base
  b. pair
  Schiff b.
  skull b.
  b. view
baseball finger fracture
baseline
  pretherapy b.
basement membrane
base-plus-fog level
base-ring tilt
basilar
  b. angiography
  b. artery
  b. femoral neck fracture
  b. impression
  b. invagination
basilic vein
basion-axial interval
basion-dens interval
basis pontis
basivertebral vein
basket
  Amplatz through-and-
    through b.
  Dormia stone b.
  b. filter
  b. fragmentation technique
  Hawkins stone b.
  Pfister-Schwartz stone b.
  Rutner stone b.
  Segura b.
  stone b.
  Universal b.
basketing technique
basocytopenia
basocytosis
basophil
  b. chemotactic factor
  b. count

basophilia
  paraneoplastic b.
basophilic
  b. adenoma
  b. erythroblast
  b. erythrocyte
  b. leukemia
  b. normoblast
  b. stippling
basophilism
  Cushing b.
basophilocytic leukemia
basosquamous
  b. carcinoma
  b. nonkeratinizing carcinoma
basosquamous carcinoma
Batanopride
Batson plexus
battered
  b. baby syndrome
  b. child syndrome
battledore placenta
batwing
  b. configuration
  b. lung consolidation
Bauer Temno biopsy needle
bauxite pneumoconiosis
Bavarian thyroid
Baxter
  B. infuser
  B. INtermate
bayesian analysis
bayonet position of fracture
Bay region concept
Bazex disease
BB
  blue bloater
BBB
  blood-brain barrier
BBD
  benign breast disease
BBs
  both bones
BCAP
  BCNU, cyclophosphamide,
    Adriamycin, prednisone
B-CAVe
  bleomycin, CCNU, Adriamycin,
    Velban
B-cell
  B-c. acute lymphoblastic
    leukemia

B-c. acute lymphocytic
leukemia
B-c. chronic lymphocytic
leukemia
B-c. differentiation factor
B-c. epitope protein
B-c. lineage antigen
B-c. lymphoma
B-c. neoplasia
B-c. neoplasm
B-c. surface antigen B7
B-c. surface immunoglobulin
B-c. tumor
B-cell-stimulating factor
BCG
Bacille Calmette-Guérin
BCG osteomyelitis
scarification of BCG
Tice BCG
bcl-1 **oncogene**
bcl-2
bcl-2 oncogene
bcl-2 protein
bcl-2 proto-oncogene
bcl-2/Ig **fusion gene**
bcl-3 **oncogene**
BCNU
bischlorethylnitrosourea
bischloronitrosurea
carmustine
**BCNU, ara-C, cyclophosphamide
(BAC)**
**BCNU, ara-C, cyclophosphamide,
6-thioguanine (BACT)**
**BCNU, cyclophosphamide,
Adriamycin, prednisone (BCAP)**
**BCNU, cyclophosphamide,
vinblastine, procarbazine,
prednisone (BCVPP)**
**BCNU, etoposide, ara-C,
cyclophosphamide (BEAC)**
**BCNU, etoposide, ara-C,
melphalan (BEAM)**
bcr/abl **DNA probe**
bcr/abl **fusion gene**
bcr/abl **transcript**

BCVPP
BCNU, cyclophosphamide,
vinblastine, procarbazine,
prednisone
bleomycin, cyclophosphamide,
vincristine, procarbazine,
prednisone
BDA
balloon dilation angioplasty
B-D bone marrow biopsy needle
BDV
balloon dilation valvuloplasty
BE1 antigen
BE2 antigen
BEAC
BCNU, etoposide, ara-C,
cyclophosphamide
bead
Dynal M450 magnetic b.'s
immunomagnetic b.
magnetic b.
packed b.'s
polyacrylamide b.
beaded
b. appearance
b. duct
b. ureter
beak
b. fracture
b. sign
beaked appearance
beaking
antral b.
tectal b.
BEAM
BCNU, etoposide, ara-C,
melphalan
beam
b. attenuation
cone b.
electron b.
b. energy
b. filtration
b. hardening
laser b.
b. limitation
b. pattern

NOTES

beam *(continued)*
    b. shaper
    b. steering
    x-ray b.
beam-hardening
    b.-h. artifact
    b.-h. effect
beam-modifying device
beam-splitting mirror
bean
    castor b.
Bearn-Kunkel-Slater syndrome
beast stromal pattern
beaten brass appearance
Beau lines
BEB
    blind esophageal brushing
Bebulin VH
Becker nevus
Beckwith-Wiedemann
    B.-W. syndrome
Becquerel
Becton
    B. Dickinson balloon
    B. Dickinson FAC scan
bed
    b. block
    Clinitron b.
    Kin Air b.
Bednar tumor
bedroom fracture
bedside radiography
beef heart antigen
Behçet
    B. disease
    B. syndrome
behenoylcytosine arabinoside
Behring law
Beiswenger disease
BELD
    bleomycin, Eldisine, lomustine, dacarbazine
Belganyl
bell-and-clapper deformity
belli
    Isopora b.
Bellini duct
Bell palsy
belly bath chemotherapy
Benadryl
Bence Jones
    B. J. body
    B. J. myeloma
    B. J. protein
    B. J. proteinuria
beneficial atrial septal defect
benign
    b. bone lesion
    b. breast disease (BBD)
    b. cyst
    b. duct ectasia
    b. fetal hamartoma
    b. fibrous histiocytoma
    b. gastric ulcer
    b. infiltrate
    b. intracranial hypertension
    b. juvenile melanoma
    b. lesion
    b. lymphadenopathy
    b. lymphocytoma cutis
    b. lymphoepithelial lesion
    b. lymphoepithelial parotid tumor
    b. lymphoma of rectum
    b. lymphoproliferative lesion
    b. mass
    b. meningeal fibrosis
    b. nevus
    b. ovarian tumor
    b. proliferation
    b. proliferative disorder
    b. prostatic hyperplasia (BPH)
    b. prostatic hypertrophy
    b. tumor
    b. vascular lesion
benignum
    lymphogranuloma b.
Bennett
    B. classification
    B. classification of lymphoma
    B. comminuted fracture
    B. fracture
benperidol
Bentley button
Bentson
    B. guidewire
    B. wire
benzamide
    substituted b.
benzene
benzoate
    methyl b.
benzodiazepine
    b. receptor

benzoic acid
benzoporphyrin derivative, monoacid
  ring A (BPD-MA)
benzquinamide
benzyamide
    4-amino-*N*-(a-
    aminophenyl) b.
benzyl guanine
benzylidene-glucose
BEP
    bleomycin, etoposide, Platinol
Berard classification for follicular
  lymphoma
bereavement services
Bergman sign
Bergquist triad
Berkefeld filter
Berkson-Gage method tumor
Berlix Oncology Foundation
Bernard-Soullier syndrome
Bernoulli
    B. equation
    B. principle
berry
    b. aneurysm
    b. cell
    B. syndrome
Berry-Dedrick phenomenon
Bertin
    cloison of B.
    column of B.
    large column of B.
    large septum of B.
berylliosis
beryllium granuloma
Bessey-Lowrey unit
best-fit smooth curve
beta
    b. camera
    b. emission
    b. emitter
    epoetin b.
    b. error
    interleukin-1 b.
beta-carotene
Betadine
beta-hCG test

beta-lapachone
beta-lipotropin
beta-2-microglobulin
beta-pleated sheet
beta-scintillation counter
Betaseron (*var. of* interferon beta,
  recombinant human)
betatron
betel cancer
Bethesda
    B. system
    B. unit
beveled-tip needle
beverage
    De Veras b.
bezoar
BFU-E
    burst-forming unit-erythroid
BGG
    bovine gammaglobulin
BG9015
B_0-gradient method
B-hCG tumor marker
bias
    detection b.
    selection b.
    time-to-treatment b.
bibasilar
BIC
bicaudate
    b. index
    b. ratio
biceps
    b. brachii
    b. brachii tendon
    b. brachii tendon reflex test
    b. femoris
    b. tendon
Bichat foramen
bicipital
    b. groove
    b. tendon sheath
bicisate
    technetium-99m b.
biclonal follicular lymphoma
biclonality

NOTES

61

bicollis
    bicornuate b.
bicondylar
    b. fracture
    b. T-shaped fracture
    b. Y-shaped fracture
bicornis
    uterus b.
bicornuate
    b. bicollis
    b. unicollis
    b. uterus
bicycle spoke fracture
bidirectional interface
Biermer anemia
Biermer-Ehrlich anemia
bifemoral graft
bifid
    b. collecting system
    b. gallbladder
    b. renal pelvis
    b. ureter
bifida
    spina b.
bifidum
    cranium b.
bifrontal
    b. index
    b. oligodendroglioma
bifunctional antibody
bifurcation
    b. aneurysm
    aortic b.
    carotid artery b.
bilateral
    b. arachnoid cyst
    b. carotid arteriography
    b. choroid plexus cyst
    b. ductal ectasia
    b. iliac crest
    b. infarction
    b. intrafacetal dislocation
    b. large kidney
    b. left-sidedness
    b. locked facets
    b. lower lobe pneumonia
    b. lymphadenectomy
    b. myocutaneous graft
    b. right-sidedness
    b. salpingo-oophorectomy
    (BSO)
    b. small kidney
Bilbao-Dotter wire guide

bile
    b. acid
    b. acid chemolitholysis
    b. canaliculum
    common b. duct
    concentrated b.
    b. duct
    b. duct carcinoma
    b. duct dilatation
    b. duct manipulation
    b. encrustation
    b. flow
    high-density b.
    b. leakage
    limy b.
    milk-of-calcium b.
    b. plug syndrome
    b. reflux gastritis
bilharzial granuloma
bilharziasis
biliary
    b. atresia
    b. calculus
    b. cirrhosis
    b. coaxial dilator
    b. colic
    b. cystadenoma
    b. decompression
    b. drainage
    b. drainage catheter
    b. duct
    b. endoprosthesis
    b. intervention
    b. lithotripsy
    b. manipulation catheter
    b. obstruction syndrome
    b. radicle
    b. sepsis
    b. stent
    b. stone
    b. stricture
    b. system
    b. tract
    b. tract cancer
    b. tract disease
    b. tract obstruction
    transhepatic b. disease
    b. tree
    b. tree obstruction
biliary-enteric, bilioenteric
    b.-e. anastomosis
    b.-e. anastomosis operation
    b.-e. fistula

Biligrafin
Biligram
bili light
Biliodyl
bilioenteric (*var. of* biliary-enteric)
    b. bypass
bilirubin
    b. test
bilirubinemia
bilithorax
Bilivistan
Billingham scale
Billroth
    cords of B.
    B. I anastomosis
    B. I gastroduodenostomy
    B. II anastomosis
    B. II gastrojejunostomy
bilobed configuration
biloma
    intrahepatic b.
Bilopaque
Biloptin
BIMAb
    I-labeled B-cell-specific anti-
      CD20 monoclonal antibody
bimalleolar fracture
B-immunoblast
binary
    b. ascariasis
    b. digit
binding
    b. assay
    b. energy
    fragment antigen b. (Fab)
    Ig b.
    iron b.
    lentil agglutination b.
    protein b.
    proteoglycan b.
    b. site
    T-lymphocyte b.
    in vivo b.
Binelli styptic
Binet
    B. staging system for

chronic lymphocytic
    leukemia
    B. system of classification
binomial pulse
Binswanger
    B. disease
    B. encephalopathy
binucleate cell
bioaccumulator
bioassay
bioavailability
biochemical
    b. epidemiology
    b. marker
    b. modulation
biochemistry
Bioclusive
    B. dressing
    B. TFD
Bio-Defense Nutritionals
Biodel
bioeffect
    thermal b.
biofeedback
bioflavonoid
biogenesis
biologic, biological
    b. effect
    b. false-positive
    b. therapy
biology
    cell b.
    molecular cell b.
    tumor b.
biomarker
biomechanics
biometry
Biopatch dressing
biophysical
    b. profile
    b. profile scoring (BPS)
    b. rhythm
biopsy
    abdominal b.
    abdominal lymph node b.
    adrenal gland b.
    aspiration b.

NOTES

biopsy *(continued)*
    automated large-core
      breast b.
    bone marrow b.
    brain b.
    breast b.
    core b.
    CT-guided b.
    cytobrush b.
    endometrial b.
    endomyocardial b.
    excisional b.
    fetal liver b.
    fetal skin b.
    fine-needle b.
    fine-needle aspiration b.
      (FNAB)
    FNA b.
    guided b.
    hilar b.
    incisional b.
    intramedullary tumor b.
    liver b.
    lung b.
    mediastinal b.
    multiple core b.
    needle b.
    b. needle
    outpatient b.
    pancreatic b.
    parathyroid b.
    pelvic b.
    pelvic aspiration b.
    percutaneous b.
    percutaneous fine-needle
      aspiration b. (PFNAB)
    percutaneous liver b.
    percutaneous needle b.
    pleural b.
    punch b.
    scalene node b.
    skeletal b.
    skin b.
    stereotactic b.
    stereotactic percutaneous
      needle b.
    surgical excision b.
    testicular b.
    thyroid needle b.
    transbronchial b.
    b. transducer
    transrectal b.
    transthoracic needle b.

    transthoracic percutaneous
      fine-needle aspiration b.
    trephine b.
    Tru-Cut needle b.
    ultrasound-guided b.
    ventricular
      endomyocardial b.
    vulvar b.
biopsy-guided attachment
Biopsys mammotome
Bioptome
Biopty gun
Biospec
biosynthesis
biotene
    b. chewing gum
    b. mouthwash
    b. toothbrush
    b. toothpaste
biotherapy
biotin
    fluoroacylated b.
biotin-labeled
    b.-l. antibody
    b.-l. anti-immunoglobulin
biotin-streptavidin peroxidase
    conjugate technique
biotinylated HPV DNA probe
biotransformation
biotryoid
Biozyme
BIP
    bleomycin, ifosfamide, Platinol
biparietal diameter (BPD)
bipartite
    b. navicula
    b. patella
biphasic
    b. malignant mesothelioma
biphosphonate
biplane
    b. angiography
    b. axial filming
    b. sector scanner
bipolar
    b. lead
    b. pacemaker
bipotential precursor cell tumor
Birbeck granule
bird
    b. beak deformity
    b. breeder's disease
birdcage coil

bird-fancier's lung
bird-of-prey sign
bird's nest filter
bird-wing joint
BI-RG-587
birth
    b. asphyxia
    b. fracture
    b. trauma
Birt-Hogg-Dube syndrome
bisacetamide
    hexamethylene b. (HMBA)
bisantrene
bischlorethylnitrosourea (BCNU)
bischloronitrosurea (BCNU)
bisexual
B-islet cell
bismuth
    b. injection
    b. toxicity
bismuth-212
bisobrin
bisphosphonate APD
bisphosponate
bispiperazinedione (ICRF)
bistrimethylsilylsulfate
bit
    parity b.
Bittner milk factor
bivariant analysis
biventricular enlargement
Bizzozero corpuscle
Björk-Shiley
    B.-S. heart valve
black
    b. blood angiograph
    b. boundary
    b. epidermoidoma
    B. nuclear staging
    b. spot artifact
"black comets" artifact
Blackfan-Diamond anemia
blackwater fever
bladder
    atonic urinary b.
    b. augmentation

    b. cancer
    b. carcinoma
    b. catheterization
    b. congenital abnormality
    b. diverticulitis
    b. diverticulum
    b. dysfunction
    b. endometriosis
    b. exstrophy
    b. flap
    b. flap hematoma
    b. hemorrhage
    b. incontinence
    kidneys, ureters, b. (KUB)
    kidneys and urinary b. (KUB)
    b. laceration
    neurogenic b.
    OncoRad for b.
    b. outlet obstruction
    shrunken b.
    spastic urinary b.
    transurethral resection of b. (TURB)
    b. tumor
    urinary b.
    b. wall thickening
    b. wall thickness
    x ray of kidneys, ureters, and b.
bladder-within-bladder sign
blade catheter
blade-of-grass lysis
Blakemore-Sengstaken tube
Blalock-Hanlon procedure
Blalock-Taussig shunt
bland thrombus
blast
    B-b.
    B-lymphocyte b.
    b. cell
    b. cell leukemia
    b. colony-forming unit
    b. crisis
    extrafollicular b.

NOTES

blast *(continued)*
    refractory anemia with
      excess b.
blastema
    metanephric b.
blastemia
blastic
    b. lesion
    b. metastasis
    b. phase
    b. transformation
    b. variant
blastocyst
Blastocystis hominis
blastocytoma
blastogenic factor
blastoma
    parenchymal b.
    pleuropulmonary b.
blastomere
blastomycosis
    European b.
    nasopharyngeal b.
    North American b.
bleb
    emphysematous b.
blebbing
    plasma membrane b.
bleeder in tumor mass
bleeding
    gingival b.
    packing for b.
    b. point
    b. site
    splenic b.
    b. time
    uterine b.
    vaginal b.
    variceal b.
Blenoxane
bleomycin
    b. sulfate
bleomycin, Adriamycin,
  cyclophosphamide, Oncovin,
  prednisone (BACOP)
bleomycin, CCNU, Adriamycin,
  Velban (B-CAVe)
bleomycin, cyclophosphamide,
  vincristine, procarbazine,
  prednisone (BCVPP)

bleomycin, Eldisine, lomustine,
  dacarbazine (BELD)
bleomycin, etoposide, Platinol
  (BEP)
bleomycin, ifosfamide, carboplatin
bleomycin, ifosfamide, Platinol
  (BIP)
bleomycin, Oncovin, lomustine,
  dacarbazine (BOLD)
bleomycin, Oncovin (vincristine),
  streptozotocin, etoposide (BOSE)
Bleonoxane
blevifolia
    the western yew, Taxus b.
blighted ovum
blind
    b. esophageal brushing
      (BEB)
    b. loop syndrome
    b. pouch syndrome
    b. segment
    b. spot
blindness
    monocular b.
B-lineage acute lymphoblastic cell
blister
    fracture b.
blistering disorder
bloater
    blue b. (BB)
bloc
    en b.
Bloch equation
block
    alcohol b.
    atrioventricular b.
    autonomic nerve b.
    bed b.
    celiac b.
    celiac ganglion b.
    Cerrobend b.
    complete heart b.
    congenital heart b.
    epidural b.
    first-degree heart b.
    heart b.
    intrathecal b.
    lung b.
    Mobitz heart b.
    nerve b.
    neurolytic b.
    neurolytic nerve b.
    peripheral nerve b.

regional neurolytic b.
second-degree heart b.
shock b.
spinal b.
splanchnic nerve b.
subarachnoid nerve b.
sympathetic b.
third-degree heart b.
b. vertebra
blockade
antrogen b.
dopamine b.
lumbar nerve root b.
receptor b.
blocker
adrenergic b.
alpha-adrenergic b.
calcium channel b.
blocking
b. antibody
b. factor
tissue b.
Bloembergen, Purcell, and Pound theory (BPP theory)
blood
b. agar plate
arterial b.
autologous b.
b. cell
citrated b.
b. clot
b. clotting factor
b. coagulation factor
b. component
b. component support
b. component therapy
cord b.
b. culture
defibrinated b.
b. doping
b. expander
fetoplacental b.
b. flow
b. flow dynamics
b. flow measurement
b. flow velocity
b. fluke

b. gas
b. group
b. group antigen
intracerebral b.
intraventricular b.
b. island
b. isotope clearance
lactescent b.
laked b.
b. lipid
occult b.
b. oxygenation level-dependent (BOLD)
b. oxygenation level-dependent contrast
b. patch
peripheral b.
platelet-poor b.
platelet-rich b.
b. pool
b. pool activity
b. pool imaging
b. pool scan
b. pool scintigraphy
b. pressure
rheology of b.
b. sample
b. sampling
b. shunting
sludged b.
b. smear
splanchnic b.
stagnant b.
b. substitute
b. sugar
b. supply
b. test
transfused b.
b. transfusion
b. tumor
b. urea nitrogen (BUN)
b. urea nitrogen test
b. velocity
venous b.
b. vessel
b. vessel invasion

NOTES

blood *(continued)*
    b. warmer
    whole b.
blood-air barrier
blood-aqueous barrier
blood-borne
blood-brain barrier (BBB)
blood-cerebrospinal fluid barrier
blood-flow index
bloodstream
blood-thymus barrier
Bloom-Richardson grade
Bloom syndrome
blot
    MTN b.
    Northern b.
    Southern b.
    b. test
    Western b.
blotting
    ligand b.
Blount
    B. disease
    B. tibia vara
blow-in fracture
blow-out fracture
blue
    Alcian b.
    b. bloater (BB)
    cresyl b.
    b. digit syndrome
    b. dome cyst
    gentian b.
    isosulfan b.
    B. Max high-pressure
      balloon
    b. nevus
    Prussian b.
    b. toe syndrome
    toluidine b.
blueberry muffin syndrome
blue-rubber-bleb-nevus syndrome
Blumer shelf
Blummenstat line
Blum syndrome
blunting
blur
    composite b.
    focal spot b.
    motion b.
    object-plane b.
blush
    choroid plexus b.

    papillary b.
    tumor b.
B-ly-7 antigen
B-lym **oncogene**
B-lymphocyte
    B-l. blast
    B-l. differentiation
    B-l. proliferation
    B-l. stimulatory factor
BM41-440
B2-microglobulin
BMMP
    bone marrow myeloid precursor
B-mode
    B.-m. echocardiography
    B.-m. ultrasonography
BMT
    bone marrow transplant
BMY-27857
BMY-28090
BMY-40900
BN acute myelocytic leukemia
   (BNML)
BNLAN cement
BNML
    BN acute myelocytic leukemia
Boari flap procedure
Bochdalek
    foramen of B.
    B. foramen
    B. hernia
Boden-Gibb staging system
body
    Amato b.
    Arnold b.
    Aschoff b.
    aspirated foreign b. (AFB)
    asteroid b.
    Auer b.
    Bence Jones b.
    Bracht-Wachter b.
    brassy b.
    Cabot ring b.
    Call-Exner b.
    cancer b.
    b. cast syndrome
    caudate b.
    Councilman b.
    Cowdry type A intranuclear
      inclusion b.
    crescent b.
    Deetjen b.
    demilune b.

Dohle b.
Donovan b.
Dutcher b.
Ehrlich hemoglobinemia b.
elementary b.
embryonal tumor of
  ciliary b.
fibrin b.
b. fluid exchange
foreign b.
gall b.
gamma-Favre b.
Gamna-Gandy b.
geniculate b.
Gordon elementary b.
Guarnieri b.
b. habitus
Hamazaki-Wesenberg b.
Harting b.
Heinz-Ehrlich b.
hematoxylin b.
Howell-Jolly b.
intraarticular b.
intraluminal foreign b.
intraocular foreign b.
intravascular foreign b.
Jaworski b.
Jolly b.
ketone b.
Lallemand b.
Lallemand-Trousseau b.
lateral geniculate b.
Leishman-Donovan b.
Lipschutz b.
loose b.
loose intraarticular b.
lyssa b.
malpighian b.
medial geniculate b.
metallic foreign b.
Michaelis-Gutmann b.
Mott b.
Müller duct b.
Negri b.
Neill-Mooser b.
osteochondral loose b.
owl's eye inclusion b.

pacchionian b.'s
b. of the pancreas
Pappenheimer b.
Paschen b.
pineal b.
Prowazek b.
Prowazek-Greeff b.
psammoma b.
pyknotic b.
radiopaque foreign b.
Reilly b.
retained foreign b.
Ross b.
Russell b.
b. scanning
Seidelin b.
b. of the stomach
b. surface area calculation
Trousseau-Lallemand b.
b. of the uterus
vertebral b.
Weibel-Palade b.
Boeck sarcoid
Boehler angle
Boerhaave syndrome
Bohr
  B. effect
  B. magneton
Boivin antigen
BOLD
  bleomycin, Oncovin, lomustine,
    dacarbazine
  blood oxygenation level-
    dependent
  BOLD contrast
bolster
  Hollister bridge suture b.
Boltzmann
  B. constant
  B. distribution
  B. factor
bolus
  barium b.
  food b.
  b. injection
  b. tagging
  b. tracking

NOTES

bolus-of-worms appearance
Bombay phenotype
bombesin
Bombriski melanoma
bond
        coordinate b.
        covalent b.
        valence b.
bone
        b. age
        b. algorithm
        both b.'s (BBs)
        bowed long b.
        cancellous b.
        b. cancer
        carpal b.
        carpal navicular b.
        b. center
        compact b.
        cortical b.
        cranial b.
        cuboid b.
        b. cyst
        dancer's b.
        b. destruction
        b. dysplasia
        ethmoid b.
        facial b.
        fencer's b.
        b. flap
        frontal b.
        gracile b.
        b. graft
        greater multangular b.
        b. hardening artifact
        heterotopic b.
        hyoid b.
        b. imaging
        b. infarct
        b. infiltration
        innominate b.
        b. island
        b. length study
        b. lesion
        lesser multangular b.
        long b.
        malar b.
        b. marrow
        b. marrow aplasia
        b. marrow aspiration
        b. marrow biopsy
        b. marrow cell
        b. marrow cellularity

b. marrow depression
b. marrow donor
b. marrow dose
b. marrow fibroblast
b. marrow fibrosis
b. marrow harvesting
b. marrow histochemistry
b. marrow hypocellularity
b. marrow hypoplasia
b. marrow immunohistology
b. marrow infiltration
b. marrow lesion
b. marrow lymphoid
  hyperplasia
b. marrow
  microenvironment
b. marrow myeloid
  precursor (BMMP)
b. marrow purging
b. marrow relapse
b. marrow rescue
b. marrow scintigraphy
b. marrow staining
b. marrow stroma
b. marrow suppression
b. marrow toxicity
b. marrow transplant (BMT)
b. marrow transplantation
metabolic b. disease
metacarpal b.
b. metastasis
metatarsal b.
b. mineral content
b. morphogenetic activity
multangular b.
navicular b.
b. neoplasm
occipital b.
omovertebral b.
b. overdevelopment
b. pain
parietal b.
petrous b.
b. plug
b. quantitative CT (BQCT)
rider's b.
b. sarcoma
b. scan
b. scintigraphy
sclerosed temporal b.
b. sclerosis
sesamoid b.
small b. enteroscopy

sphenoid b.
b. spicule
b. spur
b. strut
telephone handle b.
temporal b.
trabeculated b.
triquetral b.
b. tumor
wormian b.
bone-air interface
bone-chip allograft
bone-forming tumor
bone-on-bone contact
bone-tendon-bone graft
bone-within-bone
b.-w.-b. appearance
b.-w.-b. vertebra
Bonnevie-Ullrich syndrome
bony
b. alignment
b. ankylosis
b. bridging
b. contusion
b. erosion
b. hyperostosis
b. labyrinth
b. metastasis
b. nonunion
b. pelvis
b. projection
b. resorption
b. thorax
b. trabecular pattern
boomerang configuration
boost
b. to the oropharynx
b. technique
boot-shaped heart
boot-top fracture
border
diaphragmatic b.
irregular b.
mesenteric b.
periventricular b.
shaggy heart b.
smooth b.

borderline
b. heart size
b. malignant epithelial
neoplasm
b. malignant epithelial
ovarian neoplasm
Bordetella pertussis
Bordet-Gengou phenomenon
Boren-McKinney retriever set
boron
b. neutron-capture therapy
Borrelia burgdorferi
borreliosis
Lyme b.
Borrmann
B. classification
B. classification system
BOSE
bleomycin, Oncovin
(vincristine), streptozotocin,
etoposide
boss
carpal b.
parietal b.
Boston
B. brace
B. exanthem
Bosworth fracture
Botallo foramen
both-bone fracture
both bones (BBs)
both-column fracture
botrecetin
botryoides
sarcoma b.
botryoid sarcoma
botryomycosis
bottle
Castaneda b.
botulism
Bouchard node
bougie
bougienage
b. technique
Bouin solution
bounce point

NOTES

boundary
    air/bone/tissue b.
    artifactual black b.
    black b.
    horizontal b.
    b. layer
bounding peripheral pulse
bound water
Bourneville disease
boutonnière
    b. deformity
bovine
    b. anti-cryptosporidium
    b. arch
    b. cancer eye
    b. dialyzable leukocyte
      extract
    b. gammaglobulin (BGG)
    b. lentivirus
    b. leukemia virus
    pegademase b.
    b. red blood cells
    b. xenograft
Boving chart
bovis
    Moraxella b.
    Mycobacterium b.
    Streptococcus b.
bowed
    b. long bone
    b. micromelia
bowel
    b. cancer
    b. distention
    b. gas artifact
    herniated b.
    b. incontinence
    b. infarction
    large b.
    loop of b.
    b. obstruction
    b. preparation
    small b.
    b. sounds
    b. wall
    b. wall hematoma
    b. wall penetration
Bowen disease
bowenoid
    b. papulosis
    b. papulosis of vulva

bowing
    anterior tibial b.
    b. fracture
bowler hat sign
box
    Carpal B.
    shadow b.
    TATA b.
    view b.
boxer's fracture
boxlike cardiomegaly
Boyden
    B. chamber
    B. chamber assay
boydii
    Pseudallescheria b.
boy-in-a-bubble disease
BP
    bronchopleural
    BP fistula
    Imagent BP
BPD
    biparietal diameter
BPD-MA
    benzoporphyrin derivative,
      monoacid ring A
BPH
    benign prostatic hyperplasia
BPP theory
    Bloembergen, Purcell, and
      Pound theory
BPS
    biophysical profile scoring
    fetal BPS
BQCT
    bone quantitative CT
Braasch bulb technique
Bracco
brace
    Boston b.
    Milwaukee b.
braces artifact
brachial
    b. artery
    b. artery approach
    b. plexus
    b. plexus birth injury
    b. plexus infiltration
    b. plexus injury
    b. vein
brachialis
brachicephaly

brachii
  triceps b.
brachiocephalic
  b. artery
  b. branch
  b. trunk
  b. vessel
brachioproctic eroticism
brachioradialis tendon reflex test
brachium pontis
Bracht-Wachter body
brachycephaly
brachydactyly
brachytherapy
  high-dose-rate remote b.
  interstitial b.
  remote afterloading b.
    (RAB)
  sterotactic b.
bracing
  fracture bracing
bradycardia
bradykinin
Bragg peak
brain
  b. abscess
  b. aneurysm
  b. biopsy
  b. cancer
  b. concussion
  b. cyst
  b. death
  b. disease
  b. edema
  b. geography
  b. homeostasis
  b. imaging
  b. infection
  b. lesion
  b. mapping
  b. mass
  b. metastasis
  b. parenchyma
  b. perfusion
  b. perfusion reserve
  b. region vesicle
  b. scintigraphy

  b. stem glioma
  b. substance
  b. tumor
brainstem
  b. auditory-evoked potentials
  b. edema
  b. encephalitis
  b. ependymoma
  b. glioma
  b. infarction
  ischemic b.
  tegmentum of b.
branch
  brachiocephalic b.
  collateral b.
  geniculate b.
  b. pad
  b. pulmonary artery stenosis
branched
  b. chain
  b. decay
branchial
  b. cleft cyst
  b. sinus
branching
  anomalous b.
BRAS
  Bard rotary atherectomy system
brassy
  b. body
  b. cough
BRCA-1
BRCA1 gene
BR96-DOX
  BR96-DOX
    immunoconjugate
  BR96-DOX protocol
BrDu
  bromodeoxyuridine
BRE3
  AT90 regulated BRE3
break
  chromosome b.
breakage
  chromosome b.
breakdown
  wound b.

NOTES

break-even volume
breakpoint cluster region
breakthrough
    normal perfusion
      pressure b.
breast
    b. abnormality
    b. abscess
    adenoma of b.
    adolescent b.
    adult b.
    b. augmentation
    augmented b.
    b. biopsy
    b. calcification
    b. cancer
    b. carcinoma
    childhood b.
    b. coil
    compression of b.
    b. cyst
    b. cyst aspiration
    cystic disease of b.
    b. disease
    b. edema
    b. embryology
    fascia of b.
    b. hyperplasia
    lactating b.
    b. lesion
    male b.
    b. metastasis
    b. mucocele
    nonlactating b.
    b. parenchyma
    prepubertal development
      of b.
    b. preservation
    b. reconstruction
    b. sonography
    b. traction
breath holding
breathing
    stertorous b.
breech
    b. delivery
    b. presentation
breeder reactor
bregma
Brenner tumor
brequinar
    b. sodium

Brescia-Cimino
    B.-C. fistula
    B.-C. graft
Breslow
    B. microstaging system
    B. staging
    B. thickness in malignant
      melanoma
Breus mole
brevicollis
brevis
    adductor b.
    extensor carpi radialis b.
    extensor digitorum b.
    extensor pollicis b.
    flexor digiti minimi b.
    flexor digitorum b.
    flexor hallucis b.
    flexor pollicis b.
    palmaris b.
Brewster window
Bricker procedure
brick skin reaction
bridge
    disulfide b.
    b. graft
    nasal b.
bridging
    bony b.
    b. leaflet
    b. osteophyte
    b. syndesmophyte
    b. vein
Brief Symptom Inventory (BSI)
bright cell
bright field imaging
brightness
    b. gain
    b. mode
brim of the pelvis
brinase
bristle brush
brittle bone disease
BRM
    biological response modifier
broadband
    b. attenuation
    b. noise detection error
     artifact
broad-based
broadening
    quadripolar signal b.

quadripole b.
spectral b.
broad ligament
Broca
    B. area
    B. index
Brödel-type kidney
Broden view
Brodie abscess
Brodmann chart
bromide
    ethidium b.
    pancuronium b.
    perfluorooctyl b.
    potassium b.
brominized oil
bromocriptine
bromodeoxyuridine (BrDu)
5-bromodeoxyuridine (BUDR)
    5-b. analysis
Bromptom cocktail
bronchi (*pl. of* bronchus)
bronchial
    b. adenoma
    b. angiography
    b. arteriography
    b. artery
    b. artery embolization
    b. asthma
    b. atresia
    b. brushing
    b. carcinoid tumor
    b. carcinoma
    b. cleft cyst
    b. fracture
    b. inflammation
    b. obstruction
    b. sinus
    b. spur
    b. stenosis
    b. tract
    b. tree
bronchial-associated lymphoid tissue
bronchiectasis
    cylindrical b.

cystic b.
fusiform b.
saccular b.
tubular b.
varicose b.
bronchiolar adenocarcinoma
bronchioles
bronchiolitis
    constrictive b.
    follicular b.
    b. obliterans
    b. obliterans-organizing pneumonia
bronchitis
    asthmatic b.
    follicular b.
    lymphocytic b.
bronchoalveolar
    b. carcinoma
    b. cell adenoma
    b. lavage (BAL)
bronchocentric granulomatosis
bronchoesophageal fistula
bronchogenic
    b. carcinoma
    b. cyst
bronchogram
    air b.
    mucous b.
    Swiss chccsc air b.
bronchography
    tantalum b.
broncholithiasis
bronchoplasty
    balloon b.
bronchopleural (BP)
    b. fistula
bronchopneumonia
bronchopulmonary
    b. aspergillosis
    b. dysplasia
    b. fistula
    b. foregut
    b. neoplasm
    b. segment
    b. sequestration

NOTES

bronchorrhea
bronchoscope
    flexible b.
    rigid b.
bronchoscopy
    flexible fiberoptic b.
bronchospasm
bronchostenosis
bronchovascular pattern
bronchus, pl. bronchi
    ectatic b.
    epiarterial b.
    b. intermedius
    mainstem b.
    segmental b.
    b. sign
bronzed diabetes
Brooke tumor
bropirimine
broth
    Middlebrook b.
Broviac catheter
brown
    b. cell cyst
    B. substrate
    b. tumor
brownian motion
Brown-Roberston-Wells frame
Brown-Sequard syndrome
brown tumor
brow presentation
brucellosis
bruit
    carotid b.
    cervical b.
Brunhilde virus
Brunner
    B. gland
    B. gland hyperplasia
    B. gland hypertrophy
brush
    bristle b.
    cervical b.
brushing
    blind esophageal b. (BEB)
    bronchial b.
Bruton sex-linked
  agammaglobulinemia
bruxism
BSI
    Brief Symptom Inventory

BSO
    bilateral salpingo-oophorectomy
    buthionine sulfoximine
B/T Blue Gene Rearrangement
  test
bubbicle
bubble
    b. agent
    encapsulated gas b.
    free gas b.
    gas b.
    stomach b.
bubble-like appearance
bubbly bone lesion
bucca, pl. buccae
buccal
    b. mucosa
    b. mucosal cancer
    b. space
    b. space infection
bucket-handle
    b.-h. fracture
    b.-h. tear
buckled drainage catheter
buckle fracture
Buckley syndrome
Bucky
    B. factor
    B. grid
Buckyballs
bud
    limb b.
Budd-Chiari syndrome
budding
    viral b.
    b. yeast
Budotitane
BUD Percuflex catheter
BUDR
    5-bromodeoxyuridine
    BUDR protocol
Buerger
    B. disease
    B. prostatic needle
Buerger-Grutz disease
buffer
    D-Di b.
    Michaelis b.
    Owren-Koller b.
    Spli-Prest b.
buffy
    b. coat component

b. coat preparation
b. coat smear
buffy-coated cell
bulb
carotid b.
duodenal b.
olfactory b.
sinovaginal b.
bulbi
phthisis b.
bulbourethral artery
bulbous enlargement
bulge
annular disk b.
bulging
b. annulus
b. disk
b. fissure
bulk
b. modulus
b. water
bulky disease
bulla, pl. **bullae**
emphysematous b.
ethmoidal b.
bullet
metallic track of b.
bullet-shaped vertebra
Bullis fever
bullosa
concha b.
junctional epidermolysis b.
bullous
b. cystitis
b. dermatitis
b. disease
b. disorder
b. emphysema
b. lung disease
bull's-eye
b.-e. analysis
b.-e. lesion
b.-e. pattern
b.-e. polar map display
b.-e. technology
bumper fracture

BUN
blood urea nitrogen
bunamiodyl
bunch-of-flowers streaks
bundle
fiberoptic b.
b. of His
bundles of Probst
bunk bed fracture
Bunyavirus
buphthalmos
bupivacaine
buprenorphine
bur, burr
b. cell
b. erythrocyte
b. hole
burden
maximum permissible
body b.
tumor b.
burgdorferi
Borrelia b.
Burhenne catheter
Burkhalter-Reyes method of
phalangeal fracture
Burkitt
B. leukemia
B. lymphoma
burn
alkaline b.
caustic b.
burned-out tumor
Burnet-Talmadge-Lederberg theory
of antibody formation
burnt-out colon
burnuous
sign of the b.
burr (*var. of* bur)
bursa, pl. **bursae**
deltoid b.
b. of Fabricius
gastrocnemius b.
gastrocnemius-
semimembranosus b.
iliopsoas b.
infrapatellar b.

NOTES

bursa *(continued)*
   olecranon b.
   omental b.
   popliteus b.
   prepatellar b.
   semimembranosus b.
   subacromial b.
   subdeltoid b.
   subscapular b.
   suprapatellar b.
   synovial b.
bursa-dependent system
bursal
   b. calcification
   b. osteochondromatosis
bursitis
   calcific b.
   iliopsoas b.
   ischial b.
   pes anserinus b.
   prepatellar b.
   subacromial b.
burst
   b. fracture
   respiratory b.
burst-forming
   b.-f. cell
   b.-f. unit
   b.-f. unit-erythroid (BFU-E)
burst fracture
burst-promoting activity
Buruli ulcer
Buschke-Löwenstein tumor
buserelin
busulfan, busulphan
   b. alkylation
butanol
Butchart staging classification
buthionine sulfoximine (BSO)
Butler-Albright syndrome
butoconazole
butorphanol
   b. tartrate
butterfly
   b. coil
   b. fracture
   b. glioblastoma

   b. glioma
   b. needle
   b. pattern
   b. rash
buttock
   b. cell
button
   Bentley b.
   Panje voice b.
   patellar b.
   b. sequestrum
buttonhole fracture
tert-**butylhydroperoxide**
butyl nitrite
butyrate
   b. analog
butyrophenone
Butzler Campylobacter virus
buyo cheek cancer
BV-ara-U
BW
   bandwidth
   BW A770U
Bwamba virus
BW566C80
bypass
   aortobifemoral b.
   aortofemoral b. (AFB)
   aortovisceral b.
   bilioenteric b.
   gastric b.
   gastrojejunal b.
   b. graft
   b. procedure
   superficial temporal artery
     to posterior cerebral
     artery b.
   b. surgery
byproduct material
byssinosis
bystander effect
B-zone small lymphocytic
   lymphoma (BZSLL)
BZSLL
   B-zone small lymphocytic
   lymphoma

C

C_{max}
  maximal drug concentration
C1 inactivator
C3 receptor
CA
  cancer antigen
    CA 125 antigen
    CA 15-3 breast cancer
      tumor marker
    CA 549 breast cancer
      tumor marker
    CA 125 cross-reactivity
    CA M26 tumor marker
    CA M29 tumor marker
    CA 125 ovarian tumor
      marker
    CA 15-2 RIA test
    CA 125-11 tumor marker
    CA 19-9 tumor marker
    CA 195 tumor marker
    CA 27.29 tumor marker
    CA 50 tumor marker
    CA 72-4 tumor marker
    CA virus
CABG
  coronary artery bypass graft
c-abl proto-oncogene
Cabot ring body
cachectic
cachectin
Cache valley virus
cachexia
    paraneoplastic c.
CACS
  cancer, anorexia, cachexia
    syndrome
CAD
  common atrium, aortic atresia,
    double-outlet
  coronary artery disease
    C. right ventricle
CADD-PLUS pump
CADD-TPN
    CADD-TPN ambulatory
      infusion system
    CADD-TPN pump
cadmium
CAE
  cyclophosphamide, Adriamycin
    (doxorubicin), etoposide

CAF
    Cytoxan, Adriamycin, 5-
      fluorouracil
café-au-lait spots
caffeine
Caffey disease
Caffey-Kempe syndrome
Caffey-Silverman disease
cage
    Faraday c.
caged balloon catheter
cahedrin
    skin c.
caisson disease
cake
    c. kidney
    omental c.
calcaneal
    c. avulsion fracture
    c. displaced fracture
    c. fracture
    c. spur
calcaneocuboid joint
calcaneofibular ligament
calcaneonavicular coalition
calcaneovarus deformity
calcaneus
calcareous
calcific
    c. bursitis
    c. tendinitis
calcificans
    liponecrosis macrocystica c.
    liponecrosis microcystica c.
calcification
    abdominal diffuse c.
    abdominal vascular c.
    abdominal wall c.
    adrenal c.
    alimentary tract c.
    amorphous c.
    annular c.
    anterior spinal ligament c.
    arachnoid granulation c.
    arterial c.
    arteriovascular c.
    basal ganglia c.
    breast c.
    bursal c.
    carotid artery c.

calcification *(continued)*
    casting c.
    coarse c.
    coronary artery c.
    curvilinear c.
    dermal c.
    diffuse c.
    diffuse abdominal c.
    dystrophic c.
    eggshell c.
    falx c.
    fingertip c.
    focal alimentary tract c.
    genital tract c.
    granular c.
    granulomatous c.
    habenular commissure c.
    hepatic c.
    inadequate cranial c.
    intraabdominal c.
    intracranial c.
    intraductal c.
    intraocular c.
    ligamentous c.
    lobular c.
    malignant c.
    medullary c.
    mesenteric c.
    metastatic c.
    mitral annulus c.
    Mönckeberg c.
    multiple pulmonary c.
    neoplastic c.
    pancreatic c.
    paraspinal c.
    pathological intracranial c.
    periductal c.
    peritendinous c.
    periventricular c.
    phlebolith-like c.
    pleural c.
    popcorn like c.
    punctate c.
    renal c.
    retroperitoneal c.
    rice-like muscle c.
    scrotal c.
    sebaceous gland c.
    secondary c.
    c. sign
    skin c.
    soft tissue c.
    splenic c.
    stippled c.
    sutural c.
    thyroid c.
    tram track cortical c.
    urinary bladder wall c.
    valve leaflet c.
    vascular c.
    visceral c.
    wall c.
calcified
    c. ductus arteriosus
    c. fibroadenoma
    c. liver metastasis
    c. medullary defect
    c. metastasis
    c. renal mass
calcifying
    c. epithelial odontogenic
    c. metastasis
calcifying epithelial odontogenic
calcineurin
calcinosis
    c. circumscripta
    generalized c.
    interstitial c.
    tumoral c.
    c. universalis
calcinosis of skin, Raynaud phenomenon, esophageal dysmotility, sclerodactyly, telangiectasia (CREST)
calciphylaxis
calcis
    os c.
calcispherytes
calcitonin
Calcitrol
calcium
    c. antagonist
    c. channel blocker
    dietary c.
    fenoprofen c.
    c. heparin
    leucovorin c.
    c. leucovorin
    milk of c.
    c. oxalate calculus
    c. phosphate calculus
    c. pyrophosphate deposition disease (CPPDD)
    c. pyrophosphate dihydrate (CPPD)
    sedimented c.

c. sign
c. soap
c. tungstate
calcofluor white stain
calculation
body surface area c.
contrast-to-noise c.
signal-to-noise c.
S-method of dose c.
calculus, pl. calculi
biliary c.
calcium oxalate c.
calcium phosphate c.
intrahepatic biliary c.
nonopaque c.
obstructive c.
renal c.
staghorn c.
Steinstrasse calculi
ureteral c.
ureteric c.
uric acid c.
urinary c.
caldesmon protein
Caldwell view
calf vein thrombosis
caliber
luminal c.
tracheal c.
calibrated leak
calibration failure artifact
calibrator
dose c.
caliceal
c. abnormality
c. diverticula
c. diverticulum
c. nephrostolithotomy
calices (*pl. of* calix)
caliectasis
focal c.
California virus
californium-252 (^{252}Cf)
calix (*var. of* calyx), pl. **calices**
CALLA
common acute lymphoblastic
leukemia antigen

CALLA-negative
CALLA-positive myeloma
Call-Exner body
callosal sulcus
callosomarginal artery
callosum
splenium of corpus c.
callus formation
callus
fracture c.
Calmette-Guérin
Bacille C.-G. (BCG)
C.-G. bacillus
calmodulin
c. inhibitor
caloric intake
calusterone
calvaria, pl. calvariae
calvarial marrow
Calvé disease
Calvé-Kümmel-Verneuil disease
Calvé-Legg-Perthes disease
calvia
Calymmatobacterium
calyx, calix, pl. calyces
abortive c.
cupping of the calyces
moth-eaten c.
camalote
sign of the c.
CAM 125 antigen assay
Cambridge classification
cameloid
c. anemia
c. cell
camera
Anger c.
beta c.
cine c.
gamma c.
Isocon c.
Medx c.
Multicrystal c.
multiformat c.
Orthicon c.
pinhole c.
positron scintillation c.

NOTES

camera *(continued)*
    radioisotope c.
    scintillation c.
    triple-head c.
    video display c.
Camino intracranial pressure monitoring device
CAMP
    cyclophosphamide, Adriamycin, methotrexate, procarbazine
Campath-monoclonal antibody
campothecan
camptomelic dysplasia
camptothecin
    c. analog
Campylobacter
    C. colitis
    C. fetus
    C. jejuni
    C. pylori
Camurati-Engelmann disease
can
    can oncogene
    can proto-oncogene
canal
    acoustic c.
    adductor c.
    anal c.
    anterior condylar c.
    antropyloric c.
    atrioventricular c.
    auditory c.
    cervical c.
    Cloquet c.
    external auditory c.
    facial c.
    Hunter c.
    hyaloid c.
    hypoglossal c.
    internal auditory c.
    lumbar c.
    lumbosacral c.
    lymphatic c.
    neural c.
    nutrient c.
    obturator c.
    optic c.
    orbital c.
    persistent common atrioventricular c.
    pterygoid c.
    pyloric c.
    semicircular c.

    spinal c.
    c. stenosis
    vertebral c.
    vidian c.
canalicular immunostaining pattern
canaliculum
    bile c.
    papilloma c.
canalization
Canavan disease
cancellization
cancellous
    c. bone
    c. osteoma
Cancell therapy
cancer
    adrenal gland c.
    aerodigestive c.
    American Joint Committee on C. (AJCC)
    anal c.
    anal region c.
    androgen-independent prostate c.
    c. antigen (CA)
    appendiceal c.
    betel c.
    biliary tract c.
    bladder c.
    c. body
    bone c.
    bowel c.
    brain c.
    breast c.
    buccal mucosal c.
    buyo cheek c.
    cecal c.
    c. cell
    cervical c.
    cervical stump c.
    childhood c.
    chimney sweep's c.
    colloid c.
    colon c.
    colorectal c.
    C. Committee of College of American Pathologists
    common epithelial ovarian c.
    conjugal c.
    c. à deux
    drug-sensitive c.
    encephaloid c.

c. en cuirasse
endobronchial c.
endometrial c.
epidermoid c.
epithelial c.
epithelial ovarian c. (EOC)
esophageal c.
European Organization for
  Research and Treatment
  of C. (EORTC)
extrapulmonary small cell c.
familial c.
fulguration in bladder c.
gastric c.
gastric remnant c.
gastrointestinal c.
genitourinary c.
gingival c.
glandular c.
green c.
hard palate c.
head and neck c.
hepatic c.
hepatic flexure c.
hepatobiliary c.
hepatocellular c.
hereditary nonpolyposis
  colorectal c.
hormone-refractory breast c.
hormone-refractory
  prostate c.
hypopharyngeal c.
inflammatory breast c.
interval c.
intrahepatic biliary c.
invasive c.
iodine-131 antiferritin
  treatment for
  hepatocellular c.
Jewett-Strong-Marshall
  staging of bladder c.
c. juice
kangri c.
kidney c.
large cell lung c.
laryngeal c.
leptomeningeal c.

lip c.
liver c.
locally advanced c.
lung c.
malignant breast c.
c. map
metastatic breast c.
mouse c.
mule-spinner's c.
nasal cavity c.
nasal vestibule c.
nasopharyngeal c.
c. nest
neuroendocrine c.
node-negative c.
non-small cell lung c.
oat cell lung c.
obstructive colorectal c.
occult c.
oral c.
oropharyngeal c.
ovarian c.
palpatory T stage
  prostate c.
pancreatic c.
paraffin c.
paranasal sinus c.
perforating colorectal c.
pharyngeal wall c.
pipe-smoker's c.
pitch-worker's c.
postcricoid pharyngeal c.
primary c.
prostate c.
prostatic c.
pyriform sinus c.
rectal c.
rectosigmoid c.
recurrent c.
C. Rehabilitation Evaluation
  System (CARES)
renal c.
resectable colorectal c.
retromolar trigone c.
c. risk
Robson stage I-IV renal
  cell c.

NOTES

cancer *(continued)*
    salivary gland c.
    scar c.
    secondary c.
    skin c.
    small bowel c.
    small cell lung c. (SCLC)
    small intestine c.
    soft palate c.
    somatic mutation theory of c.
    spider c.
    splenic flexure c.
    stump c.
    C. Surveillance Program (CSP)
    suture line c.
    synchronous colorectal c.
    synchronous ipsilateral breast c. (SIBC)
    telangiectatic c.
    testicular c.
    testis c.
    thyroid c.
    tongue c.
    tonsil c.
    tonsillar area c.
    transitional cell c.
    treatment-related secondary c.
    Union Internationale Contre le C. (UICC)
    unresectable colorectal c.
    uterine c.
    uterine cervical c.
    varicoid esophageal c.
    vocal cord c.
    water c.
cancer, anorexia, cachexia syndrome (CACS)
cancer-associated
    c.-a. anemia
    c.-a. serum antigen (CASA)
Cancer Committee of College of American Pathologists
cancer-free (CF)
    c.-f. white mouse
cancericidal dose
cancerization
    field c.
candelabra artery
candela lithotripsy

Candida
    C. albicans
    C. guillermondii
    C. krusei
    C. lusitaniae
    C. parapsilosis
    C. tropicalis
candidal abscess
candidiasis
    cutaneous c.
    disseminated c.
    c. echo
    esophageal c.
    hepatic c.
    hepatosplenic c.
    oral c.
    pseudomembranous c.
candle
    c. drippings appearance
    c. flame lysis
    vaginal c.
Candlelighters Childhood Cancer Foundation (CCCF)
candle-wax-dripping streaks
candy cane appearance
Caner-Decker syndrome
canine
    c. oral papilloma
    c. venereal granuloma
canis
    Ehrlichia c.
    Microsporum c.
    Toxocara c.
cannabinoid
Cannon point
cannula
    Cohen-Eder c.
    Dotter c.
    Hassan c.
    Rutner c.
    ultrasonic lithotripter c.
cannulation
    endoscopic retrograde c.
    retrograde c.
cannulization
Cantor tube
Cantrell
    pentalogy of C.
CAP
    cyclophosphamide, Adriamycin, Platinol

cap
- cartilaginous c.
- phrygian c.

capacitance
- electric energy c.

capacitive interaction

capacity
- clonogenic c.
- diffusing c.
- functional residual c.
- iron-binding c. (IBC)
- latent iron-binding c. (LIBC)
- lung c.
- total iron-binding c. (TIBC)
- total lung c.
- vital c.

CAP-BOP
- cyclophosphamide, Adriamycin (doxorubicin), procarbazine, bleomycin, Oncovin, prednisone

capillary
- c. angioma
- c. electrophoresis
- c. endothelium
- c. hemangioblastoma
- c. hemangioma
- c. leak syndrome
- c. malformation
- c. perfusion
- c. telangiectasis

capital femoral epiphysis

capitate
- c. fracture

capitella (*pl. of* capitulum) (*pl. of* capitellum)

capitellar fracture

capitis
- fovea c.

capitulum, capitellum, pl. **capitula, capitella**
- c. radiale humeri fracture

Caplan syndrome

capreomycin

caproate
- hydroxyprogesterone c.

capsaicin

capsid

capsular thickening

capsulatum
- *Histoplasma c.*

capsule
- fibrous c.
- Glisson c.
- Heyman c.
- internal c.
- joint c.
- otic c.
- prostate c.

capsulitis
- adhesive c.

capsulolabral complex

captopril

capture
- cross-section c.
- electron c.
- gamma-ray c.
- K c.

caput
- c. medusa
- c. membranaceum
- c. succedaneum

caracemide

carazolol

Carazzi hematoxylin

carbamate
- chlorphenesin c.

carbamazepine

carbenicillin

carbethimer

carbetimer

carbimazole

carbohemoglobin

carbohydrate antigen

carbolfuchsin stain

β-carboline

carbon
- c. dioxide laser system
- c. dioxide tracer
- c. monoxide poisoning
- c. pneumoconiosis

carbon-13 spectroscopy

NOTES

carbonate
   lithium c.
carboplatin
Carbovir
carboxamide
   dimethyltriazenoimidazole c.
    (DTIC)
   imidazole c.
carboxorolone
   succinic acid ester c.
carboxyhemoglobin
carboxyimamidate
carboxymyoglobin
carboxyphosphamide
carbuncle
   renal c.
carcinoembryonic
   c. antigen (CEA)
   c. antigen doubling time
    (CEA-DT)
carcinoembryonic antigen (CEA)
carcinogen
   chemical c.
   complete c.
carcinogenesis
   chemical c.
   fiber c.
   foreign body c.
carcinogenic
carcinogenicity
carcinoid
   bronchial c. tumor
   colorectal c.
   c. crisis
   c. embryonic antigen
   c. heart disease
   intestinal c. tumor
   c. syndrome
   c. tumor
carcinolytic
carcinoma, pl. **carcinomata,**
  carcinomas
   acinar c.
   acinar cell c.
   acinic cell c.
   adenoid cystic c.
   adenoid squamous cell c.
   adnexal c.
   adrenal c.
   adrenocortical c.
   alveolar cell c.
   alveolar mucosal c.
   ampullary c.

anaplastic c.
anaplastic thyroid c.
apocrine c.
apple core c.
autolymphocyte-based
  treatment for renal cell c.
  (ALT-RCC)
Bartholin gland c.
basal cell c.
basaloid c.
basaloid nonkeratinizing c.
basaloid squamous cell c.
basosquamous c.
basosquamous
  nonkeratinizing c.
bile duct c.
bladder c.
breast c.
bronchial c.
bronchoalveolar c.
bronchogenic c.
cecal c.
cecum c.
cervical c.
cholangiocellular c.
clear cell c.
cloacogenic c.
cloacogenic
  nonkeratinizing c.
colloid c.
colonic c.
colorectal c.
contralateral synchronous c.
c. cutaneum
cylindromatous c.
cystic c.
de novo c.
differentiated c. (DC)
ductal c.
ductal papillary c.
eccrine c.
embryonal c.
endometrial c. (EC)
endometrial
  adenosquamous c.
endometrioid c.
epidermoid c.
esophageal c.
ethmoid sinus c.
c. ex pleomorphic adenoma
fallopian tube c.
false cord c.
fibrolamellar c.

fibrolamellar liver cell c.
flat colorectal c.
focal lobular c.
follicular c.
gallbladder c.
gastric c.
gastric stump c.
gastroesophageal junction c.
genital c.
giant cell c.
glandular c.
glottic c.
hepatocellular c.
Hürthle cell c.
infiltrating c.
infiltrating duct c.
infiltrating lobular c.
infiltrating small cell
  lobular c.
inflammatory c.
inflammatory breast c.
insular c.
intensive ductal c.
intermediate c.
intracystic papillary c.
intraductal c.
intraductal breast c.
intraductal papillary c.
intraepidermal c.
intraepithelial c.
invasive c.
invasive ductal c. (IDC)
invasive lobular c.
invasive squamous cell c.
jugular node metastatic c.
juvenile c.
kangri burn c.
large cell c.
large cell undifferentiated c.
latent c.
lateral aberrant thyroid c.
leptomeningeal c.
linitis plastica c.
liver cell c.
lobular c.
lobular c. in situ
lung c.

medullary c.
medullary thyroid c.
melanotic c.
meningeal c.
mesometanephric c.
mesonephric c.
metachronous c.
metaplastic c.
metastatic c.
metatypical c.
microinvasive c.
mixed type c.
morphea form basal cell c.
mucinous c.
mucin-producing c.
mucoepidermoid c.
multicentric c.
c. myxomatodes
napkin-ring c.
nasopharyngeal c.
nasopharyngeal squamous
  cell c.
nevoid basal cell c.
noninfiltrating lobular c.
nonislet cell c.
nonsquamous c.
oat cell c.
occult c.
occult papillary c.
oncoplastic c.
orofacial c.
ovarian c.
ovarian edometrioid c.
Paget c.
pancreatic c.
papillary c.
papillary serous c.
papillary thyroid c.
c. paradoxicum
parathyroid c.
periampullary c.
peripheral c.
pharyngeal wall c.
poorly-differentiated
  infiltrating duct c.
primary c.
primary hepatocellular c.

NOTES

carcinoma *(continued)*
  prostatic c.
  rectal c.
  recurrent c.
  renal c.
  renal cell c.
  renal cortical c.
  renal pelvis c.
  salivary gland c.
  sarcomatoid c.
  scar c.
  schneiderian c.
  scirrhous c.
  sebaceous c.
  secondary c.
  secretory c.
  serous c.
  signet-ring cell c.
  c. simplex
  sinonasal c.
  c. in situ (CIS)
  small cell c.
  small cell undifferentiated c.
  spindle cell c.
  squamous c.
  squamous cell c. (SCC)
  superficial spreading c.
  supraglottic c.
  sweat gland c.
  synchronous c.
  thyroid c.
  trabecular c.
  transitional cell c. (TCC)
  transverse colon c.
  tripartite duodenal c.
  tubular c.
  c. of uncertain primary site
    (CUPS)
  undifferentiated c. (UC)
  urachal c.
  ureteral c.
  uterine papillary serous c.
    (UPSC)
  V-2 c.
  vaginal c.
  varicoid c.
  verrucous c.
  villous c.
  vulvar c.
  vulvovaginal c.
  Walker c.
  well-circumscribed c.
  Wolfe classification of
    breast c.
  wolffian duct c.
carcinomatosa
  lymphangitis c.
carcinomatosis
  leptomeningeal c.
  lymphangitic c.
  lymphatic c.
  meningeal c.
  peritoneal c.
  c. peritonei
carcinomatosum
  coma c.
carcinomatous
  c. implants
  c. meningitis
  c. myelopathy
  c. myopathy
  c. neuromyopathy
  c. subacute cerebellar
    degeneration
carcinophobia
carcinosarcoma
  embryonal c.
  renal c.
  uterine c.
  Walker c.
carcinosis
carcinostatic
Cardak introducer
cardiac
  c. arrhythmia
  c. blood pool imaging
  c. catheterization
  c. cycle
  c. decompensation
  c. dilatation
  c. enlargement
  c. failure
  c. gating
  c. hypertrophy
  c. inversion
  c. irradiation
  c. output
  c. position
  c. receptor
  c. scintigraphy
  c. shadow
  c. shock
  c. silhouette
  c. status
  c. tamponade

c. toxicity
c. transplant
c. tumor
cardinal vein
cardiogenic stroke
Cardiografin
Cardiolite
  C. heart imaging scan
  technetium-tagged C.
  C. Tl-201
cardiology
cardiomegaly
  boxlike c.
  funnel-like c.
cardiomelic
  c. dysplasia
  c. syndrome
cardiomyopathy
  alcoholic c.
  anthracycline-induced c.
  congestive c.
  degenerative c.
  dilated c.
  hypertrophic c.
  obstructive c.
  restrictive c.
cardiomyoplasty
cardiophrenic
  c. angle
  c. angle mass
cardioprotectant
cardioprotective agent
cardiopulmonary
  c. abnormality
  c. disease
  c. manifestation
Cardioscint
cardiospasm
cardiosplenic syndrome
CardioTek
cardiothoracic
  c. ratio
  c. trauma
cardiothymic shadow
cardiotocogram
cardiotoxic effect

cardiotoxicity
  doxorubicin-induced c.
  mitomycin c.
cardiovascular
  c. adverse effect
  c. disease
  c. imaging technique
  c. malformation
  nuclear c. imaging
  c. radiology
  c. shadow
  c. silhouette
  c. system
cardioverter-defibrillator
  automatic implantable c.-d.
  (AICD)
carditis
  acute lethal c.
care
  comfort c.
  continuing c.
  home c.
  home health c.
  hospice c.
  institutional c.
  palliative c.
  patient c.
  supportive c.
  terminal c.
CARE Act
  Comprehensive AIDS Resources
  Emergency Act
CARES
  Cancer Rehabilitation
  Evaluation System
Carey-Coons stent
carfentanil
caries
  dental c.
carina, pl. **carinae**
carinal
  c. angle
carinii
  Pneumocystis c.
carious teeth
carisoprodol
Carlen endotracheal tube

NOTES

C-arm
    C-a. fluoroscopy
Carman meniscal sign
carmustine (BCNU)
carneous degeneration
Carney
    C. complex
    C. syndrome
    C. triad
carnitine
Caroli disease
β-carotene
carotene
carotenemia
carotenoid
caroticojugular spine
caroticotympanic artery
carotid
    c. aneurysm
    c. angiography
    c. artery
    c. artery aneurysm
    c. artery arteritis
    c. artery bifurcation
    c. artery calcification
    c. artery disease
    c. artery occlusion
    c. artery plaque
    c. artery stenosis
    c. body tumor
    c. bruit
    c. bulb
    c. cavernous sinus fistula
    c. cavernous syndrome
    c. cerebral arteriography
    c. circulation
    c. duplex ultrasonography
    c. endarterectomy
    c. foramen
    c. occlusion
    c. sheath
    c. sheath adenoma
    c. sinus
    c. siphon
    c. stenosis
    c. velocity
carotid-dural fistula
carotid-ophthalmic aneurysm
carpal
    c. angle
    c. bone
    c. bone fracture
    c. bone stress fracture

    c. boss
    C. Box
    c. navicula
    c. navicular bone
    c. tunnel
    c. tunnel release
    c. tunnel syndrome
Carpenter syndrome
Carpentier-Edwards valve
carpet
    c. lesion
    c. polyp
carpi (*pl. of* carpus)
carpomaypine
carpometacarpal joint fracture
carprofen
carpus, pl. carpi
Carrel patch
carrier-free radioisotope
carrier-mediated transport system
Carrington
    C. dermal wound gel
    C. disease
Carrion disease
Carrisyn
carrot-shaped trachea
Carr-Purcell
    C.-P. experiment
    C.-P. sequence (CP
      sequence)
Carr-Purcell-Meiboom-Gill
    C.-P.-M.-G. echo train
    C.-P.-M.-G. sequence
      (CPMG sequence)
carrying
    c. angle
Carter-Rowe view
cartesian coordinate system
cartilage
    arytenoid c.
    comiculate c.
    costal c.
    cricoid c.
    cuneiform c.
    laryngeal c.
    septal c. plate
    shark c.
    c. stroma
    thyroid c.
cartilage-containing giant cell tumor
cartilage-forming tumor
cartilage-hair hypoplasia

cartilaginous
    c. cap
    c. growth plate disorder
    c. node
    c. tumor
cartwheel fracture
Cartwright blood group
Carworth Farm mouse
CAS-200
    morphology system CAS-200
CASA
    cancer-associated serum antigen
    CASA tumor marker
cascade
    coagulation c.
    metastatic c.
    c. stomach
caseating
case-control study
casei
    Lactobacillus c.
caseous pneumonia
Casodex
Casoni skin test
Casper plate
Caspersson type B-cell
cast
    decidual c.
    plaster c.
    c. syndrome
    vascular c.
Castaneda bottle
Castañeda-Malecot catheter
castanospermine
casting calcification
Castle factor
Castleman disease
castor bean
castration
casual sex
CAT
    chloramphenicol
      acetyltransferase
    computerized axial tomography
    CAT expression gene

catabolic pathway
catadioptric lens
catamenial pneumothorax
cataract formation
catarrhalis
    Moraxella c.
catecholamine
    c. release
catenin-a protein
caterpillar sign
catfish sting
cathartic
    c. colon
    saline c.
cathepsin B
cathepsin D
cathepsin G
cathepsin L
catheter
    Abbokinase c.
    abdominal abscess
      drainage c.
    accordion c.
    afterloading c.
    afterretention c.
    Amplatz dual-stiffness
      Malecot (Stamey) c.
    Amplatz mechanical
      thrombolysis c.
    angiography c.
    angioplasty balloon c.
    Anthron heparinized c.
    Argyle c.
    Argyle Ingram trocar c.
    Auth rotablation rotational
      atherectomy c.
    balloon c.
    banana c.
    Bardex c.
    biliary drainage c.
    biliary manipulation c.
    blade c.
    Broviac c.
    buckled drainage c.

NOTES

catheter *(continued)*
BUD Percuflex c.
Burhenne c.
caged balloon c.
Castañeda-Malecot c.
central venous c.
central venous pressure c.
C-Flex c.
Chemo-Port c.
circle tube nephrostomy c.
coaxial c.
cobra c.
condom c.
Cook-Europe c.
Cope c.
Councill c.
Delcath double-balloon c.
Dialy-Nate c.
dilatation c.
directional accordion c.
Dotter coaxial Teflon c.
double-curved triangular c.
double-J polyethylene c.
double-J silicone rubber
  urinary c.
double-lumen c.
drainage c.
c. drainage
dual-stiffness Malecot c.
c. embolism
femoral arterial c.
c. fixation
Fogarty c.
Fogarty balloon c.
Fogarty balloon biliary c.
Fogarty embolectomy c.
Fogarty gallstone c.
Fogarty irrigation c.
Fogarty venous
  thrombectomy c.
Foley c.
French pigtail c.
Gensini c.
Glidewire c.
Grollman c.
Groshong c.
Grüntzig balloon c.
Hawkins accordion c.
headhunter c.
Hickman c.
Hieshima c.
hockey-stick c.

Hunter-Sessions transvenous
  balloon occlusion c.
indwelling c.
inferior vena cava c.
c. insertion
inside-the-needle infusion c.
internal double-J c.
internal-external c.
Intrasil c.
intrathoracic c.
Judkins c.
jugular c.
Kaliman atherectomy c.
Kaye tamponade c.
Kensey dynamic
  angioplasty c.
large-bore c.
long-term, U-loop
  nephrostomy c.
loop c.
Lunderquist c.
Magic c.
Malecot c.
Malecot biliary drainage c.
Mani cerebral c.
Massachusetts General
  Teflon c.
McGahan drainage c.
Mewissen infusion c.
Müller empyema c.
multifiber c.
multiple-sidehole infusion c.
multipurpose c.
mushroom c.
nasobiliary c.
nephrostomy c.
c. obstruction
Olbert balloon c.
over-the-needle infusion c.
partially-implantable c.
P.A.S. Port c.
peel-away c.
peel-away banana c.
percutaneous nephrostomy c.
percutaneous transhepatic c.
Per-Q-Cath c.
Pfeifer dynamic
  angioplasty c.
Pfeifer milling c.
pigtail c.
polyethylene c.
polyethylene balloon c.
polyvinyl chloride balloon c.

Port-A-Cath c.
c. position
pullback atherectomy c.
Quinton central venous c.
Raaf c.
rheolytic c.
rheolytic thrombectomy c.
Ring c. –
Ring biliary drainage c.
Sacks c.
Sacks-Malecot c.
shepherd's crook c.
sidewinder c.
Silastic c.
Silastic hemodialysis c.
Simmons c.
Simpson directional
  atherectomy c.
Stamey suprapubic
  Malecot c.
subclavian c.
subclavian apheresis c.
subclavian vein access c.
suction c.
SureCath port access c.
Swan-Ganz c.
Teflon c.
Tegtmeyer c.
TEGwire angioplasty c.
Tenckhoff c.
Thora-Cath c.
c. tip
Tonnesen c.
totally-implantable c.
Tracker coaxial infusion c.
Tracker-18 Unibody c.
Trac-Wright c.
transhepatic c.
transluminal
  endarterectomy c.
transluminal extraction c.
  (TEC)
triple-lumen c.
trocar c.
U-loop nephrostomy c.
valve-ended c.
Van Andel tapered c.

Vaso-Cath c.
venous c.
Walinsky c.
catheter-associated bacteremia
catheter-coiling sign
catheter-directed
  c.-d. fenestration
  c.-d. interventional
    procedure
catheter-induced
  c.-i. pulmonary artery
    hemorrhage
  c.-i. subclavian vein
    thrombosis
catheterization
  antegrade c.
  bladder c.
  cardiac c.
  central venous c.
  chronic c.
  left heart c.
  transfemoral venous c.
  transseptal c.
  transvaginal fallopian
    tube c.
catheterized barbotage specimen
catheter-securing technique
cathode ray tube (CRT)
cation
Catrix
cat-scratch fever
cat's-eye appearance
Catterall classification
Catu virus
cauda
  c. equina
  c. equina compression
  c. equina syndrome
caudal
  c. angulation
  c. direction
  c. regression
  c. regression syndrome
  c. sac
caudate
  c. body
  c. lobe

NOTES

caudate *(continued)*
    c. nucleus
    c. vein
    c. volume
cauliflower ear
causalgia
causality
caustic burn
CAV
    cyclophosphamide, Adriamycin, vincristine
cava
    collapsed inferior vena c.
    duplicated inferior vena c.
    inferior vena c. (IVC)
    membranous obstruction of inferior vena c.
    paired inferior vena c.
    persistent left inferior vena c.
    persistent left superior vena c.
    superior vena c.
    vena c.
caval opening
cave
    Meckel c.
cavernoma
cavernosa
    corpora c.
cavernosography
cavernosometry
cavernous
    c. aneurysm
    c. angioma
    c. artery
    c. hemangioma
    c. internal carotid artery
    c. lymphangioma
    c. sinus
    c. sinus aneurysm
    c. sinus fistula
    c. sinus syndrome
    c. transfer of portal vein
    c. transformation
CAVH
    continuous arteriovenous hemofiltration
cavitary
    c. lung lesion
    c. small bowel lesion
    c. tuberculosis

cavitating
    c. lung nodule
    c. metastasis
    c. neoplasm
    c. pneumonia
cavitation
    collapse c.
    stable c.
    transient c.
cavity
    abdominal c.
    abdominopelvic c.
    acetabular c.
    amniotic c.
    cranial c.
    endometrial c.
    glenoid c.
    grape skin thin-walled lung c.'s
    lung c.
    miniature uterine c.
    nasal c.
    oral c.
    peritoneal c.
    pleural c.
    sinonasal c.
    sinus c.
    syringohydromyelic c.
cavum
    c. septum pellucidum
    c. veli interpositi
    c. vergae
cavus
    pes c.
CB10-277
CB3717
C4b-BP
    Assera-Plate C4b-BP
CBF
    cerebral blood flow
CBV
    Cytoxan, BCNU, VP-16
CCAT
    conglutinating complement absorption test
CCCF
    Candlelighters Childhood Cancer Foundation
***c-cis* proto-oncogene**
CCK
    cholecystokinin

CCNU
  lomustine
  methyl CCNU
CCNU, procarbazine, methotrexate (CPM)
CCSS
  Childhood Cancer Survivor Study
CD
  cluster of differentiation
  cytarabine, daunorubicin
    CD antigen
CD1-99
CD4
    CD4 cell
    CD4 cell count
    CD4 Protein
    CD4 receptor
CD8
    CD8 cell
    CD8 cell count
CD19
CD26
    CD26 coreceptor
    CD26 protease
CD34
CD18 antigen
CD21 antigen
CD33 antigen
CD34-positive cell
CD3+ cell
CD3- cell
CD3 monoclonal antibody
CD4+ cell
CD5 marker
CD5-T lymphocyte immunotoxin
CD8+ cell
CdA
  2-chloro-2'-deoxyadenosine
CDC classification chorioretinitis
CDDP
  cis-diamminedichloroplatinum
cDNA
  complementary DNA
    cDNA cloning
    herpesvirus thymidine kinase cDNA

CDTA
  cyclohexenediaminetetraacetic acid
CE
  center-edge
  contrast-enhanced
    CE angle of Wiberg
CEA
  carcinoembryonic antigen
    CEA titer
    CEA tumor marker
CEA-DT
  carcinoembryonic antigen doubling time
CEA-Roche assay
CEA-Tc 99m
cebocephaly
cecal
  c. cancer
  c. carcinoma
  c. deformity
  c. filling defect
  c. ileus
  c. volvulus
cecostomy
  percutaneous c.
cecum
  c. carcinoma
  coned c.
  kidney-shaped distended c.
  c. mobile
cefaclor
CE-FAST
  contrast-enhanced fast-acquisition steady state
cefepime
cefoxitin
cefpodoxime proxetil
cefprozil
ceftazidime
ceftriaxone
cefuroxime axetil
ceiling dose
celery stalk sign
Celestin tube
celiac
  c. angiography

NOTES

celiac *(continued)*
    c. artery
    c. artery aneurysm
    c. axis
    c. block
    c. disease
    c. ganglion block
    c. lymph node metastasis
    c. plexus
    c. sprue
celioscopy
celiotomy
cell
    Abbe-Zeiss counting c.
    c. activation
    c. adhesion molecule
    adventitial c.
    agger nasi air c.'s
    alkaline phosphatase-
      positive c.
    allogeneic bone marrow c.
    allogeneic stem c.
    angiogenic c.
    antigen-sensitive c.
    antisheep red blood c.
    argyrophilic c.
    Aschoff c.
    autologous bone marrow c.
    autologous hematopoietic c.
    autologous red blood c.
    autologous stem c.
    B-c.
    balloon c.
    band c.
    c. bank
    berry c.
    binucleate c.
    c. biology
    B-islet c.
    blast c.
    B-lineage acute
      lymphoblastic c.
    c. block analysis
    blood c.
    bone marrow c.
    bovine red blood c.'s
    bright c.
    buffy-coated c.
    bur c.
    burst-forming c.
    buttock c.
    cameloid c.
    cancer c.

    c. carcinoma of cervix
    Caspersson type B-c.
    CD3+ c.
    CD4+ c.
    CD4 c.
    CD8 c.
    CD8+ c.
    CD3- c.
    CD34-positive c.
    central neuroepithelial c.
    centrocyte-like c.
    chromaffin c.
    Clara c.
    clonogenic myeloma c.
    clonogenic tumor c.
    club-shaped c.
    c. collection
    committed c.
    contrasuppressor c.
    counting c.
    cuboidal c.
    Custer c.
    c. cycle
    c. cycle kinetics analysis
    c. cycle stage
    c. cycling in chemotherapy
    cytotoxic c.
    Daudi c.
    daughter c.
    c. death
    dendritic c.
    dendritic reticulum c.'s
      (DRC)
    dim c.
    diploic c.
    c. division
    Dorothy Reed c.
    double c.
    double-positive c.
    Downey c.
    c. effect
    effector c.
    effusion-associated
      mononuclear c.
    embryonic c.
    endothelial c.
    end-stage c.
    enterochromaffin c.
    epithelial c.
    erythroid c.
    ethmoid air c.
    eukaryotic c.
    euoxic c.

faggot c.
Ferratea c.
flower c.
foam c.
follicular dendritic c.
follicular predominantly
  large c.
follicular predominantly
  small cleaved c.
frozen red c.
c. function
c. generation time
ghost c.
giant c.
glioma c.
glitter c.
goblet c.
grape c.
c. growth inhibitor
hairy c.
Haller c.
HeLa c.
helmet c.
helper T-c.
hematopoietic c.
hematopoietic progenitor c.
hematopoietic stem c.'s
  (HSC)
hematopoietic target c.
Hodgkin c.
Hofbauer c.
horse red blood c.'s
host c.
human interleukin for DA-
  c.'s
hybridoma c.
hyperchromatic c.
immunocompetent c.
immunohematopoietic
  stem c.
inclusion c.
indeterminate c.
inducer T-c.
c. interaction gene
interdigitating dendritic c.
intraepithelial c.
juvenile c.

K-c.
Karpas T-c.
KG-1 c.
c. kill
killer c.
c. kill log
c. kinetics
koilocytotic c.
Kulchitsky c.
Kupffer c.
L-c.
lacunar c.
LAK c.
Langerhans c.
Langhans giant c.
large noncleaved follicular
  center c.
LE-c.
Leishman chrome c.
lepra c.
leukemic c.
leuko-poor red blood c.'s
Leydig c.
L&H c.
c. line
littoral c.
liver c. adenoma
Loevit c.
low columnar c.
Lyl B-c.
lymphadenoma c.
lymphoid c.
lymphoid precursor c.
lymphoid stem c.
lymphokine-activated
  killer c.
lymphoreticular c.
M-c.
malignant c.
mammalian c.
mantle c.
Marchand c.
marginal zone c.
marrow c.
mast c.
mediator c.
c. membrane antigen

NOTES

97

cell *(continued)*
    memory c.
    mesenchymal stromal c.
    mesothelial c.
    microglial c.
    c. migration
    monocytoid B-c.
    mononuclear c.
    Mooser c.
    morular c.
    mother c.
    Mott c.
    mummified c.
    mutant c.
    myeloid c.
    myeloid precursor c.
    myeloma c.
    myocardial c.
    Nageotte c.
    natural killer c.
    neoplastic c.
    Neumann c.
    neuroendocrine c.'s
    neuroglial c.
    neutrophilic c.
    nonangiogenic c.
    nonhematopoietic stem c.
    normal hematopoietic c.
    nuclear c.
    nucleated red blood c.
    null c.
    nurse c.
    oat c.
    occult tumor c.
    c. of origin
    ox red blood c.
    c. oxygenation
    packed red blood c.'s
    Paneth c.
    peg c.
    Pelger-Huet c.
    peripheral blood
      mononuclear c.'s
    peripheral blood
      progenitor c.'s
    peripheral blood stem c.
    peripheral lymphoid c.
    peripheral stem c.
    perithelial c.
    pessary c.
    phagocytic c.
    c. phase transition
    photo c.

    physaliferous c.
    Pinocchio c.
    plaque-forming c.
    plasma c.
    pluripotent stem c.
    PNH-c.
    polychromatic c.
    polylobulated c.
    popcorn Reed-Sternberg c.
    pre-B-c.
    precursor B-c.
    precursor T-c.
    preplasma c.
    primitive stem c.
    primordial germ c.
    progenitor c.
    c. proliferation
    pulmonary endocrine c.
    Raji c.
    red blood c.
    Reed c.
    Reed-Sternberg c.
    c. repair-competent
    reticuloendothelial c.
    reticulum c.
    rhagiocrine c.
    Rieder c.
    Rindfleisch c.
    rod c.
    rosette c.
    Rouget c.
    C. Saver Haemolite
    scavenger c.
    c. sensitizer
    Sertoli c.
    Sézary c.
    Sézary lymphoma c.
    shadow c.
    sickle c.
    signet-ring c.
    c. size
    smooth muscle c.
    smudge c.
    c. sorter
    c. sorting
    spindle c.
    spur c.
    squamous c.
    stab c.
    staff c.
    stave c.
    stem c.
    stipple c.

stomach c.
stromal c.
subependymal giant c.
suppressor T-c.
c. surface
c. surface antigen
c. survival
c. suspension
syncytiotrophoblast c.
T-c.
T4-c.
tanned red c.
target c.
tart c.
T-cell-rich B c.
    T-cytotoxic c.
TDTH c.
technetium-tagged red
  blood c.
T4 helper c.
Thoma-Zeiss counting c.
thymic interdigitating
  dendritic c.
thymus-dependent c.
thymus nurse c.
Touton giant c.
tumor c.
c. tumor
tumor-derived activated c.'s
Turk c.
veiled c.
veto c.
c. viability assessment
Virchow c.
wandering c.
Warthin c.
Warthin-Finkeldy giant c.
washed red c.'s
white c.
white blood c.
wild-type c.
Cellano phenotype
cell-bound
    c.-b. antibody
    c.-b. antigen
cell-cell contact

cell-cycle
    c.-c. effect
    c.-c. parameter
cell-fixed antibody
**CELLFREE Interleukin-2 Receptor
  kit**
cell-lineage marker
cell-mediated
    c.-m. antibody
    c.-m. immunity (CMI)
cellobiose
Cell-O-Gen
cells per unit area
celltrifuge
cellular
    c. blood product transfusion
    c. cytotoxic mechanism
    c. immunity
    c. immunity deficiency
      syndrome (CIDS)
    c. immunodeficiency
    c. localization
    c. migration
    c. origin
    c. periosteal reaction
    c. pharmacology
    c. phase
    c. repolarization
    c. ribosome
    c. suspension
    c. tumor
    c. whorling
cellularity
    bone marrow c.
cellulitis
    perirectal c.
cellulose
    c. acetate
    oxidized c.
Celsite implanted port
cement
    BNLAN c.
cementifying fibroma
cementinoma
cementoblastoma
cementoma
    gigantiform c.

NOTES

cementosis
cementum
    c. fracture
CEM/HIV-1 cell line
center
    accessory ossification c.
    bone c.
    epiphyseal ossification c.
    Fred Hutchinson Cancer
      Research C.
    germinal c.
    Johns Hopkins Oncology C.
    c. line artifact
    M. D. Anderson Cancer C.
    Memorial Sloan-Kettering
      Cancer C.
    progressively transformed
      germinal c.
    pseudofollicular
      proliferation c.
    window c.
center-edge (CE)
    c.-e. angle of Wiberg
Centers for Disease Control
    classification for HIV infection
centigray (cGy, c Gy)
centistoke
Centovir
Centoxin
centracytic lymphoma
central
    c. artery
    c. axis depth dose
    c. cementifying fibroma
    c. fracture
    c. high-signal intensity
      stripe
    c. nervous system (CNS)
    c. nervous system
      lymphoma
    c. nervous system
      malformation
    c. nervous system tumor
    c. neuroepithelial cell
    c. neuroepithelial cell origin
      tumor
    c. neurologic adverse effect
    c. ossifying fibroma
    c. pontine myelinolysis
      (CPM)
    c. processing unit (CPU)
    c. sinus lipomatosis

    c. sulcus
    c. tendon
    c. venous access
    c. venous catheter
    c. venous catheterization
    c. venous drainage
    c. venous pressure catheter
    c. venous pressure line
centrally-ordered phase encoding
Centriflow membrane cone
centrifugation
    discontinuous density
      gradient c.
    Ficoll-Hypaque density
      gradient c.
centrifugum
    erythema annulare c.
centrilobular
    c. emphysema
    c. lesion
centroblast
centroblastic lymphoma
centrocyte-like
    c.-l. cell
    c.-l. type
centrocytic lymphoma
centrocytoid
centromere
centrum semiovale pattern
CEP
    cyclophosphamide, etoposide,
      Platinol
cephalad direction
cephalexin
cephalgia
cephalhematoma, cephalohematoma
cephalic
    c. index
    c. tilt view
    c. vein
Cephalin
cephalocele
    occipital c.
    oral c.
cephalohematoma (*var. of*
    cephalhematoma)
cephalomedullary nail fracture
cephalometric radiograph
cephalosporin
Cephalosporium granulomatis
cephalosyndactyly
    Vogt c.

c-erbB-2
c.-e. gene product
c.-e. oncogene, protein
cerclage
Shirodkar c.
cerebellar
c. anaplastic
c. artery
c. astrocytoma
c. atrophy
c. ectopia
c. epidermoid
c. gliosarcoma
c. hemisphere
c. hemorrhage
c. hypoplasia
c. peg
c. tonsils
c. view
c. volume
cerebelli
falx c.
tentorium c.
cerebellolabyrinthine artery
cerebellopontine
c. angle
c. angle meningioma
c. angle tumor
c. recess
cerebelloretinal
c. hemangioblastoma
c. hemangioblastomatosis
cerebellum
towering c.
cerebral
c. amyloid angiopathy
c. aneurysm
c. angiography
c. anoxia
c. aqueduct
c. arteriovenous
malformation
c. artery
c. astrocytoma
c. atrophy
c. blood flow (CBF)
c. blood vessel

c. blood volume
c. circulation
c. circulation time
c. contusion
c. convexity
c. cortex
c. death
c. edema
c. embolism
c. gumma
c. hemisphere
c. hemorrhage
c. hypoperfusion
c. infarction
c. ischemia
c. lymphoma
c. malformation
c. mantle
c. metastasis
c. nodule
c. palsy
c. palsy pathological
fracture
c. parenchyma
c. peduncle
c. perfusion study
c. revascularization
c. shunt
c. sinovenous occlusion
c. sulcus
c. syndrome
c. vascular malformation
c. vasculature
c. vasoreactivity
c. vein
c. ventricle
c. ventricular shunt
connector
c. ventriculography
c. white matter hypoplasia
cerebri
gliomatosis c.
pseudotumor c.
cerebritis
sinusitis c.
cerebrohepatorenal syndrome
cerebroside

NOTES

cerebrospinal
- c. fluid (CSF)
- c. fluid-brain barrier
- c. fluid volume

cerebrovascular
- c. accident (CVA)
- c. aneurysmal clip
- c. disease
- c. malformation

cerebrum semiovate
cerium
Cerrobend
- C. block

Cerubidine
ceruletide
ceruloplasmin
ceruminoma
cervical
- c. adenocarcinoma
- c. adenopathy
- c. artery
- c. bruit
- c. brush
- c. canal
- c. cancer
- c. carcinoma
- c. conization
- c. cord
- c. disk
- c. disk herniation
- c. disk syndrome
- c. dysplasia
- c. enlargement
- c. esophagostomy
- c. eversion
- c. fascia
- c. injury
- c. intraepithelial neoplasia (CIN)
- c. intraepithelial neoplasm
- c. lymph node
- c. meningocele
- c. myelogram
- c. neural foramen
- c. os
- c. pain syndrome
- c. plexus
- posterior c. space
- c. retention cyst
- c. rib
- c. rib syndrome
- c. sarcoma
- c. spine
- c. spine fracture
- c. spine fusion
- c. spine spondylosis
- c. stroma
- c. structure
- c. stump
- c. stump cancer
- superior c. ganglion
- c. syringomyelia
- c. tumor
- c. vertebra

cervicitis
cervicography
cervicomedullary kink
cervicotrochanteric fracture
cervix
- cell carcinoma of c.
- cone biopsy of c.
- dilated c.
- incompetent c.
- International classification of cancer of c.
- malignant tumor of c.
- c. sign
- uterine c.

cesium
- c. implant
- c. needle
- c. therapy

cesium-137 (^{137}Cs)
cessation
- smoking c.

cestoda
c-ets **oncogene**
CEV
- cyclophosphamide, etoposide, vincristine

CF
- cancer-free
- Christmas factor
- cisplatin, 5-fluorouracil
- citrovorum factor
- complement factor

^{252}Cf
- californium-252

CFA
- colony-forming assay
- complement-fixing antibody
- complete Freund adjuvant

CFD
- color-flow Doppler

CFIDS
chronic fatigue and immune
dysfunction syndrome
C-Flex
C.-F. catheter
C.-F. double-J stent
C.-F. stent
c-fms
-f. oncogene
-f. proto-oncogene
c-fos-dependent pathway
c-fos gene
c-fos-independent pathway
c-fos **oncogene**
CFT
crystal field theory
CFU
colony-forming unit
CFU$_{EOS}$
colony-forming unit-eosinophil
CFU-C
colony-forming unit-culture
CFU-E
colony-forming unit erythrocyte
CFU-F
colony-forming unit-fibroblast
CFU-GEMM
colony-forming unit granulocyte,
erythrocyte, megakaryocyte,
macrophage
CFU-GM
colony-forming unit granulocyte-
macrophage
granulocyte-macrophage colony-
forming unit
cGy, c Gy
centigray
CHAD
cyclophosphamide,
hexamethylmelamine,
Adriamycin, DDP
CHAD protocol
Chagas disease
chain
branched c.
closed c.
c. cystography

cytoplasmic μ c.
epsilon c.
gamma c.
immunoglobulin alpha c.
immunoglobulin delta c.
immunoglobulin epsilon c.
immunoglobulin gamma c.
immunoglobulin heavy c.
immunoglobulin kappa c.
immunoglobulin lambda c.
immunoglobulin mu c.
J c.
joining c.
kappa light c.
lambda light c.
ricin A c.
side c.
chair
SPECTurn c.
chalasia
chalazion
challenge
Desferal Mesylate c.
chamber
Boyden c.
c. enlargement
farmer c.
ion c.
personal ionization c.
pocket c.
sample c.
Storm Von Leeuwen c.
Chamberlain
C. line
C. procedure
Chamberlain-Towne view
CHAM-OCA
cyclophosphamide, hydroxyurea,
actinomycin D (dactinomycin),
methotrexate, Oncovin
(vincristine), citrovorum factor,
Adriamycin
champagne glass pelvis
Chance fracture
chancroid
Chandler disease

NOTES

change
  atherosclerotic c.
  cystic c.
  degenerative c.
  E:A c.
  epithelial degenerative c.
  E-to-A c.
  fibrocystic c.
  focal c.
  gender c.
  histologic c.
  pigment c.
  polyneuropathy,
    organomegaly, endocrine
    abnormalities, M-protein,
    skin c.'s (POEMS)
  postbiopsy c.
  posttherapy c.
  postthoracotomy c.
  precancerous c.
  prediverticular c.
  pseudo-Pelger-Huet c.
  redox c.
  senescent c.
  senile c.
changer
  film c.
  PUCK film c.
  rapid film c.
  Schonander film c.
  serial film c.
Chang stage
channel
  collateral venous c.
  haversian c.
  c. pyloric ulcer
  surface epithelium
    vascular c.
  thread-and-streaks
    vascular c.'s
  vascular c.
CHAP
  cyclophosphamide,
    hexamethylmelamine,
    Adriamycin, Platinol
Chaput fracture
CHAR
  continuous hyperfractionated
    accelerated radiotherapy
characteristic
  contrast transfer c.
  c. curve
  c. emission

  c. radiation
  receiver operating c.
  tip dispersion c.
  transfer c.
characterization
  immunologic c.
  tissue c.
charcoal
  dextran-coated c. (DCC)
Charcot
  C. arthropathy
  C. joint
  C. triad
Charcot-Leyden crystal
charge
  technical c.
charge-coupled device
charged-particle irradiation
Charles vacuuming needle
chart
  Boving c.
  Brodmann c.
  Segre c.
chauffeur's fracture
Chaussier line
checkerboard analysis
checker colony
Check-Flo
  C.-F. introducer
  C.-F. sheath
Chédiak-Higashi syndrome
cheilitis
  angular c.
  c. granulomatosa
chelate
  gadolinium c.
  c. immunoconjugate
chelated
  c. antibody
  c. immunoglobulin
chelating agent
chelation
chemical
  c. carcinogen
  c. carcinogenesis
  c. exchange
  c. linkage
  c. mediator
  c. pneumonitis
  c. shift
  c. shift anisotropy
  c. shift artifact
  c. shift cancellation effect

c. shift imaging (CSI)
c. shift misregistration
c. shift misregistration
  artifact (CSMA)
c. shift reference
c. shift selective (CHESS)
c. shift spatial offset
c. thrombectomy
chemical-induced hepatitis
chemistry
  anomalous serum c.
  computational c.
  radiopharmaceutical c.
  serum c.
chemoattractant
  c. cytokine
ChemoBloc vial venting system
chemodectoma
chemoembolization
  hepatic c.
  transcatheter arterial c.
    (TACE)
chemoembolotherapy
chemoendocrine therapy
chemohormonotherapy
chemolitholysis
  bile acid c.
chemolysis
chemonucleolysis
Chemo-Port catheter
chemoprevention
chemoprophylaxis
chemoprotector
chemoradiation
  marrow-ablative c.
  c. therapy
chemoradiotherapy
  high-dose c.
chemoreceptor
  c. trigger zone
  c. tumor
chemoresistant tumor
chemosensitizer
chemoserotherapy
chemotactic
  c. factor
  c. peptide

chemotaxis
chemotherapeutic
  c. agent
  c. drug
chemotherapy
  adjuvant c.
  AT-II-induced intraarterial c.
  belly bath c.
  cell cycling in c.
  combination c.
  consolidation c.
  continuous intravenous
    infusion c.
  conventional dose c.
  curative c.
  cytotoxic c.
  DACE c.
  double high-dose c.
  experimental c.
  hepatic arterial c.
  high-dose c. (HDC)
  hypertensive intraarterial c.
  induction c.
  infusion c.
  intensification c.
  intraarterial c.
  intraperitoneal c.
  intrapleural c.
  intrathecal c.
  intravenous c.
  intravenous infusion c.
  intravesical c.
  Karnofsky performance
    status of c.
  low-dose c.
  MADDOC c.
  metabolism in
    intraperitoneal c.
  multiagent c.
  multitargeted c.
  myelosuppression c.
  neoadjuvant c.
  palliative c.
  parenteral c.
  postoperative c.
  preoperative c.
  presurgical c.

NOTES

chemotherapy *(continued)*
    primary c.
    prophylactic c.
    random high-dose c.
    regional c.
    reinduction c.
    remission-induction c.
    salvage c.
    sequential c.
    sequential postremission c. (sPC)
    single c.
    single-agent c.
    single-agent high-dose c.
chemotherapy-induced
    c.-i. ischemia
    c.-i. pericarditis
    c.-i. peripheral neuropathy
    c.-i. pulmonary toxicity
chemotherapy-responsive patient
chenodeoxycholic acid
Chenuda virus
Cherenkov effect
cherry angioma
cherubism
Chesapeake
    hemoglobin C.
CHESS
    chemical shift selective
chest
    dirty c.
    c. film
    flail c.
    jail-bar c.
    narrow c.
    pneumonectomy c.
    c. radiology
    c. tube
    c. wall
    c. x-ray
Chi
    C. site
Chiari
    C. II malformation
    C. I malformation
chiasm
    optic c.
chiasmatic groove
chiasmatic/hypothalamic glioma
Chiba needle
chick-cell agglutination

chicken
    c. fat clot
    c. roosting sign
chickenpox
Chido-Rogers antigen
chignon
Chilaiditi syndrome
child
    C. cirrhosis
    C. grade
    c. lymphoblastic leukemia
childhood
    c. breast
    c. cancer
    C. Cancer Survivor Study (CCSS)
    c. granulomatous disease
    non-T, non-B acute lymphocytic leukemia of c.
    c. polycystic disease
Child-Pugh classification
chimera
    radiation c.
chimeric
    c. antibody
    c. antigen receptor gene
chimerism
    hematopoietic c.
    mixed c.
chimney-shaped high aortic arch
chimney sweep's cancer
Chinese liver fluke
chip fracture
Chiron strip
chiropractic treatment fracture
chisel fracture
chi squared test
chitin
Chlamydia
    C. psittaci
    C. trachomatis
chloracetaldehyde
chloral hydrate
chlorambucil
    pulse c.
chlorambucil, vinblastine, procarbazine, prednisone (ChlVPP)
chloramphenicol acetyltransferase (CAT)
chloranbucil
chlorazol-fast pink stain
chlordiazepoxide

Chloresium
    C. ointment
    C. solution
chlorethyl carboniom ion
chlorethylisocyanate
chlorhexidine
chloride
    magnesium c.
    manganese c.
    strontium-89 c.
    thallium-201 c.
chlormadinone
chloroacetate
    c. esterase
    c. esterase-butyrate esterase
      stain
2-chloro-2′-deoxyadenosine (CdA)
chloroethylnitrosourea (CNU)
chloroma
chloromyeloma
chlorophyllin copper complex
chlorotic anemia
chlorotrianisene
chlorozotocin
chlorphenesin carbamate
chlorpromazine
ChlVPP
    chlorambucil, vinblastine,
      procarbazine, prednisone
choanal polyp
chocolate
    c. cyst
    c. joint effusion
    c. sauce abscess
cholangiectasis
    extrahepatic c.
cholangiocarcinoma
    extrahepatic c.
    intrahepatic c.
    Klatskin c.
cholangiocellular carcinoma
cholangiodrainage
cholangiogram
    intraoperative c.
    operative c.
cholangiography
    fine-needle transhepatic c.

    intravenous c.
    percutaneous c.
    percutaneous transhepatic c.
    transhepatic c.
    T-tube c.
cholangiohepatitis
    Oriental c.
cholangiolithiasis
cholangiopancreatography
    endoscopic retrograde c.
    (ERCP)
cholangitis
    acute nonsuppurative
      ascending c.
    acute suppurative
      ascending c.
    chronic nonsuppurative
      destructive c.
    nonsuppurative ascending c.
    nonsuppurative
      destructive c.
    Oriental c.
    primary c.
    primary sclerosing c.
    pyogenic c.
    recurrent pyogenic c.
    sclerosing c.
    secondary sclerosing c.
    suppurative ascending c.
Cholebrine
cholecystectomy
    laparoscopic c.
    percutaneous c.
    surgical c.
cholecystitis
    acalculous c.
    acute c.
    chronic c.
    emphysematous c.
    gangrenous c.
    lipid c.
cholecystocholangiography
cholecystocholangitis
cholecystocolic fistula
cholecystoduodenal fistula
cholecystogram
    oral c.

NOTES

cholecystography
    oral c. (OCG)
cholecystojejunostomy
cholecystokinin (CCK)
cholecystolithiasis
cholecystomegaly
cholecystopaque
cholecystosis
    hyperplastic c.
cholecystostomy
    percutaneous c.
    surgical c.
choledochal cyst
choledochocele
choledochocholedochostomy
choledochoduodenal fistula
choledochojejunostomy stricture
choledocholithiasis
choledochoscope
cholelithiasis
cholera
    pancreatic c.
cholerae
    Vibrio c.
cholescintigraphy
cholestasis
    intrahepatic c.
cholesteatoma
    inflammatory c.
cholesterol
    c. cleft
    c. emboli
    c. gallstone
    c. pneumonia
    c. polyp
    c. stone
cholesterolosis, cholesterinosis,
    cholesterosis
Choletec
choline
    c. magnesium trisalicylate
    c. salicylate
cholinergic drug
cholioangiopancreatography
Cholografin
Cholovue
chondral fracture
chondritis
chondroblastic osteosarcoma
chondroblastoma
chondrocalcinosis
    familial c.

chondrodysplasia
    Jansen-type metaphyseal c.
    metaphyseal c.
    c. punctata
    Schmid-like metaphyseal c.
chondrodystrophia calcificans
    congenita
chondrodystrophy
chondroectodermal dysplasia
chondrofibroma
chondroid
    c. syringoma
chondroitin sulfate
chondrolysis
    posttraumatic c.
chondroma
    joint c.
    soft tissue c.
chondromalacia
    c. patellae
chondromatosis
    synovial c.
chondromyxoid fibroma
chondrosarcoma
    clear cell c.
    endosteal c.
    exostotic c.
    mesenchymal c.
    peripheral c.
    uterine c.
CHOP
    cyclophosphamide,
    hydroxydaunomycin
    (doxorubicin), Oncovin
    (vincristine), prednisone
    cyclophosphamide,
    hydroxydaunorubicin,
    Oncovin, prednisone
Chopart joint
CHOP-BLEO
    cyclophosphamide,
    hydroxydaunorubicin,
    Oncovin, prednisone,
    bleomycin
Chopper-Dixon fat suppression
    imaging
Chopper fat suppression
chordae tendineae
chorda tympani
chordoma
    sacral c.
    c. of sacrum

chorea
  Huntington c.
  Sydenham c.
chorioadenoma destruens
chorioamniotic separation
chorioangioma
choriocarcinoma
  esophageal c.
  gestational c.
  nongestational c.
  ovarian c.
choriodecidua
choriodecidual reaction
choriomeningitis
  lymphocytic c.
chorion
  c. frondosum
  c. laeve
chorionic
  c. gonadotropin
  c. plate
  c. villus
  c. villus sampling (CVS)
chorioretinitis
  CDC classification c.
choroid
  c. plexus
  c. plexus blush
  c. plexus cyst
  c. plexus neoplasm
  c. plexus papilloma
  c. point
choroidal
  c. artery
  c. fissure
  c. hemangioma
  c. melanoma
  c. osteoma
choroidal-hippocampal fissure complex
choroidea
  tela c.
choroideum
  glomus c.
CHPP
  continuous hyperthermic peritoneal perfusion

Christmas
  C. disease
  C. factor (CF)
  C. tree adapter
chromaffin
  c. cell
  c. lineage
  c. tumor
Chromagen
chromatin
  clock-face c.
  c. condensation
chromatogram
chromatography
  anti-idiotypic affinity c.
  DEAE-Sephadex A-25 c.
  gas-liquid phase c. (GLPC)
  gel filtration c.
  high-performance liquid c. (HPLC)
  high-performance size-exclusion c. (HPSEC)
  high-pressure liquid c. (HPLC)
  lentil lectin affinity c.
chromic
  c. phosphate
  c. phosphate P 32 colloidal suspension
chromium
  c. phosphate
chromium-51
chromogranin
  c. A
  c. stain
chromophilic adenoma
chromophobe adenoma
chromosomal
  c. abnormality
  c. abnormality cystic hygroma
  c. damage
  c. translocation
chromosome
  c. 2
  c. 5
  c. 7

NOTES

chromosome *(continued)*
  c. 11
  c. analysis
  banded c.
  c. banding
  c. break
  c. breakage
  deletion of c.'s
  c. deletion
  c. inversion
  c. map
  Philadelphia c.
  c. rearrangement
  c. translocation
  c. walking
  X c.
chromosome-negative
  Philadelphia c.-n.
chromosome-positive
  Philadelphia c.-p.
chromotope sodium
chronic
  c. acquired hepatic failure
  c. active hepatitis
  c. arsenism
  c. brain syndrome
  c. breast abscess
  c. catheterization
  c. cholecystitis
  c. communicating
    hydrocephalus
  c. diffuse sclerosing
    alveolitis
  c. eosinophilic pneumonia
  c. epididymitis
  c. extrinsic alveolitis
  c. fatigue and immune
    dysfunction syndrome
    (CFIDS)
  c. fibrosing alveolitis
  c. granulocytic leukemia
  c. granulomatous disease
  c. idiopathic intestinal
    pseudoobstruction
  c. infantile hyperostosis
  c. irritation
  c. leukemia
  c. lymphocytic leukemia
    (CLL)
  c. lymphocytic thyroiditis
  c. lymphoid leukemia
  c. megakaryocytic myelosis
  c. monocytic leukemia

  c. myelocytic leukemia
    (CML)
  c. myelogenous leukemia
    (CML)
  c. myeloid leukemia (CML)
  c. myelomonocytic leukemia
    (CMML)
  c. neutrophilic leukemia
  c. nonsuppurative
    destructive cholangitis
  c. obstructive pulmonary
    disease (COPD)
  c. obstructive uropathy
  c. pain syndrome
  c. pancreatitis
  c. partial epilepsy
  c. phase
  c. pluripotential
    immunoproliferative
    syndrome
  c. renal failure
  c. venous stasis
  c. venous statis syndrome
chronica
  c. et progressiva
  pityriasis lichenoides c.
chronobiology
chronotherapy
  adjuvant c.
chronotoxicology
Chrysotile
Churg-Strauss syndrome
Chvostek anemia
chyloma
chylomicron
chylothorax
chylous ascites
Chymodiactin
chymopapain
chymotrypsin
CI-921
CI-941
CIC
  circulating immune complex
cicatricial
cicatrix
cicatrizing atelectasis
CID
  cytomegalic inclusion disease
CIDS
  cellular immunity deficiency
    syndrome
cigarette smoking

ciliaris
ciliary
    c. body melanoma
    c. function
    c. ganglion
    c. muscle
ciliated cell adenocarcinoma
cimetidine
Cimino dialysis shunt
CIN
    cervical intraepithelial neoplasia
cine
    c. camera
    c. film
    c. fistulogram
    c. imaging
    c. left ventriculography
    c. magnetic resonance
      function image
    c. magnetic resonance
      imaging
    c. MRI
    c. projector
    velocity-encoded c. MR
      imaging
cineangiography
    axial c.
cinefluoroscopy
    valve c.
cinepharyngoesophagogram
cineportography
cinereum
    tuber c.
cingulate
    c. gyrus
    c. sulcus
cingulum, pl. cingula
ciprofloxacin
circadian
    c. continuous infusion
    c. pattern
    c. regimen
    c. rhythm
    c. variation
circadian-modified floxuridine
  (FUdR)

circle
    anastomotic arterial c.
    c. loop biliary drainage
    c. tube nephrostomy
      catheter
    c. of Willis
    c. wire nephrostomy
circular
    c. dichroism spectroscopy
    c. polarization wave
    submucosal c. fold
circularly-polarized coil
circulating immune complex (CIC)
circulation
    carotid c.
    cerebral c.
    collateral c.
    collateral mesenteric c.
    extracorporeal c.
    extracranial carotid c.
    fetal c.
    intracranial c.
    persistent fetal c.
    portosystemic collateral c.
    posterior c.
    posterior fossa c.
    pulmonary c.
    c. time
    uteroplacental c.
circulator
    sequential c.
circumaortic
    c. left renal vein
    c. renal vein
circumcaval ureter
circumcision
circumference
    fetal c.
    fetal abdominal c.
    fetal head c.
    head c. (HC)
    thoracic c.
circumferential
    c. coil
    c. fracture
    c. venous stenosis

NOTES

circumflex
- c. artery
- humeral c.
- c. retroesophageal arch

circummarginate placenta
circummesencephalic cistern
circumscribed mass
circumscripta
- calcinosis c.
- osteoporosis c.

circumvallate
- c. papilla
- c. placenta

cirrhosis
- alcoholic c.
- anti-hepatitis C virus-positive c.
- biliary c.
- Child c.
- diffuse c.
- Laënnec c.
- macronodular c.
- micronodular c.
- primary biliary c.

cirsoid aneurysm
CIS
- carcinoma in situ

cis-acting
cisapride
CISCA
- cisplatin, cyclophosphamide, Adriamycin

cis-**diamminedichloroplatinum (CDDP, DDP)**
cis-dichlorotranshydroxybis-isoprophylamine platinum
cisplatin
- c. analog
- c. nephrotoxicity
- c. neutralization

cisplatin, cyclophosphamide, Adriamycin (CISCA)
cisplatin, 5-fluorouracil (CF)
cis-retinoic acid
cistern
- ambient c.
- ambient wing of the quadrigeminal c.
- basal c.
- circummesencephalic c.
- perimesencephalic c.
- pontine c.
- prepontine c.
- quadrigeminal c.
- subarachnoid c.
- suprasellar subarachnoid c.
- sylvian c.

cisternal
- c. herniation
- c. puncture

cisterna magna
cisternography
- gas CT c.
- Pantopaque c.
- radionuclide c.

citrate
- clomiphene c.
- droloxifene c.
- ferric ammonium c.
- gallium c.
- gallium-67 c.
- magnesium c.
- manganese c.
- c. reaction
- tamoxifen c.

citrated
- c. blood
- c. plasma

citrovorum
- c. factor (CF)
- c. rescue factor

CK
- creatine kinase

CK-BB
- creatine kinase-BB isoenzyme
- CK-BB tumor marker

CL286558
- zeniplatin

CL287110
- enloplatin

cladribine
Clara
- C. cell
- C. cell adenocarcinoma
- C. hematoxylin

clarithromycin
Clark
- C. classification system
- C. staging system for malignant melanoma

Clark-Collip method
clasmatocyte
clasp-knife rigidity
classic carpal tunnel view

classification
Astler-Coller modification of Dukes c.
Bennett c.
Binet system of c.
Borrmann c.
Butchart staging c.
Cambridge c.
Catterall c.
Centers for Disease Control c. for HIV infection
Child-Pugh c.
dichotomous c.
Dripps c.
Dukes c.
Edmondson-Steiner c.
FAB c.
French/American/British c.
Goldman c.
Haggitt c.
Hinchey c.
immunologic c.
International C. of Diseases for Oncology (ICD-O)
Jackson and Parker c. of Hodgkin disease
Jewett and Whitmore c.
Keil tumor cell c.
Kemohan c.
Lancefield c.
Lauren c.
Linell-Ljungberg c.
Lukes and Butler c. of Hodgkin disease
Lukes and Collins c. of non-Hodgkin lymphoma
microinvasive carcinoma c.
morphologic c.
Neer c.
Potter c.
Rai c.
Rappaport c.
Rye c.
Salter-Harris c.
Snyder c.
TNM c.

tumor, node, metastasis classification
tumor, node, metastasis c. (TNM classification)
Wolfe breast carcinoma c.
World Health Organization c.
clasticus
conus c.
clathrin
c. protein
claudication
intermittent c.
Clausen method
claustrophobia
claustrum
clavicle
penciling of the distal c.
clavicular
c. birth fracture
c. fracture
c. osteitis condensans
clay
c. mineral
c. shoveler's fracture
clear
c. cell adenocarcinoma
c. cell carcinoma
c. cell chondrosarcoma
clearance
blood isotope c.
creatinine c.
immune c.
insulin c.
renal c.
cleavage fracture
Clebopride
cleft
cholesterol c.
coronal c.
c. face syndrome
facial c.
Hahn c.
c. lip
c. lip and palate syndrome
c. palate
spinal cord c.

NOTES

cleidocranial
  c. dysostosis
  c. dysplasia
Cleopatra view
Clerf cell collector
Cleveland procedure
click
  pulmonic c.
clindamycin
clinical
  c. assay
  c. correlation
  c. feature
  c. partial response (CPR)
  c. staging
  c. trial
clinicopathologic correlation
Clinitron bed
clinodactyly
clinoid
  c. process
clinoparietal line
Clinoril
clip
  aneurysmal c.
  cerebrovascular
    aneurysmal c.
  hemostatic c.
  metallic c.
  Pate c.
  sternal c.
  surgical c.
clitoris enlargement
clivus
  c. meningioma
  c. metastasis
  c. torcula line
CLL
  chronic lymphocytic leukemia
cloaca
cloacae
  Enterobacter c.
cloacal
  c. exstrophy
  c. formation
cloacogenic
  c. carcinoma
  c. carcinoma of the
    anorectum
  c. nonkeratinizing carcinoma
clock-face chromatin
clofazimine
clofibrate

cloison of Bertin
clomiphene
  c. citrate
clonal
  c. B-lymphocyte
  c. deletion theory
  c. development
  c. inhibitory factor
  c. marker
  c. selection theory
clonality
clonazepam
clone
  leukemic c.
  neoplastic c.
cloned gene
clonidine
  c. transdermal tape
cloning
  cDNA c.
  gene c.
  molecular c.
  subtraction c.
clonogenic
  c. assay
  c. capacity
  c. myeloma cell
  c. tumor cell
clonorchiasis
Cloquet
  C. canal
Clorgyline
Clorox bleach assay
closed
  c. chain
  c. fracture
closed-mouth view
closing volume
Clostridium
  C. difficile
  C. difficile enterocolitis
  C. perfringens
closure
  transcatheter c.
clot
  autologous blood c.
  blood c.
  chicken fat c.
  currant jelly c.
  fibrin c.
  fibrinous c.
  c. lysis
  c. lysis time

plasma c.
c. retraction time
sentinel c.
CLO-test
clothesline injury
clotrimazole
clotting
c. factor
c. factor VIII
clot-trapper device
Cloudman melanoma
Clough and Richter syndrome
cloverleaf
c. deformity
c. skull
clubfoot deformity
club-shaped cell
clumping
platelet c.
cluster of differentiation (CD)
Clutton painful joint
Clysodrast
CMD
corticomedullary differentiation
CMED
cyclophosphamide,
methotrexate, etoposide,
dexamethasone
CMF
cyclophosphamide,
methotrexate, 5-fluorouracil
CMFP
cyclophosphamide,
methotrexate, 5-fluorouracil,
prednisone
CMFPTH
cyclophosphamide,
methotrexate, 5-fluorouracil,
prednisone, tamoxifen,
Halotestin
CMFVP
cyclophosphamide,
methotrexate, 5-fluorouracil,
vincristine, prednisone
CMI
cell-mediated immunity

CML
chronic myelocytic leukemia
chronic myelogenous leukemia
chronic myeloid leukemia
CMML
chronic myelomonocytic
leukemia
C-MOPP
cyclophosphamide,
mechlorethamine, Oncovin,
procarbazine, prednisone
CMV
Cytomegalovirus
CMVIG
cytomegalovirus immune
globulin
c-myb
c. oncogene
c. proto-oncogene
c-myc
c. oncogene
c. protein
C/N ratio
contrast-to-noise ratio
CNS
central nervous system
CNU
chloroethylnitrosourea
^{60}Co
cobalt-60
CoA
coenzyme A
coagulation
c. cascade
disseminated intravascular c.
(DIC)
c. factor
c. profile
c. system
coagulative necrosis
coagulator
cold c.
coagulopathy
consumption c.
intravascular consumption c.
co-alcohol fractionation
coalescence

NOTES

coalition
  calcaneonavicular c.
coal worker's pneumoconiosis
Coamate antithrombin assay
coaptation
coarctation
  aortic c.
  juxtaductal aortic c.
  postductal aortic c.
  c. syndrome
coarse
  c. calcification
  c. reticulation
coast
  c. of California café-au-lait
  spots
  c. of Maine café-au-lait
  spots
coat-hanger wire
CoA-transferase
Coats disease
coaxial
  c. catheter
  c. dilator
cobalamin
  c. adenosyltransferase
cobalt
  c. megavoltage machine
  c. pneumopathy
cobalt-60 (^{60}Co)
cobblestone
  c. appearance
  c. appearance of the colon
  c. ileum
cobblestoning
Cobe double blood pump
cobra
  c. catheter
  c. head sign
cocaine granuloma
cocarcinogen
coccidioidal granuloma
Coccidioides immitis
coccidioidomycosis
  c. arthritis
coccygeal ligament
coccygeus
coccyx
  c. fracture
cochlea, pl. cochleae
cochlear
  c. aqueduct
  c. hearing loss

  c. implant
  c. lesion
  c. nerve
  c. otosclerosis
Cochran-Mantel-Haensel test
Cockayne syndrome
Cockroft method
cocktail
  Bromptom c.
  MAK-6 c.
  pain c.
coculture
cocurrent flow-related enhancement
code
  genetic c.
coded-aperture imaging
codeine
Codman
  C. triangle
  C. tumor
codominance
codominant gene
codon
  nonsense c.
coefficient
  absorption c.
  apparent diffusion c.
  attenuation c.
  diffusion c.
  reflection c.
  c. of variation
  viscosity c.
coelomic
  c. cyst
  c. epithelium
coenzyme A (CoA)
coenzyme Q (CoQ)
coeur en sabot
Coe virus
cofactor
  ristocetin c. test
  ristocetin von Willebrand c.
coffee
  c. bean appearance
  c. bean sign
  c. sign
coffee-grounds material
cognitive
  c. restructuring
  c. technique
Cohen-Eder cannula
coherence
  phase c.

Cohn fraction II
cohort study
coil
> array c.
> birdcage c.
> breast c.
> butterfly c.
> circularly-polarized c.
> circumferential c.
> crossed c.
> detector c.
> c. embolization
> endorectal c.
> field-profiling c.
> Gianturco c.
> Gianturco-Wallace-
> Anderson c.
> Gianturco-Wallace-Chuang c.
> Golay c.
> gradient c.
> Helmholtz c.
> intrarectal c.
> intravascular c.
> linearly-polarized c.
> c. loading
> local c.
> neck c.
> parallel data acquisition c.
> platinum c.
> quadrature c.
> radiofrequency c.
> radiofrequency transmitter-
> receiver c.
> receiver c.
> saddle c.
> c. selection
> shim c.
> solenoid surface c.
> stainless steel c.
> steel c.
> surface c.
> thrombogenic c.
> transmitter c.
> volume c.
> whole-volume c.
> wool c.

coiled-spring
> c.-s. appearance
> c.-s. pattern
coimmunoprecipitation
coin
> c. artifact
> c. lesion
> c. lesion of lung
coincidence loss
coinfection
coin-on-edge vertebra
Coke bottle sign
Colapinto
> C. needle
> C. sheath
colaspase
cold
> c. agglutinin
> c. antibody
> c. coagulator
> c. hemagglutinin
> c. kit
> c. nodule
> c. spot
> c. spot imaging
cold-knife conization
colectomy
Cole hematoxylin
colestipol
Coley toxin
coli
> *Escherichia c.*
> haustra c.
> melanosis c.
> pneumatosis c.
colic
> c. artery
> biliary c.
colitis
> adenovirus c.
> *Campylobacter* c.
> c. cystica profunda
> granulomatous c.
> hemorrhagic c.
> ischemic c.
> mucous c.
> pseudomembranous c.

NOTES

colitis *(continued)*
    spastic c.
    ulcerative c.
collagen
    c. cuff
    microfibrillar c.
    c. sphere
    c. stroma
    c. vascular disease (CVD)
collagenase
    c. ointment
collagenous structure
collagen-vascular disease
collapse cavitation
collapsed
    c. distal ileum
    c. inferior vena cava
    c. lung
    c. subpectoral implant
collapsing cord sign
collar button ulcer
collateral
    perirenal venous c.'s
collateral
    c. blood flow
    c. branch
    c. circulation
    cystic vein c.
    gastrorenal c.
    hemorrhoidal c.
    intestinal c.
    Kugel c.
    c. ligament
    c. mesenteric circulation
    portosystemic c.
    splenocaval c.
    splenorenal c.
    venous c.
    c. venous channel
    c. vessel
collateralization
collecting
    c. system
    c. system opacification
collection
    abdominal air c.
    air c.
    cell c.
    extraaxial fluid c.
    extracerebral fluid c.
    fluid c.
    gas c.
    pancreatic fluid c.

    periarticular fluid c.
    pericholecystic fluid c.
    perinephric fluid c.
    pleural fluid c.
    posttraumatic subcapsular
      hepatic fluid c.
collective paramagnetism
collector
    Clerf cell c.
Colles fracture
colli
    fibromatosis c.
    pterygium c.
colliculocentral point
colliculus, pl. colliculi
    facial c.
    inferior c.
    superior c.
collimating system
collimation
    secondary c.
    skin c.
    tertiary c.
collimator
    medium-energy c.
    Micro-Cast c.
collision tumor
Collison fluid
colloid
    c. adenoma
    c. cancer
    c. carcinoma
    c. cyst
    c. cyst of third ventricle
    c. goiter
    iron oxide dextran c.
    phytate c.
    radioactive c.
    c. shift
    sulfur c.
    technetium-99m c.
    technetium-99m albumin c.
    technetium-99m sulfur c.
    technetium-99m sulfur c.
    technetium sulfur c.
colloidal suspension
Collostat sponge
coloanal resection
coloboma
colocalization
colocolostomy
colocolpopoiesis
    Kun c.

colon
>   ascending c.
>   barium-filled c.
>   burnt-out c.
>   c. cancer
>   cathartic c.
>   cobblestone appearance of the c.
>   c. cutoff sign
>   descending c.
>   double-tracking of c.
>   fecal-filled c.
>   lead pipe c.
>   c. perforation
>   sigmoid c.
>   thumbprinting appearance of the c.
>   transverse c.
>   unused c.

colonic
>   c. carcinoma
>   c. diverticular hemorrhage
>   c. diverticulitis
>   c. diverticulosis
>   c. diverticulum
>   c. filling defect
>   c. ileus
>   c. narrowing
>   c. neoplasm
>   c. obstruction
>   c. perforation
>   c. polyp
>   c. stricture
>   c. ulcer
>   c. varix
>   c. volvulus

colonoscopic polypectomy
colonoscopy
colony
>   checker c.
>   daisy-head c.
>   c. formation

colony-forming
>   c.-f. assay (CFA)
>   c.-f. unit (CFU)
>   c.-f. unit-culture (CFU-C)
>   c.-f. unit-eosinophil (CFU$_{EOS}$)
>   c.-f. unit erythrocyte (CFU- E)
>   c.-f. unit-fibroblast (CFU-F)
>   c.-f. unit granulocyte, erythrocyte, megakaryocyte, macrophage (CFU-GEMM)
>   c.-f. unit granulocyte-macrophage (CFU-GM)

colony-stimulating factor (CSF)
coloproctitis
color
>   c. Doppler imaging
>   c. gain

Colorado tick fever virus
colorectal
>   c. adenoma
>   c. anastomosis
>   c. cancer
>   c. cancer endoscopy
>   c. carcinoid
>   c. carcinoma
>   c. hemorrhage
>   c. lymphoma
>   c. polyp

colorectal/ovarian (CR/OV)
color-flow
>   c.-f. Doppler (CFD)
>   c.-f. Doppler imaging
>   c.-f. Doppler sonography
>   transcranial real-time c.-f. Doppler sonography

coloscopy
>   endocervical canal c.

colostomy
>   diverting c.
>   fecal diversion c.
>   temporary diverting c.

colostomy-related problem
colostrum
>   cryptosporidium immune c.

colovaginal fistula
colovesical fistula
colpocephaly
colpocleisis
colpoperineoplasty

NOTES

colposcopy
column
    c. of Bertin
    dye c.
    immunoadsorption c.
    Prosorba c.
    vertebral c.
columnar epithelium papilla
columnization of contrast material
coma carcinomatosum
CombiBlot test
combination
    c. chemotherapy
    TAD 9/HAM c.
combined
    c. flexion-distraction injury
      and burst fracture
    c. immunotherapy with
      levamisole and bacillus
      Calmette-Guérin vaccine
    c. modality therapy
    c. modulators
    c. radial-ulnar-humeral
      fracture
combining-site antibody
comedocarcinoma
comet
    c. sign
    c. tail
    c. tail sign
Comfeel
    C. hydroolloid dressing
    C. Ulcus occlusive dressing
comfort care
comiculate cartilage
COMLA
    cyclophosphamide, Oncovin,
    methotrexate, leucovorin,
    arabinosylcytosine
comma
    c. appearance
    c. sign
comma-shaped hilum
comminuted
    c. fracture
    c. intraarticular fracture
    transverse c. fracture
commissural fiber
commissure
    anterior c.
committed cell
common
    c. acute leukemia antigen

    c. acute lymphoblastic
      leukemia antigen (CALLA)
    c. atrium
    c. atrium, aortic atresia,
      double-outlet (CAD)
    c. atrium, aortic atresia,
      double-outlet right
      ventricle
    c. bile duct
    c. bile duct diverticulum
    c. bile duct stone
    c. bile duct stricture
    c. carotid artery
    c. control design
    c. epithelial ovarian cancer
    c. femoral artery
    c. hepatic artery
    c. hepatic duct
    c. iliac artery
    c. leukocyte antigen
    c. peroneal artery
    c. variable
      agammaglobulinemia
    c. variable
      immunodeficiency
    c. variable
      immunodeficiency disease
communal
    c. needle
    c. sex
commune
    persistent ostium
      atrioventriculare c.
communicating
    c. artery
    c. artery aneurysm
    c. cavernous ectasia
    c. fistula
    c. hydrocephalus
community-acquired pneumonia
community immunity
comorbid disease
comorbidity
    illness c.
    psychiatric c.
compact
    c. bone
    c. island
companion shadow
comparison film
compartment
    extraaxial c.
    extracellular c.

extravascular c.
iliopsoas c.
intracellular c.
supramesocolic c.
vascular c.
compartmentalization
compartmental radioimmunoglobulin
  therapy
compassion fatigue
Compazine
compensation
  attenuation c.
  depth c.
  flow c.
  respiratory c.
  second-order c.
  supratentorial flow c.
  time gain c.
  time-gain c.
compensatory
  c. emphysema
  c. hypertrophy
competence
  immunologic c.
complement
  c. assay
  erythrocyte, antibody,
    and c. (EAC)
  c. factor (CF)
  c. fixation
  c. 3, 4 level
  c. lysis
  c. receptor
  c. resistance
complementary
  c. determining region
  c. DNA (cDNA)
  c. gene
complement-fixing antibody (CFA)
complement-mediated lysis
complementophil
complete
  c. carcinogen
  c. duplication
  c. fracture
  c. Freund adjuvant (CFA)
  c. heart block

c. mole
c. remission (CR)
c. response (CR)
c. transposition of great
  arteries
complex, pl. complexes
  acyclic metal chelate c.
  acylated SK-plasminogen c.
  aggregation antibody-
    antigen c.
  AIDS dementia c. (ADC)
  AIDS-related c. (ARC)
  ALD-AMN c.
  amphotericin B lipid c.
  antibody-antigen c.
  antigen-antibody c.
  anti-inhibitor coagulant c.
  avian leukemia-sarcoma c.
  avian leukosis-sarcoma c.
  avidin-biotin-peroxidase c.
  capsulolabral c.
  Carney c.
  c. chest mass
  chlorophyllin copper c.
  choroidal-hippocampal
    fissure c.
  circulating immune c. (CIC)
  Eisenmenger c.
  factor IX c.
  fibrocartilage c.
  c. fracture
  frontonasal dysplasia
    malformation c.
  gallium-transferrin c.
  Ghon c.
  Golgi c.
  growth plate c.
  histocompatibility c.
  interstitial antigen-
    antibody c.
  Kirklin meniscal c.
  labral-capsular c.
  labrum-ligament c. (LLC)
  limb-body wall c.
  macromolecular c.
  major histocompatibility c.
  mastoid c.

NOTES

complex *(continued)*
  metal chelate c.
  Michaelis c.
  Mycobacterium avium c.
    (MAC)
  nipple-areolar c.
  ostiomeatal c.
  c. periosteal reaction
  phosphorus trihydrazide c.
  preintegration c.
  Ranke c.
  renal sinus c.
  ribosome-lamella c.
  shoulder labral-capsular c.
  tetrameric antibody c.
  thrombin-antithrombin III c.
    (TAT)
  thymidylate c.
  transposition c.
  VATER c.
  VIII nerve c.
  von Meyenburg c.
compliance
  lung c.
complicated
  c. pneumoconiosis
  c. renal cyst
  c. silicosis
complication
  gonadal c.
  hematologic c.
  hepatic c.
  metabolic c.
  oral c.
  postoperative c.
  pulmonary c.
  vascular c.
component
  blood c.
  buffy coat c.
  dispersive c.
  extensive intraductal c.
  frequency c.
  leuko-poor blood c.
  secretory c.
  single-donor blood c.
composite
  c. addition technique
  c. blur
  c. fracture
  c. signal
compound
  anthraquinone c.

  c., comminuted fracture
  c. fracture
  Hurler-Scheie c.
  c. leukemia
  macromolecular nonlipid c.
  macromolecular polar c.
  nitroimidazole c.
  thorium c.
  titanium c.
compound Q
comprehensive
  C. AIDS Resources
    Emergency Act
    (CARE Act)
  c. care plan
compressed body
compression
  c. of breast
  cauda equina c.
  c. cone effect
  c. device
  external pneumatic calf c.
  extrinsic c.
  extrinsic bladder c.
  c. fracture
  image c.
  c. injury
  intrinsic c.
  c. neuropathy
  c. plate
  root c.
  c. sonography
  spinal cord c.
  spot c.
  c. ultrasonography
compressive atelectasis
Compton
  C. coherent scattering
    densitometry
  C. effect
  C. scatter
  C. scattering
computational chemistry
computed
  expiratory c. tomography
  limited-slice c. tomography
  c. radiography
  c. tomography (CT)
  c. tomography scan
computer-generated artifact
computerized axial tomography
  (CAT)
computerized patient record (CPR)

comustine
conal ventricular septal defect
concanavalin A
concatenation of shadows
concavity
concentrate
    cryptosporidium immune
      whey protein c.
    platelet c.
concentrated bile
concentration
    maximal drug c. (C_{max})
    maximum permissible c.
    serum bilirubin c.
    c. times time (C x T)
concentrator
    stem cell c.
concentric
    c. fibroma
    c. hernia
    c. hypertrophy
    c. narrowing
concentric fibroma
concept
    Bay region c.
    growth fraction c.
    line integral c.
    nonoverlapping toxicity c.
    schedule dependency c.
    self-care c.
    total dose over time c.
concha, pl. conchae
    c. bullosa
    nasal conchae
concomitant
    c. medication
    c. pneumonia
    c. therapy
concussion
    brain c.
    spinal c.
condensans
    clavicular osteitis c.
condensation
    chromatin c.
condensed phosphates
condenser discharge system

condensing osteitis
condition
    genetic c.
    inflammatory c.
    precancerous c.
    predisposing c.
    premalignant c.
    tumor-like bone c.
conditional
    c. chain terminator
    c. probability
conditioning program
condom
    c. catheter
    latex c.
    vaginal c.
conductive loop
conductivity
    tissue c.
conductor
    fiberoptic c.
    c. resistivity
conduit
    ileal c.
    intestinal c.
    urinary c.
condylar
    c. emissary vein
    c. fracture
condyle
    mandibular c.
condyloma, pl. condylomata
    c. acuminatum
    anal condylomata
condylomata
cone
    c. beam
    c. biopsy of cervix
    Centriflow membrane c.
    transvaginal c.
    c. of vignetting
coned cecum
cone-down view, coned-down view
configuration
    batwing c.
    bilobed c.
    boomerang c.

NOTES

configuration *(continued)*
    double-halo c.
    geriatric c.
    germline c.
    globular c.
    horseshoe c.
    hourglass c.
    keyhole c.
    left ventricular c.
    reverse 3 c.
    rosary bead c.
    sandwich c.
    shepherd's crook c.
    snowman heart c.
    surface c.
    T-c.
    triple-peak c.
    water bottle heart c.
    Y-c.
confinement
    regional tumor c.
confluence
    stellate c.
    c. of vascular marking
confluens sinuum
congenita
    arthrogryposis multiplex c.
    chondrodystrophia
      calcificans c.
congenital
    c. abnormality
    c. absence of pulmonary
      artery
    c. absence of pulmonary
      valve
    c. adrenal hyperplasia
    c. agammaglobulinemia
    c. amputation
    c. aneurysm of pulmonary
      artery
    c. anomaly
    c. arteriovenous fistula
    c. biliary atresia
    c. bronchogenic cyst
    c. cardiac tumor
    c. cyst
    c. cystic dilatation
    c. cystic dilatation of bile
      duct
    c. defect
    c. diaphragmatic hernia
    c. diffuse fibromatosis

    c. dilatation
    c. disease
    c. dislocation
    c. disorder
    c. duodenal obstruction
    c. dyserythropoietic anemia
    c. dyshormonogenesis
    c. dysplasia
    c. esophageal stenosis
    c. fracture
    c. generalized fibromatosis
    c. goiter
    c. heart block
    c. heart disease
    c. heart malformation
    c. hepatic cyst
    c. hepatic fibrosis
    c. hip dislocation
    c. hip dysplasia
    c. hydrocele
    c. hydrocephalus
    c. hypoplastic anemia
    c. immunity
    c. infection
    c. intestinal atresia
    c. left ventricular aneurysm
    c. lethal hypophosphatasia
    c. lobar emphysema
    c. lymphangiectasia
    c. malformation
    c. megacalices
    c. mesoblastic nephroma
    c. multiple fibromatosis
    c. muscular dystrophy
    c. nasal mass
    c. primary megaloureter
    c. renal aneurysm
    c. renal hypoplasia
    c. renal osteodystrophy
    c. stippled epiphysis
    c. syphilis
    c. tracheobiliary fistula
    c. urethral stricture
    c. vascular malformation
congenitally
    c. corrected transposition
    c. short esophagus
congestion
    c. index
    pulmonary vascular c.
    pulmonary venous c.
    venous c.

congestive
    c. cardiomyopathy
    c. heart failure
conglomerate
    c. anthracosilicosis
    c. mass
conglutinating complement
  absorption test (CCAT)
conglutination factor
conglutinogen-activating factor
conization
    cervical c.
    cold-knife c.
    LEEP c.
conjoined
    c. nerve-root anomaly
    c. twins
conjugal cancer
conjugate
    macromolecular c.
    para-iodobenzoyl c.
conjugated
    c. antigen
    c. estrogen
    c. lineoleic acid
conjunctiva
conjunctival follicular hyperplasia
connection
    atrioventricular c.
connective
    c. tissue
    c. tissue disease
    c. tissue neoplasm
    c. tissue tumor
    c. tumor
connector
    cerebral ventricular shunt c.
conniventes
    valvulae c.
Conn syndrome
conoid ligament
conotruncus
Conrad-Crosby bone marrow
  biopsy needle
Conradi-Hünermann disease
Conradi line
Conray

consensus interferon
consent
    informed c.
conservative treatment
consolidated lung
consolidating infiltrate
consolidation
    batwing lung c.
    c. chemotherapy
    fracture line of c.
    pulmonary c.
conspicuity
constant
    Boltzmann c.
    decay c.
    equilibrium dissociation c.
    equilibrium dose c.
    c. gradient
    Planck c.
    c. region
    c. segment
    time c.
    transformation c.
constitutional sclerosing bone
  disease
constrained reconstruction
constricting lesion
constrictive
    c. bronchiolitis
    c. pericarditis
constrictor
construct
    hapten-chelate c.
construction
    c. artifact
    McIndoe-Hayes c.
    stent c.
    tandem c.
consumption coagulopathy
contact
    bone-on-bone c.
    cell-cell c.
    c. dissolution therapy
    c. effect
    screen-film c.
contagiosum
    molluscum c.

NOTES

contamination
    metastatic c.
    white blood cell c.
content
    bone mineral c.
    disk water c.
    overlying bowel c.
    RNA c.
    tissue water c.
Contigen tube
contiguous
    c. organ involvement
Contin
    MS C.
continuation
    azygos c.
continuing care
continuity equation
continuous
    c. arteriovenous
      hemofiltration (CAVH)
    c. hyperfractionated
      accelerated radiotherapy
      (CHAR)
    c. hyperthermic peritoneal
      perfusion (CHPP)
    c. infusion
    c. intravenous infusion
      chemotherapy
    c. microinfusion device
    c. mode
    c. volumetric acquisition
    c. wave (CW)
continuous-wave
    c.-w. Doppler imaging
    c.-w. Doppler
      ultrasonography
    c.-w. NMR
contour
    convex-outward c.
    double-diaphragm c.
contraceptive device
contractility
    myocardial c.
contraction
    esophageal c.
    isovolumetric c.
    isovolumic c.
    kissing c.'s
    premature atrial c. (PAC)
    premature ventricular c.
      (PVC)

    c. stress test
    uterine c.
contracture
    Dupuytren c.
    flexion c.
    Volkmann c.
contralateral synchronous
  carcinoma
contrast
    c. administration
    c. agent
    c. angiography
    barium enema with air c.
    blood oxygenation level-
      dependent c.
    BOLD c.
    c. enhancement
    c. excretion
    image c.
    c. injection
    c. loading
    c. material
    c. material instillation
    c. media
    c. medium
    c. opacification
    paramagnetic c.
    phase c.
    c. ratio
    c. reaction
    c. sensitivity
    c. transfer characteristic
contrast-enhanced (CE)
    c.-e. CT
    c.-e. FAST
    c.-e. fast-acquisition steady
      state (CE-FAST)
    c.-e. MR image
contrast-improvement factor
contrast-to-noise
    c.-t.-n. calculation
    c.-t.-n. ratio (C/N ratio)
contrasuppressor cell
contrecoup
    c. fracture
    c. injury
    c. mechanism
control
    D-Di negative c.
    D-Di positive c.
    quality c.
    Spli-Prest negative c.
    Spli-Prest positive c.

controller
    IMED Gemini PC-2
    volumetric c.
contusion
    bony c.
    cerebral c.
    pulmonary c.
conus
    c. arteriosus medullaris
    c. clasticus
    c. medullaris
conventional
    c. dose chemotherapy
    c. imaging
    c. tomography
conversion
    c. defect
    c. efficiency
    hemorrhagic c.
    c. ratio
converter
    analog scan c.
    analog-to-digital c. (ADC)
    digital scan c.
    digital-to-analog c. (DAC)
    scan c.
convex array
convexity
    cerebral c.
    parietal c.
convex-outward contour
convolution
    nuclear c.
    c. process
convolutional
    c. impression
    c. marking
convulsion
Cook
    C. coaxial biliary dilator
    C. endomyocardial needle
    C. enforcer catheter dilator
    C. introducer
    C. stent
    C. urological five-wire
    helical stone extractor
Cook-Europe catheter

Cooley anemia
Coombs test
Cooper
    C. ligament
    C. regimen
    C. suspensory ligament
coordinate bond
COP
    cyclophosphamide, Oncovin,
    prednisone
COPA
    cyclophosphamide, Oncovin
    (vincristine), prednisone,
    Adriamycin
COP-BLAM
    cyclophosphamide, Oncovin
    (vincristine), prednisone,
    bleomycin, Adriamycin
    (doxorubicin), Matulane
COP-BLEO
    cyclophosphamide, Oncovin,
    prednisone, bleomycin
COPD
    chronic obstructive pulmonary
    disease
Cope
    C. biopsy needle
    C. catheter
    C. loop
    C. method
    C. retention system
    C. single-stick biliary
    drainage system
    C. suture set
    C. technique
Cope-Saddekni
    C.-S. catheter tip
    C.-S. introducer
coping style
COPP
    cyclophosphamide, Oncovin,
    procarbazine, prednisone
copper
    c. deficiency
    c. pyruvaldehyde
    thiosemicarbazone
copper-62

NOTES

coprohematology
coprolith
coproporphyria
copular point
copulation
> anal c.
> oral c.

CoQ
> coenzyme Q

cor
> c. pulmonale
> c. triatriatum

coracoacromial
> c. arch
> c. ligament

coracoclavicular
> c. bar
> c. joint
> c. ligament
> c. space

coracohumeral ligament
coracoid
> c. fracture
> c. process

coral thrombus
cord
> c.'s of Billroth
> c. blood
> cervical c.
> c. sign
> spermatic c.
> spinal c.
> split c.
> split spinal c.
> tethered c.
> tethered spinal c.
> thoracic spinal c.
> umbilical c.
> velamentous insertion of c.
> vocal c.

Cordarone
cordis
> ectopia c.

Cordis balloon expandable stent
cordocentesis
cordotomy
corduroy
> c. artifact
> c. vertebra

core
> c. biopsy
> necrotic c.

coreceptor
> CD26 c.

corepressor
Cori disease
corkscrew
> c. appearance
> c. appearance of the
> esophagus
> c. pattern
> c. ureter
> c. vessel

Cormed pump
corneae
> herpes c.

Cornelia De Lange syndrome
corner fracture
cornu, pl. cornua
corona
> c. radiata

coronal
> c. angulation
> c. cleft
> c. cleft vertebra
> c. image
> oblique c. plane
> c. plane
> c. reconstruction
> c. reconstruction view
> c. scan
> c. slit fracture
> c. suture
> c. view

coronary
> c. angiography
> c. artery
> c. artery aneurysm
> c. artery angioplasty
> c. artery bypass graft
> (CABG)
> c. artery bypass surgery
> c. artery calcification
> c. artery disease (CAD)
> c. balloon angioplasty
> c. heart disease
> c. ligament
> c. occlusion
> c. sinus
> c. thrombosis
> c. vessel anatomy

Coronavirus
coronoid
> c. fossa

c. process
c. process fracture
corpectomy
corpora
    c. amylacea
    c. cavernosa
corpulence
corpus
    c. callosum
    c. callosum agenesis
    c. hemorrhagicum
    c. luteum cyst
    c. spongiosum
    c. striatum
    c. uterus
corpuscle
    Bizzozero c.
    Eichhorst c.
    Lostorfer c.
    malpighian c.
    Norris c.
corrected transposition of great arteries
correction
    adaptive c.
    attenuation c.
    scatter c.
correlation
    clinical c.
    clinicopathologic c.
    c. time
correlational study
correlative Doppler study
corrosive gastritis
corset balloon
Cortef
cortex
    adrenal c.
    cerebral c.
    renal c.
cortical
    c. abrasion
    c. artery
    c. atrophy
    c. bone
    c. defect
    c. desmoid

c. fracture
c. hyperintensity
c. hyperostosis
c. hypointensity
c. infarction
c. necrosis
c. nephrocalcinosis
c. rest
c. rim nephrogram
c. thinning
c. vein
c. vein thrombosis
corticobulbar tract
corticomedullary
    c. differentiation (CMD)
    c. junction
corticospinal tract
corticosteroid
corticotrophic adenoma
corticotropin-releasing factor (CRF)
cortisone
    c. acetate
Cortisporin Otic
Cortrosyn
    C. stimulating test
Corynebacterium
    C. infantisepticum
    C. parvum
Coryzavirus
Cosmegen
costal
    c. cartilage
    c. margin
costocervical trunk
costochondral junction
costodiaphragmatic
    c. margin
    c. recess
costophrenic
    c. angle
    c. sulcus
costotransverse joint
costovertebral joint
cost-to-benefit
    c.-t.-b. analysis
    c.-t.-b. ratio
cothromboplastin

NOTES

cotrimoxazole
Cotton ankle fracture
cotton ball appearance
cotton-wool
    c.-w. appearance
    c.-w. skull
    c.-w. spot
cough
    brassy c.
coulombs/kg
Coulter
    C. counter
    C. volume
Coumadin
coumadinize
coumarin
coumestrol
Councill catheter
Councilman body
count
    Addis c.
    Arneth c.
    basophil c.
    CD4 cell c.
    CD8 cell c.
    differential c.
    filament-nonfilament c.
    granulocyte c.
    HIV-positive low CD4 c.
    interfollicular mitotic c.
    lymphocyte c.
    nadir c.
    neutrophil c.
    neutrophil lobe c.
    nucleated cell c.
    platelet c.
    c. rate
    reticulocyte c.
    sperm c.
    T4 c.
    WBC c.
    white blood cell c.
counter
    beta-scintillation c.
    Coulter c.
    gamma c.
    Linson electronic cell c.
    well c.
countercurrent
    c. exchanger
     immunoelectrophoresis
    c. flow-related enhancement
    c. immunoelectrophoresis

counterelectrophoresis
counterflow centrifugal elutriation
counterimmunoelectrophoresis
counterpulsation
    balloon c.
    intraaortic balloon c.
counterstimulation
counting cell
coup
coupled spin
coupling
    dipole c.
    dipole-dipole c.
    dynamic c.
    electric quadrupole c.
    hyperfine c.
    magnetic dipole-dipole c.
    scalar c.
    spin-spin c.
    static c.
Cournand arteriography needle
Cournand-Grino angiography needle
Covaderm
    C. plus dressing
    C. plus VAD
covalent bond
covered stent-graft
coverslipping
covitary TB
Cowden disease
Cowdry type A intranuclear
   inclusion body
Cowper gland
Cox
    C. life-table regression
     analysis
    C. proportional hazards
     model
    C. regression
coxa
    c. magna
    c. plana
    c. valga
    c. vara
coxarthropathy
    Postel destructive c.
coxitis fugax
Coxsackievirus
CP
    cyclophosphamide, Platinol
CPB
    cyclophosphamide, Platinol,
    BCNU

3BR

CPK
creatine phosphokinase
CPM
CCNU, procarbazine,
methotrexate
central pontine myelinolysis
cyclophosphamide
CPMG sequence
Carr-Purcell-Meiboom-Gill
sequence
CPPD
calcium pyrophosphate
dihydrate
CPPDD
calcium pyrophosphate
deposition disease
CPR
clinical partial response
computerized patient record
CP sequence
Carr-Purcell sequence
CPT-11
CPT-11 irinotecan
CPTR
cyproterone
CPU
central processing unit
CPV
cyclophosphamide, Platinol
(cisplatin), VP-16
CR
complete remission
complete response
CR103
OncoScint CR103
CR372
OncoScint CR372
13-CRA
13-cis-retinoic acid
cracked walnut appearance
cradle
Spectrum DG-P pediatric c.
Cragg
C. filter
C. wire
Craig needle
Crampton line

cranial
c. bone
c. cavity
c. fossa
c. granulomatous arteritis
c. irradiation
c. nerve
c. nerve neoplasm
c. nerve rhizotomy
c. neuropathy
c. osteopetrosis
c. suture
c. vault
craniectomy
keyhole-shaped c.
craniocaudal view
craniofacial
c. anomaly
c. dysjunction
c. synostosis
craniolacunia
craniopagus
craniopharyngioma
ectopic c.
cranioschisis
craniospinal irradiation
craniostenosis
craniosynostosis
craniotabes
craniotomy
c. defect
craniovertebral junction
cranium
c. bifidum
split c.
Crasnitin
crater
CRDS
curdlan sulfate
CRE
cumulative radiation effect
C-reactive protein
crease
simian c.
creatine
c. kinase (CK)

NOTES

131

creatine *(continued)*
    c. kinase-BB isoenzyme (CK-BB)
    c. kinase-MB isoenzyme fraction
    c. phosphokinase (CPK)
creatinine
    c. clearance
    c. level
    serum c.
    c. test
creation
    McIndoe vaginal c.
creeping
    c. fat
    c. substitution
cremaster
cremasteric artery
Cremophor
crenated erythrocyte
crenation
crenocytosis
crepitation
crescent
    c. artifact
    c. body
    c. cell anemia
    c. sign
crescentic
    c. submucosal fold
CREST
    calcinosis of skin, Raynaud phenomenon, esophageal dysmotility, sclerodactyly, telangiectasia
    CREST syndrome
crest
    anterior iliac c.
    bilateral iliac c.
    c.'s of the ilia
    iliac c.
    c. of the ilium
    intertrochanteric c.
    posterior iliac c.
    pubic c.
cresyl blue
cretinism
    goitrous c.
Creutzfeldt-Jakob disease
CRF
    corticotropin-releasing factor
CRF-187

criblé
    état c.
cribriform
    c. form
    c. pattern
    c. plate
cribriform plate
cricoarytenoid
cricohyoidepiglottopexy
cricoid cartilage
cricopharyngeal, cricopharyngeus
    c. achalasia
    c. bar
    c. diverticulum
cricothyroid
cri-du-chat syndrome
crinkle artifact
crisis
    blast c.
    carcinoid c.
    sickle cell c.
    vasoocculsive c.
crisnatol mesylate
crista supraventricularis
criteria
    Jones c.
    National Prostatic Cancer Project c.
    radiographic c.
    Schumacher c.
criterion
    Nyquist c.
Critikon oximeter
CritSpin
CRL
    crown-rump length
Crocidolite
Crohn disease
cromolyn
Cronkhite-Canada syndrome
Crookes-Hittorf tube
cross
    c. immunity
    c. reactivity
    c. section
cross-agglutination
crossed
    c. coil
    c. ectopia
    c. immunoelectrophoresis
cross-filling
cross-fused ectopy
cross-linking reagent

crossmatch
crossover
    c. design
    c. trial
cross-reactive protein (CRP)
cross-reactivity
    CA 125 c.-r.
cross-relaxation
cross-resistance
cross-section
    c.-s. capture
cross-sensitization
cross-table
    c.-t. lateral projection
    c.-t. lateral view
    c.-t. view
cross-talk
    c.-t. effect artifact
cross-term
croup
croup-associated virus
Crouzon disease
CR/OV
    colorectal/ovarian
    OncoScint CR/OV
crow-foot sign
Crow-Fukase syndrome
crown artifact
crown-rump length (CRL)
crow's teet bands
CRP
    cross-reactive protein
CRT
    cathode ray tube
cruces (*pl. of* crux)
cruciate ligament
crus, pl. crura
    c. of the diaphragm
    displaced c.
crush
    c. artifact
    c. fracture
    c. preparation
    c. syndrome
    thoracic c.
"crushed eggshell" fracture
Crutchfield tongs

Cruveilhier-von Baumgarten
    syndrome
crux, pl. cruces
cruzi
    Trypanosoma c.
cryoanalgesia
cryobath
cryocrit
cryoelectrom microscopy
cryofibrinogen
cryogen
cryoglobulin
cryoglobulinemia
cryomagnet
cryoprecipitate
cryopreservation
    autograft c.
cryopreserved tissue banking
cryoprotectant
cryoprotein
cryostat
    c. section
cryosurgery
cryotherapy
    oral c.
cryotome
crypt
    Lieberkühn c.
cryptococcal
    c. meningitis
    c. spondylitis
cryptococcoma
cryptococcosis
    intracranial c.
Cryptococcus neoformans
cryptoleukemia
cryptorchidism, cryptorchism
cryptoscope
cryptosporidiosis
    c. antibody
    c. enteritis
Cryptosporidium
    C. baileyi
    C. listeria
    C. meleagridis
    C. muris
    C. parvum

NOTES

cryptosporidium
    c. immune colostrum
    c. immune whey protein
      concentrate
crystal
    Charcot-Leyden c.
    c. deposition disorder
    c. field theory (CFT)
    leukocytic c.
    Reinke c.
    sodium iodide c.
    Teichmann c.
CrystalEYES video system
crystal-induced chemotactic factor
crystalline iron oxide
crystallography
    Laue x-ray c.
    x-ray c.
crystalloid of Reinke
^{137}**Cs**
    cesium-137
CSF
    cerebrospinal fluid
    colony-stimulating factor
      hematopoietic CSF
      human urinary CSF (HU-CSF)
csf1R1 **gene**
CSI
    chemical shift imaging
CSLEX1 monoclonal antibody
CSMA
    chemical shift misregistration
      artifact
CSP
    Cancer Surveillance Program
CT
    computed tomography
    cytarabine, 6-thioguanine
      bone quantitative CT
        (BQCT)
      contrast-enhanced CT
      dynamic CT
      CT gantry
      helical CT
      CT scan
      spiral CT
      spiral volumetric CT
      stable xenon CT
      twin-beam CT
      xenon-enhanced CT
CT-aided volumetry

CT-guided
    CT-g. biopsy
    CT-g. needle aspiration
CTX
    Cytoxan
C-type retrovirus
cubitus valgus deformity
cuboid
    c. bone
cuboidal cell
cuff
    c. arthropathy
    collagen c.
    Dacron c.
cuffing
    peribronchial c.
cuirasse
    cancer en c.
cul-de-sac
culpocephaly
culture
    blood c.
    hanging-block c.
    hanging-drop c.
    Rotalex c.
    Rubacell II c.
    c. and sensitivity
cumulative
    c. dose
    c. radiation effect (CRE)
cumulus oophorus
cuneatus
cuneiform cartilage
cuneus, pl. cunei
cuniculi
    Encephalitozoon c.
cunnilingus
cupping of the calyces
cupremia
CUPS
    carcinoma of uncertain primary
    site
curacin A
curative
    c. chemotherapy
    c. intent
    c. treatment
curcumin
curdlan sulfate (CRDS)
cured patient
curettage
    dilatation and c.

endocervical c.
suction c.
curette, curet
Curie
C. effect
C. law
Curling ulcer
currant
c. jelly clot
c. jelly stool
current
direct c. (DC)
eddy c.
Curry intravascular retriever set
curvature
c. lymph-mode
curve
area under the c. (AUC)
best-fit smooth c.
characteristic c.
dose-survival c.
elimination c.
flow volume c.
fractionated dose-survival c.
Frank-Starling c.
full-width-at-half-maximum
of lorentzian c.
gompertzian growth c.
H and D c.
Hunter and Driffield curve
H & D c.
Hunter and Driffield c. (H
and D curve)
isodose c.
Kaplan-Meier survival c.
lordotic c.
lorentzian c.
receiver operating
characteristic c.
ROC c.
stress-strain c.
survival c.
curved radiolucent line
curvilinear
c. calcification
c. threshold shoulder (Dq)

Curvularia
Cushing
C. basophilism
C. disease
C. syndrome
cushingoid appearance
cusp
valve c.'s
Custer cell
cutanea
cutaneous
c. adverse drug effect
c. angiocentric T-cell
lymphoma
c. aspergillosis
c. bacterial infection
c. B-cell lymphoma
c. candidiasis
c. dissemination
c. eruption
c. graft-versus-host disease
c. infection
c. lesion
c. lymphocyte antigen
c. lymphoid hyperplasia
c. lymphoma
c. melanoma
c. Merkel cell tumor
c. neoplasm
c. pneumocystosis
c. T-cell lymphoma
c. tumor
c. viral infection
cutaneum
carcinoma c.
cutdown
cutis
aplasia c.
benign lymphocytoma c.
leiomyoma c.
leukemia c.
cut locus
cutoff
c. frequency
c. sign
Cuvier duct

NOTES

CVA
cerebrovascular accident
CVD
collagen vascular disease
CVP
cyclophosphamide, vincristine, prednisone
CVS
chorionic villus sampling
CW
continuous wave
CW Doppler ultrasonography
CW NMR
C x T
concentration times time
CY223
cyamella
cyanemia
cyanhemoglobin
cyanmetmyoglobin
cyanoacrylate
isobutyl c. (IBCA)
cyanocobalamin
cyanosis
cyanotic
c. heart disease
cycle
cardiac c.
cell c.
division c.
duty c.
estrogen-progestin artificial c.
imaging c.
menstrual c.
nasal c.
ovarian c.
respiratory c.
c. time
cycle-nonspecific agent
cycle-specific agent
cyclic-SoSo
cyclin D protein
cycling
phase c.
cyclobutane dicarboxylation ring structure
cyclodextrin
Cyclodisone
cyclohexenediaminetetraacetic acid (CDTA)

cycloheximide
α-cyclohexitrin
cyclohydrolase
cyclooxygenase
c. enzyme
c. enzyme inhibition
c. inhibitor
cyclophilin
cyclophosphamide (CPM)
cyclophosphamide, Adriamycin (doxorubicin), etoposide (CAE)
cyclophosphamide, Adriamycin (doxorubicin), procarbazine, bleomycin, Oncovin, prednisone (CAP-BOP)
cyclophosphamide, Adriamycin, methotrexate, procarbazine (CAMP)
cyclophosphamide, Adriamycin, Platinol (CAP)
cyclophosphamide, Adriamycin, vincristine (CAV)
cyclophosphamide, etoposide, Platinol (CEP)
cyclophosphamide, etoposide, vincristine (CEV)
cyclophosphamide, Halotestin, Oncovin, prednisone (CyHOP)
cyclophosphamide, hexamethylmelamine, Adriamycin, DDP (CHAD)
cyclophosphamide, hexamethylmelamine, Adriamycin, Platinol (CHAP)
cyclophosphamide, hydroxydaunomycin (doxorubicin), Oncovin (vincristine), prednisone (CHOP)
cyclophosphamide, hydroxydaunorubicin, Oncovin, prednisone (CHOP)
cyclophosphamide, hydroxydaunorubicin, Oncovin, prednisone, bleomycin (CHOP-BLEO)
cyclophosphamide, hydroxyurea, actinomycin D (dactinomycin), methotrexate, Oncovin (vincristine), citrovorum factor, Adriamycin (CHAM-OCA)
cyclophosphamide, mechlorethamine,

Oncovin, procarbazine,
prednisone (C-MOPP)
cyclophosphamide, methotrexate,
etoposide, dexamethasone
(CMED)
cyclophosphamide, methotrexate, 5-
fluorouracil (CMF)
cyclophosphamide, methotrexate, 5-
fluorouracil, prednisone (CMFP)
cyclophosphamide, methotrexate, 5-
fluorouracil, prednisone,
tamoxifen, Halotestin
(CMFPTH)
cyclophosphamide, methotrexate, 5-
fluorouracil, vincristine,
prednisone (CMFVP)
cyclophosphamide, Oncovin,
methotrexate, leucovorin,
arabinosylcytosine (COMLA)
cyclophosphamide, Oncovin,
prednisone (COP)
cyclophosphamide, Oncovin,
prednisone, bleomycin (COP-
BLEO)
cyclophosphamide, Oncovin,
procarbazine, prednisone (COPP)
cyclophosphamide, Oncovin
(vincristine), prednisone,
bleomycin, Adriamycin
(doxorubicin), Matulane (COP-
BLAM)
cyclophosphamide, Oncovin
(vincristine), prednisone,
Adriamycin (COPA)
cyclophosphamide, Platinol (CP)
cyclophosphamide, Platinol, BCNU
(CPB)
cyclophosphamide, Platinol
(cisplatin), VP-16 (CPV)
cyclophosphamide, vincristine,
Adriamycin,
dimethyltriazenoimidazole
carboxamide (CY-VA-DIC,
CyVADIC)
cyclophosphamide, vincristine,
prednisone (CVP)

cyclopia
Cycloplatam
cyclops
cycloserine
cyclosporin A
cyclosporine
    c. therapy
    c. toxicity
CYFRA 21-1 tumor marker
CyHOP
    cyclophosphamide, Halotestin,
    Oncovin, prednisone
Cyklokapron
cylindrical bronchiectasis
cylindroma
cylindromatous carcinoma
cylindrosarcoma
cyproterone (CPTR)
    c. acetate
cyroprecipitate-depleted plasma
cyst
    adnexal c.
    adrenal c.
    allantoic duct c.
    ampulla of Vater c.
    aneurysmal bone c.
    apocrine c.
    arachnoid c.
    aryepiglottic c.
    c. aspiration
    Baker c.
    benign c.
    bilateral arachnoid c.
    bilateral choroid plexus c.
    blue dome c.
    bone c.
    brain c.
    branchial cleft c.
    breast c.
    bronchial cleft c.
    bronchogenic c.
    brown cell c.
    cervical retention c.
    chocolate c.
    choledochal c.
    choroid plexus c.

NOTES

137

cyst *(continued)*
   coelomic c.
   colloid c.
   complicated renal c.
   congenital c.
   congenital bronchogenic c.
   congenital hepatic c.
   corpus luteum c.
   cysticercus c.
   Dandy-Walker c.
   dentigerous c.
   dermoid c.
   dermoid ovarian c.
   c. drainage
   duodenal duplication c.
   duplication c.
   ecchinococcal c.
   Eggers c.
   ejaculatory duct c.
   endometriotic c.
   enteric c.
   enterogenous c.
   ependymal c.
   epidermal inclusion c.
   epidermidoma c.
   epidermoid c.
   epidermoid inclusion c.
   epididymal c.
   epidural arachnoid c.
   epithelial c.
   esophageal duplication c.
   follicular c.
   functional ovarian c.
   ganglionic c.
   Gartner duct c.
   gastric duplication c.
   gastrointestinal c.
   hemorrhagic c.
   hepatic c.
   hydatid c.
   implantation c.
   inclusion c.
   interhemispheric c.
   intracranial c.
   intracranial dermoid c.
   intraduodenal choledochal c.
   intrameniscal c.
   intraosseous keratin c.
   intrapulmonary
    bronchogenic c.
   intraspinal enteric c.
   intratesticular c.
   intrathoracic c.

Kimura-type choledochal c.
leptomeningeal c.
lipid c.
lumbar synovial c.
luteal c.
lymphoepithelial c.
mediastinal c.
mediastinal bronchogenic c.
mediastinal dorsal enteric c.
mesenteric c.
mesothelial c.
müllerian duct c.
multilocular c.
multilocular renal c.
multiple c.
multiple thyroid c.
nabothian c.
nasopharyngeal mucus
  retention c.
neurenteric c.
nuchal c.
odontogenic c.
oil c.
omental c.
omphalomesenteric c.
ovarian c.
pancreatic c.
parameniscal c.
paramesonephric duct c.
paraovarian c.
parapelvic c.
parapharyngeal space c.
paratubal serous c.
paraurethral c.
parovarian c.
pericaliceal c.
pericardial c.
perineural sacral c.
peripelvic c.
peritoneal inclusion c.
pineal c.
placental c.
placental septal c.
pleural c.
pleuropericardial c.
pontine hydatid c.
popliteal c.
porencephalic c.
postmenopausal adnexal c.
posttraumatic spinal cord c.
primordial c.
prostatic c.
pulmonary c.

pyelogenic c.
racemose c.
radicular c.
Rathke cleft c.
reactive c.
reactive spinal c.
renal c.
retention c.
retrocerebellar arachnoid c.
retroperitoneal c.
sebaceous c.
seminal vesicle c.
serous c.
simple c.
simple bone c.
simple cortical c.
solitary bone c.
splenic c.
subarachnoid c.
subchondral c.
subependymal c.
synovial c.
talar dome c.
Tarlov c.
tension c.
testicular c.
theca-lutein c.
thoracic c.
thoracic duct c.
Thornwaldt c.
thymic c.
thyroglossal duct c.
thyroid c.
Tornwaldt c.
traumatic bone c.
traumatic lipid c.
traumatic lung c.
tunica albuginea c.
umbilical cord c.
unicameral bone c.
urachal c.
utricle c.
cystadenocarcinoma
mucinous c.
mucous c.
ovarian c.

pseudomucinous c.
serous c.
cystadenofibroma
cystadenoma
biliary c.
glycogen-rich c.
c. lymphomatosum
macrocystic c.
mucinous c.
ovarian c.
ovarian proliferative c.
papillary epididymal c.
serous c.
thyroid c.
cystectomy
ovarian c.
radical c.
cysteine
c. proteinase
secreted protein, acidic and
rich in c.
cystic
acquired renal c. disease
c. adenocarcinoma
c. adenoma
c. adenomatoid
malformation
c. adrenal mass
c. angiomatosis
c. appearance
c. arachnoiditis
c. artery
c. astrocytoma
c. bronchiectasis
c. carcinoma
c. change
c. chest mass
c. dilatation
c. disease
c. disease of breast
c. duct
c. duct remnant
c. duct stone
c. dysplasia
c. fibrosis
c. fluid
c. ganglioglioma

NOTES

cystic *(continued)*
    c. glandular hyperplasia
    c. glioma
    c. hemangioblastoma
    c. hygroma
    c. hyperplasia
    c. hyperplasia
      photomicrograph
    c. intraparenchymal
      meningioma
    c. kidney disease
    c. lymphangioma
    c. mastitis
    c. medial necrosis
    c. metastasis
    c. myelomalacia
    c. myelopathy
    c. neoplasm
    c. nephroblastoma
    c. nephroma
    c. ovarian disease
    c. partially-differentiated
      nephroblastoma
    c. pelvic mass
    c. pituitary adenoma
    c. process
    c. renal disease
    c. structure
    c. teratoma
    c. tumor
    c. vein collateral
cystica
    cystitis c.
    mastitis fibrosa c.
    osteitis fibrosa c.
    pyelitis c.
    pyeloureteritis c.
    ureteritis c.
cysticercosis
    parenchymal c.
    subarachnoid c.
cysticercus cyst
cysticus
    Echinococcus c.
cystine stone
cystinosis
    nephropathic c.
cystinuria
cystitis
    bullous c.
    c. cystica
    emphysematous c.
    eosinophilic c.

    c. follicularis
    c. glandularis
    granulomatous c.
    hemorrhagic c.
    interstitial c.
    radiation c.
    tuberculous c.
cystocarcinoma
cystocele
cystofibroma
Cystografin
cystography
    chain c.
Cystokon
cystomyoma
cystoplasty
    ileocecal c.
cystoprostatectomy
cystoradiogram
cystosarcoma
    c. phyllodes
cystoscopy
cystostomy
cystourethrogram
    voiding c. (VCUG, VCU)
Cyt
    cytosine
CytaBOM (*See* ProMACE-
    CytaBOM)
Cytadren
cytapheresis
cytarabine (ara-C, ARA-C)
    c. hydrochloride
    mitoxantrone, c. (MC)
cytarabine, daunorubicin (CD)
cytarabine, 6-thioguanine (CT)
Cytidine
cytobrush biopsy
cytocentrifugation
cytocentrifuge preparation
cytochalasin
cytochemistry
cytochrome
    c. P450
    c. P450 enzyme
cytocide
cytocrit
CytoGam
cytogenetic analysis
cytogenetics
    interphase c.
cytogenic anemia
CytoGuard aerosol protector device

cytohybridization
cytokeratin
    c. membrane antigen
cytokine
    chemoattractant c.
    pleiotropic c.
    c. synthesis inhibitory factor
cytokinetic resistance
cytologic maturity
cytology
    aspiration c.
    exfoliative c.
    c. and histology
    histology and c.
    nipple aspiration c.
    peritoneal c.
cytolysin
cytolytic T-cell
cytoma
cytomatrix
cytomegalic inclusion disease
  (CID)
Cytomegalovirus **(CMV)**
cytomegalovirus
    c. immune globulin
    (CMVIG)
    c. infection
    c. interstitial pneumonitis
    c. pneumonia
    c. with microcephaly
Cytomel
cytometer
cytometry
    DNA flow c.
    flow c.
    image c.
    Krishan procedure for DNA
      analysis by flow c.
cytomorphology
cytopathicity
cytopenia
cytophagocytosis
cytophilic antibody
cytophotometry
    DNA c.
cytoplasm

cytoplasmic
    c. basophilic granule
    c. CD3 antigen
    c. μ chain
    c. filaments
    c. granularity
    c. Ig
    c. immunoglobulin
    c. inclusion
    c. organelle
    c. protein kinase
    c. vacuolization
cytoreductive
    c. surgery
    c. therapy
Cytorhodin S
Cytosar
Cytosar-U
cytosine (Cyt)
    c. arabinoside (ara-C, ARA-
      C)
    c. arabinoside-liposome
    c. arabinosine hydrochloride
    arabinosyl c.
cytoskeletal antigen
cytosol
cytosolic
cytospin
    c. smear
cytotoxic
    c. agent
    c. antibody
    c. antibody-mediated disease
    c. cell
    c. chemotherapy
    c. drug
    c. edema of the gray
      matter
    c. effect
    c. factor
    c. T-lymphocyte
cytotoxicity
    antibody-dependent cell c.
    (ADCC)
    antibody-dependent cell-
      mediated c.
    immunotoxin-mediated c.

NOTES

cytotrophoblast
Cytovene
Cytoxan (CTX)
Cytoxan, Adriamycin, 5-fluorouracil
  (CAF)
Cytoxan, BCNU, VP-16 (CBV)

CY-VA-DIC, CyVADIC
  cyclophosphamide, vincristine,
  Adriamycin,
  dimethyltriazenoimidazole
  carboxamide

2D
two-dimensional
2D phase measurement
3D
three-dimensional
D5 1/2 normal saline
DAB
3,3'-diaminobenzidine
tetrahydrochloride dihydrate
10-DAB
DAB389 antibody
DABIS maleate
DAC
deoxyazacytidine
digital-to-analog converter
dacarbazine (DTIC)
DACE
dexamethasone, ara-C,
carboplatin, etoposide
DACE chemotherapy
dacrocyte
Dacron
D. aortic bifurcation graft
D. aortobifemoral graft
D. cuff
D. tail
D. velour graft
dacryocystocele
dacryocystography
DACT
dactinomycin
dactinomycin (DACT)
dactinomycin-loaded liposome
dactinomycin, methotrexate,
cyclophosphamide (DMC)
dactylitis
dactylolysis spontanea
DADAG
1,2:5,6-
diacetyldianhydrogalactitol
dAdo
deoxyadenosine
dADP
deoxyadenosine diphosphate
daisy-head colony
Dalacin C
Dale-Laidlaw clotting time
Dale reaction
Dalkon shield
dalton

dam
dental d.
latex d.
damage
chromosomal d.
endothelial d.
genetic d.
projection fiber d.
seminiferous tubular d.
dammini
Ixodes d.
dAMP
deoxyadenosine monophosphate
Dana-Farber Cancer Institute
(DFCI)
danazol
dancer's bone
Dandy-Walker
D.-W. cyst
D.-W. malformation
D.-W. syndrome
D.-W. variant
Dane particles
Danis-Weber fracture
Danysz phenomenon
dapsone
Daraprim
darkfield
d. imaging
d. microscopy
Darrach procedure
dartos muscle
dashboard fracture
Dasher guide wire
DAT
daunorubicin, ara-C
(cytarabine), thioguanine
data
d. acquisition window
d. analysis
epidemiological d.
imaginary d.
d. management
d. matrix
d. reordering
d. sampling
d. spike detection error
artifact
d. system

data-clipping
    d.-c. artifact
    d.-c. detection error artifact
Datelliptium
dating
    second trimester
      gestational d.
    third trimester gestational d.
dATP
    deoxyadenosine triphosphate
DATTA
    Diagnostic and Therapeutic
      Technology Assessment
DATVP
    daunomycin, ara-C, thioguanine,
      vincristine, prednisone
Daudi cell
daughter
    d. cell
    d. isotope
daunomycin (DNM)
    d. hydrochloride
**daunomycin, ara-C, thioguanine,
vincristine, prednisone (DATVP)**
daunomycin, cytarabine, thioguanine
**daunomycin, cytosine, arabinoside,
VP-16**
daunorubicin (DNR)
    d. hydrochloride
    liposomal d.
**daunorubicin, ara-C (cytarabine),
thioguanine (DAT)**
daunorubicin, ara-C, VP-16 (DAV)
**daunorubicin, cytarabine,
thioguanine (DCT)**
DaunoXome
DAV
    daunorubicin, ara-C, VP-16
DAVA
    desacetyl vinblastine amide
DAVH
    dibromodulcitol, Adriamycin,
      vincristine, Halotestin
Davidsohn test
DAVTH
    dibromodulcitol, Adriamycin
      (doxorubicin), vincristine,
      tamoxifen, Halotestin
dawn phenomenon
Day factor
Dayhoff model
dB
    decibel

DC
    differentiated carcinoma
    direct current
      DC offset artifact
DCC
    dextran-coated charcoal
DCF
    2'-deoxycoformycin
DCIS
    ductal carcinoma in situ
DCT
    daunorubicin, cytarabine,
      thioguanine
DDC
    dideoxycytidine
D-Di
    Asserachrom D-D.
    D-D. buffer
    D-D. latex
    D-D. negative control
    D-D. plate
    D-D. positive control
    D-D. test
D-dimer
DDL
    dideoxyinosine
DDP
    cis-diamminedichloroplatinum
de
    D. Haas Van Alphen effect
    d. Morsier syndrome
    d. novo
    d. novo carcinoma
    d. Quervain disease
    d. Quervain fracture
    d. Quervain tenosynovitis
    d. Quervain thyroiditis
    D. Veras beverage
dead time
DEAE
    diethylaminoethyl
**DEAE-Sephadex A-25
chromatography**
deafferentation pain
deaminase
    adenosine d. (ADA)
    deoxycytidine d.
    polyethylene glycol-modified
      adenosine d. (PEG-ADA)
Dean and Webb titration
death
    apoptotic cell d.
    brain d.

cell d.
cerebral d.
fetal d.
necrotic cell d.
pathologic cell d.
physiologic cell d.
programmed cell d.
deazaguanine mesylate
DeBakey aortic dissection
debris
debrisoquine metabolic phenotype
Debrosan
Debrun
D. balloon
D. latex balloon preparation
debulking
d. surgery
d. of tumor
Decadron
decalcified bone marrow sample
decarboxylase
ornithine d.
decarboxylation
decay
branched d.
d. constant
d. equation
free induction d.
d. scheme
d. time
decay-activating factor
decibel (dB)
decidua
decidual
d. cast
d. reaction
decision
d. analysis
d. theory
d. tree
decitabine
decompensation
cardiac d.
decomplementize

decomposition
linear prediction with
singular value d.
three-level Haar wavelet d.
decompression
biliary d.
endoscopic d.
d. sickness
deconditioned exercise response
deconvolution
decoupling
heteronuclear d.
decubitus
d. film
d. radiograph
d. view
deep
d. to the nipple
d. tumor
d. vein thrombosis (DVT)
d. venous thrombosis
(DVT)
deep-seated infection
Deetjen body
defecography
defect
abdominal wall d.
atrial septal d. (ASD)
atrioventricular septal d.
beneficial atrial septal d.
calcified medullary d.
cecal filling d.
colonic filling d.
conal ventricular septal d.
congenital d.
conversion d.
cortical d.
craniotomy d.
dehalogenase d.
deiodinase d.
duodenal filling d.
Eisenmenger d.
electron transport chain d.
endocardial cushion d.
endocardial cushion type
ventricular septal d.
esophageal filling d.

NOTES

defect *(continued)*
  extrinsic d.
  extrinsic filling d.
  extrinsic ureteral d.
  fetal abdominal wall d.
  fibrous cortical d.
  fibrous medullary d.
  fibrous metaphyseal-
    diaphyseal d.
  filling d.
  fixed perfusion d.
  gastric filling d.
  gouge d.
  hatchet d.
  Hill-Sachs d.
  incisura d.
  interatrial septal d.
  interventricular septal d.
  intraluminal filling d.
  intramural filling d.
  intravascular filling d.
  intrinsic d.
  intrinsic filling d.
  inverted umbrella d.
  junctional cortical d.
  mass d.
  neural tube d. (NTD)
  organification d.
  ostium primum atrial
    septal d.
  ostium secundum atrial
    septal d.
  pars d.
  perfusion d.
  pericardial d.
  perimembranous ventricular
    septal d.
  postcricoid d.
  punched-out bony d.
  radiolucent d.
  radiolucent linear filling d.
  resolving ischemic
    neurologic d.
  reversible perfusion d.
  septal d.
  septum transversum d.
  sinus venosus atrial
    septal d.
  slash d.
  subperiosteal cortical d.
  subsegmental perfusion d.
  supracristal ventricular
    septal d.

  trapping d.
  tumor d.
  ventilation d.
  ventricular septal d.
defense
  host d.
  phagocytic d.
deferens
  vas d.
deferential artery
deferoxamine
defibrinated blood
defibrination syndrome
deficiency
  adenosine deaminase d.
  alpha antitrypsin d.
  antigen d.
  antitrypsin d.
  arylsulfatase A d.
  copper d.
  disaccharidase d.
  factor IX d.
  fatty acyl-Co-A
    synthetase d.
  fibrinolytic factor d.
  galactosylamide β-
    galactosidase d.
  G6PD d.
  growth hormone d. (GHD)
  idiopathic growth
    hormone d.
  immune d.
  iron d.
  leukocyte adhesion d.
  selenium d.
  thymic-dependent d.
  vitamin A d.
  vitamin B_{12} d.
deficit
  motor d.
  neurologic d.
  reversible ischemic
    neurologic d. (RIND)
  self-care d.
deflector
  tip d.
deformans
  arthritis syphilitica d. (ASD)
  osteitis d.
  spondylosis d.
deformity
  Arnold-Chiari d.
  bell-and-clapper d.

bird beak d.
boutonnière d.
calcaneovarus d.
cecal d.
cloverleaf d.
clubfoot d.
cubitus valgus d.
equinovalgus d.
equinovarus d.
Erlenmeyer flask d.
flexion d.
foot d.
funnel chest d.
garden spade d.
gibbous d.
gooseneck d.
hammertoe d.
Hill-Sachs d.
kleeblatschädel d.
lanceolate d.
Madelung d.
pectus carinatum d.
pectus excavatum d.
pencil-in-cup d.
phrygian cap d.
pigeon-breast d.
ping-pong ball d.
rat tail d.
rotoscoliotic d.
round back d.
saber-shin d.
saddle nose d.
shepherd's crook d.
silver fork d.
spondylitic d.
Sprengel d.
swan-neck d.
thoracic d.
varus d.
DEFT
driven equilibrium Fourier
transform
DEFT technique
degenerated fibroadenoma
degeneration
acquired hepatocerebral d.

carcinomatous subacute
cerebellar d.
carneous d.
disk d.
hepatocerebral d.
hepatolenticular d.
hypertrophic olivary d.
intrameniscal mucoid d.
microcystic d.
olivary d.
spongiform d.
wallerian d.
degenerative
d. arthritis
d. brain disease
d. cardiomyopathy
d. change
d. dementia
d. disease
d. disk
d. disk disease
d. joint disease
d. narrowing
d. nuclear pattern
deglutition
muscle of d.
degradable starch microsphere
degradation
image d.
d. of image
degranulation
histamine d.
degree of inspiration
dehalogenase defect
dehalogenation
dehiscence
Killian d.
dehydration
dehydroepiandrosterone (DHEA)
d. sulfate (DHEAS)
dehydrogenase
aldehyde d.
20-α-dihydroprogestin d.
dihydropyrimidine d.
glucose-6-phosphate d.
(G6PD)
lactic d. (LDH)

NOTES

dehydrotest sterone
deiodinase defect
Deisting
    D. prostatic dilation
      technique
    D. prostatic dilator
deivisum
    pancreatic d.
Déjérine-Sottas hypertrophic
  polyneuropathy
dek
    dek oncogene
    dek proto-oncogene
Deladiol
Delalutin
Delatest
Delatestryl
delavirdine
delay
    developmental d.
    echo d.
    readout d.
    d. time
    d. time selection
delayed
    d. engraftment
    d. hypersensitivity
    d. small bowel transit
    d. vomiting
Delcath double-balloon catheter
Delestrogen
deletion
    allelic d.
    chromosome d.
    d. of chromosomes
    DNA d.
delirium
delivered total dose (DTD)
delivery
    breech d.
    drug d.
    intracavitary d.
    oxygen d.
    preterm d.
delta
    d. antigen
    d. function
    d. protein
    d. sign
Delta-Cortef
Deltanyne
Deltasone
delta-9-tetrahydrocannabinol (THC)

Deltec-Pharmacia CADD pump
Deltec portable external infusion
  device
deltoid
    d. bursa
    d. ligament
demand
    oxygen d.
dementia
    degenerative d.
    HIV-associated d.
Demerol
4-demethoxydaunorubicin
4-demethylepipodophyllotoxin
demilune body
demineralization
Demodex folliculorum
demodicidosis
demodulation
demodulator
demyelinating disease
demyelination
    intramedullary d.
DeMyer system of cerebral
  malformation
denaturing
dendritic
    d. cell
    d. reticulum cells (DRC)
dendrocytoma
    disseminated dermal d.
dengue
    Philippine d.
    d. virus
Denis Browne classification of
  sacral fractures
Dennis tube
Denonvilliers fascia
dens
    d. aplasia
    d. fracture
    d. view of cervical spine
dense
    d. brain mass
    d. metaphyseal bands
    d. rib
densitometer
densitometry
    Compton coherent
      scattering d.
density
    areal d.
    arterial linear d.

double d.
energy flux d.
fat d.
heterogenous d.
hydrogen d. (N(H))
hydrogen spin d.
information d.
integrated optical d. (IOD)
lung d.
magnetic flux d.
optical d. (OD)
patchy area of d.
proton d.
reticulogranular
 pulmonary d.
spin d.
streaky d.
urographic d.
water d. line
dental
 d. caries
 d. dam
 d. disorder
 d. granuloma
 d. material
 d. radiography
DentaScan multiplanar reformation
dentate
 d. ligament
 d. nucleus
dentigerous cyst
dentin, dentine, dentinum
dentinogenesis imperfecta
denuded connective tissue
Denver
 D. ascites shunt
 D. Pak
 D. peritoneovenous shunt
Denys-Leclef phenomenon
deodorant artifact
deossification
deoxyadenosine (dAdo)
 d. diphosphate (dADP)
 d. monophosphate (dAMP)
 d. triphosphate (dATP)
deoxyazacytidine (DAC)
2′-deoxycoformycin (DCF)

deoxycytidine
 d. deaminase
 d. kinase
2-deoxyglucose
deoxyhemoglobin
deoxynojirimycin
deoxynucleotidyl transferase
deoxyribonuclease (DNAse)
deoxyribonucleic acid (DNA)
deoxyribonucleoside
 5-FU d.
deoxyribonucleotide
 total adenine d.
deoxyspergualin (DSG)
deoxythymidine kinase
dependence
 nicotine d.
 quadratic d.
 relaxation rate frequency d.
 solvent water TI
 frequency d.
dependency
 schedule d.
**dephase-rephase magnitude
 subtraction technique**
dephasing
 odd-echo d.
 spin d.
depletion
 lymphocyte d.
 myeloid d.
 plasma d.
 white blood cell d.
Depo-Medrol
depo-medroxyprogesterone
 d.-m. acetate (DMPA)
Depo-Provera
deposit
 amyloid d.
deposition
 antibody d.
 fibrin d.
 iron d.
 perivillous fibrin d.
 reticulin d.
 subchorionic fibrin d.
 d. of tracer

NOTES

Depot
> Lepron D.
Depotest
depressed
> d. fracture
> d. skull fracture
depression
> bone marrow d.
> d. fracture
> pacchionian d.
depth
> d. compensation
> d. pulse
> d. pulse technique
> scatterer d.
> signal d.
> skin d.
depth-dose distribution
depth-resolved surface coil spectroscopy (DRESS)
de Quervain
DER
> dual-energy radiograph
derangement
derepressed gene
Derifil
derivative
> diphenhydramine d.
> hematoporphyrin d.
> purified protein d.
dermal
> d. calcification
> d. duct tumor
> d. sinus tract
dermatitis
> allergic contact d.
> atopic d.
> bullous d.
> erythematous d.
> exfoliative d.
> d. herpetiformis
> photosensitivity d.
> seborrheic d.
dermatofibroma
dermatofibrosarcoma
> pigmented d.
> d. protuberans
dermatographism
dermatologic toxicity
dermatology
dermatomal zoster
dermatomyoma

dermatomyositis
> paraneoplastic d.
dermatopathic
> d. lymphadenitis
> d. lymphadenopathy
Dermatophagoides
> *D. farinae*
> *D. pteronyssimus*
dermatophyte
dermatophytosis
dermatosis
> acantholytic d.
> transient acantholytic d.
Dermiform hypo-allergenic knitted tape
dermis
dermoid
> d. cyst
> intracranial d. cyst
> d. ovarian cyst
> d. plug
> d. tumor
DES
> diethylstilbestrol
> DES task force
desacetyl
> vinblastine amide d.
> d. vinblastine amide (DAVA)
DESAD
> National Collaborative Diethylstilbestrol Adenosis Project
desamino-D-arginine vasopressin
descending
> d. aorta
> d. colon
> left anterior d. (LAD)
descent
> basal d.
> epididymal d.
Deschamps needle
Descot fracture
desensitization
desetope
desexualize
Desferal Mesylate challenge
desferosamine
desferrioxamine B
desferrioxancine
design
> common control d.
> crossover d.

3-D pulse d.
factorial d.
pulse d.
designer drug
Desilets-Hoffman introducer
desipramine
desmins
desmoid
cortical d.
periosteal d.
subperiosteal d.
d. tumor
desmoplasia
desmoplastic
d. fibroma
d. infantile ganglioglioma
d. melanoma
desmopressin
desmosome
despeciated serum
desquamated epithelial hyperplasia
desquamation
desquamative
d. fibrosing alveolitis
d. interstitial pneumonia
destruction
bone d.
moth-eaten bone d.
mucosal d.
destructive bone lesion
destruens
chorioadenoma d.
detachable balloon
detachment
retinal d.
detail
intraluminal d.
rib d.
detection
d. bias
early d.
indirect d.
d. pulse
quadrature d.
d. system
detective quantum efficiency

detector
d. artifact
d. coil
flame ionization d.
fluorescence d.
mass spectrophotometric d.
nitrogen-phosphorus d.
phase-sensitive d.
quadrature d.
d. response
solid-state d.
d. transfer function
ultraviolet d.
detergent effect
determinant
antigen d.
antigenic d.
d. group
immunogenic d.
isoallotypic d.
isotypic d.
sequential d.
determination
immunoglobulin clonality d.
DeToni-Debré-Fanconi syndrome
detrorubicin
detrusor
d. hyperreflexia
d. muscle
detrusor-sphincter dyssynergia
deuterium
deux
cancer à d.
devascularized
developer
d. artifact
development
clonal d.
drug d.
endocardial cushion d.
pubertal d.
developmental
d. delay
d. variation
deviation
genetic d.
standard d.

NOTES

Devic disease
device
Arnoff external fixation d.
atherectomy d.
atherolytic reperfusion
wire d.
beam-modifying d.
Camino intracranial pressure
monitoring d.
charge-coupled d.
clot-trapper d.
compression d.
continuous microinfusion d.
contraceptive d.
CytoGuard aerosol
protector d.
Deltec portable external
infusion d.
electrooptical d.
Günther aspiration
thromboembolectomy d.
halo d.
Hysterocath
hysterosalpingography d.
Ilizarov d.
implantable vascular
access d.
intrauterine contraceptive d.
(IUD)
Mediport infusion access d.
nail-plate d.
orthopedic fixation d.
Ponomar transjugular clot-
trapper d.
prosthetic d.
Rashkind ductus occluder d.
reperfusion d.
Sideris buttoned double-
disk d.
Simpson atherectomy d.
suction d.
vascular access d.
venous access d.
DeVilbiss nebulizer
dexamethasone
high-dose methotrexate,
bleomycin, Adriamycin,
cyclophosphamide,
Oncovin, d. (M-BACOD)
moderate-dose methotrexate,
bleomycin, Adriamycin,
cyclophosphamide,
Oncovin, d. (m-BACOD)

dexamethasone, ara-C, carboplatin,
etoposide (DACE)
dexniguldipine
dextra
dextran
d. sulfate
dextran-coated charcoal (DCC)
dextroamphetamine
dextrocardia
dextroconcave
dextrogastria
dextronomer
dextroposition
dextroscoliosis
dextroversion
dezocine
DF3 antigen
DFA
direct fluorescent antibody
D factor
DFA-TP
direct fluorescent antibody
staining for *Treponema*
pallidum
DFCI
Dana-Farber Cancer Institute
DFMO
difluoromethylornithine
2DFr
two-dimensional Fourier
imaging
3DFr
three-dimensional Fourier
imaging
DFT
discrete Fourier transform
2DFT
two-dimensional Fourier
transform
2DFT time-of-flight MR
angiography
3DFT
three-dimensional Fourier
transform
3DFT gradient-echo MR
imaging
DHAD
mitoxantrone
DHE
dihematoporphyrin ether
dihydroergocryptine
dihydroergotamine

DHEA
dehydroepiandrosterone
DHEAS
dehydroepiandrosterone sulfate
DHFR
dihydrofolate reductase
DHPG
ganciclovir
DI
dose intensity
diabetes
bronzed d.
gestational d.
d. inositus
d. insipidus
Lancereaux d.
lipoplethoric d.
d. mellitus
phosphate d.
diabetic
d. foot
d. gastroparesis
diabeticorum
gastroparesis d.
1,2:5,6-diacetyldianhydrogalactitol (DADAG)
diacylglycerol
diagnosis
differential d.
intrauterine sonographic d.
laparoscopic abdominal tumor diagnosis
laparoscopic abdominal tumor d.
noninvasive d.
ultrasound d.
diagnostic
d. imaging
D. and Therapeutic Technology Assessment (DATTA)
diagnostic-related group (DRG)
diagram
pulse-timing d.
Dialy-Nate catheter
dialysis
d. fistula
peritoneal d.
renal d.
d. tubing
dialyze
dialyzer
Dow hollow fiber d.
hollow fiber d.
parallel plate d.
diamagnetic substance
diamagnetism
Landau d.
diameter
anterior sagittal d. (ASD)
biparietal d. (BPD)
film d.
lumen d.
minimal port d. (MPD)
diametric pelvic fracture
diamide
d. dimercaptide
d. dithiolate
diaminetetraacetate
ethylene d.
3,3′-diaminobenzidine tetrahydrochloride dihydrate (DAB)
diaminoditholate
diamniotic pregnancy
diamond sign
diamond-tip needle
diapedesis
leukocyte d.
diaphanography
diaphragm
antral mucosal d.
aperture d.
crus of the d.
duodenal d.
eventration of the d.
d. eventration
excursion of the d.
gastric d.
leaf of the d.
Potter-Bucky d.
d. sign
traumatic rupture of the d. (TRD)

NOTES

diaphragma sellae
diaphragmatic
    d. border
    d. crural repair
    d. echo
    d. elevation
    d. esophageal hiatus
    d. eventration
    d. fascia
    d. hernia
    d. lymph node
    d. paralysis
    d. rupture
    d. slip
diaphyseal
    d. aclasis
    d. dysplasia
    d. fracture
    d. ossification
diaphysis, pl. diaphyses
diaphysitis
    luetic d.
diarrhea
diarthrosis
diastasis
    sutural d.
diastatic fracture
diastematomyelia
    spinal d.
diastolo
diastolic
    d. notch impedance
    d. pseudogating
    d. velocity ratio
diastrophic
    d. dwarfism
    d. dysplasia
diathermic
    d. snare
    d. vascular occlusion
diathesis, pl. diatheses
diatrizoate
    meglumine d.
    d. meglumine
    d. meglumine radiopaque
      medium
diatrizoic acid
Diatube-H
diazepam
diaziquone
diazohydroxide
    pyrazine d.
dibenzanthracene

dibenzyline
dibromodulcitol
dibromodulcitol, Adriamycin
    (doxorubicin), vincristine,
    tamoxifen, Halotestin (DAVTH)
dibromodulcitol, Adriamycin,
    vincristine, Halotestin (DAVH)
dibromodulcitol, doxorubicin,
    vincristine
DIC
    disseminated intravascular
      coagulation
dichorionic
    d. diamniotic twin
      pregnancy
    d. twin
dichorionic-diamniotic twin
dichotomous classification
Dick test
diclazuril
dicondylar fracture
dicoumarol
dicrotic notch
didanosine
didehydrodeoxythymidine (d4T)
didelphys
    uterus d.
didemnin B
dideoxycytidine (DDC)
dideoxyinosine (DDL)
Didiee projection
DIDOX
    dihydroxybenzohydroxamic acid
Dieffenbach serrifine forceps
Diego blood group
dielectric loss
diencephalon
die punch fracture
diet
    high-fiber d.
    low-residue d.
    Minot-Murphy d.
    Zen macrobiotic d.
dietary
    d. calcium
    d. fat
    d. intervention
    d. therapy
diethylamide
    N1-alkyl-2-iodo-lyseric
      acid d.
diethylaminoethyl (DEAE)

diethyldithiocarbamate
diethylenetriamine pentaacetic acid
  (DTPA)
diethylstilbestrol (DES)
  d. diphosphate
DiFerrante syndrome
difference
  field-echo d.
differential
  d. count
  d. density sign
  d. diagnosis
  d. linearity
  manual d.
  d. uniformity
differentiated carcinoma (DC)
differentiation
  adenocarcinoma with
    squamous d.
  d. antigen
  B-lymphocyte d.
  cluster of d. (CD)
  corticomedullary d. (CMD)
  minimal d.
  plasmacytoid d.
  T-lymphocyte d.
difficile
  Clostridium d.
Diff-Quik
  D.-Q. stain
  D.-Q. staining
diffuse
  d. abdominal calcification
  d. aggressive lymphoma
  d. air space disease
  d. alveolar hemorrhage
  d. bacterial nephritis
  d. calcification
  d. cerebral histiocytosis
  d. cirrhosis
  d. fatty infiltration
  d. fibrocystic disease
  d. fibrosis type
  d. fine reticulation
  d. goiter
  d. hepatic enlargement

  d. idiopathic skeletal
    hyperostosis (DISH)
  d. intermediate lymphocytic
    lymphoma
  d. large cell lymphoma
    (DLCL)
  d. lung disease
  d. lymphocytic lymphoma
  d. lymphoma
  d. mixed small and large
    cell lymphoma
  d. osteosclerosis
  d. panbronchiolitis
  d. pancreatitis
  d. pattern
  d. pulmonary alveolar
    hemorrhage
  d. pulmonary hemorrhage
  d. reflector
  d. sarcomatosis
  d. scleroderma
  d. sclerosing alveolitis
  d. sclerosis
  d. small cell lymphocytic
    lymphoma
  d. small cleaved cell
    lymphoma
  d. thickening
  d. thymic enlargement
  d. toxic goiter
  d. ulcerative lesion
diffusely swollen hemisphere
diffusing capacity
diffusion
  anisotropic d.
  anisotropically-rotational d.
    (ARD)
  d. coefficient
  directional d.
  exchange d.
  d. factor
  d. imaging
  molecular d.
  passive d.
  restricted d.
  d. spectroscopy
  spin d.

NOTES

diffusion *(continued)*
  d. time (T_d)
  translational d.
diffusion-sensitive sequence
diffusion-weighted scanning
diffusum
  papilloma d.
Diflucan
diflunisal
difluorodeoxycytidine
difluoromethylornithine (DFMO)
DiGeorge syndrome
digestion
  exonucleolytic d.
digestive system
digiscope
  Direx d.
digit *(var. of* digitus)
  binary d.
digital
  d. arteriography
  d. artery
  d. beam attenuation
  d. celiac trunk angiography
  d. examination
  d. free hepatic venography
  d. gray scale
  d. markings
  d. neuroma
  d. radiography
  d. rectal examination (DRE)
  d. road mapping
  d. sampling rate
  d. scan converter
  d. subtraction
  d. subtraction angiography
    (DSA)
  d. subtraction arteriography
    (DSA)
  d. vascular imaging
  d. video gastrointestinal
    radiography
digitalis
  fetus d.
  herpes d.
digital-to-analog converter (DAC)
digiti (*pl. of* digitus)
digitization
digitizer
digitorum
  extensor d.
digitus, digit, pl. **digiti**
  digiti minimi

diGugliemo disease
dihematoporphyrin ether (DHE)
dihydrate
  calcium pyrophosphate d.
    (CPPD)
  3,3'-diaminobenzidine
    tetrahydrochloride d.
    (DAB)
dihydro-5-azacytidine
dihydroergocryptine (DHE)
dihydroergotamine (DHE)
  d. mesylate plus sodium
    heparin
dihydrofolate reductase (DHFR)
20-α-dihydroprogestin
  dehydrogenase
dihydropyrimidine
  d. dehydrogenase
dihydrotestosterone
dihydroxybenzohydroxamic
  d. acid (DIDOX)
diisopropyliminodiacetic acid
  (DISIDA)
dilatans
  pneumosinus d.
dilatation
  aneurysmal d.
  bile duct d.
  cardiac d.
  d. catheter
  congenital d.
  congenital cystic d.
  d. and curettage
  cystic d.
  ductal d.
  ex vacuo d.
  fusiform d.
  gaseous d.
  junctional d.
  pancreatic duct d.
  poststenotic d.
  prestenotic d.
  pupillary d.
  transurethral balloon d.
  Virchow-Robin space d.
dilated
  d. bile duct
  d. cardiomyopathy
  d. cervix
  d. collateral vein
  d. intercavernous sinus
dilation, dilatation
  balloon d.

tract d.
ventricular d.
dilator
Amplatz long tapered
Teflon d.
Amplatz renal d.
Amplatz tapered-tip
coaxial d.
angiographic Teflon d.
balloon d.
biliary coaxial d.
coaxial d.
Cook coaxial biliary d.
Cook enforcer catheter d.
Deisting prostatic d.
esophageal balloon d.
fascial d.
Grüntzig d.
Grüntzig-type nephrostomy
tract d.
Jackson d.
Mercier urethral d.
metal d.
nephrostomy d.
Olbert d.
over-the-guidewire d.
d. pupillae
renal d.
Savary-Gilliard d.
semirigid d.
tapered-tip d.
Teflon d.
vessel d.
Dilaudid
Dilaudid-HP
dilutional hyponatremia
dim cell
dimeglumine
gadopentetate d. (Gd-DTPA)
dimenhydrinate
dimer
thymine d.
dimercaptide
diamide d.
dimercaptosuccinic acid (DMSA)
dimerization
growth factor d.

Dimertest EIA
dimethyl
d. iminodiacetic acid
d. sulfoxide (DMSO)
dimethylbusulfan
**dimethyltriazenoimidazole
carboxamide (DTIC)**
dimethylxanthine
dimorphic anemia
dimple
pretibial d.
d. sign
dinitrochlorobenzene
dinitrofluorobenzene
dinucleotide
nicotinamide adenine d.
diode module
diodine
diodone
Diodrast
Dionosil Oily
dioxide
sulfur d.
thorium d.
DIP
distal interphalangeal joint
diphallus
diphenhydramine
d. derivative
d. hydrochloride
diphenoxylate
diphenylhydantoin
diphosphate
adenosine d.
deoxyadenosine d. (dADP)
diethylstilbestrol d.
5'-diphosphate
adenosine 5'-d. (ADP)
diphosphonate
methylene d.
diphtheria antigen
Diplococcus pneumoniae
diploic cell
diploid
diploidy
diplomyelia
diplopia

NOTES

dipole
    d. coupling
    electric d.
    d. field
    magnetic d.
dipole-dipole
    d.-d. coupling
    d.-d. interaction
    d.-d. relaxation rate
diprenorphine
diprotrizoate
dipyridamole
    d. technetium-99m-2-
      methoxy isobutyl
    d. technetium-99m-2-
      methoxy isobutyl isonitrile
    d. thallium-201
dipyridamole/thallium stress test
direct
    d. current (DC)
    d. fluorescent antibody
      (DFA)
    d. fluorescent antibody
      staining for *Treponema*
      pallidum (DFA-TP)
    d. Fourier transformation
      imaging
    d. immunofluorescence
      analysis
    d. needle puncture
direction
    caudal d.
    cephalad d.
    phase-encoding d.
    Z d.
directional
    d. accordion catheter
    d. atherectomy
    d. diffusion
directive
    advance d.
directly observed therapy (DOT)
Direx
    D. digiscope
    D. Thermex
    D. Tripter
Dirkum disease
dirty
    d. chest
    d. fat
    d. necrosis
disaccharidase deficiency
disappearance frequency

disappearing fetus
disarticulation
    hip d.
disc (*var. of* disk)
discharge
    nipple d.
    d. planning
    vaginal d.
disciformis
    granulomatosis d.
discission needle
discitis
discogenic disease
discoid atelectasis
discontinuous
    d. density gradient
    d. density gradient
      centrifugation
discordance
    atrioventricular d.
discordant
    d. thyroid nodule
    d. twin
discounting
Discrene breast form
discrete
    d. Fourier transform (DFT)
    d. lesion
disease
    acyanotic heart d.
    Addison d.
    adrenal medullary d.
    adrenocortical d.
    adult polycystic kidney d.
    ainhum d.
    air space d.
    Albers-Schönberg d.
    Alexander d.
    allergic d.
    allogeneic d.
    alloimmune d.
    alpha heavy-chain d.
    alveolar d.
    Alzheimer d.
    amyloid oral cavity d.
    Anderson d.
    angiomatous d.
    anterior horn cell d.
    aortic valvular d.
    aortoiliac d.
    apatite deposition d.
    arterial d.
    arteriosclerotic occlusive d.

arteriosclerotic renal d.
asbestos-related pleural d.
atheroembolic renal d.
atherosclerotic d.
autosomal dominant
  polycystic kidney d.
autosomal recessive
  polycystic kidney d.
Ayerza d.
Banti d.
Bazex d.
Behçet d.
Beiswenger d.
benign breast d. (BBD)
biliary tract d.
Binswanger d.
bird breeder's d.
Blount d.
Bourneville d.
Bowen d.
boy-in-a-bubble d.
brain d.
breast d.
brittle bone d.
Buerger d.
Buerger-Grutz d.
bulky d.
bullous d.
bullous lung d.
Caffey d.
Caffey-Silverman d.
caisson d.
calcium pyrophosphate
  deposition d. (CPPDD)
Calvé d.
Calvé-Kümmel-Verneuil d.
Calvé-Legg-Perthes d.
Camurati-Engelmann d.
Canavan d.
carcinoid heart d.
cardiopulmonary d.
cardiovascular d.
Caroli d.
carotid artery d.
Carrington d.
Carrion d.
Castleman d.

cat scratch d.
celiac d.
cerebrovascular d.
Chagas d.
Chandler d.
childhood granulomatous d.
childhood polycystic d.
Christmas d.
chronic granulomatous d.
chronic obstructive
  pulmonary d. (COPD)
Coats d.
collagen-vascular d.
collagen vascular d. (CVD)
common variable
  immunodeficiency d.
comorbid d.
congenital d.
congenital heart d.
connective tissue d.
Conradi-Hünermann d.
constitutional sclerosing
  bone d.
Cori d.
coronary artery d. (CAD)
coronary heart d.
Cowden d.
Creutzfeldt-Jakob d.
Crohn d.
Crouzon d.
Cushing d.
cutaneous graft-versus-
  host d.
cyanotic heart d.
cystic d.
cystic kidney d.
cystic ovarian d.
cystic renal d.
cytomegalic inclusion d.
  (CID)
cytotoxic antibody-
  mediated d.
degenerative d.
degenerative brain d.
degenerative disk d.
degenerative joint d.
demyelinating d.

NOTES

159

disease *(continued)*
    de Quervain d.
    Devic d.
    diffuse air space d.
    diffuse fibrocystic d.
    diffuse lung d.
    diGugliemo d.
    Dirkum d.
    discogenic d.
    disk d.
    diverticular d.
    duodenal peptic ulcer d.
    duodenal ulcer d.
    dysmyelinating d.
    dysplasia cystic d.
    embolic d.
    end-stage renal d.
    Engelmann d.
    Engelmann-Camurati d.
    Erdheim-Chester d.
    Evans stage IV-S d.
    extensive-stage d.
    extracranial carotid
     artery d.
    extramammary Paget d.
    Fabry d.
    Fairbank d.
    Fallot d.
    Farber d.
    Fenwick d.
    fibrocystic d.
    field d.
    fifth d.
    Filatori d.
    focal intestinal
     inflammatory d.
    focal lung d.
    Fong d.
    Forestier d.
    Freiberg d.
    Friedrich d.
    Gaisbock d.
    gamma heavy-chain d.
    Gaucher d.
    gay-related
     immunodeficiency d.
     (GRID)
    Gee-Thaysen d.
    gestational nonmetastatic
     trophoblastic d.
    gestational trophoblastic d.
    glycogen storage d.
    Gorham d.

    graft-versus-host d. (GVHD)
    granulomatous d.
    Graves d.
    Günther d.
    Hajdu-Cheney d.
    Hallervorden-Spatz d.
    Hand-Schüller-Christian d.
    Hansen d.
    Hartnup d.
    Hashimoto d.
    heart d.
    heavy-chain d.
    hemoglobin S-C d.
    hemoglobin S-O-Arab d.
    hemoglobin S-thalassemia d.
    hepatic vein d.
    hepatic venoocclusive d.
     (HVOD)
    hepatocellular d.
    hepatocerebral d.
    Hers d.
    Hippel-Lindau d.
    Hirschsprung d.
    Hodgkin d. (HD)
    Hoffa d.
    homologous d.
    Hong Kong d.
    Huntington d.
    hyaline membrane d.
    hyaline-vascular
     Castleman d.
    hydatid d.
    hydroxyapatite deposition d.
     (HADD)
    hypertensive
     cardiovascular d.
    iatrogenic d.
    I cell d.
    immune complex d.
    immunoproliferative small
     intestinal d.
    infantile polycystic d.
    infantile Refsum d.
    infantile type polycystic
     kidney d.
    inflammatory d.
    inflammatory bowel d.
    interstitial lung d.
    intradural inflammatory d.
    intrahepatic pigment
     stone d.
    intramedullary d.
    intramedullary bony d.

intrarenal arterial d.
iron storage d.
ischemic d.
ischemic bowel d.
ischemic heart d.
Jagziekte d.
Jakob-Creutzfeldt d.
Jeune d.
juvenile autosomal recessive
  polycystic d.
Kashin-Bek d.
Kawasaki d.
Kellgren d.
Kienböck d.
Kikuchi d.
Kimura d.
Köhler d.
Krabbe d.
Kugelberg-Welander d.
Kümmel d.
labyrinthine d.
Langer-Saldino d.
Larsen-Johannson d.
Legg-Calvé-Perthes d.
Legionnaire's d.
Leiner d.
Letterer-Siwe d.
lichenoid graft-versus-host d.
Lichtenstein-Jaffe d.
limited-stage d.
lipid storage d.
Lobstein d.
locoregional d.
Lyme d.
lymphocyte-depletion
  Hodgkin d.
lymphocyte-predominant
  Hodgkin d.
lymphocytic and histiocytic
  nodular Hodgkin d.
lysosomal storage d.
macronodular lung d.
Maffucci d.
Majewski d.
mammary proliferative d.
maple bark d.
marble bone d.

March d.
Marchiafava-Bignami d.
Marchiafava-Micheli d.
Marek herpesvirus d.
Marie-Strumpell d.
mast cell d.
medullary cystic d.
Ménétrier d.
Ménière d.
metabolic d.
metabolic bone d.
Meyer-Betz d.
micronodular lung d.
microvascular d.
Mikulicz d.
minimal residual d. (MRD)
mixed cellularity
  Hodgkin d.
mixed connective tissue d.
  (MCTD)
Mondor d.
Mounier-Kuhn d.
moyamoya d.
Mucha-Habermann d.
mu heavy-chain d.
multicentric Castleman d.
multiple gland d.
Murri d.
myeloid d.
myocardial deposition d.
Naumoff d.
neonatal lung d.
neonatal wet lung d.
Newcastle d.
Niemann-Pick d.
nodal d.
nodular sclerosing
  Hodgkin d.
nodular thyroid d.
no evidence of disease-
  stationary d. (NED-SD)
nonatherosclerotic d.
nonneoplastic d.
Norrie d.
obstructive d.
obstructive lung d.
obstructive pulmonary d.

NOTES

161

disease *(continued)*
 occlusive cerebrovascular d.
 occlusive vascular d.
 Ollier d.
 olycystic ovarian d.
 Ormond d.
 Osgood-Schlatter d.
 Paget d.
 pancreatic d.
 Panner d.
 Parenti-Fraccaro d.
 Parkinson d.
 Pelizaeus-Merzbacher d.
 Pellegrini-Stieda d.
 pelvic inflammatory d.
  (PID)
 peptic ulcer d.
 pericardial d.
 periodontal d.
 peripheral arterial d.
 peripheral vascular d.
 perirectal d.
 periureteral d.
 Peyronie d.
 Pfeiffer d.
 Pick d.
 pigment stone d.
 pleural d.
 Plummer d.
 polycystic kidney d.
 polycystic ovarian d.
  (PCOD)
 polycystic renal d.
 Pompe d.
 Pott d.
 precancerous d.
 prediverticular d.
 progressive d.
 pseudo-Hodgkin d.
 pulmonary embolic d.
 pulmonary interstitial d.
 pulmonary
  thromboembolic d.
 pulmonary venoocclusive d.
 Pyle d.
 Refsum d.
 renal d.
 renal artery d.
 renal cystic d.
 Rendu-Osler-Weber d.
 renovascular d.
 residual d.
 restrictive lung d.

rheumatic d.
rheumatic heart d.
ribbing d.
Rosai-Dorfman d.
Royal Free d.
runt d.
Rye classification of
 Hodgkin d.
Sandhoff d.
Scheuermann d.
Schilder d.
Schimmelbusch d.
Schönlein d.
sclerodermoid graft-versus-
 host d.
secretory d.
Sever d.
severe combined
 immunodeficiency d.
 (SCID)
sexually-transmitted d.
 (STD)
Shaver d.
sickle cell d.
sickle-Thal d.
silo-filler's d.
Simmond d.
Sinding-Larsen-Johansson d.
sixth d.
slim d.
stable d. (SD)
Stickler d.
Still d.
Sturge-Weber d.
Taussig-Bing d.
T-gamma proliferative d.
thromboembolic d.
thyroid d.
Touraine-Solente-Gole d.
transhepatic biliary d.
transient
 myeloproliferative d.
Trevor d.
trophoblastic d.
ulcer d.
uremic medullary cystic d.
valvular heart d.
Vaquez-Osler d.
vascular d.
venoocclusive d. (VOD)
von Gierke d.
von Hippel-Lindau d.
 (VHL)

von Recklinghausen d.
von Willebrand d.
Weber-Christian d.
Werdnig-Hoffmann d.
Werlhof d.
wet lung d.
Whipple d.
white matter d.
Wilson d.
Winckel d.
Wolman d.
disease-free survival
disease-modifying antirheumatic drug (DMARD)
disequilibrium
linkage d.
Disetronic infuser syringe pump
DISH
diffuse idiopathic skeletal hyperostosis
dish
Lux culture d.
panning d.
DISI
dorsal intercalated segment instability
disialoganglioside Gd2
DISIDA
diisopropyliminodiacetic acid
disintegration rate
disk, disc
bulging d.
cervical d.
d. degeneration
degenerative d.
d. disease
d. extrusion
fibrocartilaginous d.
herniated d.
d. herniation
intervertebral d.
lumbar d.
d. margin
Molnar d.
occult residual herniated d.
d. protrusion
sequestered d.

d. sequestration
d. space
d. space infection
d. space narrowing
thoracic d.
d. water content
diskectomy
lumbar d.
diskitis
septic d.
diskography
dislocation
atlantooccipital d.
bilateral intrafacetal d.
congenital d.
congenital hip d.
dysplasia d.
d. fracture
lunate d.
midcarpal d.
milkmaid's elbow d.
perilunar d.
perilunate d.
radiocarpal d.
rotational d.
scapholunate d.
shoulder d.
transscaphoid perilunate d.
unilateral intrafacetal d.
wrist d.
dismutase
superoxide d.
disodium
etidronate d.
pamidronate d.
disofenin
technetium-99m d.
disorder
acid-base d.
allergic lung d.
angiitis-granulomatosis d.
angiocentric immunoproliferative d.
articular d.
atypical lymphoproliferative d.
autoimmune d.

NOTES

disorder *(continued)*
    benign proliferative d.
    blistering d.
    bullous d.
    cartilaginous growth plate d.
    congenital d.
    crystal deposition d.
    dental d.
    drug-induced bullous d.
    electrolyte d.
    facial d.
    granulomatous d.
    granulomatous slack skin d.
    hematologic d.
    hematopoietic d.
    hereditary d.
    infiltrative d.
    lymphoproliferative d.
    malignant
      lymphoproliferative d.
    mandibular d.
    metabolic bone d.
    motility d.
    myelinoclastic d.
    myeloproliferative d.
    myotonic d.
    neurocutaneous d.
    nodular d.
    nutritional d.
    patellofemoral d.
    personality d.
    PIE d.
    posttransplantation
      lymphoproliferative d.
    proliferative d.
    pulmonary d.
    pulmonary lymphoid d.
    sexual differentiation d.
    skin d.
    systemic
      lymphoproliferative d.
    T-cell d.
    T-gamma
      lymphoproliferative d.
    tongue d.
    vascular d.
dispersing agent
dispersion
    amphotericin B colloidal d.
      (ABCD)
    gradient-induced phase d.
    intravoxel phase d.
    d. mode

dispersive component
displaced
    d. crus
    d. crus sign
    d. fracture
    d. gallbladder
displacement
    d. ghost
    inferior d.
    palmar d.
    retroperitoneal fat stripe d.
    superolateral d.
display
    bull's-eye polar map d.
    image d.
    d. matrix
    multiplanar d. (MPD)
disruption
    traumatic aortic d.
dissecans
    osteochondritis d.
dissecting
    d. aneurysm
    d. basilar artery aneurysm
    d. hematoma
    d. intramural hematoma
dissection
    aortic d.
    arterial d.
    arterial wall d.
    axillary d.
    DeBakey aortic d.
    elective lymph node d.
      (ELND)
    groin d.
    medial d.
    pelvic lymph node d.
      (PLND)
    postradical neck d.
    radical axillary d.
    radical neck d.
    retroperitoneal lymph
      node d.
    Stanford-type aortic d.
disseminata
    leiomyomatosis
      peritonealis d.
    osteopathia condensans d.
disseminated
    d. candidiasis
    d. CNS histoplasmosis
    d. dermal dendrocytoma

d. intravascular coagulation (DIC)
d. lipogranulomatosis
d. necrotizing leukoencephalopathy
dissemination
cutaneous d.
hematogenous d.
d. pattern
peritoneal d.
dissociation
scapholunate d.
dissolution
distal
d. common bile duct obstruction
d. femoral epiphyseal fracture
d. femur
d. humoral fracture
d. interphalangeal joint (DIP)
d. predominantly sensory polyneuropathy
d. radial fracture
d. shift
d. splenorenal shunt
distance
interuncal d.
distant
d. metastasis
d. spread
distention, distension
abdominal d.
bowel d.
gaseous d.
hydraulic d.
venous d.
distraction of fracture
distress syndrome
distribution
Boltzmann d.
depth-dose d.
loop d.
spectral d.

disturbance
architectural d.
gait d.
disulfide
d. bridge
glutathione d.
disuse
d. atrophy
d. syndrome
dithiocarbamate
dithiolate
diamide d.
diuretic
divergent
d. ray projection
d. spiculated pattern
diversion
urinary d.
diversity
gene d.
d. segment
diverticula (*pl. of* diverticulum)
esophageal d.
diverticular
d. abscess
d. disease
diverticulation abnormality
diverticulitis
acute d.
bladder d.
colonic d.
diverticulosis
colonic d.
intramural d.
jejunal d.
tracheal d.
diverticulum, pl. diverticula
bladder d.
caliceal d.
common bile duct d.
cricopharyngeal d.
ductus d.
duodenal d.
epinephric d.
epiphrenic d.
esophageal d.
gallbladder d.

NOTES

diverticulum *(continued)*
    gastric d.
    giant sigmoid d.
    Hutch d.
    interaorticobronchial d.
    interbronchial d.
    intraluminal d.
    intraluminal duodenal d.
    inverted d.
    jejunoileal d.
    Kommerell d.
    Meckel d.
    penile urethra d.
    pulsion d.
    pyelocaliceal d.
    sigmoid d.
    small bowel d.
    thoracic pulsion d.
    thoracic root sleeve d.
    traction d.
    urethral d.
    urinary d.
    urinary bladder d.
    Zenker d.
diverting colostomy
division
    cell d.
    d. cycle
    maxillary d.
    ophthalmic d.
divisum
    pancreas d.
Dixon
    D. fat suppression method
    D. method
    D. technique
dizygotic twin
Djian Annonier angle
DLCL
    diffuse large cell lymphoma
D,L-leucovorin
DLT
    dose-limiting toxicity
DMARD
    disease-modifying antirheumatic
      drug
DMC
    dactinomycin, methotrexate,
      cyclophosphamide
DMFO
    eflornithine

DMPA
    depo-medroxyprogesterone
      acetate
DMSA
    dimercaptosuccinic acid
DMSO
    dimethyl sulfoxide
DNA
    deoxyribonucleic acid
    DNA aneuploidy
    DNA chain terminator
    complementary DNA
      (cDNA)
    DNA content analysis
    DNA cytophotometry
    DNA deletion
    double-stranded DNA
      (dsDNA)
    DNA fingerprinting
    DNA flow cytometry
    DNA footprinting
    genomic DNA
    germline DNA
    DNA hybridization study
    DNA index
    DNA intercalator
    DNA library
    DNA microinjection
      technique
    minisatellite DNA
    nuclear DNA
    DNA ploidy
    DNA polymerase
    recombinant DNA
    DNA replication
    DNA sequencing
    telemeric DNA
    DNA topoisomerase type II
      enzyme
    DNA transfection
    DNA transfection assay
    DNA virus transforming
      gene
DNA-ploidy
DNAse
    deoxyribonuclease
    DNAse footprinting
DNM
    daunomycin
DNP
    dynamic nuclear polarization
DNR
    daunorubicin

Dobbhoff feeding tube
dobutamine
doctor-patient relationship
documentary arteriogram
dog-ear sign
dogleg fracture
Dohle body
dolasetron
dolichocephaly
dolichoectasia
Dolobid
domain
    frequency d.
    HLH d.
    magnetic d.
    time d.
Dombrock blood group
dome fracture
dominant
    d. artery
    autosomal d.
    d. gene
    d. lethal mutation
    d. mass
Donath-Landsteiner antibody
donor
    allogenic d.
    alternative d.
    autologous d.
    bone marrow d.
    d. graft
    histocompatible d.
    HLA-identical d.
    HLA-nonidentical d.
    matched related d.
    matched unrelated d.
      (MUD)
    mismatched related d.
    d. site
    twin d.
    d. twin
    unrelated d. (URD)
    unrelated bone marrow d.
donor-cleavage reaction
Donovan body
donut
    sonolucent d.

dopamine
    d. blockade
    d. D1 receptor
    d. D2 receptor
    d. receptor
dopaminergic receptor
doping
    blood d.
Doppler
    D. angle
    D. assessment
    color-flow D. (CFD)
    duplex D.
    D. effect
    D. enhancement
    D. equation
    D. flow index
    D. flowmetry
    D. frequency
    D. image
    D. interrogation
    periorbital D.
    D. phenomenon
    D. physics
    pulsed D.
    D. shift frequency
    D. signal
    D. sonography
    transcranial D.
    transcranial real-time color-
      flow D. sonography
    D. ultrasonography
    D. waveform
d'orange
    peau d.
Dormia stone basket
Dornier
    D. HM3 lithotripter
    D. HM4 lithotripter
Dorothy Reed cell
dorsal
    d. artery
    d. aspect
    d. column stimulation
    d. induction
    d. induction error

NOTES

dorsal *(continued)*
    d. intercalated segment
      instability (DISI)
    d. interossei
    d. penile vein
    d. rim
    d. route entry zone lesion
    d. scapular
    d. spine
    d. tubercle
dorsalis
    d. pedis
    d. pedis pulse
    tabes d.
dorsum sella
dose
    absorbed d.
    average radiation d.
    bone marrow d.
    d. calibrator
    cancericidal d.
    ceiling d.
    central axis depth d.
    cumulative d.
    delivered total d. (DTD)
    d. equivalent
    equivalent d.
    d. escalation
    exposure d.
    d. fractionation
    gonad d.
    gonadal d.
    integral d.
    d. intensification
    d. intensity (DI)
    d. intensity analysis
    isoeffect d.
    lethal d. (LD)
    loading d.
    maximal permissible d.
    maximum permissible d.
    maximum tolerated d.
      (MTD)
    medical internal
      radiation d.
    minimum effective d.
      (MED)
    nominal standard d. (NSD)
    optimum biologic d. (OBD)
    d. per fraction
    protocol-specified d.
    radiation d.
    radiation absorbed d. (rad)

    d. rate effect
    d. response
    tandem double d.
dose-limiting
    d.-l. factor
    d.-l. myelosuppression
    d.-l. toxicity (DLT)
dose-response relationship
dose-survival curve
dosimeter
    Gardray d.
    thermoluminescent d.
dosimetristradiation beam monitor
dosimetry
    medical internal
      radiation d. (MIRD)
    phantom d.
Dos Santos needle
DOT
    directly observed therapy
dot
    d. blot analysis
    Maurer d.
    Schuffner d.
DOTA
    tetraazacyclododecanetetraacetic
      acid
DOTP
    tetraazacyclododecanetetraacetic
      tetramethylene phosphonate
Dotter
    D. cannula
    D. coaxial Teflon catheter
    D. intravascular retrieval set
    D. stiffener
double
    d. aortic arch
    d. autograft
    d. blind study
    d. cell
    d. decidual sac
    d. density
    d. emission
    d. exposure drift artifact
    d. fracture
    d. gallbladder
    d. high-dose chemotherapy
    d. inversion recovery
      sequence
    d. lumen
    d. Malecot prostatic stent
    d. minute
    d. transplant

double-arc
    d.-a. shadow
    d.-a. shadow sign
double-ball sign
double-barbed Gianturco stent
double-barrel
    d.-b. aorta
    d.-b. esophagus
    d.-b. shotgun sign
double-bleb sign
double-bubble sign
double-bulb appearance
double-channel endoscope
double-contrast
    d.-c. barium study
    d.-c. enema
    d.-c. examination
    d.-c. radiograph
double-curved triangular catheter
double-decidual sign
double-diaphragm contour
double-duct sign
double-exposed rib
double-exposure drift artifact
double-freeze technique
double-halo configuration
double-helix prostatic stent
double-inlet
    d.-i. single ventricle
    d. i. ventricle anomaly
double-J
    internal d.-J catheter
    d.-J polyethylene catheter
    d.-J silicone rubber urinary
      catheter
    d.-J stent
    d.-J ureteral stent
double-line sign
double-lumen catheter
double-outlet
    common atrium, aortic
      atresia, d.-o. (CAD)
    d.-o. right ventricle
double-pigtail stent
double-positive cell
double-stick technique
double-stranded DNA (dsDNA)

double-target sign
double-tracking of colon
double-track sign
doubling time
doughnut sign
Douglas
    pouch of D.
dounce glass homogenizer
Dow
    D. hollow fiber analyzer
    D. hollow fiber dialyzer
dowager's hump
down
    malignant d.
Downey cell
downhill varices
downsloping activity
Down syndrome
doxazosin
doxepin
Doxil
doxorubicin, dacarbazine (AD)
doxorubicin hydrochloride
doxorubicin-induced cardiotoxicity
doxycycline
DPA
    dual-photon absorptiometry
DPS Plus
DPTA CSF flow study
Dq
    curvilinear threshold shoulder
Drabkin solution
dracunculiasis, dracunculosis
drain
    Jackson-Pratt d.
    Penrose d.
    radiopaque d.
    retroperitoneal d.
    rubber d.
    sump d.
drainage
    abscess d.
    biliary d.
    catheter d.
    d. catheter
    central venous d.
    circle loop biliary d.

NOTES

drainage *(continued)*
    cyst d.
    gravity d.
    guided d.
    internal biliary d.
    lymphatic d.
    lymph node d.
    nephrostomy d.
    pancreatic pseudocyst d.
    percussion and postural d.
     (PPD)
    percutaneous d.
    percutaneous biliary d.
    percutaneous catheter d.
    percutaneous transhepatic d.
    percutaneous transhepatic
     biliary d. (PTBD)
    perinephric abscess d.
    spontaneous d.
    suction d.
    transhepatic d.
    venous d.
Dramamine
draping sign
DRC
    dendritic reticulum cells
DRE
    digital rectal examination
drepanocytemia
drepanocytic anemia
Dresbach
    D. anemia
    D. syndrome
DRESS
    depth-resolved surface coil
    spectroscopy
dressing
    Allevyn hydrophilic
     polyurethane d.
    Bard absorption d.
    Bioclusive d.
    Biopatch d.
    Comfeel hydroolloid d.
    Comfeel Ulcus occlusive d.
    Covaderm plus d.
    DuoDerm hydrocolloid d.
    Geliperm gel d.
    Hydragran absorption d.
    hydrocolloid d.
    Lipisorb d.
    Nu-Derm foam island d.
    Nu Gauze d.
    Op-Site d.

    Restore hydrocolloid d.
    Tegaderm d.
    thin-film d. (TFD)
    Uniflex d.
    vascular access d. (VAD)
    Vigilon gel d.
Dressler syndrome
DRG
    diagnostic-related group
Driffield
    Hunter and D. (H and D)
drift
    antigenic d.
    field d.
drink
    effervescent d.
drip
    Reno-M d.
Dripps classification
driven
    d. equilibrium Fourier
     transform (DEFT)
    d. equilibrium Fourier
     transform technique
Drolban
droloxifene
    d. citrate
dromedary hump
dromostanolone propionate
dronabinol
droop
    lid d.
drooped shoulder
drooping lily sign
drop metastasis
dropout
    myofibrillar d.
drowning
    dry d.
    fresh water d.
    near d.
    sea water d.
    secondary d.
drug
    d. absorption
    d. action
    adjuvant analgesic d.
    d. administration
    anticancer d.
    anticholinergic d.
    antihelminthic d.
    antineoplastic d.
    antiretroviral d.

antitumor d.
chemotherapeutic d.
cholinergic d.
cytotoxic d.
d. delivery
designer d.
d. development
disease-modifying
  antirheumatic d.
  (DMARD)
d. formulation
d. fraction
d. handling
illicit d.
immunosuppressive d.
intravenous cytotoxic d.
investigational d.
investigational new d.
  (IND)
marrow toxic d.
myelotoxic d.
nonsaturable d.
nonsteroidal anti-
  inflammatory d. (NSAID)
parent d.
psychomimetic d.
recreational d.
d. resistance
d. resistance protein
d. resistant tumor
d. tolerance
d. toxicity
drug-induced
  d.-i. alopecia
  d.-i. bone marrow
    suppression
  d.-i. bullous disorder
  d.-i. drug resistance
  d.-i. immune hemolytic
    anemia
drug-sensitive cancer
Drummond
  artery of D.
  marginal artery of D.
drumstick
  d. appearance
  d. phalanges

drusen
  optic d.
dry
  d. drowning
  d. ice
DS
  Bactrim DS
  Septra DS
DSA
  digital subtraction angiography
  digital subtraction arteriography
dsDNA
  double-stranded DNA
DSG
  deoxyspergualin
D-S-S-laxative
d4T
  didehydrodeoxythymidine
DTD
  delivered total dose
DTIC
  dacarbazine
  dimethyltriazenoimidazole
    carboxamide
DTIC-Dome
DTPA
  diethylenetriamine pentaacetic
    acid
  indium-111 DTPA
  ytterbium-169 DTPA
D-transposition
dual-energy
  d.-e. linear accelerator
  d.-e. radiograph (DER)
  d.-e. radiography
  d.-e. subtraction
  d.-e. x-ray absorptiometry
    (DXA)
dual-isotope SPECT
dual-photon absorptiometry (DPA)
dual-stiffness Malecot catheter
dual transverse linear-array
  sonogram
Dubin-Johnson phenomenon
Duchenne muscular dystrophy
duck
  d. embryo vaccine

NOTES

duck *(continued)*
    d. virus hepatitis yolk
      antibody
ducreyi
    Haemophilus d.
duct
    aberrant intrahepatic bile d.
    alveolar d.
    anicteric bile d.
    asymmetric bile d.
    Bartholin d.
    beaded d.
    bile d.
    biliary d.
    d. cell adenocarcinoma
    common bile d.
    common hepatic d.
    congenital cystic dilatation
      of bile d.
    dilated bile d.
    endolymphatic d.
    extrahepatic bile d.
    focally dilated d.
    hepatic d.
    intrahepatic d.
    intrahepatic bile d.
    lactiferous d.
    main pancreatic d. (MPD)
    main papillary d. (MPD)
    mammary d.
    mesonephric d.
    müllerian d.
    nasofrontal d.
    omphalomesenteric d.
    pancreatic d.
    parotid d.
    percutaneous dilatation of
      biliary d.
    Rivinus d.'s
    solitary dilated d.
    Stensen d.
    submandibular d.
    vitelline d.
    Wharton d.
    wolffian d.
ductal
    d. adenoma
    d. carcinoma
    d. carcinoma in situ (DCIS)
    d. dilatation
    d. ectasia
    d. hyperplasia
    d. microcalcification

    d. papillary carcinoma
    d. papilloma
ductectatic
    d. mucinous cystic
      neoplasm
    d. mucinous tumor
ductography
ductule
ductus, pl. **ductus**
    d. aneriosus
    d. arch
    d. arteriosus
    d. diverticulum
    d. infundibulum
    d. venosus
Duffy
    D. antibody
    D. antigen
    D. blood group
Duhamel operation
Duke bleeding time
Dukes classification
Dulong and Petit law
dumbbell
    d. mass
    d. tumor
dumbbell-shaped spinal cavernous
  hemangioma
Dumdum fever
dumping syndrome
Duncan syndrome
Dunnet test
duodenal
    d. artery
    d. atresia
    d. bulb
    d. diaphragm
    d. diverticulum
    d. duplication cyst
    d. filling defect
    d. hernia
    d. loop
    d. narrowing
    d. obstruction
    d. papilla
    d. peptic ulcer disease
    d. stricture
    d. sweep
    d. ulcer
    d. ulcer disease
    d. varices
duodenal-gastric outlet obstruction
duodenitis

duodenogastroesophageal reflux
duodenography
duodenojejunitis
duodenum
DuoDerm
    D. hydrocolloid dressing
Duografin
DuP 785
DuP 937
duplex
    d. Doppler
    d. echocardiography
    d. scanner
    d. sonography
    d. ultrasonography
duplicated inferior vena cava
duplication
    d. anomaly
    complete d.
    d. cyst
    esophageal d.
    gallbladder d.
    partial d.
    renal d.
Dupuytren
    D. contracture
    D. fracture
dura
    lamina d.
    d. mater
Duragen
Duragesic
Duragesic C
dural
    d. arteriovenous fistula
    d. sinus
    d. sinus occlusion
    d. sinus thrombosis
    d. sinus thrombosis
      infarction
    d. tail
    d. venous sinus
Duralutin
Duran-Reynals factor
Duratest
Durathate
Duret hemorrhage

Duroliopaque
durum
    papilloma d.
Dutcher body
duty
    d. cycle
    d. factor
Duverney
    D. foramen
    D. fracture
DVT
    deep vein thrombosis
    deep venous thrombosis
dwarfism
    achondroplastic d.
    acromelic d.
    Amsterdam d.
    diastrophic d.
    late-onset d.
    lethal d.
    mesomelic d.
    metatrophic d.
    micromelic d.
    nonlethal d.
    pituitary d.
    rhizomelic d.
    thanatophoric d.
dwell time
DXA
    dual-energy x-ray absorptiometry
dye
    d. column
    Evans blue d.
    d. exclusion assay
    d. laser system
    lipophilic d.
    d. reduction spot test
Dyke-Davidoff-Masson syndrome
Dynabead
Dynal M450 magnetic beads
dynalyzer equipment
dynamic
    blood flow d.'s
    d. bolus tracking technique
    d. computed tomography
    d. coupling
    d. CT

NOTES

dynamic *(continued)*
    d. enhancement
    flow d.'s
    d. image
    d. magnetic resonance
      imaging
    d. nuclear polarization
      (DNP)
    d. range
dynein protein
dysarthria syndrome
dysautonomia
dysbaric osteonecrosis
dyschondroplasia
dyschondrosteosis
dyschromia
dyscrasia
    plasma cell d.
dyscrasic fracture
dysdiadochokinesia
dyselectrolytemia
dysembroma
dysentery
    amebic d.
    bacillary d.
dysequilibrium
dyserythropoiesis
dyserythropoietic anemia
dysesthesia
dysfibrinogenemia
dysfunction
    bladder d.
    erectile d.
    gonadal d.
    hepatocellular d.
    male sexual d.
    neurogenic bladder d.
    neuromuscular d.
    organic erectile d.
    oropharyngeal d.
    postoperative bladder d.
    renal d.
    salivary gland d.
    testis d.
dysgenesis
    epiphyseal d.
    gonadal d.
    mixed gonadal d.
    ovarian d.
    renal d.
    renal tubular d.
    tubular d.

dysgenetic
    d. kidney
    d. syndrome
dysgerminoma
    ovarian d.
    ovarian pediatric d.
    pineal d.
dyshematopoiesis
dyshormonogenesis
    congenital d.
dysjunction
    craniofacial d.
dyskeratosis
dyskeratotic keratinocyte
dyskinesis
dysmaturity
    pulmonary d.
dysmenorrhea
dysmorphism
    lobar d.
dysmotile cilia syndrome
dysmotility
    esophageal d.
dysmyelinating disease
dysmyelination
dysmyelopoietic syndrome
dysostosis
    cleidocranial d.
    epiphyseal d.
    mandibulofacial d.
    metaphyseal d.
    mutational d.
dyspareunia
dysphagia
dysplasia
    acetabular residual d.
    acromelic d.
    asphyxiating thoracic d.
    bone d.
    bronchopulmonary d.
    camptomelic d.
    cardiomelic d.
    cervical d.
    chondroectodermal d.
    cleidocranial d.
    congenital d.
    congenital hip d.
    cystic d.
    d. cystic disease
    diaphyseal d.
    diastrophic d.
    d. dislocation
    ectodermal d.

ectrodactyly-ectodermal d.
epiphyseal d.
d. epiphysealis hemimelica
d. epiphysealis multiplex
fetal musculoskeletal d.
fetal skeletal d.
fibromuscular d.
fibrous d.
frontonasal d.
hip d.
lethal bone d.
lethal musculoskeletal d.
mammary d.
mesodermal d.
mesomelic d.
metaphyseal d.
metatrophic d.
Meyer d.
micromelic d.
monostotic fibrous d.
multicystic d.
multiple epiphyseal d.
  (MED)
neuroectodermal d.
nonlethal d.
osseous d.
osteofibrous d.
periapical cemental d.
periosteal d.
polyostotic fibrous d.
Potter d.
progressive diaphyseal d.
renal d.
rhizomelic d.
septooptic d.
short limb d.

skeletal d.
spondyloepiphyseal d.
testis d.
thanatophoric d.
thoracic d.
dysplastic nevus
dyspnea
dyspneic
dysprosium
dysproteinemia
  angioimmunoblastic
    lymphadenopathy with d.
    (AILD)
dysraphism
  spinal d.
dysregulation
dysrhythmia
  fetal cardiac d.
dyssynergia
  detrusor-sphincter d.
dystonia
dystonic reaction
dystrophic calcification
dystrophy
  congenital muscular d.
  Duchenne muscular d.
  Fukuyama-type congenital
    muscular d.
  limb-girdle muscular d.
  muscular d.
  neuraxonal d.
  reflex sympathetic d.
  Sudeck d.
  sympathetic d.
  X-linked Duchenne
    muscular d.

NOTES

175

E
  erythrocyte
    E antigen
    E rosette
    E rosette assay
    E rosette negative
    E rosette receptor
E.
    E. coli ASN-ase
    E. coli L-asparaginase
E_1
    prostaglandin E_1
E_2
  estradiol
E2A
    E2A oncogene
    E2A proto-oncogene
E2A/PBX1 **fusion gene**
EA
    erythrocyte and antibody
      EA rosette
EAC
    erythrocyte, antibody, and
      complement
      EAC rosette assay
EACA
    epsilon-aminocaproic acid
E:A change
Eagle-Barrett syndrome
EAP
    etoposide, Adriamycin, Platinol
ear
    cauliflower e.
    e. implant
    inner e.
Earle
    E. L fibrosarcoma
    E. salts
early
    e. amnion rupture sequence
    e. antigen
    e. detection
    e. echo
    e. osteoarthritis
    e. stromal invasion
Eaton agent
Eaton-Lambert syndrome
EBER protein
    Epstein-Barr early region protein
Ebola-Marburg virus

Ebola virus
Ebstein
    E. anomaly
    E. malformation of
      tricuspid valve
eburnation
EBV
    epirubicin, bleomycin,
      vinblastine
    Epstein-Barr virus
EC
    endometrial carcinoma
ecalculia
ECBO virus
eccentric narrowing
ecchinococcal cyst
ecchymosis, pl. ecchymoses
    lap-belt e.
ecchymotic
eccrine
    e. carcinoma
    e. hidradenitis
ECG
    electrocardiogram
Echinacea angustifolia
echinocandin
    c. analog
echinococcosis
    alveolar e.
Echinococcus
    E. alveolaris
    E. cysticus
    E. granulosus
    E. multilocularis
echinomycin
echo
    asymmetric e.
    candidiasis e.
    e. delay
    diaphragmatic e.
    early e.
    fast field e.'s
    fast spin e.
    field e.
    generation e.
    gradient e.
    Hahn spin e.
    hepatic pattern e.
    high-amplitude e.
    highly reflective e.

echo *(continued)*
    e. imaging
    multiplanar gradient-recalled e.
    offset RF spin e.
    e. planar
    radiofrequency spin e.
    renal e.
    e. rephasing
    sludge-like intraluminal e.
    spin e.
    spin-e.
    spin-echo using repeated gradient e.'s
    stimulated e.
    supraventricular venous e.
    symmetric e.
    e. texture
    e. time
    e. train
    T1-weighted spin e.
echocardiography
    aortic valve e.
    B-mode e.
    duplex e.
    fetal e.
    M-mode e.
    supine bicycle stress e.
    transesophageal e.
echodense pattern
echoendoscope
    Olympus GF-UM2, GF-UM3 e.
echo-free area
echogenic
    e. nodule
    e. plug
echogenicity
echolalia
echolucent
    e. pattern
EchoMark
echopenic liver metastasis
echo-planar imaging (EPI)
ECHO virus
Echovist
eclampsia
eclamptic
ECMO
    extracorporeal membrane oxygenation

extracorporeal membrane oxygenator
    ECMO virus
econazole
ECT
    emission computed tomography
ectasia
    annuloaortic e.
    benign duct e.
    bilateral ductal e.
    communicating cavernous e.
    ductal e.
    renal tubular e.
    vascular e.
ectatic
    e. bronchus
    e. carotid artery
ecthyma gangrenosum
ectocervix
ectocyst
ectodermal dysplasia
ectomesenchyme
ectopia
    cerebellar e.
    e. cordis
    crossed e.
    gallbladder e.
    posterior pituitary gland e.
    renal e.
    testicular e.
    e. testis
ectopic
    e. ACTH syndrome
    e. adenoma
    e. anus
    e. craniopharyngioma
    e. kidney
    e. nevus
    e. ossification
    e. pancreas
    e. parathormone production
    e. parathyroid
    e. parathyroid adenoma
    e. pinealoma
    e. pregnancy
    e. spleen
    e. tissue
    e. ureterocele
ectopy
    cross-fused e.
ectrodactyly-ectodermal dysplasia
EDAM

10-EDAM
  10-ethyl-10-diazaaminopterin
edatrexate
eddy
  e. current
  e. current artifact
  e. ringing artifact
Edelmann anemia
edema
  alveolar pulmonary e.
  brain e.
  brainstem e.
  breast e.
  cerebral e.
  fetal scalp e.
  frank pulmonary e.
  gut e.
  interstitial e.
  interstitial pulmonary e.
  noncardiogenic pulmonary e.
  ovarian e.
  periorbital e.
  placenta e.
  pulmonary e.
  stasis e.
  subcutaneous e.
  testicular posttraumatic e.
  umbilical cord e.
  unilateral pulmonary e.
  vasogenic e.
edematous pancreatitis
edentulous
edge
  e. artifact
  e. enhancement
  e. ringing
  shelving e.
  e. spread function
Edinger-Westphal nucleus
Edmondson-Steiner classification
EDTA
  ethylenediaminetetraacetic acid
Edwards hypothetical double aortic arch system
EEG
  electroencephalography
eel wire

EES
  endometrial stromal sarcoma
effaced collecting system
effacement
  architectural e.
effect
  Auger e.
  autocrine e.
  bag-of-bones e.
  bag-of-worms e.
  beam-hardening e.
  biologic e.
  Bohr e.
  bystander e.
  cardiotoxic e.
  cardiovascular adverse e.
  cell e.
  cell-cycle e.
  central neurologic adverse e.
  chemical shift cancellation e.
  Cherenkov e.
  compression cone e.
  Compton e.
  contact e.
  cumulative radiation e. (CRE)
  Curie e.
  cutaneous adverse drug e.
  cytotoxic e.
  De Haas-Van Alphen e.
  detergent e.
  Doppler e.
  dose rate e.
  engraftment e.
  Fahraeus-Lindqvist e.
  flow-void e.
  gastrointestinal adverse e.
  genitourinary adverse e.
  graft-versus-immunocompetent cell e.
  graft-versus-leukemia e. (GVL)
  graft-versus-lymphoma e.
  graft-versus-tumor e.
  granulocyte priming e.
  heel e.

NOTES

179

effect *(continued)*
  hematologic adverse e.
  immune-mediated
    antileukemia e.
  isotope e.
  ladder e.
  log e.
  lymphangiography e.
  Mach band e.
  macromolecular hydration e.
  magic angle e.
  magnetohydrodynamic e.
  mass e.
  missile e.
  multilog e.
  neurologic adverse e.
  nozzle e.
  nuclear Overhauser e.
  Overhauser e.
  pad e.
  partial volume e.
  peripheral neurologic
    adverse e.
  piezoelectric e.
  priming e.
  pulmonary adverse e.
  radiation e.
  reverse dose e.
  scalar e.
  sink e.
  skin e.
  snowplow e.
  star e.
  susceptibility e.
  systematic relaxation e.
  teratogenic e.
  thermal e.
  time-of-flight e.
  topical e.
  tumoricidal e.
  Venturi e.
effective
  e. half-life
  e. renal plasma flow
  e. transverse relation time
effectiveness
  relative biologic e. (RBE)
effector cell
effector/target cell interaction
effeminate
efferent loop

effervescent
  e. citrocarbonate granules
  e. drink
efficacy
  e. study
efficiency
  conversion e.
  detective quantum e.
  quantum detection e.
  window e.
efficient relaxation time
effluvium
  anagen e.
  telogen e.
effort
  inspiratory e.
  shallow inspiratory e.
effusion
  chocolate joint e.
  epidural e.
  exudative pleural e.
  knee joint e.
  loculated e.
  malignant e.
  parapneumonic e.
  pericardial e.
  pleural e.
  serous e.
  subdeltoid bursal e.
  subdural e.
  subpulmonic e.
  transient pleural e.
  transudative pleural e.
  tuberculous e.
  unilateral pleural e.
effusion-associated mononuclear cell
eflornithine (DMFO)
EFP
  etoposide, 5-fluorouracil,
    Platinol
Efudex
EG
  esophagogastric
    EG junction
EGFR
  epidermal growth factor receptor
egg
  e. lecithin
  e. lecithin lipid
Eggers cyst
egg-on-its-side
  heart

EggsAct
eggshell calcification
EGI
    endogenous GAD inhibitor
egophony
EGS
    extragonadal seminoma
EH
    endometrial hyperplasia
EHL
    electrohydraulic lithotripsy
Ehlers-Danlos syndrome
Ehrlich
    E. hemoglobinemia body
    E. side chain theory
    E. theory of antibody
      formation
Ehrlichia canis
ehrlichosis
EIA
    enzyme immunoassay
    Dimertest EIA
Eichelter sleeve
Eichhorst corpuscle
eicosapentaenoic acid
eighth nerve tumor
EIN
    endometrial intraepithelial
    neoplasia
Einstein equation
einsteinium-255 (^{255}Es)
Eisenmenger
    E. complex
    E. defect
    E. reaction
    E. syndrome
ejaculatory duct cyst
ejection fraction
EKG
    electrocardiogram
    EKG trigger
Eklund
    E. technique
    E. view
elafin gene
El-Ahwany classification of
    humeral supracondylar fractures

Elase ointment
elastica Van Gieson
elastic recoil
elasticum
    pseudoxanthoma e.
elastofibroma
elbow
    e. coronal scan
    e. fracture
    e. joint
    Little Leaguer's e.
    nursemaid's e.
    tennis e.
Eldisine
elective lymph node dissection
    (ELND)
electric
    e. dipole
    e. energy capacitance
    e. induction
    e. interaction
    e. quadrupole coupling
    e. stimulation
    e. syringe
electrically activated implant
electrocardiogram (ECG, EKG)
electrocardiography
electrocautery
    endoluminal
    radiofrequency e.
electrocoagulation
electroconvulsive therapy
electrode
    monitoring e.
electrodesiccation
electroejaculation
electroencephalography (EEG)
electrohydraulic
    e. fragmentation
    e. lithotripsy (EHL)
electrolyte
    e. disorder
    e. imbalance
electromagnet
electromagnetic
    e. absorption
    e. field

NOTES

electromagnetic *(continued)*
   e. radiation
   e. radiation exposure
   e. spectrum
   e. wave
electromotive force
electromyogram
electron
   e. arc technique
   Auger e.
   e. beam
   e. beam boost field
   e. capture
   K e.
   L e.
   e. microscopy
   e. paramagnetic resonance
   e. spin
   e. spin resonance (ESR)
   e. therapy
   transition e.
   e. transport chain defect
   e. volt (eV)
electroneuromyography
electronic magnification
electrooptical device
electropherogram
electrophoresis
   agar gel e.
   capillary e.
   field inversion gel e.
   moving boundary e.
   Paragon immunofixation e.
   protein e.
   pulsed-field gel e.
electrospray ionization mass spectroscopy
electrostatic
   e. imaging
   e. imaging system
electrostimulation for nonunion of fracture
element
   fibroglandular e.'s
   glandular e.'s
   myeloid blood e.
   nonhematopoietic e.
   promoter e.
   stromal e.'s
elementary
   e. body
   e. fracture
elephantiasis neuromatosa

elevation
   diaphragmatic e.
   periosteal e.
   prolactin e.
   unilateral diaphragmatic e.
elfin facies
ELIEDA
   enzyme-linked immunoelectrodiffusion assay
elimination
   e. curve
   e. half-life ($t_{1/2}$elim)
Elipten
ELISA
   enzyme-linked immunoabsorbent assay
   Asserachrom D-Di ELISA
Elliot B solution
elliptical
ellipticine
elliptocytotic anemia
Ellis technique for Barton fracture
Ellis-van Creveld syndrome
ELND
   elective lymph node dissection
Elobromol
elongation factor
Elsamicin
elsamitrucin
Elspar
El Tor vibrio
eluate factor
elutriation
   counterflow centrifugal e.
EMA-CO
   etoposide, methotrexate-leucovorin, actinomycin D, cyclophosphamide, Oncovin
Embden-Meyerhof pathway
embedding
   paraffin block e.
   plastic block e.
embolectomy
   pulmonary e.
emboli (*pl. of* embolus)
embolic
   e. disease
   e. infarction
   e. phenomenon
   e. reflux
   e. stroke
embolism
   amniotic fluid e.

catheter e.
cerebral e.
fat e.
paradoxical cerebral e.
pulmonary e.
septic pulmonary e.
therapeutic e.
tumor e.
venous thrombosis e.
embolization
bronchial artery e.
coil e.
foreign body e.
hepatic artery e.
internal mammary artery e.
Ivalon e.
metallic fragment e.
particulate e.
renal e.
splenic e.
therapeutic e.
thoracic vascular e.
transarterial platinum coil e.
transcatheter e.
transcatheter splenic e.
embolize
embolotherapy
balloon e.
ethanol e.
Gelfoam e.
Gelfoam/Sotradecol e.
vascular e.
embolus, pl. emboli
cholesterol emboli
foreign body e.
Gianturco spring e.
intravascular metallic
fragment e.
e. migration
pulmonary emboli
saddle e.
embryo
adnexal e.
e. transfer
embryogenesis
embryology
breast e.

genital tract e.
reproductive tract e.
urogenital e.
embryonal
e. adenoma
e. carcinoma
e. carcinosarcoma
e. hematopoiesis
e. leukemia
e. rhabdomyosarcoma
e. sarcoma
e. teratoma
e. tumor
e. tumor of ciliary body
embryonic
e. cell
e. period
e. tumor
embryopathy
HIV e.
Emcyt
emedullate
emergency
metabolic e.
oncologic e.
surgical e.
urologic e.
**Emerson-Segal Medimizer demand
nebulizer**
emesis
emetogenic
EMG
examphalos, macroglossia,
gigantism
EMG syndrome
eminence
intercondylar e.
malar e.
parietal e.
EMI scan
emissary sphenoidal foramen
emission
beta e.
characteristic e.
e. computed tomography
(ECT)
double e.

NOTES

emission *(continued)*
    filament e.
    gamma e.
    photoelectric e.
    e. range
    spectral e.
    thermonic e.
EMIT
    enzyme-multiplied immunoassay
    technique
emitter
    beta e.
    gamma e.
EMLA
    eutectic mixture of local
    anesthetics
Emmet operation
emotional
    e. state
    e. support services
emperipolesis
emphysema
    bullous e.
    centrilobular e.
    compensatory e.
    congenital lobar e.
    gastric e.
    increased markings of e.
    interstitial e.
    intramural gastric e.
    lobar e.
    mediastinal e.
    nonbacterial gastric e.
    obstructive e.
    orbital e.
    panacinar e.
    panlobular e.
    pulmonary e.
    pulmonary interstitial e.
    (PIE)
    restrictive pulmonary e.
    subcutaneous e.
    unilateral lobar e.
emphysematous
    e. bleb
    e. bulla
    e. cholecystitis
    e. cystitis
    e. gastritis
    e. pyelonephritis
empiric therapy
empty
    e. delta sign

    e. gestational sac
    e. sella syndrome
    e. triangle sign
emptying
    gastric e.
    oropharyngeal e.
empyema
    epidural e.
    Hawkins accordion-type e.
    Müller e.
    subdural e.
emulsion
    ethiodized oil e.
    lipid e.
    oil e.
en
    e. bloc
    e. bloc excision
    e. bloc resection
    e. face
enalaprilat
enalaynil
ENANB hepatitis
enanthate
    testosterone e.
enarthrosis
encapsidation
encapsulated
    e. fluid
    e. gas bubble
encapsulation
encephalic angioma
encephalitis
    brainstem e.
    herpes e.
    herpes simplex e.
    listeria e.
Encephalitozoon cuniculi
encephalocele
    frontoethmoidal e.
encephalography
    air e.
encephaloid cancer
encephalomalacia
    macrocystic e.
    microcystic e.
encephalomyelitis
    acute disseminated e.
    paraneoplastic e.
    postinfectious e.
encephalomyelopathy
encephalomyopathy
    mitochondrial e.

encephalopathia subcorticalis
  progressiva
encephalopathy
    anoxic e.
    Binswanger e.
    HIV e.
    hypertensive e.
    ischemic e.
    subcortical e.
    subcortical arteriosclerotic e.
    subcortical atherosclerotic e.
encephalotrigeminal
    e. angiomatosis
    e. syndrome
enchondroma
enchondromatosis
    multiple e.
enchondrosarcoma
encoding
    centrally-ordered phase e.
    frequency e.
    gradient e.
    one-dimensional phase e.
    ordered phase e.
    phase e.
    position e.
    reordering of phase e.
    respiratory ordered phase e.
    respiratory sorted phase e.
    spatial e.
    e. velocity
    wavelet e.
encroachment
encrustation
    bile e.
endarterectomy
    carotid e.
    surgical e.
endarteritis obliterans
end-diastolic velocity measurement
endemic Burkitt lymphoma
endemicum
    granuloma e.
end-exhalation
end-expiration
end-inhalation
Endobile

endobronchial
    e. cancer
    e. tuberculosis
endocardial
    e. cushion defect
    e. cushion development
    e. cushion type ventricular
      septal defect
    e. fibroelastosis
endocarditis
    bacterial e.
    Libman-Sacks e.
    Löffler fibroplastic e.
    marantic e.
    nonbacterial e.
    paraneoplastic e.
    thrombotic e.
endocardium
endocatheter ruler
endocervical
    e. canal coloscopy
    e. curettage
    e. mucosa
endochondral ossification
endochondroma
endocrine
    e. abnormality
    e. cell micronest
    e. exophthalmos
    e. factor
    e. fracture
    e. imaging
    e. neoplasia
    e. system
    e. therapy
    e. toxicity
    e. tumor
endocyst
endodermal
    e. sinus
    e. sinus tumor
endodermal sinus tumor
endofluoroscopic technique
endofluoroscopy
    flexible e.
    percutaneous e.
    rigid e.

NOTES

endogenous
- e. antigen
- e. bacteria
- e. biotin activity
- e. flora
- e. GAD inhibitor (EGI)
- e. hormones
- e. lipid pneumonia
- e. peroxidase activity

endoglycosidase
Endografin
endoluminal
- e. radiofrequency electrocautery
- e. sonography

endolymphatic
- e. duct
- e. stromal myosis

endometrial
- e. adenoacanthoma
- e. adenosquamous carcinoma
- e. biopsy
- e. cancer
- e. carcinoma (EC)
- e. cavity
- e. chemical shift imaging
- e. hyperplasia (EH)
- e. intraepithelial neoplasia (EIN)
- e. island
- e. jet washing
- e. polyp
- e. sarcoma
- e. secretory adenocarcinoma
- e. stromal sarcoma (EES)
- e. thickness

endometrioid
- e. carcinoma
- e. tumor

endometrioma
endometriosis
- bladder e.

endometriotic cyst
endometritis
- inflammatory e.

endometrium
- inactive e.
- postmenopausal e.
- thickened irregular e.

endomyelography
endomyocardial
- e. biopsy

- e. fibroplasia
- e. fibrosis

endoneural
endoneurium
endonuclease
Endopap endometrial sampler
endopeptidase
- neutral e.

endophthalmitis
- granulomatous e.
- sclerosing e.
- *Toxocara canis* e.

endoprosthesis
- biliary e.
- Wallstent biliary e.

endopyelotomy
endorectal
- e. coil
- e. ultrasonography

end organ resistance
endorphins
endoruler
endosalpingosis
endoscope
- double-channel e.

endoscopic
- e. decompression
- e. laser
- e. procedure
- e. retrograde cannulation
- e. retrograde cholangiopancreatography (ERCP)
- e. sinus surgery
- e. sonography
- e. ultrasonography

endoscopy
- colorectal cancer e.
- gastrointestinal e.
- lung imaging fluorescent e. (LIFE)
- percutaneous e.
- upper gastrointestinal e.

endosome
endosonography
- anal e.
- rectal e.
- transduodenal e.
- transgastric e.
- vaginal e.

endosteal chondrosarcoma
endosteum

endothelial
    e. barrier
    e. cell
    e. damage
    e. factor
    e. injury
    e. localization of antigen
    e. myeloma
endothelialization
endothelin-1
endothelium
    capillary e.
endothelium-derived relaxing factor
endothorax
    tension e.
endotoxin
endotracheal (ET)
    e. intubation
    e. tube
endourological therapy
endovaginal
    e. sonography
    e. ultrasonography
endovascular technique
Endoxan
endplate, end-plate
    e. sclerosis
endpoint, end-point
    biological e.
    stress e.
    e. of stress
end-stage
    e.-s. cell
    e.-s. renal disease
end-to-end anastomosis
end-to-side
    e.-t.-s. anastomosis
    e.-t.-s. portacaval shunt
end-viewing transducer
enelapnil
enema
    air contrast barium e.
    (ACBE)
    barium e.
    double-contrast e.
    E-Z-EM balloon e.
    Gastrografin e.

    Hypaque e.
    Rowasa e.
    small bowel e.
energy
    beam e.
    binding e.
    e. fluence
    e. flux density
    laser e.
    e. level
    quantum e.
    e. resolution
    e. spectra
    e. window
Engel alkalinity
Engelmann-Camurati disease
Engelmann disease
engineering
    genetic e.
engraftment
    delayed e.
    e. effect
    hematologic e.
    hematopoietic e.
    myeloid e.
    neutrophil e.
    trilineage e.
    white blood cell e.
enhancement
    acoustic e.
    antibody-dependent e.
    cocurrent flow-related e.
    contrast e.
    countercurrent flow-
      related e.
    Doppler e.
    dynamic e.
    edge e.
    e. factor
    flow-related e.
    immune e.
    immunologic e.
    leptomeningeal e.
    multislice flow-related e.
    nodular e.
    paradoxical e.
    paramagnetic contrast e.

NOTES

enhancement *(continued)*
    proton relaxation e.
    radiation e.
    rapid acquisition with
      relaxation e.
    sulcal e.
enhancing
    e. brain lesion
    e. lesion
    e. ventricular margins
enlargement
    adenomyosis in uterine e.
    air space e.
    azygos vein e.
    biventricular e.
    bulbous e.
    cardiac e.
    cervical e.
    chamber e.
    clitoris e.
    diffuse hepatic e.
    diffuse thymic e.
    epiglottic e.
    extraocular muscle e.
    global renal e.
    papilla of Vater e.
    parathyroid gland e.
    sulcal e.
    thymic e.
    ventricular e.
enloplatin (CL287110)
Enneking staging system
enolase
    neuron-specific e.
enostosis
Enovid
enoxacin
ensiform process
Ensure
    E. HN
    E. nutritional supplement
Entamoeba histolytica
enteral
    e. feeding
    e. feeding tube
    e. nutrition
    e. nutritional supplement
enteric
    e. cyst
    e. cytopathogenic bovine
      orphan
    e. cytopathogenic human
      orphan

    e. cytopathogenic monkey
      orphan
    e. fistula
    e. stricture
enteritidis
    Salmonella e.
enteritis
    cryptosporidiosis e.
    e. follicularis
    granulomatous e.
    Mycobacterium avium-
      intracellulare e.
    regional e.
Enterobacter
    E. aerogenes
    E. agglomerans
    E. cloacae
    E. gergoviae
    E. liquefaciens
    E. vermicularis
Enterobacteriaceae
enterochromaffin cell
enteroclysis
enterococcus
enterocolic fistula
enterocolitica
    Yersinia e.
enterocolitis
    Clostridium difficile e.
    necrotizing e.
    yersinia e.
enterocutaneous fistula
enterogenous cyst
enterolith
enteropathica
    acrodermatitis e.
enteropathy
    AIDS e.
    gluten-sensitive e.
    protein-losing e.
enteropathy-associated
    e.-a. lymphoma
    e.-a. T-cell lymphoma
enteroscopy
    small bowel e.
enterostomy
    percutaneous e.
enterovaginal fistula
enthesis
entry phenomenon
enucleation
enuresis
Envacor test

envelope
fascial e.
e. feedback
e. gene
e. gene product
gp 160 e.
environment
protective e.
social e.
environmental
e. factor
E. Protection Agency
enzymatic pathway
enzyme
angiotensin-converting e.
(ACE)
cyclooxygenase e.
cytochrome P450 e.
DNA topoisomerase type
II e.
e. immunoassay (EIA)
lipoxygenase e.
metalloproteinase-
proteolytic e.
O-glycanase e.
proteolytic e.
recombinant N-glycanase e.
recombinant N-glycanase
glycerol-free e.
restriction e.
enzyme-linked
e.-l. immunoabsorbent assay
(ELISA)
e.-l. immunoelectrodiffusion
assay (ELIEDA)
enzyme-multiplied immunoassay
technique (EMIT)
Enzymune test
EOC
epithelial ovarian cancer
EORTC
European Organization for
Research and Treatment of
Cancer
EORTC index
EORTC QLQ-C30
European Organization for
Research and Treatment of
Cancer Core Quality of Life
Questionnaire-C30
eosinophil
e. chemotactic factor
eosinophilia
Löffler e.
e. myalgia syndrome
paraneoplastic e.
pulmonary infiltration
with e. (PIE)
tropical e.
eosinophilic
e. adenoma
e. cystitis
e. endomyocardial
fibroplasia
e. fibrohistiocytic lesion
e. fibrohistiocytosis
e. gastroenteritis
e. granuloma
e. leukemia
e. myelocyte
e. pneumonia
eosin stain
ependymal cyst
ependymitis
bacterial e.
e. granularis
ependymoblastoma
ependymoma
brainstem e.
myxopapillary e.
sacrococcygeal
myxopapillary e.
subcutaneous sacrococcygeal
myxopapillary e.
EPI
echo-planar imaging
epiarterial bronchus
EPIblot
E. HIV-1 test
E. HIV Western blot test
epicardial fat pad
epicenter
epicondylar fracture
epicondyle

NOTES

189

epidemic parotitis
epidemiological
    e. data
    e. study
epidemiology
    biochemical e.
    molecular e.
epidermal
    e. growth factor
    e. growth factor receptor
    (EGFR)
    e. growth factor rector
    (EGFR)
    e. inclusion cyst
    e. necrolysis
epidermidis
    Staphylococcus e.
epidermidoma cyst
epidermis
epidermodysplasia verruciformis
epidermoid
    e. cancer
    e. carcinoma
    e. carcinoma of vulva
    cerebellar e.
    e. cyst
    e. inclusion cyst
    e. tumor
epidermoidoma
    black e.
    incisural e.
    intradural e.
    prepontine white e.
epididymal
    e. cyst
    e. descent
    e. fibrosarcoma
epididymis, pl. epididymides
    e. lesion
    postvasectomy change in e.
epididymitis
    chronic e.
epididymoorchitis
epidophyllotoxin
epidural
    e. abscess
    e. analgesia
    e. anesthesia
    e. anesthetic
    e. angiolipoma
    e. arachnoid cyst
    e. block
    e. cavernous hemangioma

    e. effusion
    e. empyema
    e. extramedullary lesion
    e. fibrosis
    e. hematoma
    e. infusion
    e. injection
    e. lipomatosis
    e. meningitis
    e. pneumatosis
    e. runoff
    e. scar
    e. space
    e. steroid injection
epigastric
    e. region
    e. vein
epigastrium
epiglottic
    e. enlargement
    e. fold
epiglottis
epiglottitis
    bacterial e.
epiglycanin
epignathus
epilarynx
epilation
epilepsy
    chronic partial e.
    intractable e.
    temporal lobe e.
epiligrin
epinephric diverticulum
epinephrine
epinine
epiphrenic diverticulum
epiphyseal
    e. dysgenesis
    e. dysostosis
    e. dysplasia
    e. fracture
    e. growth plate
    e. growthplate fracture
    e. line
    e. ossification center
    e. overgrowth
    e. plate fracture
    e. plate injury
    e. slip fracture
    e. tibial fracture
epiphyseolysis
epiphysis, pl. epiphyses

ball-and-socket e.
balloon e.
congenital stippled e.
femoral e.
ossifying e.
ring e.
slipped e.
slipped capital femoral e.
stippled e.
epiphysitis
juvenile e.
epiploia
epiploic
e. foramen
epipodophyllotoxin
epiroprim
epirubicin
epirubicin, bleomycin, vinblastine
(EBV)
episodic spells
epispadia
epistaxis
Gull renal e.
epithalamus
epithelial
e. cancer
e. cell
e. colonic polyp
e. cyst
e. degenerative change
e. hyperplasia
e. membrane antigen
e. neoplasm
e. ovarian cancer (EOC)
e. polyp
e. toxicity
e. tumor
epithelialization
epithelioid
e. angiomatosis
e. hemangioendothelioma
e. hemangioma
e. leiomyoma
e. malignant mesothelioma
e. osteosarcoma
e. sarcoma

epitheliotropism
epithelium
atypical e.
Barrett e.
coelomic e.
germinal e.
papilla of columnar e.
squamous metaplasia
white e.
surface e.
white e.
epitope
shared e.
epoetin
e. alfa
e. beta
Epogen
epoöphoron
epsilon-aminocaproic acid (EACA)
epsilon chain
Epstein-Barr
E.-B. early region protein
(EBER protein)
E.-B. infection
E.-B. virus (EBV)
E.-B. virus-associated
lymphoproliferative
syndrome
Epstein method
E-PTFE
expanded
polytetrafluoroethylene
E-PTFE graft
E-PTFE shunt
equalization
scan e.
equation
Bernoulli e.
Bloch e.
continuity e.
decay e.
Doppler e.
Einstein e.
Holen-Hatle e.
Larmor e.

NOTES

equation *(continued)*
Solomon-Bloembergen e.'s
Ussing e.
equi
Rhodococcus e.
equianalgesic
equilibrium
e. dissociation constant
e. dose constant
e. magnetization
secular e.
state e.
thermal e.
transient e.
equina
cauda e.
equinovalgus deformity
equinovarus
e. deformity
talipes e.
equipment
e. artifact
dynalyzer e.
static gray scale
ultrasound e.
equipoise
equivalent
dose e.
e. dose
meconium ileus e.
radiobiologic e. (RBE)
equivocal
e. finding
eradication
leukemia e.
Erb
E. palsy
E. paralysis
erb A
erb A protein
erb A proto-oncogene
erb B
erb B oncogene
erb B proto-oncogene
Erb-Duchenne
E.-D. palsy
E.-D. paralysis
E.-D. plexus injury
Erb-Duchenne-Klumpke paralysis
erbium-171
erbium-YAG

ERCP
endoscopic retrograde
cholangiopancreatography
Erdheim-Chester disease
Erdheim tumor
erect
e. radiograph
erecta
luxatio e.
erectile
e. dysfunction
e. function
erectile dysfunction
Ergamisol
erg 1 gene
ergometer
ergonovine
Erlenmeyer flask deformity
Ernst angle
erosion
bony e.
infraspinatus insertion e.
marginal e.
tumor e.
varioliform e.
erosive
e. gastritis
e. gingivitis
e. osteoarthritis
eroticism
anal e.
brachioproctic e.
Erpalfa
error
alpha e.
beta e.
dorsal induction e.
flow-related phase e.
interobserver e.
intraobserver e.
preparation e.
quantization e.
relative e.
erucic acid
eruption
cutaneous e.
Kaposi varicelliform e.
lichenoid drug e.
rhythmic paradoxical e.
eruptive
Erwinia **ASN-ase**
Erwinia **ʟ-asparaginase**

erythema
    acral e.
    e. annulare centrifugum
    e. gyratum repens
    heliotrope e.
    e. migrans
    e. multiforme
    necrolytic migratory e.
    e. nodosum
    paraneoplastic e.
erythematosus
    lupus e. (LE)
    systemic lupus e. (SLE)
erythematous
    e. dermatitis
    e. papulonodule
erythremic myelosis
erythroblast
    basophilic e.
    orthochromatic e.
    polychromatophilic e.
erythroblastopenia
erythroblastosis fetalis
erythrocyte (E)
    achromic e.
    e. and antibody (EA)
    e., antibody, and
      complement (EAC)
    basophilic e.
    bur e.
    colony-forming unit e.
      (CFU-E)
    crenated e.
    hypochromic e.
    e. maturation factor
    Mexican hat e.
    mucleated e.
    normochromic e.
    orthochromic e.
    packed e.'s
    polychromic e.
    target e.
    e. transfusion
    e. volume
erythrocythemia
erythrocytopenia

erythrocytosis
    paraneoplastic e.
erythrodermatous
    e. lesion
    e. variant
erythrodermic follicular mucinosis
erythroid
    e. activity
    e. burst-forming unit
    e. cell
    e. marker
    e. organ
    e. precursor
    e. progenitor
erythroleukemia
erythromycin
erythron
erythronormoblastic anemia
**erythrophagocytic T-gamma
  lymphoma**
erythrophagocytosis
erythroplasia
    Queyrat e.
erythropoiesis
erythropoietic-stimulating factor
erythropoietin
    e. gene
    recombinant human e.
^{255}Es
    einsteinium-255
escalation
    dose e.
escape
    phenotypic e.
eschar
Escherichia coli
Escobar syndrome
eskimoma
esophageal
    e. atresia
    e. balloon dilator
    e. cancer
    e. candidiasis
    e. carcinoma
    e. choriocarcinoma
    e. contraction
    e. diverticula

NOTES

esophageal *(continued)*
- e. diverticulum
- e. duplication
- e. duplication cyst
- e. dysmotility
- e. filling defect
- e. hiatus
- e. inflammation
- e. intramural
  pseudodiverticulosis
- e. leiomyosarcoma
- e. narrowing
- e. neoplasm
- e. opening
- e. perforation
- e. peristalsis
- e. ring
- e. rupture
- e. stricture
- e. tear
- e. tumor
- e. ulcer
- e. varices
- e. vein
- e. vestibule
- e. web

esophagectomy
- transhiatal e. (THE)
- transthoracic e.

esophagitis
- peptic e.
- reflux e.

esophagogastric (EG)
- e. junction

esophagogastrostomy
esophagojejunostomy
esophagoscopy
- Lugol dye e.

esophagostomy
- cervical e.
- palliative e.

esophagotracheal fistula
esophagram
- air e.
- barium-water e.
- radionuclide e.

esophagus
- Barrett e.
- congenitally short e.
- corkscrew appearance of
  the e.
- double-barrel e.
- shish kebab e.

esorubicin
Esperatrucin
ESR
- electron spin resonance

essential
- e. osteolysis
- e. thrombocythemia

Essex-Lopresti
- E.-L. fracture
- E.-L. joint depression
  fracture

ester
- glutathione monoethyl e.
- iodipamide ethyl e.
- midobenzoyl-*N*-
  hydroxysuccinimide e.
- phorbol e.
- quinuclidinyl e.

esterase
- alpha-naphthyl acetate e.
- alpha-naphthyl butyrate e.
- aminocaproate e.
- chloroacetate e.
- nonspecific e.
- serine e.

esterified estrogen
esthesioneuroblastoma
esthesioneurocytoma
esthesioneuroepithelioma
estimation
- frequency e.

Estinyl
Estrace
estracyte
estradiol (E_2)
- ethinyl e.

Estradurin
Estra-L
estramustine phosphate sodium
Estratab
Estraval
Estren-Damashek anemia
Estrinyl
estrogen
- conjugated e.
- esterified e.
- e. rebound regression
- e. receptor
- e. replacement therapy

estrogen-progestin artificial cycle
estrone

ESWL
extracorporeal shock-wave
lithotripsy
ET
endotracheal
ET tube
etanidazole
état
état criblé
état lacunaire
état pre-criblé
ethacrynic acid
ethambutol
ethanesulfonate
meta-azidopyrimethamine e.
ethanol
e. ablation
absolute e.
e. embolotherapy
ether
methyl-*tert*-butyl e.
ethesioneuroblastoma
Ethibloc
ethidium bromide
ethinyl estradiol
Ethiodane
ethiodized
e. oil
e. oil emulsion
Ethiodol
ethiofos (WR-2721)
ethionamide
ethmocephaly
ethmoid
e. air cell
e. bone
e. foramen
e. sinus
e. sinus carcinoma
ethmoidal
e. artery
e. bulla
ethnic variation
ethoxysclerol
10-ethyl-10-diazaaminopterin (10-EDAM)

ethylene
e. diaminetetraacetate
e. hydroxydiphosphonate
ethylenediaminetetraacetate
ethylenediaminetetraacetic acid (EDTA)
ethylenehydroxyphenylglycine
ethylester
glutathione e.
ethyliodophenylundecyl
Ethyol
etidronate
e. disodium
rhenium-186 e.
technetium-99m e.
etiology
E-to-A change
ET-18-OCH/d3/D
etodolac
etoglucid
etoposide (VePesid, VP-16)
dexamethasone, ara-C,
carboplatin, e. (DACE)
ifosfamide, carboplatin, e.
(ICE)
e. phosphate
etoposide, Adriamycin, Platinol (EAP)
etoposide, doxorubicin, Platinol
etoposide, 5-fluorouracil, Platinol (EFP)
etoposide, methotrexate, actinomycin, cyclophosphamide, Oncovin
etoposide, methotrexate-leucovorin, actinomycin D, cyclophosphamide, Oncovin (EMA-CO)
etoposide, vinblastine, Adriamycin (EVA)
ets-1 **proto-oncogene**
ets-2 **proto-oncogene**
EU
excretory urography
euchromatin
euglobulin
e. lysis time

NOTES

195

eukaryotic cell
Eulexin
euoxic cell
European
    E. blastomycosis
    E. Kaposi sarcoma
    E. mistletoe
    E. Organization for
    Research and Treatment
    of Cancer (EORTC)
    E. Organization for
    Research and Treatment
    of Cancer Core Quality of
    Life Questionnaire-C30
    (EORTC QLQ-C30)
    E. yew
eustachian tube
eutectic mixture of local
  anesthetics (EMLA)
euthanasia
eV
    electron volt
EVA
    etoposide, vinblastine,
    Adriamycin
evacuation
evaluation
    neurodiagnostic e.
    pretreatment e.
    quantitative e.
    real-time acquisition and
    velocity e.
    roentgenographic e.
    stent e.
    Wright-Giemsa e.
Evans
    E. blue dye
    E. stage IV-S disease
    E. stages of neuroblastoma
    E. syndrome
even-echo rephasing
event
    life e.
eventration
    diaphragm e.
    e. of the diaphragm
    diaphragmatic e.
Everone
eversion
    cervical e.
evidence
    scintigraphic e.

Ewing
    extraosseous E.
    E. sarcoma
    E. tumor
ex
    e. vacuo dilatation
    e. vivo
    e. vivo gene therapy
    e. vivo marrow treatment
exacerbation
exaggerated craniocaudal view
examination
    barium e.
    digital e.
    digital rectal e. (DRE)
    double-contrast e.
    gray scale e.
    limited e.
    physical e.
    proctoscopic e.
    self-breast e. (SBE)
    small bowel follow-
    through e.
    suboptimal e.
    T1-weighted spin-echo e.
    T2-weighted spin-echo e.
examphalos, macroglossia,
  gigantism (EMG)
exanthem
    Boston e.
exanthematous drug rash
Excalibur introducer
Excel
    Simplastin E.
excess
    soluble antigen e.
excessive callus formation
exchange
    air e.
    body fluid e.
    chemical e.
    e. diffusion
    proton-proton
    magnetization e.
    sister chromatid e.
    spin e.
exchanger
    heat e.
Excimer
    E. dye laser
    E. laser system
excision

en bloc e.
large loop e.
local e.
excisional biopsy
excitation
fast acquisition multiple e.
(FAME)
nonuniform e.
number of e.'s
quadrature e.
selective e.
slice-selective e.
tailored e.
volume-selective e.
exclusion
allelic e.
excretion
contrast e.
urinary e.
excretory urography (EU)
excursion of the diaphragm
exenteration
anterior e.
orbital e.
pelvic e.
pyelonephritis in e.
stress reaction in e.
total e.
exercise
flexion and extension e.'s
Kegel e.'s
e. radionuclide
angiocardiography
exfoliative
e. cytology
e. dermatitis
existential pain
exocytosis
exogenous
e. antigen
e. flora
e. hormones
exon
exonuclease
exonucleolytic digestion

exophthalmos, exophthalmus
endocrine e.
pulsating e.
exophytic
e. glioblastoma
e. gut mass
exostosis, pl. exostoses
hereditary multiple exostoses
osteocartilaginous e.
pelvic e.
exostotic chondrosarcoma
exotoxin
Pseudomonas e.
expanded
e. plasma
e. polytetrafluoroethylene
(E- PTFE)
expander
blood e.
plasma e.
expansile
e. lesion
e. unilocular well-
demarcated bone lesion
expenditure
resting energy e.
experiment
Carr-Purcell e.
multiple quantum e.
rotating-frame e.
surface coils in rotating-
frame e.
experimental
e. chemotherapy
e. therapy
e. treatment
expiratory
e. computed tomography
e. view
explosion fracture
explosive follicular hyperplasia
exponential kinetics
expoSURE
exposure
e. dose
electromagnetic radiation e.
magnetic radiation e.

NOTES

exposure *(continued)*
    operator e.
    radiation e.
expression
    anomalous antigen e.
    antigen e.
    gene e.
    phospholipase cyl-1 e.
    PRAD-1 gene e.
    thymidylate synthase e.
exsanguination
exstrophy
    bladder e.
    cloacal e.
extended
    e. field irradiation therapy
    e. field of view
    e. radical mastectomy
extension
    extranodal tumor e.
    extrascleral e.
    radiolucent operating room table e.
    e. teardrop fracture
    thrombus e.
    e. view
extensive
    e. bilateral pneumonia
    e. intraductal component
extensive-stage disease
extensor
    e. carpi radialis brevis
    e. carpi radialis longus
    e. carpi ulnaris
    e. digitorum
    e. digitorum brevis
    e. digitorum longus
    e. hallucis longus
    e. indicis
    e. pollicis brevis
    e. pollicis longus
    e. retinaculum
    e. tendon
    e. tensor pollicis brevis
externa
    otitis e.
external
    e. acoustic foramen
    e. auditory canal
    e. auditory meatus
    e. beam irradiation
    e. beam radiation
    e. carotid

    e. carotid artery
    e. ear neoplasm
    e. elastic lamina
    e. iliac artery
    e. oblique muscle
    e. orthovoltage irradiation
    e. os
    e. pneumatic calf compression
    e. rotation view
    e. scanning
    e. sphincter
    e. urethral sphincter
    e. x-ray therapy
extirpation
extraarachnoid, extraarachnoid
    e. injection
    e. myelography
extraaxial, extra-axial
    e. cavernous hemangioma
    e. compartment
    e. fluid collection
extracapsular
    e. fracture
    e. metastasis
extracardiac mass
extracellular
    e. compartment
    e. fluid
    e. matrix
extracerebral
    e. cavernous angioma
    e. fluid collection
extrachorialis
    placenta e.
extrachorial placenta
extracorporeal
    e. circulation
    e. irradiation
    e. membrane oxygenation (ECMO)
    e. membrane oxygenator (ECMO)
    e. shock wave
    e. shock-wave lithotripsy (ESWL)
extracranial
    e. carotid artery disease
    e. carotid circulation
    e. cerebral vasculature
    e. mass lesion
    e. vasculature

extract
  bovine dialyzable
  leukocyte e.
  pine cone e.
  sea algae e.
extractable nuclear antigen
extraction
  first-pass e.
  liquid e.
  micro liquid e.
  solid phase e.
  vacuum e.
extractor
  Cook urological five-wire
  helical stone e.
  removable sheath helical e.
extradural hematoma
extrafascial hysterectomy
extrafollicular blast
extragonadal seminoma (EGS)
extrahepatic
  e. bile duct
  e. binary obstruction
  e. cholangiectasis
  e. cholangiocarcinoma
  e. hypertension
  e. lesion
  e. obstruction
  e. portal hypertension
  e. primary malignant tumor
  e. stone
extralobar sequestration
extraluminal
  e. gas
  e. hemorrhage
extramammary Paget disease
extramedullary
  e. hematopoiesis
  e. hemopoiesis
  e. involvement
  e. leukemic plasmacytoma
  e. plasmacytoma
  e. toxicity
extranodal
  e. follicular lymphoma
  e. lymphoma
  e. proliferation

  e. site
  e. tumor extension
extraoctave fracture
extraocular
  e. muscle
  e. muscle enlargement
extraosseous
  e. Ewing
  e. osteosarcoma
extrapelvic malignancy
extraperitoneal
extrapolate
extrapulmonary
  e. sequestration
  e. small cell cancer
extrapyramidal
  e. reaction
  e. system
extrarenal renal pelvis
extrascleral extension
extraskeletal osteosarcoma
extra-stiff guidewire
extratesticular
  e. lesion
  e. tumor
extrathoracic metastasis
extrauterine pelvic mass
extravaginal testicular torsion
extravasation
  urinary e.
extravascular
  e. compartment
  e. mass
extraventricular
  e. hydrocephalus
  e. obstructive hydrocephalus
extravesical infrasphincteric ectopic ureter
extremely low-frequency field
extreme micromelia
extremity
  e. abnormality
  e. hemangioma
  lower e.
  e. malformation
  e. osteosarcoma
  e. rhabdomyosarcoma

NOTES

extrinsic
  e. allergic alveolitis
  e. alveolitis
  e. asthma
  e. bladder compression
  e. cellular parameter
  e. compression
  e. defect
  e. esophageal impression
  e. field uniformity
  e. filling defect
  e. impression
  e. ureteral defect
extruded disk fragment
extrusion
  disk e.

exudative
  e. pleural effusion
  e. tuberculosis
eye
  bovine cancer e.
  e. exposure limit
  fetal e.
  intraconal portion of the e.
E-Z-CAT
E-Z-EM
  E-Z-EM balloon enema
  E-Z-EM cut biopsy needle
  E-Z-EM needle

F18
fludeoxyglucose F18
FAA
flavone acetic acid
FAB
French/American/British
FAB classification
Fab
fragment antigen binding
Fab fragment
Fab-DTPA
antimyosin F.-D.
fabella
os f.
Faber anemia
Fabian prostatic stent
Fabricius
bursa of F.
Fabry disease
FAC
5-fluorouracil, Adriamycin, cyclophosphamide
face
en f.
facet, facette
f. arthropathy
articular f.
bilateral locked f.'s
f. joint
f. joint arthritis
f. joint injection
facetectomy
faceted gallstone
facette (*var. of* facet)
facial
f. abnormality
f. artery
f. bone
f. canal
f. cleft
f. colliculus
f. disorder
f. fracture
f. hemangioma
f. hypesthesia
f. lymph node
f. marrow
f. nerve
f. neurofibroma

f. neuroma
f. paralysis
faciale
granuloma f.
facialis
herpes f.
facies, pl. **facies**
elfin f.
rodent f.
FACT
Functional Assessment of Cancer Therapy
factor
accelerator f.
activation f.
antianemia f.
antiangiogenesis f.
anticomplementary f.
antihemophilic f.
antihemorrhagic f.
antinuclear f.
autocrine growth f.
automotility f.
basophil chemotactic f.
B-cell differentiation f.
B-cell-stimulating f.
Bittner milk f.
blastogenic f.
blocking f.
blood clotting f.
blood coagulation f.
B-lymphocyte stimulatory f.
Boltzmann f.
Bucky f.
Castle f.
chemotactic f.
Christmas f. (CF)
citrovorum f. (CF)
citrovorum rescue f.
clonal inhibitory f.
clotting f.
coagulation f.
colony-stimulating f. (CSF)
complement f. (CF)
conglutination f.
conglutinogen-activating f.
contrast-improvement f.
corticotropin-releasing f. (CRF)

factor *(continued)*
  crystal-induced
    chemotactic f.
  cytokine synthesis
    inhibitory f.
  cytotoxic f.
  D f.
  Day f.
  decay-activating f.
  diffusion f.
  dose-limiting f.
  Duran-Reynals f.
  duty f.
  elongation f.
  eluate f.
  endocrine f.
  endothelial f.
  endothelium-derived
    relaxing f.
  enhancement f.
  environmental f.
  eosinophil chemotactic f.
  epidermal growth f.
  erythrocyte maturation f.
  erythropoietic-stimulating f.
  factor VIII:C heat-treated
    antihemophilic f.
  fibrin-stabilizing f.
  fibroblast growth f.
  filling f.
  Fitzgerald f.
  Fletcher f.
  gamma f.
  geometry f.
  glass f.
  granulocyte colony-
    stimulating f. (G-CSF)
  granulocyte-macrophage
    colony-stimulating f.
    (GM- CSF)
  growth f.
  growth hormone releasing f.
  H f.
  Hageman f.
  helper f.
  hematologic f.
  hematopoietic colony-
    stimulating f.
  hematopoietic growth f.
  hematopoietic stem cell f.
  hepatocyte-stimulating f.
  host f.
  host-related f.

  human granulocyte-
    stimulating f.
  human growth f.
  human macrophage-
    monocyte chemotactic and
    activating f. (rhMCAF)
  humoral f.
  insulin-like growth f. (IGF,
    ILGF)
  intrinsic f.
  f. IX antigen
  f. IX complex
  f. IX deficiency
  Lactobacillus casei f.
  Lactobacillus lactis
    Dorner f.
  Laki-Lorand f.
  LE f.
  leucovorin-citrovorum f.
    (L- CF)
  leucovorin rescue f.
  leukemia inhibitory f. (LIF)
  limulus anti-DPS f.
  lymphocyte-activating f.
  lymphocyte mitogenic f.
  macrophage-activating f.
  macrophage chemotactic f.
  macrophage colony-
    stimulating f. (M-CSF)
  macrophage growth f.
  macrophage-inhibition f.
  mast cell growth f.
  megakaryocyte colony-
    stimulating f. (MEG-CSF)
  migration inhibitory f.
  milk f.
  mitogenic f.
  monocyte colony-
    stimulating f.
  monocyte tissue f.
  mouse mammary tumor f.
  multicolony-stimulating f.
  murine granulocyte-
    macrophage colony-
    stimulating growth f.
  myeloid growth f.
  neutrophil chemotactic f.
  neutrophil migration-
    inhibition f.
  nonhematopoietic growth f.
  nuclear f.
  osteoclast-activating f.
  P f.

p40 T-cell growth f.
Passovoy f.
P-cell stimulating f.
plasmacytoma growth f.
platelet-activating f.
platelet-derived growth f.
pre-B-cell growth f.
prognostic f.
protection f. (PF)
protein f.
Prower f.
psychological f.
Q f.
quality f.
radiation weighting f.
recombinant hematopoietic growth f.
recombinant human colony-stimulating f.
recombinant human granulocyte colony-stimulating f. (rhG-CSF)
recombinant human granulocyte-macrophage colony-stimulating f. (rGM-CSF, rhGM-CSF)
recombinant human granulocyte-stimulating f.
recombinant human growth f.
recombinant human macrophage colony-stimulating f. (rhM-CSF)
recruitment f.
relative conversion f.
releasing f.
r-GM-colony-stimulating f.
Rh f.
Rhesus f.
rheumatoid f.
risk f.
scatter degradation f.
Simon septic f.
skin reactive f.
social f.
specific macrophage-arming f.

Steel f.
stem cell f.
Stuart f.
Stuart-Prower f.
T-cell growth f.
T-cell replacement f.
technical f.
thymus-replacing f.
thyrotropin-releasing f.
tissue weighting f.
transcription f.
transfer f.
transforming growth f.
tumor angiogenesis f.
tumor angiogenic f.
tumor autocrine mobility f.
tumor-limiting f.
tumor necrosis f. (TNF)
V f.
f. VII antigen (VII:Ag)
f. VIII coagulation function
f. VIIIR
f. VIII-related antigen
von Willebrand f. (factor VIIIR, vWF)
Wills f.
X f.
f. X antigen (X:Ag)

factor-α
transforming growth f.
tumor necrosis f.
factor-β
transforming growth f.
factor-1
insulin-like growth f. (IGF-1)
factor-2
insulin-like growth f. (IGF-2)
factor-4
recombinant platelet f. (rPF4)
factor-AA
platelet-derived growth f.-A.
factor-acidic
fibroblast growth f.-a.

NOTES

factor-alpha
    tumor necrosis f.-a.
Factorate
factor-basic
    fibroblast growth f.-b.
factor-BB
    platelet-derived growth f.-B.
factorial design
fadrozole
faecalis
    Streptococcus f.
faggot cell
Fahraeus-Lindqvist effect
Fahraeus method
FAIDS
    feline AIDS
failed back surgery syndrome
failing ovary syndrome
failure
    adrenal f.
    cardiac f.
    chronic acquired hepatic f.
    chronic renal f.
    congestive heart f.
    frank congestive f.
    graft f.
    heart f.
    hepatic f.
    kidney f.
    left ventricular f.
    leptomeningeal f.
    locoregional f.
    multisystem organ f.
    neonatal cardiac f.
    organ f.
    ovarian f.
    ovulatory f.
    passive congestive f.
    postrenal f.
    prerenal f.
    renal f.
    respiratory f.
    time-to-treatment f. (TTF)
failure-free survival
Fairbank disease
falces (*pl. of* falx)
falciform ligament
fallen
    f. fragment sign
    f. lung sign
fallopian
    f. tube carcinoma

    f. tube mass
    f. tubes
Fallot
    F. disease
    pentalogy of F.
    F. syndrome
    tetralogy of F.
    trilogy of F.
false
    f. aneurysm
    f. cord carcinoma
    f. frequency
    f. hypoechogenicity
    f. knot
    f. lumen
    f. negative ratio
    f. pelvis
    f. positive ratio
false-positive
    biologic f.-p.
falx, pl. falces
    f. artery
    f. calcification
    f. cerebelli
    f. cerebri
    f. meningioma
FAM
    5-fluorouracil, Adriamycin,
      mitomycin
FAME
    fast acquisition multiple
      excitation
FAMe
    5-fluorouracil, Adriamycin,
      methyl-CCNU
familial
    f. acro-osteolysis
    f. adenomatous polyposis
      (FAP)
    f. atypical multiple mole
      melanoma syndrome
      (FAMMM)
    f. cancer
    f. chondrocalcinosis
    f. dysplastic nevus
      syndrome (FDNS)
    f. hemophagocytic
      lymphohistiocytosis
    f. hypophosphatemic rickets
    f. immunity
    f. Mediterranean fever
    f. multiple polyposis
    f. onychoosteodysplasia

f. polyposis syndrome
f. xanthomatosis
famine osteomalacia
FAMMM
familial atypical multiple mole
melanoma syndrome
FAMP
fludarabine monophosphate
fan beam projection
Fanconi
F. anemia
F. syndrome
Fansidar
F₂ antibody
FAP
familial adenomatous polyposis
Faraday
F. cage
F. law
F. shield
F. shielded resonator
Farber disease
far field
farinae
Dermatophagoides f.
farmarubicin
farmer chamber
farmer's lung
Farr test
fascia
f. of breast
cervical f.
Denonvilliers f.
diaphragmatic f.
Gerota f.
obturator f.
pharyngobasilar f.
rectal f.
renal f.
spigelian f.
supraanal f.
thoracolumbar f.
transversalis f.
umbilicovesical f.
vesical f.
fascial
f. dilator

f. envelope
f. incisor
f. plane
fascicular sarcoma
fasciculata
zona f.
fasciculation
tongue f.
fasciculus
longitudinal f.
mamillothalamic f.
medial longitudinal f.
occipitofrontal f.
superior longitudinal f.
superior occipitofrontal f.
fasciitis
necrotizing f.
nodular f.
palmar f.
f. panniculitis
plantar f.
pseudosarcomatous f.
FAST
Fourier-acquired steady-state
technique
contrast-enhanced FAST
FAST pulse sequence
reduced-acquisition matrix
FAST
RF-spoiled FAST
T1-weighted FAST
fast
f. acquisition multiple
excitation (FAME)
f. adiabatic trajectory in
steady state (FATS)
f. array processor
f. exchange-cellular
suspension
f. exchange-soft tissue
f. field echos
f. Fourier imaging (FFr)
f. Fourier transform
f. hemoglobin
f. imaging
f. imaging with steady-state
free precession (FISP)

NOTES

fast *(continued)*
    f. low-angle shot (FLASH)
    f. neutron
    f. neutron radiation therapy
    f. scan magnetic resonance
    f. scan magnetic resonance
      imaging
    f. spin echo
fast-breeder reactor
fat
    autologous f.
    creeping f.
    f. density
    dietary f.
    dirty f.
    f. embolism
    f. graft
    f. herniation
    Hoffa f. pad
    infrapatellar f. pad
    intratumoral f.
    f. island
    f. line
    lipid content of storage f.'s
    f. lobule
    mediastinal f.
    f. necrosis
    f. pad
    f. pad sign
    perigastric f.
    f. plane
    f. presaturation
    renal sinus f.
    subcutaneous f.
    f. suppression
    unsaturated f.
    ventral epidural f.
fat-density
    f.-d. area
    f.-d. line
fat-fluid
    f.-f. density interface
    f.-f. level
fatigue
    compassion f.
    f. fracture
FATS
    fast adiabatic trajectory in steady
      state
fat-suppression MR imaging
fatty
    f. acyl-Co-A synthetase

    f. acyl-Co-A synthetase
      deficiency
    f. dysplastic regenerative
      hepatic nodule
    f. halo
    f. infiltration
    f. liver
    f. marrow
    f. meal sonography
    f. pancreas
    f. prostatic tissue
    f. tissue
    f. tumor
fat/water
    f. chemical shift imaging
    f. signal separation
faucial pillar
**faulty radiofrequency shielding
  artifact**
fawn tail sign
fazarabine
FbDP
    fibrin degradation product
      Fibrinostika FbDP
FBM
    fetal breathing movement
Fc
    F. fragment
    F. portion
    F. receptor
FCA
    Freund complete adjuvant
FDA
    Food and Drug Administration
FDNS
    familial dysplastic nevus
      syndrome
5-FdUMP
    5-fluorodeoxyuridylate
feature
    clinical f.
    pathologic f.
features
    mongoloid f.
febrile
    f. neutropenia
    f. patient
febrilis
    herpes f.
fecal
    f. carcinoembryonic antigen
    f. diversion colostomy
    f. impaction

f. material
f. occult blood testing
f. stone
f. tumor
fecal-filled colon
fecalith
fecapentaene
feces
    inspissated f.
    semiliquid f.
feedback
    envelope f.
feeding
    enteral f.
    enteral f. tube
    f. tube
Fe-EHPG
    Fe- ethylenehydroxy-
      phenylglycine
Fe-ethylenehydroxyphenylglycine
  (Fe-EHPG)
Feiba VH Immuno
Feist-Mankin position
Felbatol
feline
    f. AIDS (FAIDS)
    f. ataxia virus
    f. leukemia
    f. leukemia-sarcoma virus
    f. leukemia virus
fellatio
Felson
    silhouette sign of F.
Felton syndrome
Felty syndrome
female pseudohermaphroditism
feminization
    testicular f.
feminizing
    f. adrenal tumor
    f. testes syndrome
Feminone
femora (*pl. of* femur)
femoral
    f. arterial catheter
    f. artery
    f. artery approach

f. canal
f. condyle
f. epiphysis
f. fracture
f. hernia
f. intertrochanteric fracture
f. length (FL)
f. neck fracture
f. nerve
f. pulse
f. ring
f. runoff angiography
f. runoff arteriography
f. septum
f. shaft
f. shaft fracture
f. sheath
f. supracondylar fracture
f. triangle
f. vein
femoris
    biceps f.
    quadriceps f.
    rectus f.
    tensor fascia f.
femorocerebral catheter angiography
femoropatellar joint
femoropopliteal
    f. bypass graft
    f. outflow system
    f. vessel
femur, pl. **femura, femora**
    distal f.
    head of the f.
    proximal f.
fen
    tian hau f.
fencer's bone
fender fracture
fenestration
    catheter-directed f.
fenfluramine
fenoldopam mesylate
fenoprofen
    f. calcium
fenretinide
fentangle patch

NOTES

fentanyl
Fenwick disease
Fe₃O₄
   magnetite
Ferguson angle
Feridex
fermium-255 (^{255}Fm)
ferpentetate
   technetium-99m f.
Ferratea cell
Ferrein foramen
ferric
   f. ammonium citrate
   f. subsulfate
Ferris bone marrow aspiration
   needle
ferrite
ferritin
   rabbit antirat f.
ferritin-labeled yttrium
ferrohemoglobin
ferromagnetic
   f. artifact
   f. material
   f. microembolization
   f. microembolization
      treatment
   f. microsphere
ferromagnetism
ferropolysaccharide
ferrosome
ferrotherapy
ferrous iron
fertility
fertilization
   in vitro f.
FES
   flame emission spectroscopy
fes **proto-oncogene**
FESS
   functional endoscopic sinus
      surgery
fetal
   f. abdominal circumference
   f. abdominal wall
   f. abdominal wall defect
   f. adenoma
   f. age
   f. anomaly
   f. aortic flow volume
   f. arrhythmia
   f. ascites
   f. asphyxia

f. behavioral state
f. biophysical profile scoring
f. blood analysis
f. bone fracture
f. BPS
f. breathing movement
   (FBM)
f. cardiac anomaly
f. cardiac dysrhythmia
f. cardiosplenic syndrome
f. chest anomaly
f. circulation
f. circumference
f. cystic adenomatoid
   malformation
f. cystic fibrosis
f. death
f. death in utero
f. echocardiography
f. eye
f. femoral length
f. foot-length measurement
f. gastrointestinal anomaly
f. gender
f. growth acceleration
f. hamartoma
f. head circumference
f. heart
f. heart rate acceleration
f. hemoglobin
f. hydrops
f. liver biopsy
f. lobation
f. lobulation
f. long bone measurement
f. lymphoid tissue
f. measurement
f. mensuration
f. movement (FM)
f. musculoskeletal dysplasia
f. musculoskeletal system
f. period
f. renal function
f. renal hamartoma
f. renal obstruction
f. scalp edema
f. skeletal dysplasia
f. skin biopsy
f. spine
f. swallowing
f. tissue sampling
f. tone

f. urogenital tract
f. weight
fetalis
erythroblastosis f.
hydrops f.
nonimmune hydrops f.
fetal movement (FM)
feticide
fetishism
fetoglobin
fetomaternal transfusion
fetoplacental blood
fetoprotein
α-fetoprotein
fetus
Campylobacter f.
f. digitalis
disappearing f.
multiple f.'s
small-for-gestational-age f.
trisomic f.
fever
Argentinian hemorrhagic f.
blackwater f.
Bullis f.
cat scratch f.
cat-scratch f.
Dumdum f.
familial Mediterranean f.
fracture f.
Katayama f.
Korin f.
Lone Star f.
Mediterranean f.
neutropenic f.
nine-mile f.
Pel-Ebstein f.
polymer fume f.
Q f.
Rift Valley f.
San Joaquin Valley f.
scarlet f.
unexplained f.
yellow f.
FFr
fast Fourier imaging
fgr **proto-oncogene**

fiber
annular f.
asbestos f.'s
association f.
bare f.
f. carcinogenesis
commissural f.
Nutren with f.
optical f.
proprioception nerve f.
Purkinje f.'s
Rosenthal f.
Sharpey f.'s
f. tip modification
fiberglass pneumoconiosis
fiberoptic
f. bundle
f. conductor
Fibonacci search scheme
fibrillary
f. astrocytic neoplasm
f. astrocytoma
fibrillation
atrial f.
fibrin
f. body
f. clot
f. degradation product (FbDP)
f. deposition
Henle f.
f. plate method
f. split products
fibrinogen
f. equivalent unit
f. split products
fibrinogenemia
fibrinogenopenia
fibrinolysin
fibrinolysis
fibrinolytic
f. factor deficiency
f. system
f. therapy
fibrinopeptide A
fibrinoplatelet aggregate
Fibrinostika FbDP

NOTES

fibrinous clot
fibrin-stabilizing factor
fibroadenolipoma
fibroadenoma
    calcified f.
    degenerated f.
    giant f.
    hyalinized f.
    juvenile f.
fibroadenomatosis
fibroblast
    bone marrow f.
    f. growth factor
    f. growth factor-acidic
    f. growth factor-basic
    stromal f.
fibroblastic
    f. osteosarcoma
    f. variant
fibrocalcareous
fibrocarcinoma
fibrocartilage complex
fibrocartilaginous
    f. disk
fibrocaseous
fibrochondrogenesis
fibrocystic
    f. change
    f. disease
fibrodysplasia ossificans progressiva
fibroelastosis
    endocardial f.
fibroepithelial
    f. papilloma
    f. polyp
fibroepithelioma
fibrofatty breast tissue
fibrogenesis imperfecta ossium
fibroglandular elements
fibrohemosideric
fibrohistiocytic lesion
fibrohistiocytoma
fibrohistiocytosis
    eosinophilic f.
fibroid
    f. adenoma
    parasitic f.
    f. polyp
    f. tumor
    uterine f.
fibrolamellar
    f. carcinoma

    f. liver cell carcinoma
    f. variant
fibroleiomyoma
fibrolipomatosis
    pelvic f.
fibroma
    ameloblastic f.
    aponeurotic f.
    cementifying f.
    central cementifying f.
    central ossifying f.
    chondromyxoid f.
    concentric f.
    desmoplastic f.
    giant cell f.
    irritation f.
    juvenile aponeurotic f.
    f. molle
    f. molle gravidarum
    f. molluscum
    f. myxomatodes
    nonossifying f.
    nonosteogenic f.
    odontogenic f.
    ossifying f.
    osteogenic f.
    ovarian f.
    peripheral ossifying f.
    periungual f.
    polypoid f.
    psammomatoid ossifying f.
    rabbit f.
    recurrent digital f.
    scrotal f.
    senile f.
    Shope f.
    sinonasal psammomatoid
      ossifying f.
    telangiectatic f.
    ungual f.
fibromatoid
fibromatosis
    abdominal f.
    aggressive f.
    aggressive infantile f.
    f. colli
    congenital diffuse f.
    congenital generalized f.
    congenital multiple f.
    infantile digital f.
    juvenile f.
    juvenile hyalin f.
    juvenile palmoplantar f.

palmar f.
penile f.
plantar f.
fibromatous
fibromuscular dysplasia
fibromyoma
fibromyositis
fibronectin
    Asserachrom f.
fibronodular
fibroplasia
    adventitial f.
    endomyocardial f.
    eosinophilic
        endomyocardial f.
    intimal f.
    medial f.
    perimedial f.
    retrolental f.
fibroproductive tuberculosis
fibrosa
    area hepatica f.
    osteitis f.
fibrosarcoma
    ameloblastic f.
    Earle L f.
    epididymal f.
    infantile f.
    inflammatory f.
    f. variant
fibrosing
    f. alveolitis
    f. mediastinitis
    f. mesenteritis
fibrosis
    annular f.
    benign meningeal f.
    bone marrow f.
    congenital hepatic f.
    cystic f.
    endomyocardial f.
    epidural f.
    fetal cystic f.
    focal f.
    hepatic f.
    horseshoe f.

idiopathic interstitial f.
interstitial pulmonary f.
    (IPF)
lymph node f.
mediastinal f.
meningeal f.
myocardial f.
pancreatic cystic f.
periductal f.
perineural f.
perivascular f.
progressive massive f.
pulmonary f.
radiation f.
retroperitoneal f.
fibrosum
    adenoma f.
    molluscum f.
fibrosus
    annulus f.
fibrothorax
fibrotic scarring
fibrous
    f. bone lesion
    f. capsule
    f. connective tissue
    f. cortical defect
    f. dysplasia
    f. hamartoma
    f. histiocytoma
    f. mastitis
    f. medullary defect
    f. metaphyseal-diaphyseal
        defect
    f. nodular pattern
    f. osteoma
    f. polypoid lesion
    f. septa
    f. union
fibroxanthoma
    pediatric f.
fibula, pl. fibulae
    proximal f.
fibular
    f. fracture
    f. notch

NOTES

fibular notch
Fick
    F. law
    F. method
    F. position
    F. principle
Ficoll-Hypaque
    F.-H. density gradient
      centrifugation
fidelity
    lineage f.
fiducial alignment system
field
    f. cancerization
    dipole f.
    f. disease
    f. drift
    f. echo
    electromagnetic f.
    electron beam boost f.
    f. emission tube
    extremely low-frequency f.
    far f.
    f. gradient
    gradient f.
    gradient magnetic f.
    high-power f. (hpf)
    f. inversion gel
      electrophoresis
    f. lock
    low-power f. (lpf)
    lung f.
    magnetic f.
    near f.
    radiofrequency f.
    shrinking f.
    skimming of magnetic f.
    static magnetic f.
    f. strength
    time-varying magnetic f.
    f. uniformity
    f. of view (FOV)
field-echo
    f.-e. difference
    f.-e. imaging
    f.-e. sum
Fielding-Magliato classification of
  subtrochanteric fractures
field-profiling coil
Fiessinger-Leroy-Reiter syndrome
Fiessinger-Leroy syndrome
fifth disease
fighter's fracture

FIGO
    International Federation of
      Gynecology and Obstetrics
    FIGO nomenclature
    FIGO staging system
figure
    mitotic f.
figure-3 sign
figure-8 sign
figure-of-eight abnormality
filaggrin
filament
    cytoplasmic f.'s
    f. emission
filament-nonfilament count
filariasis
Filatori disease
filgrastim
filling
    f. defect
    f. factor
    subintimal f.
    zero f.
film
    abdominal plain f.
    f. changer
    chest f.
    cine f.
    comparison f.
    decubitus f.
    f. diameter
    f. fog
    horizontal beam f.
    latitude f.
    left lateral decubitus f.
    occlusal f.
    overhead f.
    PA chest f.
    plain f.
    Polaroid f.
    portable chest f.
    postevacuation f.
    postvoiding f.
    right lateral decubitus f.
    scout f.
    silver halide f.
    f. speed
    spot f.
    survey f.
    wide-latitude f.
filming
    biplane axial f.
    sequential f.

filter
Amplatz-Lund retrievable f.
band-pass f.
basket f.
Berkefeld f.
bird's nest f.
Cragg f.
flattening f.
Gianturco bird's nest f.
Gianturco-Roehm bird's nest vena cava f.
Greenfield f.
Greenfield titanium inferior vena cava f.
Günther f.
Hanning window-type low-pass f.
helix f.
high-pass f.
inferior vena cava f.
inferior vena cava umbrella f.
inherent f.
Kim-Ray Greenfield caval f.
leukocyte f.
low-pass f.
Lund-Amplatz retrievable f.
Millipore f.
Mobin-Uddin f.
Mobin-Uddin umbrella f
MU f.
Nitinol f.
Nitinol inferior vena cava f.
Palestrant/Simon f.
Pall f.
Pall ELD-96 Set Saver f.
Pall leukocyte removal f.
Pall transfusion f.
rhodium f.
sigma f.
Simon f.
Simon-Nitinol inferior vena cava f.
superior vena cava f.
temporal f.
Thoreau f.

titanium Greenfield vena cava f.
umbrella f.
vena cava f.
Vena Tech dual vena cava f.
wall f.
filtered back projection
filtering
low-pass f.
phase f.
filtration
beam f.
gel f.
filum terminale
fimbriated
finasteride
finding
equivocal f.
laboratory f.
roentgenographic f.
fine-needle
f.-n. aspiration (FNA)
f.-n. aspiration biopsy (FNAB)
f.-n. biopsy
f.-n. transhepatic cholangiography
finger
hypocratic f.'s
tapered f.'s
finger-in-the-glove mucous plug
fingerized hypoplastic thumb
finger-like mucous plug
fingerprinting
DNA f.
fingerstick blood sample
fingertip calcification
firearm injury
Firooznia
threshold of F.
first
f. carpal row
f. echelon lymph node
f. generation regimen
first-degree heart block

NOTES

first-pass
    f.-p. cardiac perfusion
    f.-p. extraction
first-set phenomenon
First Temp Genius tympanic
    thermometer
FISH
    fluorescence in situ
    hybridization
Fisher exact test
Fisher-Race theory
fishmouth fracture
fishtail vertebra
Fisk and Subbarow method
Fisons nebulizer
FISP
    fast imaging with steady-state
    free precession
    FISP pulse sequence
fissure
    accessory f.
    azygos f.
    bulging f.
    choroidal f.
    f. fracture
    inferior accessory f.
    interlobar f.
    ligamentum venosum f.
    longitudinal f.
    lung f.
    major f.
    minor f.
    nasopalatal f.
    oblique f.
    f. of Rolando
    f. sign
    superior orbital f.
    sylvian f.
    f. of Sylvius
fist fornication
fisting
    anal f.
    rectal f.
fistula, pl. fistulae
    aortoenteric f.
    arterial-arterial f.
    arterial-portal f.
    arteriobiliary f.
    arterioportobiliary f.
    arteriosinusoidal f.
    arteriosinusoidal penile f.
    arteriovenous f. (AVF)
    AV f.

    biliary-enteric f.
    BP f.
    Brescia-Cimino f.
    bronchoesophageal f.
    bronchopleural f.
    bronchopulmonary f.
    carotid cavernous sinus f.
    carotid-dural f.
    cavernous sinus f.
    cholecystocolic f.
    cholecystoduodenal f.
    choledochoduodenal f.
    colovaginal f.
    colovesical f.
    communicating f.
    congenital arteriovenous f.
    congenital tracheobiliary f.
    dialysis f.
    dural arteriovenous f.
    enteric f.
    enterocolic f.
    enterocutaneous f.
    enterovaginal f.
    esophagotracheal f.
    gastrocutaneous f.
    gastrointestinal f.
    gastrojejunocolic f.
    hepatic artery-portal vein f.
    hepatoportal biliary f.
    H-type f.
    H-type tracheoesophageal f.
    iatrogenic arteriovenous f.
    intracranial arteriovenous f.
    intrahepatic arterial-portal f.
    labyrinthine f.
    postbiopsy renal AV f.
    pulmonary arteriovenous f.
    rectovaginal f.
    spinal dural arteriovenous f.
    TE f.
    tracheobiliary f.
    tracheobronchoesophageal f.
    tracheoesophageal f. (TEF)
    ureteral f.
    ureteroperitoneal f.
    ureterovaginal f.
    urinary f.
    venobiliary f.
    vesicovaginal f.
fistular formation
fistulogram
    cine f.
    venous f.

fistulous tract
fit
    smoothed curve f.
Fitzgerald factor
Fitz-Hugh and Curtis syndrome
FIVB
    5-fluorouracil, imidazole
    (dacarbazine), vincristine,
    BCNU (carmustine)
five L analysis
five-year cure rate
fixation
    catheter f.
    complement f.
    metallic rod f.
    microwave f.
    open reduction and
      internal f. (ORIF)
fixative
    B5 f.
    tannic acid f.
fixed
    f. macrophage
    f. perfusion defect
FK-506
FL
    femoral length
flabrata
    Torulopsis f.
flaccid
flaccidity
flag
    Rudick red f.'s
    f. sign
flagellantism
flagellate pigmentation
FLAG-ida
    fludarabine, ara-C, G-CSF,
      idarubicin
flail
    f. chest
    f. mitral valve
FLAIR
    fluid attenuated inversion
    recovery
    FLAIR pulse sequence

FLAK
    flow artifact killer
    FLAK technique
flame
    f. emission spectroscopy
    (FES)
    f. ionization detector
flammeus
    nevus f.
    osteohypertrophic nevus f.
flange
    shaft f.
flank
    f. pain
    f. stripe
flap
    bladder f.
    bone f.
    foramen ovale f.
    intimal f.
    Karapandzic f.
    Limberg f.
    McFarlane skin f.
    myocutaneous f.
    postangioplasty intimal f.
    rectus abdominis
      musculocutaneous f.
    rectus abdominis
      myocutaneous f.
    f. tear
flare
    hormonal f.
    optical f.
    f. phenomenon
FLASH
    fast low-angle shot
    FLASH magnetic resonance
    imaging
    FLASH pulse sequence
flash
    f. photolysis
flat colorectal carcinoma
flatfoot
flattening filter
flatulence
flava
    ligamenta f.

NOTES

flavone
f. acetic acid (FAA)
flavoprotein
flavum
ligamentum f.
flavus
Aspergillus f.
Fleckinger view
Fleischner
F. line
F. sign
FLEP
5-FU, leucovorin, Platinol
Fletcher
F. factor
F. rule of irradiation
tolerance
**Fletcher-Suit system for radium
therapy**
flexible
f. biopsy needle
f. bronchoscope
f. endofluoroscopy
f. fiberoptic bronchoscopy
f. forceps
f. nephroscope
flexion
f. contracture
f. deformity
f. and extension exercises
f. and extension views
f. teardrop fracture
f. view
flexneri
Shigella f.
Flexner-Wintersteiner rosette
flexor
f. carpi radialis
f. carpi ulnaris
f. digiti minimi
f. digiti minimi brevis
f. digitorum brevis
f. digitorum longus
f. digitorum profundus
f. digitorum superficialis
f. hallucis brevis
f. hallucis longus
f. pollicis brevis
f. pollicis longus
f. retinaculum
f. superficialis
f. tendon

flexure
hepatic f.
splenic f.
FLIC
Functional Living Index-Cancer
flight
time of f.
flinic acid rescue
Flint Colon Injury Scale
flip
f. angle
spin f.
flip-angle image
flip-flop phenomenon
floating
f. gallbladder
f. gallstone
f. kidney
f. teeth
flocculation
Ramon f.
floor
f. of mouth
f. of the orbit
floppy
f. mitral valve
f. thumb sign
f. valve syndrome
floppy-tip wire
flora
endogenous f.
exogenous f.
intestinal f.
microbial f.
florid follicular hyperplasia
flos-aquae
Aphanizomenon f.-a.
flow
absolute blood f.
antegrade f.
f. artifact
axoplasmic f.
bile f.
blood f.
cerebral blood f. (CBF)
collateral blood f.
f. compensated image
f. compensation
f. of contrast material
f. cytometric analysis
f. cytometric DNA
measurement
f. cytometry

f. cytometry sample preparation
f. cytometry technique
f. dynamics
f. effect artifact
effective renal plasma f.
helical blood f.
hepatofugal f.
hepatopedal f.
hypothalamic blood f.
intrarenal arterial f.
laminar f.
laminar air f.
f. mode ultrafast computed tomography
myocardial blood f.
f. pattern
peritrophoblastic f.
pharmacologic maintenance erection f.
f. phenomenon
plug f.
portal f.
f. portion of bone scan
f. profile
pulmonary blood f.
f. rate
regional cerebral blood f.
turbulent f.
unequal pulmonary blood f.
f. velocity
f. velocity waveform
f. void
f. volume curve
f. volume loop
zero net f.
flow artifact killer (FLAK)
flower cell
flowmetry
Doppler f.
flow-on gradient-echo image
flow-related
f.-r. enhancement
f.-r. enhancement artifact
f.-r. phase error
flow-sensitive MR imaging

flow-void effect
floxuridine (FUDR)
circadian-modified f. (FUdR)
f. in hepatic metastases
intraarterial f.
fluconazole
flucytosine
Fludara
fludarabine
f. monophosphate (FAMP)
f. phosphate
fludarabine, ara-C, G-CSF, idarubicin (FLAG-ida)
fludeoxyglucose F18
fluence
energy f.
flufenamic acid
fluffy periosteal reaction
fluid
amniotic f.
ascitic f.
f. attenuated inversion recovery (FLAIR)
cerebrospinal f. (CSF)
f. collection
Collison f.
cystic f.
f. embolic agent
encapsulated f.
extracellular f.
free peritoneal f.
f. intake
intravenous f.
f. level
loculated pleural f.
loculation of f.
f. overload
pericardial f.
pericholecystic f.
perigraft f.
peritoneal f.
peritoneal cavity f.
pleural f.
f. retention
silicone f.
straw-colored f.

NOTES

fluid *(continued)*
    subphrenic f.
    f. vascular-occluding agent
fluid-filled
fluid-fluid level
fluke
    blood f.
    Chinese liver f.
    liver f.
    Oriental lung f.
flumazenil
fluorenylacetamide
    N-2 f.
fluorescein isothiocyanate
fluorescence
    f. detector
    f. polarization
    f. in situ hybridization
      (FISH)
    f. yield
fluorescence-activated cell sorter
fluorescens
    Pseudomonas *f.*
fluorescent
    f. antibody
    f. antibody technique
    f. auramine-rhodamine stain
    f. cytoprint assay
    f. shift
    f. treponemal antibody virus
      (FTA-ABS)
fluoride
    f. therapy
    yttrium lithium f. (YLF)
fluorine
fluorine-18
fluorine-19
    f.-19 spectroscopy
fluormethane
fluoro-6-thia-heptadecanoic acid
fluoroacylated biotin
fluorobenzyl-ABV
fluorocaptopril
fluorochrome
fluorodeoxyglucose
fluorodeoxyglucose-6-phosphate
fluorodeoxyuridine (FUdR)
5-fluoro-2-deoxyuridine (FUdR)
5-fluorodeoxyuridylate (5-FdUMP)
fluorodopa
6-fluorodopa
fluoroestradiol
fluoro-16α-ethyl-19-norprogesterone

fluorometer
    96-well scanning f.
β-fluoromethylene-m-tyrosine
fluoromibolerone
fluoromisonidazole
Fluoroplex
fluoropropylepidepride
fluoropyrimidine
Fluoroscan C-arm fluoroscopy
fluoroscopic
    f. guidance
    f. pushing technique
    f. technique
fluoroscopy
    C-arm f.
    Fluoroscan C-arm f.
    rapid scan f.
    video f.
fluorosis
fluorotropapride
fluorotyrosine
fluorouracil
5-fluorouracil (5-FU)
5-fluorouracil, Adriamycin,
    cyclophosphamide (FAC)
5-fluorouracil, Adriamycin, methyl-
    CCNU (FAMe)
5-fluorouracil, Adriamycin,
    mitomycin (FAM)
5-fluorouracil, imidazole
    (dacarbazine), vincristine, BCNU
    (carmustine) (FIVB)
fluorouridine
FluoroVision
Fluosol
Fluosol-DA
fluoxetine
fluoxymesterone
flurbiprofen
flush
    serotonin f.
flushing technique
flutamide
flutter
    atrial f.
flux
    magnetic f.
FM
    fetal movement
^{255}Fm
    fermium-255
FMD

FMISO
F-misonidazole
F-misonidazole (FMISO)
FMLP
N-formyl-1-methionyl-1-leucyl-1-
phenylalamine
fms **oncogene**
FNA
fine-needle aspiration
FNA biopsy
FNAB
fine-needle aspiration biopsy
FNH
focal nodular hyperplasia
foam
f. cell
polyvinyl alcohol f.
foamy histiocyte
focal
f. adhesion kinase protein
f. alimentary tract
calcification
f. atelectasis of the
newborn
f. atrophy
f. bacterial nephritis
f. caliectasis
f. cerebral ischemia
f. cerebral syndrome
f. change
f. cortical hyperplasia
f. fibrosis
f. gallbladder wall
thickening
f. intestinal inflammatory
disease
f. ischemia
f. length
f. limb abnormality
f. lobular carcinoma
f. lung disease
f. nodular hyperplasia
(FNH)
f. pancreatitis
f. parenchymal brain lesion
f. pathology
f. pyloric hypertrophy

f. renal hypertrophy
f. sclerosis
f. splenic lesion
f. spot
f. spot blur
f. spot size
f. zone
focally dilated duct
foculin protein
focus, pl. foci
multizone transmit-receive f.
Simon f.
focused grid
focused, segmented, ultrasound
machine (FSUM)
focusing
zone f.
fog
f. artifact
film f.
Fogarty
F. balloon biliary catheter
F. balloon catheter
F. catheter
F. embolectomy catheter
F. gallstone catheter
F. irrigation catheter
F. venous thrombectomy
catheter
fogging phenomenon
folate
f. antagonist
f. polyglutamylation system
f. uptake pathway
fold
aryepiglottic f.
crescentic submucosal f.
epiglottic f.
gastric f.
glossoepiglottic f.
hidebound small bowel f.
Kerckring f.
mucosal f.
rugal f.
semilunar f.
skin f.
small bowel f.

NOTES

fold *(continued)*
    submucosal f.
    submucosal circular f.
    thickened f.
    uteric f.
folded lung
foldover
    image f.
Folex
Foley catheter
folic
    f. acid
    f. acid antagonist
Folin
    F. method
    F. and Wu method
folinic acid
follicle
    geographic f.
    graafian f.
    inverse f.
    lollipop f.
    luteinized unruptured f.
    f. lysis
    neoplastic f.
    ovarian f.
follicle-stimulating hormone
follicular
    f. adenocarcinoma of
      thyroid
    f. adenoma
    f. bronchiolitis
    f. bronchitis
    f. carcinoma
    f. cyst
    f. dendritic cell
    f. dendritic sarcoma
    f. gastritis
    f. hyperplasia
    f. involution
    f. lymphoma
    f. mucinosis
    f. pattern
    f. predominantly large cell
    f. predominantly small
      cleaved cell
follicularis
    cystitis f.
    enteritis f.
folliculitis
    staphylococcal f.
folliculorum
    Demodex f.

follow-through
    GI series and small
      bowel f.-t.
followup (noun, adjective),
    follow up (verb)
folylpolyglutamate synthetase
Fong disease
Fonio solution
Fontan
    F. patient
    F. procedure
    F. repair
fontanel, fontanelle
Food
    F. and Drug Administration
      (FDA)
food bolus
foot
    f. deformity
    diabetic f.
    rocker-bottom f.
football sign
foot-drop
footprinting
    DNA f.
    DNAse f.
foramen, pl. foramina
    alveolar foramina
    anterior condyloid f.
    anterior palatine f.
    anterior sacral f.
    aortic f.
    Bichat f.
    f. of Bochdalek
    Bochdalek f.
    Botallo f.
    carotid f.
    cervical neural f.
    Duverney f.
    emissary sphenoidal f.
    epiploic f.
    ethmoid f.
    external acoustic f.
    Ferrein f.
    Huschke f.
    Hyrtl f.
    interventricular f.
    jugular f.
    f. lacerum
    f. of Luschka
    Magendie f.
    f. magnum
    mandibular f.

mastoid f.
f. of Monro
neural f.
nutrient f.
obturator f.
optic f.
f. ovale
f. ovale flap
palatine f.
parietal f.
petrosal f.
Retzius f.
f. rotundum
sacral f.
f. spinosum
Stenson f.
stylomastoid f.
supraorbital f.
f. transversarium
f. venosum
vertebral f.
f. of Vesalius
Weitbrecht f.
f. of Winslow
zygomaticofacial f.
foraminal stenosis
force
DES task f.
electromotive f.
repulsive f.
shearing f.
forced expiratory volume
forceps
alligator f.
Dieffenbach serrifine f.
flexible f.
laryngeal f.
Mazzariello-Caprini f.
Randall f.
rigid f.
forearm
f. fracture
forebrain
forefoot
foregut
bronchopulmonary f.

foreign
f. body
f. body carcinogenesis
f. body embolization
f. body embolus
f. body granuloma
f. material artifact
forensic radiology
foreshortened
Forestier disease
form
band f.
cribriform f.
Discrene breast f.
Nearly Me breast f.
ring-shaped f.
formaldehyde
formalin
formation
antiantibody f.
Burnet-Talmadge-Lederberg
theory of antibody f.
callus f.
cataract f.
cloacal f.
colony f.
Ehrlich theory of
antibody f.
excessive callus f.
fistular f.
heterotopic bone f.
image f.
Jerne theory of antibody f.
neointima f.
osteophyte f.
pannus f.
Pauling theory of
antibody f.
periosteal new bone f.
pseudopod f.
reticular f.
forme fruste
formula
Glendenin-Coryell f.
rapid dissolution f. (RDF)
Somacin f.

NOTES

formulation
drug f.
lyophilized recombinant
interferon f.
fornication
fist f.
fornix, pl. fornices
vaginal f.
forskolin
Forssman
F. antibody
F. antigen
Fortaz
fortuitum
Mycobacterium f.
Forty
Model F.
forward angle light scatter
foscarnet sodium
fos **proto-oncogene**
fossa, pl. fossae
acetabular f.
antecubital f.
coronoid f.
cranial f.
glenoid f.
hypoglossal f.
infratemporal f.
intratemporal f.
mandibular f.
meningioma of posterior f.
mesentericoparietal f.
middle cranial f.
f. navicularis
ovarian f.
paraduodenal f.
pararectal f.
paravesical f.
pituitary f.
popliteal f.
posterior f.
posterior pituitary f.
pterygoid f.
pterygopalatine f.
rectouterine f.
rhomboid f.
f. of Rosenmüller
supraclavicular f.
temporal f.
uterovesical f.
Waldeyer f.
Foster-Kennedy syndrome
fotemustine

Fouchet test
Foundation
Berlix Oncology F.
Candlelighters Childhood
Cancer F. (CCCF)
Fourier
F. analysis
F. imaging
F. imaging technique
F. optical theory
F. transfer
F. transform
F. transformation
F. transform imaging
Fourier-acquired steady-state
technique (FAST)
Fournier
F. gangrene
four-part fracture
four-point assay
four-quadrant bar pattern
FOV
field of view
fovea capitis
Fowler position
FPA
Asserachrom FPA
fraction
f. 5
creatine kinase MB
isoenzyme f.
dose per f.
drug f.
ejection f.
growth f.
left ventricular ejection f.
plasma f.
plasma protein f.
quiescent f.
regurgitant f.
shunt f.
S-phase f.
fractional cell kill
fractionated
f. dose-survival curve
f. external beam irradiation
f. irradiation
f. radiation therapy
fractionation
accelerated f.
co-alcohol f.
dose f.
S-phase f.

fracture
- abduction-external rotation f.
- acetabular f.
- acetabular posterior wall f.
- acetabular rim f.
- acute f.
- Aebi-Etter-Coscia fixation dens f.
- agenetic f.
- anatomic f.
- Anderson-Hutchins tibial f.
- angulated f.
- ankle f.
- ankle mortise f.
- anterior column f.
- anterolateral compression f.
- apophyseal f.
- arch f.
- articular mass separation f.
- articular pillar f.
- Ashhurst-Bromer classification of ankle f.'s
- Atkin epiphyseal f.
- atlas f.
- atrophic f.
- avulsion f.
- avulsion stress f.
- axis f.
- backfire f.
- banana f.
- Bankart f.
- Barton f.
- Barton-Smith f.
- basal neck f.
- baseball finger f.
- basilar femoral neck f.
- bayonet position of f.
- beak f.
- bedroom f.
- Bennett f.
- Bennett comminuted f.
- bicondylar f.
- bicondylar T-shaped f.
- bicondylar Y-shaped f.
- bicycle spoke f.
- bimalleolar f.

- birth f.
- f. blister
- blow-in f.
- blow-out f.
- boot-top f.
- Bosworth f.
- both-bone f.
- both-column f.
- bowing f.
- boxer's f.
- f. bracing
- bronchial f.
- bucket-handle f.
- buckle f.
- bumper f.
- bunk bed f.
- Burkhalter-Reyes method of phalangeal f.
- burst f.
- butterfly f.
- buttonhole f.
- calcaneal f.
- calcaneal avulsion f.
- calcaneal displaced f.
- f. callus
- f. callus loading
- capitate f.
- capitellar f.
- capitulum radiale humeri f.
- carpal bone f.
- carpal bone stress f.
- carpometacarpal joint f.
- cartwheel f.
- cementum f.
- central f.
- cephalomedullary nail f.
- cerebral palsy pathological f.
- cervical spine f.
- cervicotrochanteric f.
- Chance f.
- Chaput f.
- chauffeur's f.
- chip f.
- chiropractic treatment f.
- chisel f.
- chondral f.
- circumferential f.

NOTES

fracture *(continued)*
clavicular f.
clavicular birth f.
clay shoveler's f.
cleavage f.
closed f.
coccyx f.
Colles f.
combined flexion-distraction
  injury and burst f.
combined radial-ulnar-
  humeral f.
comminuted f.
comminuted intraarticular f.
complete f.
complex f.
composite f.
compound f.
compound, comminuted f.
compression f.
condylar f.
congenital f.
contrecoup f.
coracoid f.
corner f.
coronal slit f.
coronoid process f.
cortical f.
Cotton ankle f.
crush f.
"crushed eggshell" f.
Danis-Weber f.
dashboard f.
Denis Browne classification
  of sacral f.'s
dens f.
depressed f.
depressed skull f.
depression f.
de Quervain f.
Descot f.
diametric pelvic f.
diaphyseal f.
diastatic f.
dicondylar f.
die punch f.
dislocation f.
displaced f.
distal femoral epiphyseal f.
distal humoral f.
distal radial f.
distraction of f.
dogleg f.

dome f.
double f.
Dupuytren f.
Duverney f.
dyscrasic f.
El-Ahwany classification of
  humeral supracondylar f.'s
elbow f.
electrostimulation for
  nonunion of f.
elementary f.
Ellis technique for
  Barton f.
f. en coin
endocrine f.
f. en rave
epicondylar f.
epiphyseal f.
epiphyseal growthplate f.
epiphyseal plate f.
epiphyseal slip f.
epiphyseal tibial f.
Essex-Lopresti f.
Essex-Lopresti joint
  depression f.
explosion f.
extension teardrop f.
extracapsular f.
extraoctave f.
facial f.
fatigue f.
femoral f.
femoral intertrochanteric f.
femoral neck f.
femoral shaft f.
femoral supracondylar f.
fender f.
fetal bone f.
f. fever
fibular f.
Fielding-Magliato
  classification of
  subtrochanteric f.'s
fighter's f.
fishmouth f.
fissure f.
flexion teardrop f.
forearm f.
four-part f.
f. fragment
f. frame
frontal f.
Gaenslen f.

Galeazzi f.
f. gap
Garden femoral neck f.
Gartland classification of
  humeral supracondylar f.
glenoid f.
glenoid rim f.
Gosselin f.
Grantham classification of
  femoral f.
greater trochanteric
  femoral f.
greater tuberosity f.
greenstick f.
gunshot f.
Gustilo-Anderson open
  clavicular f.
Hahn-Steinthal f.
hairline f.
hamate f.
hamate tail f.
hangman's f.
Hansen classification of f.'s
Hawkins classification of
  talar f.'s
head-splitting humeral f.
healing f.
hemicondylar f.
Henderson f.
Hormodooon f.
hickory-stick f.
Hoffa f.
Holstein-Lewis f.
hook of the hamate f.
hoop stress f.
horizontal f.
humeral f.
humeral head-splitting f.
humeral physeal f.
humeral supracondylar f.
Hutchinson f.
ice skater's f.
ileofemoral wing f.
impacted f.
implant f.
impression f.
incomplete f.

inflammatory f.
infraction f.
Ingram-Bachynski
  classification of hip f.'s
insufficiency f.
intercondylar f.
intercondylar femoral f.
intercondylar humeral f.
intercondylar tibial f.
internal fixation f.
interperiosteal f.
intertrochanteric f.
intertrochanteric four-part f.
intraarticular f.
intraarticular proximal
  tibial f.
intracapsular f.
intraoperative f.
inverted-Y f.
ipsilateral femoral neck f.
ipsilateral femoral shaft f.
irreducible f.
Jefferson f.
Jeffery classification of
  radial f.'s
joint f.
joint depression f.
Jones f.
juxtacortical f.
Key-Conwell classification of
  pelvic f.'s
Kilfoyle classification of
  condylar f.'s
knee f.
Kocher f.
LaGrange classification of
  humeral supracondylar f.'s
laminar f.
lap seatbelt f.
lateral condylar humeral f.
lateral malleolar f.
lateral tibial plateau f.
Lauge-Hansen classification
  of ankle f.'s
Laugier f.
lead pipe f.
Le Fort f.

NOTES

fracture *(continued)*
Le Fort fibular f.
Le Fort mandibular f.
Le Fort-Wagstaffe f.
lesser trochanteric f.
f. line
linear f.
f. line of consolidation
Lisfranc f.
Lloyd-Roberts open
  reduction of Monteggia f.
long oblique f.
loose f.
lorry driver's f.
low-energy f.
lumbar spine f.
lumbar spine burst f.
Maisonneuve f.
Maisonneuve fibular f.
malar f.
Malgaigne f.
Malgaigne pelvic f.
malleolar f.
mallet f.
malunited f.
March f.
marginal f.
Mathews classification of
  olecranon f.'s
maxillofacial f.
metacarpal f.
metaphyseal f.
metatarsal f.
Meyers-McKeever
  classification of tibial f.'s
midfoot f.
midshaft f.
Milch classification of
  humeral f.'s
milkman's f.
minipilon f.
Moberg-Gedda f.
molar tooth f.
monomalleolar f.
Monteggia f.
Montercaux f.
Moore f.
Mouchet f.
multangular ridge f.
multiray f.
nasoorbital f.
navicular f.
naviculocapitate f.

f. of necessity
neck f.
Neer-Horowitz classification
  of humeral f.'s
neoplastic f.
neurogenic f.
neuropathic f.
Newman classification of
  radial neck and head f.'s
nightstick f.
noncontiguous f.
nondisplaced f.
nonphyseal f.
nonrotational burst f.
f. nonunion
nonunited f.
nutcracker f.
oblique f.
O'Brien classification of
  radial f.'s
obturator avulsion f.
occipital condyle f.
occult f.
odontoid f.
odontoid condyle f.
Ogden classification of
  epiphyseal f.'s
olecranon f.
one-part f.
open-book f.
open-break f.
orbital f.
osteochondral f.
osteochondral slice f.
Pais f.
Papavasiliou classification of
  olecranon f.'s
paratrooper's f.
pars interarticularis f.
patellar f.
patellar sleeve f.
pathologic f.
Pauwels f.
pedicle f.
pelvic f.
pelvic ring f.
pelvic straddle f.
penetrating f.
periarticular f.
periprosthetic f.
peritrochanteric f.
phalangeal f.
phalangeal diaphyseal f.

physeal f.
Piedmont f.
pillion f.
pillow f.
pilon f.
pilon ankle f.
ping-pong f.
Pipkin classification of
  femoral f.'s
pisiform f.
plafond f.
plastic bowing f.
Poland classification of
  epiphyseal f.'s
Posada f.
posterior arch f.
posterior element f.
posterior ring f.
posterior wall f.
postirradiation f.
postoperative f.
Pott f.
Pott ankle f.
pronation-abduction f.
pronation-eversion f.
proximal femoral f.
proximal humeral f.
proximal tibial f.
proximal tibial
  metaphyseal f.
pyramidal f.
Quinby classification of
  pelvic f.'s
radial f.
radial head f.
radial neck f.
radial styloid f.
f. reduction
reverse Barton f.
reverse Colles f.
reverse Monteggia f.
rib f.
ring f.
ring-disrupting f.
Riseborough-Radin
  classification of
  intercondylar f.

Rockwood classification of
  clavicular f.
Rolando f.
rotational f.
rotational burst f.
sacral f.
sacroiliac f.
Sakellarides classification of
  calcaneal f.'s
Salter-Harris f.
Salter-Harris classification of
  epiphyseal f.'s
Salter I-IV f.
scaphoid f.
scottie dog f.
seatbelt f.
secondary f.
Segond f.
Seinsheimer classification of
  femoral f.'s
sentinel f.
SER-IV f.
shaft f.
shear f.
Shepherd f.
short oblique f.
sideswipe f.
f. site
skier's f.
Skillern f.
skull f.
sleeve f.
Smith f.
Sorbie classification of
  calcaneal f.
spinal f.
spinous process f.
spiral f.
spiral oblique f.
split f.
split-heel f.
splitting f.
spontaneous f.
sprain f.
sprinter's f.
stability of f.
stairstep f.

NOTES

fracture *(continued)*
  stellate f.
  Stieda f.
  straddle f.
  stress f.
  strut f.
  subcapital f.
  subperiosteal f.
  subtrochanteric f.
  supination-adduction f.
  supination-eversion f.
  supination-external rotation
    IV f.
  supracondylar humeral f.
  supracondylar Y-shaped f.
  T-f.
  talar f.
  talar avulsion f.
  talar neck f.
  talar osteochondral f.
  T-condylar f.
  teacup f.
  teardrop f.
  temporal bone f.
  tension f.
  testis f.
  Thompson-Epstein
    classification of
    femoral f.'s
  thoracic spine f.
  thoracolumbar spine f.
  three-part f.
  through-and-through f.
  thrower's f.
  tibial f.
  tibial bending f.
  tibial condyle f.
  tibial diaphyseal f.
  tibial open f.
  tibial plafond f.
  tibial plateau f.
  tibial shaft f.
  tibial triplane f.
  tibial tuberosity f.
  Tillaux f.
  Tillaux-Chaput f.
  Tillaux-Kleiger f.
  toddler's f.
  tongue f.
  torsional f.
  torus f.
  tracheal f.
  traction f.

  trampoline f.
  transcaphoid f.
  transcapitate f.
  transcervical femoral f.
  transchondral f.
  transcondylar f.
  transepiphyseal f.
  transhamate f.
  transiliac f.
  transsacral f.
  transscaphoid dislocation f.
  transtriquetral f.
  transverse f.
  transversely oriented
    endplate compression f.
  transverse process f.
  trapezium f.
  trimalleolar f.
  trimalleolar ankle f.
  triplane f.
  tripod f.
  triquetral f.
  Tronzo classification of
    intertrochanteric f.'s
  trophic f.
  tuft f.
  two-part f.
  ulnar f.
  uncinate process f.
  undisplaced f.
  unicondylar f.
  unimalleolar f.
  unstable f.
  ununited f.
  vertebral body f.
  vertebral compression f.
  vertebra plana f.
  vertebral wedge
    compression f.
  vertical sheer f.
  Volkmann f.
  Vostal classification of
    radial f.'s
  wagon wheel f.
  Wagstaffe f.
  Walther f.
  Watson-Jones classification
    of tibial tubercle
    avulsion f.'s
  wedge f.
  wedge compression f.
  "western boot" in open f.

Wilkins classification of
  radial f.'s
willow f.
Wilson f.
Winquist-Hansen
  classification of
  femoral f.'s
Y-f.
Y-T f.
zygomaticomaxillary f.
fracture-dislocation
  Galeazzi f.-d.
  pedicolaminar f.-d.
fractured kidney
fragilitas ossium
fragilocytosis
fragment
  f. antigen binding (Fab)
  avulsed f.
  extruded disk f.
  Fab f.
  Fc f.
  fracture f.
  free disk f.
  iodine-125-labeled f.
  Klenow f.
  metallic f.
  overriding of fracture f.'s
  retropulsion of posterior f.
  Spengler f.
  trap door f.
fragmentation
  electrohydraulic f.
  nuclear f.
frame
  Brown-Roberston-Wells f.
  fracture f.
  nonferromagnetic MR-
    compatible f.
  f. of reference
  stereotaxic localization f.
  Stryker f.
framework region
frank
  f. congestive failure
  f. pulmonary edema
  f. pus

Fränkel
  F. classification system
  F. white line
Franklin-Silverman biopsy needle
Frank-Starling curve
Franseen needle
fraternal twin
Fraunfelder technique
Fraunhofer zone
frayed
  f. metaphyses
  f. string appearance
F reagent
Frederick-Miller tube
Fred Hutchinson Cancer Research
  Center
free
  f. air
  f. disk fragment
  f. fragment herniation
  f. gas bubble
  f. induction decay
  f. macrophage
  f. peritoneal fluid
  f. precession
  f. radical
  f. radical scavenging system
  f. thyroxine index
  f. water
freehand method
freeze-dried paraffin-embedded
  tissue
freezing process
Frei antigen
Freiberg
  F. disease
  F. infraction
fremitus
French
  F. pigtail catheter
  F. spring-eye needle
French/American/British (FAB)
  FAB classification
frequency
  angular f.
  f. component
  cutoff f.

NOTES

frequency *(continued)*
   disappearance f.
   f. domain
   Doppler f.
   Doppler shift f.
   f. encoding
   f. estimation
   false f.
   f. intensification
   Larmor f.
   Nyquist f.
   precessional f.
   pulse repetition f.
   f. range
   resonance f.
   resonant f.
   rotational f.
   f. separation
   spatial f.
   f. spectrum
   f. synthesizer
frequency-following response
frequency-selective
   f.-s. inversion
   f.-s. pulse
Frerich theory
fresh
   f. cell suspension
   f. frozen plasma
   f. thrombotic occlusion
   f. tissue allocation
   f. water drowning
fresh-frozen tissue section
Fresnel zone plate
Freund
   F. adjuvant
   F. complete adjuvant (FCA)
fribroadenoma
Friedländer bacillus
Friedrich disease
Friend
   F. leukemia virus
   F. virus
FRODO technique
frog-leg
   f.-l. lateral projection
   f.-l. view of the hips
frondosum
   chorion f.
frontal
   f. abscess
   f. arteriovenous
     malformation

   f. artery
   f. bone
   f. bossing of Parrot
   f. fracture
   f. horn
   f. lobe
   f. nerve
   f. sinus
   f. sinus mucocele
frontier ulcer
frontoethmoidal
   f. encephalocele
   f. mucocele
frontonasal
   f. dysplasia
   f. dysplasia malformation
     complex
frontoparietal arteriovenous
  malformation
frontopolar artery
Frostberg-3 sign
Frostberg inverted-3 sign
frostbite
frozen
   f. red cell
   f. shoulder
   f. tissue section
fruste
   forme f.
FS test
FSUM
   focused, segmented, ultrasound
     machine
Ft
   ftorafur
FTA-ABS
   fluorescent treponemal antibody
     virus
ftorafur (Ft)
FT tumor marker
5-FU
   5-fluorouracil
     5-FU deoxyribonucleoside
     leucovorin-modulated 5-FU
     5-FU, leucovorin, Platinol
      (FLEP)
     LV + 5-FU
Fuchs
   F. adenoma
   F. odontoid view
   F. position
   F. principle

FUDR
floxuridine
FUdR
circadian-modified floxuridine
fluorodeoxyuridine
5-fluoro-2-deoxyuridine
fugax
amaurosis f.
coxitis f.
Fukuyama-type congenital muscular dystrophy
fulguration
f. in bladder cancer
nephroscopic f.
full-column view
Fuller earth pneumoconiosis
fullerene
full-intensity needle
full-width-at-half-maximum of lorentzian curve
fulminant hepatitis
fumarate
liarozole f.
fumigatus
Aspergillus f.
function
cell f.
ciliary f.
delta f.
detector transfer f.
edge spread f.
erectile f.
factor VIII coagulation f.
fetal renal f.
gaussian f.
gonadal f.
hematopoietic f.
left ventricular f.
line spread f.
MALT f.
menstrual f.
modulation transfer f.
myocardial f.
neuromuscular f.
ovarian f.
point spread f.
renal f.

Salmon-Durie staging f.
sexual f.
survival f.
systolic f.
thyroid f.
time activity f.
tubular f.
ventricular f.
white blood cell f.
functional
f. activation
f. asplenia
F. Assessment of Cancer Therapy (FACT)
f. bowel syndrome
f. endoscopic sinus surgery (FESS)
f. imaging
f. independent measurement score
F. Living Index-Cancer (FLIC)
f. neuroimaging
f. ovarian cyst
f. residual capacity
fundoplication
Nissen f.
fundus, pl. fundi
saddle-shaped uterine f.
fungal infection
fungating tumor
fungoides
mycosis f.
tumor d'emblee mycosis f.
fungus, pl. fungi
f. ball
funiculi gracilis
funnel chest deformity
funnel-like cardiomegaly
Fura
furazolidone
furfur
Malassezia f.
furifosmin
technetium-99m f.
furosemide
furunculosis

NOTES

Fusarium
fused
    f. kidney
    f. vertebrae
fusiform
    f. aneurysm
    f. bronchiectasis
    f. dilatation

fusion
    cervical spine f.
    interbody f.
    müllerian duct formation
      and f.
    f. peptide
    spinal f.
Fy antigen

G

    gauss
        G cell hyperplasia
        G cell tumor
        G protein
        G proto-oncogene

G1

    immunoglobulin G1

Ga

    gallium

^{67}Ga

    gallium-67

gabapentin
gadodiamide
gadolinium

    g. chelate
    g. cyclohexanediaminetetraacetic acid (Gd-CDTA)
    g. ethylenediaminetetraacetic acid (Gd-EDTA)
    g. iron
    g. sucralfate
    g. tetraazacyclododecanetetraacetic acid (Gd-DOTA)

gadolinium 153
gadolinium-diethylenetriamine pentaacetic acid (Gd-DTPA)
gadolinium-DTPA (Gd-DTPA)
gadolinium-enhanced MR imaging
gadopentetate

    g. dimeglumine (Gd-DTPA)

gadopentetic acid
gadopentolate-polylysine
gadoteridol (Gd-HP-DO3A)
Gaenslen fracture
gag

    g. gene
    g. protein

Gage sign
gain

    accelerated phase g.
    brightness g.
    color g.
    phase g.
    power g.
    quadratic phase g.
    swept g.
    time-compensated g.
    time-varied g.

Gaisbock disease
gait

    antalgic g.
    g. disturbance

galactitol
galactocele
galactoglycoprotein
galactogram
galactography
galactophoritis
galactosemia
galactosyl
galactosylamide β-galactosidase deficiency
galactosylation
Galeazzi

    G. fracture
    G. fracture-dislocation

Galen

    vein of G.

galenic venous malformation
gallbladder

    bifid g.
    g. carcinoma
    displaced g.
    g. diverticulum
    double g.
    g. duplication
    g. ectopia
    floating g.
    g. gravel
    g. hydrops
    g. hypoplasia
    multiseptated g.
    pearl necklace g.
    g. perforation
    porcelain g.
    porcine g.
    g. septation
    g. sludge
    g. stone
    strawberry g.
    g. torsion
    g. wall

gallbladder-vena cava line
gall body

gallinarum
  Haemophilus g.
gallium (Ga)
  g. citrate
  g. imaging
  g. nitrate
  g. scan
  g. scanning
  g. scintigraphy
gallium-67 (^{67}Ga)
  g. citrate
gallium-67-labeled leukocytes
gallium-avid thymic hyperplasia
gallium-PAT
gallium-transferrin complex
gallstone
  cholesterol g.
  faceted g.
  floating g.
  gas-containing g.
  g. ileus
  laminated g.
  layered g.
  solitary g.
gamekeeper's thumb
gamete interfallopian transfer (GIFT)
Gamimune N
gamma
  g. camera
  g. chain
  g. counter
  g. emission
  g. emitter
  g. factor
  g. heavy-chain disease
  g. interferon (IFN-G)
  g. irradiation
  g. radiation
  g. ray
  g. ray knife
  recombinant interferon g. (rIFN-gamma)
  g. signal
  g. Y immunoglobulin
gamma-2a
  interferon g.
gamma-1b
  interferon g.
gamma-emitting isotope
gamma-Favre body
Gammagard
Gammagee

gammaglobulin
  bovine g. (BGG)
gammaglobulinopathy
gammagram
Gammar
gamma-ray capture
gammopathy
  monoclonal g.
  monoclonal g. of undetermined significance
Gamna-Gandy
  G.-G. body
  G.-G. nodule
Gamulin Rh
ganciclovir (DHPG)
ganglia (*pl. of* ganglion)
gangliocytoma
ganglioglioma
  cystic g.
  desmoplastic infantile g.
  infantile g.
  intracerebral g.
ganglioma
  intracerebral g.
ganglion, pl. ganglia
  basal ganglia
  g. cell tumor
  ciliary g.
  gasserian g.
  geniculate g.
  intraosseous g.
  pterygopalatine g.
  submandibular g.
  superior cervical g.
ganglioneuroblastoma
ganglioneuroma
ganglionic
  g. cyst
  g. lineage
ganglioside
gangliosidosis
gangrene
  Fournier g.
gangrenescens
  granuloma g.
gangrenosum
  ecthyma g.
gangrenous cholecystitis
gantry
  CT g.
gap
  air g.

anion g.
fracture g.
interslice g.
Garden
    G. femoral neck fracture
garden spade deformity
Gardnerella vaginalis
Gardner-Rasheed sarcoma virus
Gardner syndrome
Gardray dosimeter
gargoylism
Garland
    G. syndrome
    G. triangle
garland
    g. sign
Garré
    sclerosing osteomyelitis
      of G.
Garth view
Gartland classification of humeral supracondylar fracture
Gartner duct cyst
gas
    blood g.
    g. bubble
    g. collection
    g. CT cisternography
    extraluminal g.
    intrauterine g. (IUG)
    overlying bowel g.
    g. pattern
    portal venous g.
gas-containing gallstone
gaseous
    g. dilatation
    g. distention
gasless abdomen
gas-liquid phase chromatography (GLPC)
gasserian ganglion
gastrectomy
gastric
    g. antrum
    g. artery
    g. atony
    g. bypass

g. bypass procedure
g. cancer
g. carcinoma
g. diaphragm
g. diverticulum
g. duplication cyst
g. emphysema
g. emptying
g. emptying scan
g. filling defect
g. fold
g. hernia
g. hypersecretion
g. lavage
g. leiomyosarcoma
g. lumen
g. lymphoma
g. narrowing
g. outlet obstruction
g. pneumatosis
g. polyp
g. pouch
g. pull-through procedure
g. remnant
g. remnant cancer
g. rugae
g. stump carcinoma
g. ulcer
g. vein
g. volvulus
gastrica
    area g.
gastrinoma
gastrin-releasing peptide
gastrins
gastritis
    alcoholic g.
    bile reflux g.
    corrosive g.
    emphysematous g.
    erosive g.
    follicular g.
    granulomatous g.
    hemorrhagic g.
    hypertrophic g.
    phlegmonous g.
gastrocnemius bursa

NOTES

gastrocnemius-semimembranosus bursa
gastrocutaneous fistula
gastroduodenal
    g. artery
    g. junction
    g. mucosal prolapse
gastroduodenostomy
    Billroth I g.
gastroenteritis
    eosinophilic g.
gastroenterogenous rickets
gastroenterostomy
    percutaneous g.
    g. stoma
gastroepiploic
gastroesophageal (GE)
    g. angle
    g. junction
    g. junction carcinoma
    g. junction stricture
    g. reflux
Gastrografin
    G. enema
    G. swallow
gastrointestinal
    g. adverse effect
    g. cancer
    g. complication of radiation therapy
    g. cyst
    g. endoscopy
    g. fistula
    g. hemorrhage
    g. lymphoma
    g. malignancy
    g. obstruction
    g. series
    g. syndrome
    g. toxicity
    g. tract
    g. tract adenocarcinoma
    g. tract obstruction
    g. tube
    upper g. (UGI)
gastrointestinal-associated lymphoid tissue
gastrojejunal
    g. bypass
    g. mucosal prolapse
gastrojejunocolic fistula
gastrojejunostomy
    Billroth II g.

gastroparesis
    diabetic g.
    g. diabeticorum
gastropathy
    hyperplastic g.
gastropexy
gastroplasty
gastroptosis
gastrorenal collateral
gastroschisis
gastroscopy
gastrostomy
    palliative g.
    percutaneous g.
    percutaneous endoscopic g. (PEG)
    g. tube
gastrotomy
Gastrozepine
gastrulation
gated
    g. blood pool imaging
    g. blood pool study
    g. radionuclide angiocardiography
gating
    cardiac g.
    peripheral g.
    respiratory g.
    retrospective g.
Gaucher disease
gauss (G)
gaussian
    g. function
    g. line
gay
    g. bowel infection
    g. bowel syndrome
    g. lymph node syndrome
gay-related immunodeficiency disease (GRID)
G-banding
GBM
    glioblastoma multiforme
    glomerular basement membrane
    GBM antibody
G cell
    G c. tumor
G-CFU
    granulocyte colony-forming unit
G-CSF
    granulocyte colony-stimulating factor

granulocyte recombinant G-CSF
recombinant G-CSF
Gd2
disialoganglioside Gd2
GD2T herpes vaccine
Gd-CDTA
gadolinium cyclohexanediaminetetraacetic acid
Gd-DOTA
gadolinium tetraazacyclododecanetetraacetic acid
Gd-DTPA
gadolinium-diethylenetriamine pentaacetic acid
gadolinium-DTPA
gadopentetate dimeglumine
Gd-DTPA-bismethylamide (Gd-DTPA-BMA)
Gd-DTPA-BMA
Gd-DTPA-bismethylamide
Gd-EDTA
gadolinium ethylenediaminetetraacetic acid
Gd-HP-DO3A
gadoteridol
GE
gastroesophageal
GE junction
GE reflux
Gee-Thaysen disease
gel
acoustic g.
Carrington dermal wound g.
g. filtration
g. filtration chromatography
gelatin
g. sphere
g. sponge
gelatinase
gelatin-encapsulated nitrogen microsphere
gelatinous ascites
Gelfoam
G. embolotherapy

G. powder
G. torpedoes
Gelfoam/Sotradecol embolotherapy
Geliperm
G. agar
G. gel dressing
gel-shift assay
GEM
gemcitabine
GEM 91
gemcitabine (GEM)
gemellus
gemistocytic astrocytoma
gemistocytoma
Gemzar
genavense
Mycobacterium g.
gender
g. assignment
g. change
g. dysphoria syndrome
fetal g.
gene (oncogene)
allelic g.
g. amplification
antigen receptor g.
autosomal g.
g. bank
bcl-2/Ig fusion g.
bcr/abl fusion g.
BRCA1 g.
CAT expression g.
cell interaction g.
c-fos g.
chimeric antigen receptor g.
cloned g.
g. cloning
codominant g.
complementary g.
g. construct RevM10
csf1R1 g.
derepressed g.
g. diversity
DNA virus transforming g.
dominant g.
E2A/PBX1 fusion g.
elafin g.

NOTES

gene *(continued)*
 envelope g.
 erg 1 g.
 erythropoietin g.
 g. expression
 gag g.
 globin g.
 H g.
 hairy g.
 histocompatibility g.
 holandric g.
 H-ras g.
 Ig g.
 immune response g.
 immune suppressor g.
 immunoglobulin g.
 g. induction
 inhibiting g.
 Ir g.
 Is g.
 Ki-ras g.
 leaky g.
 lethal g.
 g. library
 lineage-associated g.
 major g.
 g. mapping
 masfin g.
 MCC g.
 mdr g.
 mdr-1 g.
 met g.
 modifying g.
 multiple-drug resistance g.
 mutant g.
 MyoD g.
 nef g.
 nm23 g.
 nonstructural g.
 operator g.
 PGY1 g.
 PGY3 g.
 pleiotropic g.
 pol g.
 g. pool
 g. product (gp)
 g. promoter
 proneural g.
 RAG-1 g.
 RAG-2 g.
 Rb g.
 g. rearrangement
 rearrangement of g.'s
 g. rearrangement study
 recessive g.
 reciprocal g.
 g. regulation
 g. replacement therapy
 reporter g.
 repressed g.
 repressor g.
 retinoblastoma g.
 rev g.
 g. sequence
 g. sequencing
 sex-conditioned g.
 sex-linked g.
 sex-reversal g.
 silent g.
 g. splicing
 structural g.
 sublethal g.
 suicide g.
 suppressor g.
 g. switching
 syntenic g.
 tal-1/SIL fusion g.
 tat g.
 tax g.
 g. therapy
 T-lymphocyte receptor g.
 g. transcription
 g. transfection
 g. transfer
 g. transfer transcription
  assay
 transforming g.
 tumor suppressor g.
 vpa g.
 vpr g.
 vpu g.
 vpx g.
 wild-type g.
 X-linked g.
 Y-linked g.
GeneAmp PCR test
general
 g. anesthesia
 g. anesthetic
generalisata
 platyspondyly g.
generalized
 g. calcinosis
 g. cortical hyperostosis
 g. lymphangiectasia
generation echo

generator
 high-voltage g.
 piezoelectric g.
 radionuclide g.
 spark gap g.
 video signal g.
 x-ray g.
gene-silencing phenomenon
genetic
 g. approach
 g. code
 g. condition
 g. damage
 g. deviation
 g. engineering
 g. immunity
 g. lability
 g. lesion
 g. linkage map
 g. marker
 g. marking
 g. masking tape
 molecular g.'s
 g. mutation
 g. polymorphism
 g. probe
 reverse g.'s
 g. screening
 g. susceptibility
 g. switch
Gengou phenomenon
geniculate
 g. body
 g. branch
 g. ganglion
 g. ganglion schwannoma
genioglossus muscle
genistein
genital
 g. carcinoma
 g. tract calcification
 g. tract embryology
 g. wart
genitalia
 lymphatic drainage of g.

genitalis
 herpes g.
genitourinary (GU)
 g. adverse effect
 g. anomaly
 g. cancer
 g. reflex
 g. rhabdomyosarcoma
 g. toxicity
 g. tract
genome
 helper g.
 vector g.
genomic DNA
genotoxic
Gensini catheter
gentamicin
gentian
 g. blue
 g. violet
genu
 g. valgum
 g. varum
geode
geographic
 g. follicle
 g. skull
 g. variation
geography
 brain g.
geometry factor
geophagia
 g. artifact
gergoviae
 Enterobacter g.
geriatric configuration
germ
 g. cell neoplasm
 g. cell tumor
 g. tube test
germinal
 g. aplasia
 g. center
 g. center pattern
 g. epithelium
 g. matrix hemorrhage
 g. matrix related-hemorrhage

NOTES

germinolysis
    subependymal g.
germinoma
    multicentric g.
Germistan virus
germline
    g. band
    g. configuration
    g. DNA
Gerota fascia
gestation
    intrauterine g.
    multiple g.
    normal g.
    triplet g.
gestational
    g. age
    g. choriocarcinoma
    g. diabetes
    g. nonmetastatic
      trophoblastic disease
    g. sac
    g. trophoblastic disease
    g. trophoblastic neoplasia
    g. trophoblastic neoplasm
    g. trophoblastic tumor
gestationis
    herpes g.
Gesterol
gestranol hexanoate
geyser sign
GFR
    glomerular filtration rate
GH
    growth hormone
GHD
    growth hormone deficiency
Ghon
    G. complex
    G. lesion
    G. node
ghost
    g. artifact
    g. cell
    displacement g.
    g. image
    red cell g.
    separation of g.'s (SEP)
    g. vertebra
GHRH
    growth hormone-releasing
    hormone

GHz
    gigahertz
GI
    Imagent GI
    GI series and small bowel
      follow-through
giant
    g. aneurysm
    g. cell
    g. cell aortitis
    g. cell arteritis
    g. cell astrocytoma
    g. cell carcinoma
    g. cell carcinoma of thyroid
      gland
    g. cell fibroma
    g. cell granuloma
    g. cell myeloma
    g. cell reaction
    g. cell reparative granuloma
    g. cell sarcoma
    g. cell tumor
    g. cell tumor of tendon
      sheath
    g. duodenal ulcer
    g. fibroadenoma
    g. limb of Robertson
    g. lymph node hyperplasia
    g. melanocytic nevus
    g. sigmoid diverticulum
Gianturco
    G. bird's nest filter
    G. coil
    G. self-expanding metallic
      stent
    G. self-expanding Z stent
    G. spring embolus
    G. stent
    G. zigzag stent
**Gianturco-Roehm bird's nest vena
cava filter**
Gianturco-Rösch stent
Gianturco-Roubin
    G.-R. balloon
    G.-R. balloon expandable
      stent
Gianturco-Wallace-Anderson coil
Gianturco-Wallace-Chuang coil
Giardia
    G. lamblia
giardiasis
gibbon ape lymphosarcoma virus
Gibbons ureteral stent

gibbous deformity
Gibbs
    G. phenomenon
    G. phenomenon artifact
    G. sampling
Gibbs-Donnan law
gibbus
Gibson sign
Giemsa stain
Giemsa-trypsin banding procedure
Gieson
    elastica Van G.
GIFT
    gamete interfallopian transfer
gigahertz (GHz)
gigantiform
    g. cementoma
gigantism
Gignotti-Crosti syndrome
Gilbert phenomenon
Gill
    G. lesion
    G. procedure
gingiva
gingival
    g. bleeding
    g. cancer
    g. mucosa
gingivitis
    erosive g.
    necrotizing ulcerative g.
gingivostomatitis
    herpetic g.
ginseng
    Panax g.
gip2 **proto-oncogene**
girdle
    pectoral g.
    pelvic g.
    shoulder g.
Girdlestone arthroplasty
glabella
glactose oxidase-Schiff reaction
gladiatorum
    herpes g.
gladiolus
gladiomanubrial

gland
    adrenal g.
    Brunner g.
    Cowper g.
    giant cell carcinoma of
      thyroid g.
    lacrimal g.
    mammary g.
    mixed tumor of salivary g.
    Montgomery g.'s
    mucosal g.
    parathymus g.
    parathyroid g.
    parotid g.
    periurethral g.
    pineal g.
    pituitary g.
    prostate g.
    salivary g.
    Stensen g.
    sublingual g.
    submandibular g.
    submaxillary g.
    substernal thyroid g.
    thymus g.
    thyroid g.
    Wharton g.
Glandosane
glandular
    g. cancer
    g. carcinoma
    g. elements
    g. hyperplasia
    g. parenchyma
    g. structure
    g. tissue
glandularis
    cystitis g.
Glanzmann syndrome
glare
    imaging chain veiling g.
    veiling g.
Glasgow Coma Scale
glass
    g. eye artifact
    g. factor

NOTES

glaucoma
    angle-closure g.
Glazunov tumor
Gleason
    G. score
    G. tumor grading system
Glendenin-Coryell formula
Glenn
    G. anastomosis
    G. shunt
glenohumeral ligament
glenoid
    g. cavity
    g. fossa
    g. fracture
    g. labrum
    g. labrum injury
    g. rim fracture
glial
    g. acidic protein
    g. brain tumor
    g. fibrillary acidic protein
Glidewire
    G. catheter
glioblastoma
    butterfly g.
    exophytic g.
    multicentric g.
    g. multiforme (GBM)
glioma
    brain stem g.
    brainstem g.
    butterfly g.
    g. cell
    chiasmatic/hypothalamic g.
    cystic g.
    hypothalamic g.
    malignant g.
    optic g.
    optic nerve g.
    pontine g.
    supratentorial g.
gliomatosis cerebri
gliosarcoma
    cerebellar g.
gliosis
    isomorphic g.
Glisson capsule
glitter cell
global renal enlargement
globe cell anemia
globin gene

globoid cell leukodystrophy
globular
    g. configuration
    g. meningioma
globulin
    anti-HIV immune serum g.
    (HIVIG)
    antihuman g.
    antithymocyte g. (ATG)
    cytomegalovirus immune g.
    (CMVIG)
    hepatitis B immune g.
    horse antihuman thymus g.
    hyperimmune g.
    immune g.
    immune gamma g.
    Pseudomonas
     hyperimmune g.
    rabies immune g.
    Rh0D immune g.
    tetanus immune g.
    thyroxin-binding g.
    varicella-zoster immune g.
    (VZIG)
    zoster immune g. (ZIG)
globus
    g. hystericus
    g. major
    g. pallidus
glomangioma
glomerular
    g. basement membrane
    (GBM)
    g. filtration rate (GFR)
    g. lesion
    g. mesangial hyperplasia
    g. nephritis
glomeruli (*pl. of* glomerulus)
glomerulonephritis
glomerulopathy
glomerulosa
    zona g.
glomerulosclerosis
glomerulus, pl. glomeruli
glomus
    g. body tumor
    g. caroticum tumor
    g. choroideum
    g. of choroid plexus
    g. jugulare
    g. jugulare tumor
    g. tumor

g. tympanicum
g. vagale
glossectomy
total g.
glossitis
Hunter g.
glossoepiglottic fold
glossopharyngeal nerve
glottic
g. carcinoma
g. narrowing
glottis, pl. glottides
gloved-finger sign
GLPC
gas-liquid phase chromatography
GLQ223
glucagon
glucagonoma
glucamoma
glucarate
glucepate
technetium-99m g.
glucocerebrosidase
glucocorticoid
glucoheptanate
gluconate
trimetrexate g.
gluconurate
trimetrexate g.
glucopyranoside moiety
glucose
hypertonic g.
g. metabolism
glucose-6-phosphate dehydrogenase (G6PD)
glucose-6-phosphatase
glucuronide
glutamine-supplemented total parenteral nutrition
glutamylcysteine synthetase
glutaraldehyde
glutaric acid
glutaric aciduria type I
glutathione
g. disulfide
g. ethylester
g. modification

g. monoethyl ester
g. S-transferase
g. transferase
glutathione-depleting agent
gluteal
g. line
g. region
gluten enteropathy-associated T-cell lymphoma
gluten-sensitive enteropathy
gluteus
g. maximus
g. medius
g. minimus
glycerol
glycinate
aphidicolin g.
glycogen
g. acanthosis
g. storage disease
glycogenosis
glycogen-rich cystadenoma
glycol
polyethylene g. (PEG)
glycophorin A and C
glycoprotein
gp 48 g.
SPARC g.
tumor-associated g. (TAG)
glycoprotein-72
tumor-associated g. (TAG-72)
glycosaminoglycan
glycosylated hemoglobin
glycosyltransferase
glycyrrhetinic acid
Gm antigen
GM-CSF
granulocyte-macrophage colony-stimulating factor
rMu GM-CSF
GMN
gradient moment nulling
GMR
gradient moment reduction
gradient moment rephasing

NOTES

GNRH
GNRH agonist
GnRH (*var. of* GRH)
GnRH analog
goblet
g. cell
g. sign
goblet-shaped pelvis
Godwin tumor
goiter
adenomatous g.
colloid g.
congenital g.
diffuse g.
diffuse toxic g.
iodine-deficiency g.
multinodular g.
retrotracheal g.
toxic nodular g.
goitrous cretinism
Golay coil
gold
radioactive g.
g. seed
g. therapy
gold-198 (^{198}Au)
g. wire
golden
motility of G.
g. pneumonia
g. showers
S-sign of G.
Goldie-Coldman
G.-C. hypothesis
G.-C. model
Goldman classification
Goldstein hematemesis
Golgi
G. apparatus
G. complex
G. stack
Golgi-specific protein
Goltz syndrome
Gomori
G. methenamine silver
G. methenamine silver stain
gompertzian
g. growth
g. growth curve
gonad
g. dose
indifferent g.'s
maternal g.

gonadal
g. artery
g. complication
g. dose
g. dysfunction
g. dysgenesis
g. function
g. stroma
g. toxicity
g. venography
gonadoblastoma
ovarian g.
gonadotrope
gonadotropin
chorionic g.
human chorionic g. (hCG)
human menopausal g.
(hMG)
menopausal g.
gonadotropin-producing
gonadotropin-releasing
g.-r. hormone (GRH,
GnRH)
g.-r. hormone agonist
gondii
Toxoplasma g.
Gongylonema neoplasticum
gonorrhea
gonorrhoeae
Neisseria g.
Gonzales blood group
Goodpasture syndrome
Good syndrome
gooseneck deformity
gordonae
Mycobacterium g.
Gordon elementary body
GORE-TEX
G.-T. graft
G.-T. patch
Gorham
G. disease
G. syndrome
Gorham-Stout syndrome
Gorlin-Pindborg syndrome
Gorlin syndrome
goserelin
g. acetate
Gosselin fracture
Gottron papule
gouge defect
gout
tophaceous g.

gouty
> g. arthritis
> g. arthropathy

Gower
> hemoglobin G.

Gowers solution

gp
> gene product
> gp 160 envelope
> gp 48 glycoprotein

gp 120

gp 160

G6PD
> glucose-6-phosphate
> dehydrogenase
> G6PD deficiency

G$_0$ period

GR 63178A

graafian follicle

gracile bone

gracilis
> funiculi g.
> g. tendon

grade
> Bloom-Richardson g.
> Child g.
> histologic g.
> g. I-IV astrocytoma
> nuclear g.

graded compression sonography technique

Gradenigo syndrome

gradient
> g. acquisition
> g. amplitude
> g. bandwidth
> g. coil
> constant g.
> discontinuous density g.
> g. echo
> g. encoding
> field g.
> g. field
> linear g.
> g. linearity
> magnetic field g.
> g. magnetic field

> g. method
> g. moment nulling (GMN)
> g. moment reduction (GMR)
> g. moment rephasing (GMR)
> oscillating g.
> phase-encoding g.
> portosystemic g.
> pullback pressure g.
> g. pulse
> readout g.
> g. rephasing
> rephasing g.
> g. reversal
> g. scheme
> g. selection
> sensitizing g.
> spoiler g.
> g. system
> thoracoabdominal g.
> g. timing
> transstenotic g.
> velocity g.
> X g.
> Y g.
> Z g.

gradient-echo
> g.-e. imaging
> g.-e. method
> g.-e. MR imaging
> g.-e. sequence
> g.-e. technique

gradient-induced phase dispersion

gradient-recalled echo image

gradient-refocused acquisition in the steady state (GRASS)

gradient-reversal fat suppression method

gradient-to-noise imaging

Graffi virus

graft
> g. anastomosis
> aortic g.
> aorticorenal g.
> aortofemoral g.
> aortofemoral bypass g.

NOTES

graft *(continued)*
    aortoiliac bypass g.
    arterial bypass g.
    autogenous vein bypass g.
    autologous g.
    autologous vein g.
    axillobifemoral bypass g.
    bifemoral g.
    bilateral myocutaneous g.
    bone g.
    bone-tendon-bone g.
    Brescia-Cimino g.
    bridge g.
    bypass g.
    coronary artery bypass g.
      (CABG)
    Dacron aortic bifurcation g.
    Dacron aortobifemoral g.
    Dacron velour g.
    donor g.
    E-PTFE g.
    g. failure
    fat g.
    femoropopliteal bypass g.
    GORE-TEX g.
    heterologous g.
    interbody bone g.
    interposition g.
    g. interstices
    isogeneic g.
    patch g.
    polytetrafluoroethylene g.
    g. rejection
    reversed vein g.
    Sauvage filamentous
      velour g.
    in situ vein g.
    soybean lectin T-
      lymphocyte-depleted
      marrow g.
    Sparks mandrel g.
    g. stenosis
    subcutaneous arterial
      bypass g.
    suprailiac aortic
      mesenteric g.
    synthetic vascular bypass g.
    vascular g.
    vascular bypass g.
    venous interposition g.
graft-versus-host
    g.-v.-h. disease (GVHD)

graft-versus-immunocompetent cell effect
graft-versus-leukemia effect (GVL)
graft-versus-lymphoma effect
graft-versus-tumor effect
Graham-Cole test
Gram-negative, gram-negative
    G.-n. bacteria
    G.-n. organism
    G.-n. pneumonia
    G.-n. rod
Gram-positive, gram-positive
    G.-p. bacteria
    G.-p. organism
Gram stain
Granger
    G. line
    G. projection
granisetron
    g. HCl
Grantham classification of femoral fracture
granular
    g. acute lymphoblastic
      leukemia
    g. calcification
    g. cell myoblastoma
    g. cell tumor
granularis
    ependymitis g.
granularity
    cytoplasmic g.
granulation
    pacchionian g.'s
granule
    azurophilic g.
    Birbeck g.
    cytoplasmic basophilic g.
    effervescent
      citrocarbonate g.'s
    Neisser g.
    specific cytoplasmic g.
    sulfur g.'s
Granulex
granulocyte
    g. colony-forming unit
      (G- CFU)
    g. colony-stimulating factor
      (G-CSF)
    g. count
    g. phagocytosis
    g. priming effect

g. recombinant G-CSF
g. transfusion
granulocyte-macrophage
colony-forming unit g.-m. (CFU-GM)
g.-m. colony-forming unit (CFU-GM)
g.-m. colony-stimulating factor (GM-CSF)
granulocytic
g. leukemia
g. marker
g. sarcoma
granulocytopenia
granulocytosis
paraneoplastic g.
granuloma, pl. granulomata
actinic g.
amebic g.
g. annulare
apical g.
beryllium g.
bilharzial g.
canine venereal g.
cocaine g.
coccidioidal g.
dental g.
g. endemicum
eosinophilic g.
g. faciale
foreign body g.
g. gangrenescens
giant cell g.
giant cell reparative g.
g. gravidarum
hyalinizing g.
infectious g.
g. inguinale
laryngeal g.
lethal midline g.
lipoid g.
lipophagic g.
Majocchi g.
malignant g.
midline g.
g. multiforme
oily g.

paracoccidioidal g.
parasitic g.
periapical g.
plasma cell g.
pseudopyogenic g.
g. pudendi
pulmonary hyalinizing g.
pyogenic g.
g. pyogenicum
reparative giant cell g.
root end g.
sarcoidal g.
schistosome g.
sea urchin g.
silicon g.
sperm g.
swimming pool g.
g. telangiectaticum
g. tropicum
g. venereum
zirconium g.
granulomatis
Cephalosporium g.
granulomatosa
cheilitis g.
granulomatosis
allergic g.
bronchocentric g.
g. disciformis
lipid g.
lipoid g.
lipophagia g.
lymphocytic angiitis and g.
lymphomatoid g.
mainline g.
Miescher g.
pulmonary mainline g.
g. siderotica
Wegener g.
granulomatous
g. abscess
g. angiitis
g. arteritis
g. calcification
g. colitis
g. cystitis
g. disease

NOTES

granulomatous *(continued)*
   g. disorder
   g. endophthalmitis
   g. enteritis
   g. gastritis
   g. infection
   g. inflammation
   g. mastitis
   g. meningitis
   g. nocardiosis
   g. process
   g. prostatitis
   g. slack skin
   g. slack skin disorder
   g. slack skin syndrome
   subacute g.
granulopoiesis
granulosa
   g. cell tumor
   pyoderma g.
granulosa-stromal cell tumor
granulosus
   Echinococcus g.
grape
   g. cell
   g. skin thin-walled lung cavities
graph
   spin-phase g.
Graseby pump
Grashey view
grasping technique
GRASS
   gradient-refocused acquisition in the steady state
   GRASS pulse sequence
   spoiled GRASS (SPGR)
gravel
   gallbladder g.
Graves disease
gravidarum
   fibroma molle g.
   granuloma g.
   hyperemesis g.
gravis
   myasthenia g.
gravity drainage
Grawitz tumor
gray
   g. matter
   g. platelet syndrome
   g. scale
   g. scale examination

   g. scale image
   g. scale imaging
   g. scale ultrasonography
   g. unit
gray-white junction
greater
   g. curvature of the stomach
   g. multangular bone
   g. omentum
   g. petrosal
   g. saphenous vein
   g. sphenoid wing
   g. trochanter
   g. trochanteric femoral fracture
   g. tuberosity fracture
great vessels
green cancer
Greene
   G. biopsy set
   G. needle
Greenfield
   G. filter
   G. titanium inferior vena cava filter
greenstick
   g. fracture
Greenwald and Lewman method
GRE imaging
Grenz zone
Grey Turner sign
GRH, GnRH
   gonadotropin-releasing hormone
GRID
   gay-related immunodeficiency disease
grid
   Bucky g.
   focused g.
   g. ratio
   g. technique
Grisel syndrome
griseofulvin
Grocott methenamine silver
groin
   g. dissection
   g. mass
Grollman catheter
groove
   bicipital g.
   chiasmatic g.
   meningeal artery g.
   middle meningeal artery g.

Groshong catheter
gross
- G. cell surface antigen
- G. leukemia
- G. leukemia virus
- g. specimen

ground
- g. glass appearance
- g. itch anemia
- g. state

ground-glass pattern
group
- ABO blood g.
- Auberger blood g.
- blood g.
- g. B streptococcal infections
- Cartwright blood g.
- determinant g.
- diagnostic-related g. (DRG)
- Diego blood g.
- Dombrock blood g.
- Duffy blood g.
- Gonzales blood g.
- high frequency blood g.
- I blood g.
- iodinated tyrosine g.
- Kell blood g.
- Kell-Cellano blood g.
- Kidd blood g.
- Lewis blood g.
- low frequency blood g.
- Lutheran blood g.
- MN blood g.
- MNSs blood g.
- P blood g.
- Rh blood g.
- self-help g.
- sulfhydryl g.
- TORCH blood g.
- tyrosine phenolic g.

growth
- g. abnormality
- g. acceleration
- g. arrest line
- g. factor
- g. factor dimerization
- g. factor receptor
- g. fraction
- g. fraction concept
- gompertzian g.
- g. hormone (GH)
- g. hormone deficiency (GHD)
- g. hormone-producing adenoma
- g. hormone releasing factor
- g. hormone-releasing hormone (GHRH)
- g. impairment
- morphologic g.
- nutrient artery g.
- g. parameters
- g. plate
- g. plate complex
- g. recovery lines of Harris
- g. retardation
- spinal g.
- tumor g.

growth-related tumor markers ALP isoenzyme
Greulich and Pyle bone age standard
Grüntzig
- G. balloon catheter
- G. dilator

Grüntzig-type nephrostomy tract dilator
gsp proto-oncogene
GSW
- gunshot wound

GTP
- guanosine triphosphate

GTP-binding protein
GU
- genitourinary

guaiac
- g. needle
- g. negative
- g. positive stool
- g. testing

Guama virus

NOTES

guanine
 benzyl g.
 methyl g.
guanosine triphosphate (GTP)
Guarnieri body
Guaroa virus
gubernaculi
 pars infravaginalis g.
Gubler
 G. line
 G. tumor
guidance
 angioscopic g.
 fluoroscopic g.
 indirect ultrasound g.
 sonographic g.
 g. system selection
guide
 Bilbao-Dotter wire g.
 hollow needle g.
 Lunderquist wire g.
 g. wire
guided
 g. biopsy
 g. coaxial balloon catheter
  system
 g. drainage
 g. fine-needle aspiration
guidewire, guide wire
 angiographic g.
 Bentson g.
 g. exchange technique
 extra-stiff g.
 hydrophilic g.
 g. manipulation
 open-ended g.
 Rosen g.
 Terumo g.
 through-and-through g.
 torque control g.
 torsional attenuating
  diameter g.
 Wholey steerable g.
Guillain-Barré syndrome
guillermondii
 Candida g.
Gull renal epistaxis
gum
 biotene chewing g.

gumma
 cerebral g.
gun
 Biopty g.
Gunderson-Sosin modification
Gun Hill hemoglobin
gunshot
 g. fracture
 g. wound (GSW)
Günther
 G. aspiration
  thromboembolectomy
  device
 G. disease
 G. filter
Gustave-Roussy
 Institut G.-R.
Gustilo-Anderson open clavicular
 fracture
gut
 g. edema
 primitive g.
 g. signature
gut-associated lymphoid tissue
Guthrie bacterial inhibition assay
gutter
 paracolic g.
GVHD
 graft-versus-host disease
GVL
 graft-versus-leukemia effect
gyanandromorphism
gynander
gynandroblastoma
gynecologic
 g. cancer patient
 g. malignancy
 g. tumor
gynecomastia, gynecomasty
Gynogen
gyri (*pl. of* gyrus)
gyriform pattern
gyromagnetic ratio
gyrus, pl. gyri
 cingulate g.
 hippocampal g.
 inferior temporal g.
 postcentral g.
 precentral g.

H
    H antigen
    H & D curve
    H and D curve
    H factor
    H gene
hv
H-2 antigen
HAA
    hepatitis-associated antigen
Haaginsen staging
haarscheibe tumor
habenular commissure calcification
Haber toxicologic principle
habitus
    body h.
HADD
    hydroxyapatite deposition
        disease
Hadlock table
Haemate-P
Haemolite
    Cell Saver H.
Haemonetics Cell Saver
haemophilum
    Mycobacterium h.
Haemophilus, Hemophilus
    H. aegyptius
    H. aphrophilus
    H. ducreyi
    H. gallinarum
    H. influenzae
    H. influenzae meningitis
    H. influenzae pneumonia
Haemophilus influenzae type B
Hafnia alvei
Hagedorn
    H. and Jansen method
    H. needle
Hageman factor
Haggitt classification
Hagie pin
Hahn
    H. cleft
    H. spin echo
Hahn-Steinthal fracture
hair
    h. loss
    Schridde cancer h.'s
hairline fracture

hair-on-end periosteal reaction
hairpin vessel
hair-standing-on-end appearance
hairy
    h. cell
    h. cell index
    h. cell leukemia (HCL)
    h. gene
    h. leukopenia
    h. leukoplakia
Hajdu-Cheney disease
Hakim
    H. syndrome
    H. valve and pump
halazepam
Halbrecht syndrome
Haldol
    Ativan, Benadryl, H. (ABH)
half
    h. axial view
    h. Nex imaging
half-axial projection
half-Fourier
    h.-F. imaging (HFI)
    h.-F. transformation
        technique
half-intensity needle
half-life
    biological h.-l.
    effective h.-l.
    elimination h.-l. ($t_{1/2}$elim)
    h.-l. layer
    physical h.-l.
    radioactive h.-l.
half-moon artifact
half-time
    pressure h.-t.
half-value layer (HVL)
Hall antidote
Haller cell
Hallervorden-Spatz disease
hallucis
    adductor h.
    extensor h. longus
    flexor h. brevis
    flexor h. longus
hallux
    h. rigidus
    h. valgus
    h. varus

halo
> h. device
> fatty h.
> h. melanoma
> h. sign
> sonolucent h.
> subendometrial h.

halogenated pyrimidine
halo melanoma
haloperidol
halopyrimidine
Halotestin
halothane
> h. anesthesia

halstedian concept of tumor spread
Halsted paradigm
HAM
> hexazomacrocycles

HAMA
> human antimouse antibody

hamartoma
> angiomatous lymphoid h.
> astrocytic h.
> benign fetal h.
> fetal h.
> fetal renal h.
> fibrous h.
> leiomyomatous h.
> mesenchymal h.
> renal h.

hamartomatous polyp
hamate
> h. fracture
> h. tail fracture

Hamazaki-Wesenberg body
hamburger
> H. phenomenon
> h. vertebrae

Hamman-Rich syndrome
Hammarsten test
hammered
> h. brass appearance
> h. silver appearance

Hammerschlag method
hammertoe deformity
hammock-like posterior bowing of mitral valve
Hampton
> H. hump
> H. line
> H. maneuver
> H. view

hamstring

Hancock procedure
hand
> spade-like h.
> trident h.

hand-foot syndrome
hand-held nebulizer
handicap
> physical h.

hand-instilled contrast material
handle
> Amplatz radiolucent h.
> Universal h.

handling
> drug h.
> sample h.

hand-mirror
> h.-m. cell leukemia
> h.-m. cell type
> h.-m. lymphocyte

Hand-Schüller-Christian disease
Hangar-Rose skin test antigen
Hanger test
hanging-block culture
hanging-drop culture
hangman's fracture
Hanks balanced salt solution
Hanning window-type low-pass filter
Hansel stain
Hansemann macrophage
Hansen
> H. classification of fractures
> H. disease

haploidentical
haploidy
haplotype
hapten
hapten-chelate construct
hapten X
haptoglobin
hard
> h. palate
> h. palate cancer
> h. papilloma
> h. pulse

hard-copy image
hardening
> beam h.

Harding-Passey melanoma (HPM)
Hardy-Zuckerman 2 feline sarcoma virus
harlequin appearance

harness
  Pavlik h.
Harrington-Allison repair
Harrington rod
Harris
  growth recovery lines of H.
  H. lines
Harting body
Hartmann pouch
Hartnup disease
Harvard mouse
harvesting
  bone marrow h.
Harvey sarcoma virus
Hashimoto
  H. disease
  H. thyroiditis
Hassan cannula
hatchet
  h. defect
  h. sign
HAT medium
haustra
  h. coli
haustra (*pl. of* haustrum)
haustral pattern
haustration
haustrum, pl. haustra
haversian channel
Hawkins
  H. accordion catheter
  H. accordion-type empyema
  H. breast lesion localization
    needle
  H. classification of talar
    fractures
  H. inside-out nephrostomy
    set
  H. inside-out nephrostomy
    technique
  H. method
  H. needle
  H. one-stick needle
  H. single-stick technique
  H. stone basket
  H. technique
Hawkins-Akins needle

Hayem solution
HB
  hepatitis B
HBsAg
  hepatitis B surface antigen
HC
  head circumference
  hydrocortisone
    Sustacal HC
4-HC
  4-hydroperoxycyclophosphamide
HCFA
  Health Care Financing
    Administration
hCG
  human chorionic gonadotropin
hck **proto-oncogene**
HCL
  hairy cell leukemia
HCl
  granisetron HCl
  hydromorphone HCl
  losoxantrone HCl
HCV
  hepatitis C virus
H and D
  Hunter and Driffield
HD
  Hodgkin disease
HDARA-C
  high-dose ara-C
HDC
  high-dose chemotherapy
HDL
  high-density lipoprotein
HDMTX
  high-dose methotrexate
HDR
  high-dose rate
    HDR intracavitary radiation
      therapy
head
  h. of the caudate nucleus
  h. circumference (HC)
  h. of the femur
  h. of the humerus
  h. and neck cancer

NOTES

head *(continued)*
    h. of the pancreas
    pancreatic h.
headhunter catheter
head-splitting humeral fracture
Heaf test
healing fracture
Health Care Financing
  Administration (HCFA)
heart
    h. anomaly
    apex of the h.
    h. block
    boot-shaped h.
    h. disease
    egg-on-its-side h.
    h. failure
    fetal h.
    h. murmur
    right h.
    h. silhouette
    single outlet of h.
    h. sounds
    squared-off h.
    swinging h.
    Taussig-Bing h.
    h. transplant
    univentricular h.
    h. valve
    h. valve leaflet
    h. volume
heat
    h. exchanger
    h. shock protein
    h. transfer mechanism
heat-killed Listeria monocytogenes
heat-stable alkaline phosphatase
heavy
    h. charged particle
    h. ion
    h. metal injection
heavy-chain
    h.-c. disease
    h.-c. immunoglobulin
Heberden node
Hedley procedure
heel
    h. effect
    h. pad thickening
heel-stick hematocrit
Heerfordt syndrome
Heidenhain iron hematoxylin stain
Heimlich valve

Heinig view
Heinz body hemolytic anemia
Heinz-Ehrlich body
Heister
    valve of H.
Hektoen, Kretschmer, and Welker
  protein
Hektoen phenomenon
HeLa cell
helical
    h. blood flow
    h. computed tomography
    h. CT
    h. scanning
helices (*pl. of* helix)
helicine artery
Helicobacter pylori
Helios laser system
heliotrope erythema
helium-cadmium laser
helix, pl. helices
    h. filter
    H. multihead nuclear
      imaging system
    h. pomatia agglutinin (HPA)
helix-loop-helix (HLH)
    h.-l.-h. structure
helix-turn-helix (HTH)
Hellmer sign
HELLP
    H. syndrome
Helmes 3 antigen
helmet cell
Helmholtz coil
helminthic infection
helminthoma
helper
    h. factor
    h. genome
    h. T-cell
    h. T-lymphocyte
hemachrome
hemacytometer
hemadynamometer
hemafacient
Hemagard collection tube
hemagglutination
    indirect h.
    h. titer
hemagglutinin
    cold h.
hemangioblastoma
    capillary h.

cerebelloretinal h.
cystic h.
third ventricular h.
hemangioblastomatosis
cerebelloretinal h.
hemangioendothelial sarcoma
hemangioendothelioma
epithelioid h.
infantile h.
hemangioendotheliosis
hemangioepithelioma
hemangiofibroma
juvenile h.
hemangiolymphangioma
hemangioma
arteriovenous h.
capillary h.
cavernous h.
choroidal h.
dumbbell-shaped spinal
cavernous h.
epidural cavernous h.
epithelioid h.
extraaxial cavernous h.
extremity h.
facial h.
hepatic h.
pediatric h.
splenic h.
subglottic h.
vertebral h.
hemangiomatosis
hemangiopericytoma
hemangiosarcoma
hemapheresis
hemarthrosis
hematemesis
Goldstein h.
hematobilia (*var. of* hemobilia)
hematocele
scrotal h.
hematochezia
hematocrit
heel-stick h.
h. phenomenon
hematocyte

hematogenous
h. dissemination
h. metastasis
h. osteomyelitis
hematogone
hematologic
h. adverse effect
h. complication
h. disorder
h. engraftment
h. factor
h. malignancy
h. reconstitution
h. recovery time
h. toxicity
hematoma
axillary h.
basal ganglia h.
bladder flap h.
bowel wall h.
dissecting h.
dissecting intramural h.
epidural h.
extradural h.
interhemispheric h.
interhemispheric subdural h.
interstitial loculated h.
intracerebral h.
intraparenchymal h.
isodense subdural h.
nasopharyngeal h.
paraaortic h.
parenchymal h.
periaortic mediastinal h.
pericardial h.
peridiaphragmatic h.
perigraft h.
perinephric h.
perirenal h.
rectal sheath h.
retroperitoneal h.
retroplacental h.
subcapsular h.
subcapsular renal h.
subchorionic h.
subdural h.
subdural interhemispheric h.

NOTES

hematoma *(continued)*
  subfascial h.
  subgaleal h.
  submembranous placental h.
  subperiosteal h.
  umbilical cord h.
hematometra
hematometrocolpos
hematomyelia
hematophagia
hematopoiesis, hemopoiesis
  embryonal h.
  extramedullary h.
  extramedullary h.
  Ogawa model for h.
  trilineage h.
hematopoietic
  h. cell
  h. chimerism
  h. colony-stimulating factor
  h. CSF
  h. disorder
  h. engraftment
  h. function
  h. growth factor
  h. marrow
  h. microenvironment
  h. precursor
  h. progenitor
  h. progenitor cell
  h. recovery
  h. stem cell factor
  h. stem cells (HSC)
  h. system
  h. target cell
hematopoietic-inductive
  microenvironment model
hematopoietin-1
hematoporphyrin
  h. derivative
  h. therapy
hematoxylin
  h. body
  Carazzi h.
  Clara h.
  Cole h.
  h. and eosin stain
  Lillie h.
hematuria
heme synthesis
hemianopsia, hemianopia
  homonymous h.

hemiatrophy
hemiazygous vein
hemibody irradiation
hemic
hemichorea-hemiballismus syndrome
hemicondylar fracture
hemicranium
hemidesmosome
hemidiaphragm
  accessory h.
  h. rupture
hemifacial spasm
hemiglossectomy
hemimandibulectomy
hemimeganencephaly
hemimelia
hemimelica
  dysplasia epiphysealis h.
hemimyelocele
hemiparesis
hemiparkinsonism
hemipelvectomy
hemisensory syndrome
hemisphere
  cerebellar h.
  cerebral h.
  diffusely swollen h.
  swollen h.
hemispheric vein
hemithorax, pl. hemithoraces
hemithyroidectomy
hemitruncus
hemivertebra
hemizygosity
hemobilia, hematobilia
  tropical h.
hemoblastic leukemia
Hemoccult test
hemochromatosis
hemoclip
HemoCue photometer
hemocyanin
  keyhole limpet h.
hemocytoblastic leukemia
hemocytoblastoma
Hemo-Dial dialysate additive
hemodialysis
  h. access
  h. arthropathy
hemodialyze
hemodialyzer
hemodilution

hemodynamic
hemodynamically significant
hemodynamics
Hemofil M
hemofiltration
  continuous arteriovenous h.
  (CAVH)
hemoglobin
  h. A_2
  h. A_{IC}
  Bart h.
  h. Chesapeake
  fast h.
  fetal h.
  glycosylated h.
  h. Gower
  Gun Hill h.
  high-affinity h.
  h. Lepore
  mean corpuscular h.
  muscle h.
  nitric oxide h.
  h. oxidation
  oxidized h.
  oxygenated h.
  h. Portland
  pyridoxilated stroma-free h.
  h. Rainier
  rHb1.1 recombinant h.
  h. S-C disease
  h. Seattle
  slow h.
  h. S-O-Arab disease
  h. S-thalassemia disease
  h. Yakima
hemoglobin A, C, D, E, H, I,
  M, S
hemoglobinemia
hemoglobineria
  PCH-paroxysmal cold h.
hemoglobin M
hemoglobinopathy
hemoglobinuria
  paroxysmal nocturnal h.
  (PNH)
hemograft
hemogram

hemolysin
  hot-cold h.
hemolysis
  intravascular h.
hemolysis, elevated liver enzymes,
  low platelets
hemolytic
  h. anemia
  h. complement assay
  h. plaque assay
  h. uremic syndrome
hemonectin
hemoperitoneum
hemophagocytic
  h. histiocytic hyperplasia
  h. lymphohistiocytosis
  h. syndrome
hemophilia
  h. A
  h. B
  h. B Leyden
  h. C
  h. neonatorum
hemophilia-associated AIDS
hemophiliac
  h. arthropathy
Hemophilus (*var. of Haemophilus*)
hemopoiesis (*var. of*
  hematopoiesis)
hemoptysis
Hemopump
hemorrhage
  abdominal h.
  adrenal h.
  alveolar h.
  antepartum h.
  bladder h.
  catheter-induced pulmonary
  artery h.
  cerebellar h.
  cerebral h.
  colonic diverticular h.
  colorectal h.
  diffuse alveolar h.
  diffuse pulmonary h.
  diffuse pulmonary
  alveolar h.

NOTES

hemorrhage *(continued)*
    Duret h.
    extraluminal h.
    gastrointestinal h.
    germinal matrix h.
    germinal matrix related-h.
    intraabdominal arterial h.
    intracerebral h.
    intracranial h.
    intraluminal h.
    intramural h.
    intraparenchymal h.
    intraventricular h.
    mediastinal h.
    neonatal intracranial h.
    neonatal intraventricular h.
    nonaneurysmal
      perimesencephalic
      subarachnoid h.
    perinephric h.
    perinephric space h.
    petechial h.
    posttraumatic h.
    preplacental h.
    pulmonary artery h.
    retroperitoneal h.
    retropharyngeal h.
    small bowel h.
    spontaneous renal h.
    subarachnoid h.
    subchorial h.
    subchorionic h.
    subdural h.
    subependymal h.
    subperiosteal h.
hemorrhagic
    h. colitis
    h. conversion
    h. cyst
    h. cystitis
    h. cystitis prophylaxis
    h. gastritis
    h. infarction
    multiple idiopathic h.
    h. neuroblastoma
    h. pancreatitis
    h. telangiectasia
hemorrhagicum
    corpus h.
hemorrhoidal
    h. artery
    h. collateral

hemosiderin
    h. ring
hemosiderosis
    idiopathic pulmonary h.
    pulmonary h.
hemostasis
hemostatic clip
Hemostix
hemothorax
Henderson fracture
Henle
    H. fibrin
    loop of H.
Henoch-Schonlein purpura
Henry test
henselae
    Rochalimaea h.
Henson node
HEPA
    high-efficiency, particulate air
Hepaclot
Hepanorm LMWH
heparin
    calcium h.
    dihydroergotamine mesylate
      plus sodium h.
    h. lock
    low-dose h.
    low molecular weight h.
      (LMWH)
    Rotachrom h.
    sodium h.
    Stachrom h.
heparinization
    h. procedure
hepatectomy
hepatic
    h. abscess
    h. adenoma
    h. anaplastic sarcoma
    h. angiography
    h. angiosarcoma
    h. angle
    h. angle sign
    h. arterial chemotherapy
    h. arterial therapy
    h. artery
    h. artery aneurysm
    h. artery embolization
    h. artery infusion
    h. artery ligation
    h. artery-portal vein fistula
    h. artery pseudoaneurysm

h. artery stenosis
h. calcification
h. cancer
h. candidiasis
h. chemoembolization
h. complication
h. cyst
h. 2,6-dimethyliminodiacetic acid (HIDA)
h. duct
h. echo pattern
h. failure
h. fibrosis
h. flexure
h. flexure cancer
h. fungal infection
h. hemangioma
h. lobe
h. metabolism
h. metastasis
h. necrosis
h. neoplasm
h. parenchyma
h. pattern echo
h. resection
h. steatosis
subcapsular h. necrosis
h. transplant
h. tumor
h. vein
h. vein disease
h. venography
h. venoocclusive disease (HVOD)
h. venous system

hepatis
bacillary peliosis h.
peliosis h.
porta h.
sagittal porta h.

hepatitis
acute h.
h. A virus
h. B (HB)
h. B immune globulin
h. B surface antigen (HBsAg)

h. B virus
chemical-induced h.
chronic active h.
h. C virus (HCV)
h. delta virus
ENANB h.
h. E virus
fulminant h.
herpes simplex h.
infectious h.
neonatal h.
non-A, non-B h.
peliosis h.
radiation h.
recurrent pyogenic h.
viral h.
hepatitis-associated antigen (HAA)
hepatobiliary
h. cancer
h. contrast agent
h. imaging
h. scan
hepatoblastoma
hepatocarcinogenesis
hepatocarcinoma
hepatocellular
h. adenoma
h. cancer
h. carcinoma
h. disease
h. dysfunction
hepatocerebral
h. degeneration
h. disease
hepatocyte
hepatocyte-stimulating factor
hepatoduodenal ligament
hepatofugal flow
hepatogram
hepatoid adenocarcinoma
hepatojejunal anastomosis
hepatolenticular degeneration
hepatoma
malignant h.
hepatomegaly
hepatopathy
paraneoplastic h.

NOTES

hepatopedal flow
hepatoportal biliary fistula
hepatosplenic
    h. candidiasis
    h. lymphoma
hepatosplenomegaly (HSM)
hepatotoxicity
hep lock
hepsulfam
heptamer/nonamer sequence
Heptavax B
heptoglobin
HER-2/neu **oncogene**
herbal
    h. remedy
    h. tea
herbalism
Herbst registry
herd immunity
hereditary
    h. chronic nephritis
    h. disorder
    h. hemorrhagic telangiectasia
    h. hemorrhagic telangiectasis
    h. hyperphosphatasia
    h. leptocytosis
    h. multiple exostoses
    h. nephritis
    h. nonpolyposis colorectal
    cancer
    h. pancreatitis
    h. spherocytosis
heredity
Hermansky-Pudlak syndrome
hermaphrodite
hermaphroditism
Hermodsson
    H. fracture
    H. tangential projection
hernia
    abdominal wall h.
    axial h.
    Bochdalek h.
    concentric h.
    congenital diaphragmatic h.
    diaphragmatic h.
    duodenal h.
    femoral h.
    gastric h.
    hiatal h.
    incarcerated h.
    incisional h.
    inguinal h.

    internal h.
    lesser sac h.
    lumbar h.
    h. metastasis
    Morgagni h.
    h. neoplasm
    paraduodenal h.
    paraesophageal h.
    parahiatal h.
    h. paralysis
    peritoneopericardial
    diaphragmatic h.
    rolling hiatal h.
    h. rupture
    short esophagus type
    hiatal h.
    sliding hiatal h.
    spigelian h.
    transient hiatal h.
    traumatic diaphragmatic h.
    umbilical h.
    ventral h.
hernial sac
herniated
    h. bowel
    h. disk
    h. nucleus pulposus (HNP)
herniation
    cervical disk h.
    cisternal h.
    disk h.
    fat h.
    free fragment h.
    intercervical disk h.
    nucleus pulposus h.
    h. pit
    thoracic disk h.
heroin
Herp-Check antibody test
herpes
    anal h.
    anorectal h.
    h. corneae
    h. digitalis
    h. encephalitis
    h. facialis
    h. febrilis
    h. genitalis
    h. gestationis
    h. gladiatorum
    h. labialis
    h. menstrualis
    ocular h.

pharyngeal h.
h. progenitalis
h. simplex (HS)
h. simplex encephalitis
h. simplex hepatitis
h. simplex infection
h. simplex virus (HSV)
h. simplex virus infection
h. virus
h. virus-2
h. whitlow
wrestler's h.
h. zoster
h. zoster ophthalmicus
Herpesvirus
H. hominis
H. saimiri
H. simiae
herpesvirus
human h. type 6 (HHV-6)
h. pneumonia
h. thymidine kinase cDNA
herpetic
h. gingivostomatitis
h. neuritis
h. proctitis
herpetiformis
dermatitis h.
Herrick anemia
Herring tube
Hers disease
hertz (Hz)
Hespan
heteroagglutination
heteroantibody
heteroantigen
heterochromatin
heterodimer
heteroduplex analysis
heterogeneic
h. antigen
heterogeneity
lineage h.
heterogeneous
heterogenetic antibody
heterogenous density
heterograft

heterohemagglutination
heteroimmune
heterokaryon
heterologous
h. antigen
h. graft
h. tumor
heterolysin
heteronuclear decoupling
heterophil
h. antibody
h. antigen
heteroploid index
heteroserotherapy
heterosexual
heterotaxy, heterotaxia, heterotaxis
visceral h.
heterotopia
incomplete band h.
heterotopic
h. bone
h. bone formation
h. gray matter
h. ossification
heterotransplantation
heterozygosity
heterozygous
h. achondroplasia
Heubner
recurrent artery of H.
Hexabrix
Hexa-CAF
hexamethylmelamine,
cyclophosphamide,
amphotericin B, 5-fluorouracil
hexadecylphosphocholine
Hexalen
hexametazime
hexamethylene bisacetamide (HMBA)
hexamethylmelamine
hexamethylmelamine, cyclophosphamide, amphotericin B, 5-fluorouracil (Hexa-CAF)
hexamethylpropyleneamine oxime (HMPAO)

NOTES

hexanoate
gestranol h.
Hexastat
hexazomacrocycles (HAM)
Heyman capsule
Heymann nephritis
HF
Mamm-Aire H.
HFI
half-Fourier imaging
HGH
human growth hormone
HGPT locus
HHV-6
human herpesvirus type 6
5-HIAA
5-hydroxyindoleacetic acid
hiatal hernia
hiatus
diaphragmatic esophageal h.
esophageal h.
h. semilunaris
hibernoma
hiccup, hiccough
Hickman
H. catheter
H. line
hickory-stick fracture
**Hicks-Pitney thromboplastin
generation test**
HIDA
hepatic 2,6-
dimethyliminodiacetic acid
HIDA scan
technetium-99m HIDA
HI-DAC
high-dose cytosine arabinoside
hidebound small bowel fold
hidradenitis
eccrine h.
neutrophilic eccrine h.
hierarchy of terms
Hieshima
H. balloon
H. catheter
high
h. endothelial venule
h. frequency blood group
h. index of suspicion
h. linear energy transfer
radiation
h. output state
h. signal

h. spin
h. velocity
high-affinity
h.-a. antibody
h.-a. hemoglobin
high-amplitude echo
high-attenuation
mediastinal h.-a. mass
high-density
h.-d. bile
h.-d. lipoprotein (HDL)
high-dose
h.-d. ara-C (HDARA-C)
h.-d. chemoradiotherapy
h.-d. chemotherapy (HDC)
h.-d. cytosine arabinoside
(HI-DAC)
h.-d. methotrexate
(HDMTX)
h.-d. methotrexate,
bleomycin, Adriamycin,
cyclophosphamide,
Oncovin, dexamethasone
(M-BACOD)
h.-d. radiotherapy
h.-d. rate (HDR)
h.-d. therapy
**high-dose-rate remote
brachytherapy**
**high-efficiency, particulate air
(HEPA)**
high-energy
h.-e. accelerator
h.-e. phosphate reaction
high-fiber diet
high-frequency
h.-f. transducer
high-grade
h.-g. B-cell lymphoma
h.-g. neutropenia
h.-g. proximal stenosis
high-intensity
h.-i. lesion
h.-i. signal
high-kV technique
high-lying patella
highly reflective echo
high-osmolar
h.-o. contrast agent (HOCA)
h.-o. contrast medium
(HOCM)
high-pass filter

high-performance
 h.-p. liquid chromatography (HPLC)
 h.-p. size-exclusion chromatography (HPSEC)
high-power field (hpf)
high-pressure liquid chromatography (HPLC)
high-resolution
 h.-r. bone algorithm technique
 h.-r. computed tomography (HRCT)
 h.-r. 3DFT MR imaging
 h.-r. imaging
 h.-r. multisweep
 h.-r. transducer
high-riding third ventricle
high-risk
 h.-r. patient
 h.-r. sex
high-speed imaging
high-velocity
 h.-v. flow pattern
 h.-v. signal loss
high-voltage
 h.-v. generator
 h.-v. pulsed galvanic stimulation (HVPGS)
hila (*pl. of* hilum)
Hilal
 H. embolization apparatus
 H. microcoil
hilar
 h. adenopathy
 h. biopsy
 h. cell tumor of ovary
 h. comma sign
 h. lip
 h. mass
 h. shadow
 h. shadows
 h. tumor
 h. vessel
 h. waterfall sign

Hill-Sachs
 H.-S. defect
 H.-S. deformity
hilum, pl. **hila**
 comma-shaped h.
Himalayan yew
Hinchey classification
hindbrain
Hine-Duley phantom
hinge region
Hinton test
hip
 h. disarticulation
 h. dysplasia
 frog-leg view of the h.'s
 h. joint
 h. pinning
 h. pointer
 h. prosthesis
 transient osteoporosis of h.
 transient synovitis of h.
Hippel-Lindau disease
hippocampal
 h. atrophy
 h. gyrus
 h. sclerosis
 h. sulcus
hippocampus
Hippuran
hippuric acid
Hirschsprung disease
hirsutism
hirudin
His line
histamine
 h. degranulation
 h. H1 receptor
histaminemia
Histerone
histioblast
histiocyte
 foamy h.
 sea-blue h.
 sinus h.
 sinusoidal h.
histiocytic
 h. lymphoma

NOTES

histiocytic *(continued)*
    h. medullary reticulosis
    h. necrotizing lymphadenitis
    h. neoplasm
    h. proliferation
    h. tissue
histiocytoma
    angiomatoid malignant
      fibrous h.
    benign fibrous h.
    fibrous h.
    malignant h.
    malignant fibrous h.
    myxoid malignant fibrous h.
    scrotal h.
histiocytosis
    diffuse cerebral h.
    Langerhans cell h.
    malignant h.
    regressing atypical h.
    sinus h.
    h. X
histobath
histochemical method
histochemistry
    bone marrow h.
histocompatibility
    h. antigen
    h. complex
    h. gene
histocompatible donor
histofluorescence
histogram
    integrated optical density h.
histoid
    h. neoplasm
    h. tumor
histoincompatibility
histologic
    h. analysis
    h. architecture
    h. change
    h. grade
    h. subdivision
histology
    cytology and h.
    h. and cytology
    lymph node h.
histolytica
    Entamoeba h.
histone
    h. acetylation

histopathologic
    h. abnormality
    h. validation
Histoplasma capsulatum
histoplasmosis
    disseminated CNS h.
history
    natural h.
hitchhiker's thumb
HIV
    human immunodeficiency virus
    H. bands
    H. embryopathy
    H. encephalopathy
    H. envelope protein
    HIVAGEN test for H.
    H. infection
    NSI variant of H.
    H. p24 antigen
    H. phenotype test
    H. receptor
    SI variant of H.
    Tat protein of H.
    transfusion-acquired H.
    H. vaccine
    H. wasting syndrome
HIV-1
    human immunodeficiency virus
    1
    HIV-1 infection
    HIV-1 specific primer pair
    SUDS HIV-1
HIV-2
    human immunodeficiency virus
    2
    HIV-2 infection
HIV-AB
    human immunodeficiency virus
    antibody
HIVAGEN
    HIVAGEN test
    HIVAGEN test for HIV
HIV-associated dementia
HIVIG
    anti-HIV immune serum
    globulin
HIV-positive low CD4 count
HIV-related follicular involution
HLA
    human leukocyte antigen
    HLA antigen
    HLA sensitization
HLA-A1 antigen

HLA-B27
HLA-B antigen
HLA-C antigen
HLA-D antigen
HLA-DR
    HLA-DR antigen
    HLA-DR 1 antigen
    HLA-DR 5 antigen
HLA-identical
    HLA-i. donor
    HLA-i. sibling transplant
HLA-L antigen
HLA-nonidentical donor
HLH
    helix-loop-helix
        HLH domain
HLI
    human leukocyte interferon
HLTV-I antibody-positive
HMB45
    homatropine methylbromide
HMB-45 antibody
HMBA
    hexamethylene bisacetamide
hMG
    human menopausal
      gonadotropin
HMPAO
    hexamethylpropyleneamine
    oxime
HN
        Ensure HN
        Osmolite HN
        TwoCal HN
HN$_2$
    nitrogen mustard
HNP
    herniated nucleus pulposus
HOCA
    high-osmolar contrast agent
hockey-stick
        h.-s. appearance of the
          ureters
        h.-s. catheter
HOCM
    high-osmolar contrast medium

Hodgkin
    H. cell
    H. disease (HD)
    H. lymphoma
Hodgkin-related
Hodson-type kidney
HOE-BAY 964
Hoechst
    H. 33342
    H. dye method
Hoerr rule
Hofbauer cell
Hoffa
    H. disease
    H. fat pad
    H. fracture
Hoffmeister series
holandric gene
holding
    breath h.
holdup in flow of barium
hole
    bur h.
Holen-Hatle equation
hole-within-hole appearance
holistic medicine
Hollenhorst plaques
Holliday junction
Hollister
    H. bridge suture holster
    H. wound exudate absorber
hollow
    h. fiber dialyzer
    h. needle guide
holmium
    166 h.
holmium-166
holmium-YLF
holoacardia
holography
holoprosencephaly
    alobar h.
    lobar h.
    semilobar h.
Holoxan
Holstein-Lewis fracture
Holt-Oram syndrome

NOTES

Homans sign
homatropine methylbromide
  (HMB45)
home
    h. care
    h. health care
    h. nutritional support
homeobox
homeodomain
homeopathy
homeostasis
    brain h.
    immunologic h.
Homerlok needle
Homer Mammalok needle
Homer Wright rosette
homing
    h. mechanism
    h. molecule
    h. receptor
    T-lymphocyte h.
hominis
    Blastocystis h.
    Herpesvirus h.
homocholic acid
homocysteic acid
homocystinemia
homocystinuria
homodimer
homoerotic
homogenates
homogeneity
homogenizer
    dounce glass h.
homogenously staining region
homograft
homoharringtine
homoharringtonine
homolog
homologous
    h. antigen
    h. disease
    h. tumor
homonymous hemianopsia
homophobe
homophobic
homosexuality
homosexual panic
homospoil
Homo-Tet
homotransplantation
homozygosity
homozygous achondroplasia

honeycomb
    h. pattern
    h. vertebra
honeycombed appearance
honeycombing
Hong Kong disease
Honvan
hooked acromion
hook of the hamate fracture
hookwire
    Kopan breast lesion
    localization h.
hookworm
    h. anemia
hoop
    h. stress
    h. stress fracture
Hoover sign
HOP
    hydroxydaunorubicin, Oncovin,
    prednisone
Hopmann papilloma
Hoppe-Seyler test
hordeolum
horizontal
    h. beam film
    h. boundary
    h. fracture
    h. overframing
    h. transmission of virus
hormesis
hormonagogue
hormonal
    h. ablative therapy
    h. agent
    h. assay
    h. flare
    h. prevention
    h. therapy
hormone
    adrenocorticotropic h.
      (ACTH)
    angiotensin-converting h.
    antidiuretic h. (ADH)
    endogenous h.'s
    exogenous h.'s
    follicle-stimulating h.
    gonadotropin-releasing h.
      (GRH, GnRH)
    growth h. (GH)
    growth hormone-releasing h.
      (GHRH)
    human growth h. (HGH)

luteinizing h. (LH)
luteinizing hormone-
   releasing h. (LHRH)
lymphocyte-stimulating h.
parathyroid h. (PTH)
h. receptor
serum parathyroid h.
sex h.
steroidal h.
syndrome of inappropriate
   secretion of antidiuretic h.
   (SIADH)
h. therapy
thyroid h.
thyroid-stimulating h. (TSH)
thyrotropin-releasing h.
   (TRH)
hormone-refractory
   h.-r. breast cancer
   h.-r. prostate cancer
hormone-releasing
horn
   frontal h.
   iliac h.
   occipital h.
   temporal h.
Horner syndrome
Horner-Wright rosette
horse
   h. antihuman thymus
      globulin
   h. red blood cells
horseradish peroxidase
horseshoe
   h. configuration
   h. fibrosis
   h. kidney
   h. lung
hospice
   h. care
Hospital
   H. for Sick Children pain
      scale
   St. Jude Children's
      Research H.
hospital-based registry

host
   h. cell
   h. defense
   h. defense mechanism
   h. factor
   h. reaction
   h. rescue
   h. response
   h. response mechanism
   h. vector system
host-related factor
hot
   h. appendix
   h. caudate lobe
   h. contrast medium
   h. spot
   h. spot imaging
   h. thyroid nodule
hot-cold hemolysin
hot-cross-bun appearance
hot-tip probe
hot-water circulating suit
Hounsfield unit (HU)
hourglass
   h. configuration
   h. membrane
   h. phalanges
   h. stenosis
   h. ventricle
Howell-Jolly body
HOX11
   HOX11 oncogene
   HOX11 proto-oncogene
HPA
   helix pomatia agglutinin
   hypothalamic-pituitary-adrenal
   axis
   HPA suppression
HPA-23
   antimonium tungstate
HPD
   hypothalamic-pituitary-gonadal
HpD phototherapy
HPETE
   hydroperoxyeicosatetraenoic
   acid

NOTES

hpf
    high-power field
hPL
    human placental lactogen
HPLC
    high-performance liquid
      chromatography
    high-pressure liquid
      chromatography
HPM
    Harding-Passey melanoma
HPSEC
    high-performance size-exclusion
      chromatography
HPV
    human papillomavirus
    human parvovirus
HPV-16
H-ras
    H -r. oncogene
    H -r. proto-oncogene
H-ras gene
HRCT
    high-resolution computed
      tomography
HS
    herpes simplex
HSAP
      HSAP phosphatase
      HSAP tumor marker
HSC
    hematopoietic stem cells
HSG
    hysterosalpingogram
H-shape vertebrae
HSM
    hepatosplenomegaly
***hst (K-fgf)* proto-oncogene**
HSV
    herpes simplex virus
HTH
    helix-turn-helix
HTLV
    human T-cell leukemia virus
    human T-cell lymphotropic virus
    human T-lymphotropic
      retrovirus
H-type
    H.-t. fistula
    H.-t. tracheoesophageal
      fistula

HU
    Hounsfield unit
    hydroxyurea
Huber needle
HU-CSF
    human urinary CSF
Hudson nebulizer
Hughston view
HuIFN
    human interferon
hum
    venous h.
human
    h. AML cell line
    h. antimouse antibody
      (HAMA)
    h. chorionic gonadotropin
      (hCG)
    h. granulocyte-stimulating
      factor
    h. growth factor
    h. growth hormone (HGH)
    h. herpesvirus type 6
      (HHV-6)
    h. immunodeficiency virus
      (HIV)
    h. immunodeficiency virus
      1 (HIV-1)
    h. immunodeficiency virus
      2 (HIV-2)
    h. immunodeficiency virus
      antibody (HIV-AB)
    h. interferon (HuIFN)
    interferon beta,
      recombinant h., Betaseron
    h. interleukin
    interleukin-1-alpha,
      recombinant h.
    h. interleukin for DA-cells
    interleukin-1 receptor
      antagonist, recombinant h.
    interleukin-3, recombinant h.
    h. leukemia-associated
      antigen
    h. leukocyte antigen (HLA)
    h. leukocyte Cw5 antigen
    h. leukocyte interferon
      (HLI)
    h. macrophage-monocyte
      chemotactic and activating
      factor (rhMCAF)
    h. menopausal gonadotropin
      (hMG)

h. papillomavirus (HPV)
h. parvovirus (HPV)
h. placental lactogen (hPL)
h. serum albumin
h. T-cell leukemia virus (HTLV)
h. T-cell leukemia virus type 1-5
h. T-cell lymphotropic virus (HTLV)
h. T-lymphotropic retrovirus (HTLV)
h. T-lymphotropic virus
h. tumor
h. urinary CSF (HU-CSF)
humanized antibody
human-leukocyte-antigen-identical transplant
human-murine xenograft
Humaplastin
Humatin
humeral
h. avulsion of the glenohumeral ligament
h. circumflex
h. fracture
h. head-splitting fracture
h. length
h. line
h. physeal fracture
h. supracondylar fracture
humeroradial articulation
humerus
head of the h.
humoral
h. antibody
h. factor
h. immunity
hump
dowager's h.
dromedary h.
Hampton h.
Humphry
H. ligament
ligament of H.
Humulin

Hunter
H. canal
H. and Driffield (H and D)
H. and Driffield curve (H and D curve)
H. glossitis
H. syndrome
Hunter-Sessions
H.-S. balloon
H.-S. transvenous balloon occlusion catheter
Huntington
H. chorea
H. disease
H. rod insertion
Hurler-Scheie compound
Hurler syndrome
Hurst phenomenon
Hürthle
H. cell adenoma
H. cell carcinoma
H. cell neoplasia
H. cell tumor
Huschke foramen
HUTCH-1 antigen
Hutch diverticulum
Hutchinson
H. fracture
H. syndrome
H. triad
Huygens principle
H-vertebrae
HVL
half-value layer
HVOD
hepatic venoocclusive disease
HVPGS
high-voltage pulsed galvanic stimulation
hyaline
h. leukocyte
h. membrane disease
hyaline-vascular
h.-v. Castleman disease
h.-v. variant
hyalinized fibroadenoma
hyalinizing granuloma

NOTES

hyaloid
    h. artery
    h. canal
hyaloserositis
hyaluronan marker
hyaluronic acid
H-Y antigen
Hyate
hybrid
    h. imaging
    h. magnet
    h. probe
    h. regimen
    h. subtraction technique
hybridization
    fluorescence in situ h.
    (FISH)
    Northern h.
    nucleic acid h.
    h. probe
    in situ h.
    Southern blot h.
    in vitro h.
hybridization-subtraction technique
hybridized orbital
hybridoma
    h. antibody
    h. cell
    h. technique
hybridon
hycamptamine
Hycodan
hydatid
    h. cyst
    h. disease
    Morgagni h.
    h. sand
hydatidiform mole
hydatidosis
Hydragran absorption dressing
hydralazine
hydramnios
hydranencephaly
hydrate
    chloral h.
hydration
    h. layer water
    h. water
hydraulic distention
hydrazine sulfate
Hydrea
hydrocalicosis
hydrocalyx

hydrocarbon inhalation
hydrocele
    congenital h.
    idiopathic h.
hydrocephalus
    chronic communicating h.
    communicating h.
    congenital h.
    extraventricular h.
    extraventricular
      obstructive h.
    h. ex vacuo
    infantile h.
    intraventricular h.
    intraventricular
      obstructive h.
    low-pressure h.
    noncommunicating h.
    nonobstructive h.
    normal-pressure h.
    normal pressure h. (NPH)
    obstructive h.
    posttraumatic h.
    unilateral h.
hydrochloride
    cytarabine h.
    cytosine arabinosine h.
    daunomycin h.
    daunorubicin h.
    diphenhydramine h.
    doxorubicin h.
    hydroxydaunomycin h.
    lidocaine h.
    mechlorethamine h.
    melphalan h.
    meperidine h.
    mitoxantrone h.
    nalbuphine h.
    procarbazine h.
    rubidomycin h.
    tolazoline h.
    tripelennamine h.
    zorubicin h.
hydrocodone
hydrocolloid dressing
hydrocolpos, hydrocolpocele
hydrocortisone (HC)
    h. sodium succinate
hydrogen
    h. density (N(H))
    h. peroxide
    h. spin density
hydrogen-1

hydrogen-2
hydrolase
    S-adenosylhomocysteine h.
    (AdoHcyase)
hydrolysis
hydrometer
hydrometra
hydrometrocolpos
hydromorphone
    h. HCl
hydromyelia
hydromyoma
hydronephrosis
4-hydroperoxycyclophosphamide (4-HC)
    4-h. acid
hydroperoxyeicosatetraenoic acid (HPETE)
hydrophilic guidewire
hydrophone
hydropneumothorax
    loculated h.
hydrops
    fetal h.
    h. fetalis
    gallbladder h.
    immune h.
    nonimmune h.
    h. tubae profluens
hydropyonephrosis
hydroquinone
hydrosalpinx
hydrostatic reduction
hydrosyringomyelia
hydrothorax
hydroureter
hydroxamamide
4-hydroxyandrostenedione
hydroxyapatite
    h. deposition disease (HADD)
    h. rheumatism
hydroxycobalamin
17-hydroxycorticosteroid
hydroxydaunomycin hydrochloride
hydroxydaunorubicin, Oncovin, prednisone (HOP)

hydroxydiphosphonate
    ethylene h.
hydroxyethyl starch
4-hydroxyifosfamide (4-OHIPA)
hydroxylase
    tyrosine h.
hydroxylation
    microsomal h.
    ring h.
hydroxyprogesterone
    h. caproate
hydroxyurea (HU)
hydroxyzine
Hy-Gestrone
hygiene
    oral h.
hygroma
    chromosomal abnormality
    cystic h.
    cystic h.
hylic tumor
Hylutin
Hymenolepis nana
Hymlek portable chest tube
hyoglossus muscle
hyoid
    h. bone
Hypaque
    H. enema
    H. swallow
Hyperab
hyperabduction syndrome
hyperactive peristalsis
hyperactivity
hyperacute rejection
hyperaeration
hyperalbuminemia
hyperaldosteronism
hyperalimentation
hyperammonemia
hyperamylasemia
hyperandrogenism
hyperargininemia
hyperbaric oxygen
hyperbeta-alaninemia
hyperbetalipoproteinemia
hyperbilirubinemia

NOTES

hyperbradykininemia
hypercalcemia
    h. of infancy
    h. of malignancy
    paraneoplastic h.
hypercalcuria
hypercapnia
hypercarotenemia
hypercellularity
hypercementosis
hyperchlorhydria
hyperchromatic cell
hypercoagulability
    paraneoplastic h.
hypercorticism
hypercortisolemia
hypercortisolism
hypercystinuria
hyperdense
    h. brain lesion
    h. lesion
hyperdiploid
    h. tumor
hyperdiploidy
hyperechogenicity
hyperechoic
    h. renal medulla
hyperemesis gravidarum
hyperemia
    reactive h.
hypereosinophilia
hypereosinophilic syndrome
hypererythrocythemia
hyperextension
hyperfibrinogenemia
hyperfine coupling
Hyperforat
hyperfractionated
    h. total body irradiation
hyperfractionation
hypergammaglobulinemia
hyperglycemia
hypergranular acute promyelocytic
  leukemia
hyperhemoglobinemia
Hyper-Hep
hyperhomocystinemia
hypericin
hyperimmune globulin
hyperinflation
hyperintense
    h. brain lesion
    h. lesion

hyperintensity
    cortical h.
    incidental punctate white
      matter h.
    punctate white matter h.
hyperkeratosis
hyperleukocytosis
hyperlipidemia
hyperlipoproteinemia
hyperlucent
hypermobile joint
hypermotility
hypermutation
    somatic h.
hypernephroma
hyperosmolality
hyperosmolar
hyperosmolarity
hyperostosis
    ankylosing h.
    bony h.
    chronic infantile h.
    cortical h.
    diffuse idiopathic skeletal h.
    (DISH)
    h. frontalis interna
    generalized cortical h.
    infantile h.
    infantile cortical h.
    skeletal h.
    vertebral h.
hyperoxaluria
hyperparathyroidism
    persistent h.
    primary h.
    recurrent h.
    secondary h.
hyperpathia
hyperperistalsis
hyperphenylalaninemia
hyperphosphatasia
    hereditary h.
hyperpigmentation
    nail h.
    oral h.
hyperpigmented lesion
hyperpituitarism
hyperplasia
    adenomatoid h.
    adenomatous h.
    adrenal h.
    alveolar epithelial h.
    angiofollicular h.

angiofollicular lymph
  node h.
angiolymphoid h.
atypical regenerative h.
benign prostatic h. (BPH)
bone marrow lymphoid h.
breast h.
Brunner gland h.
congenital adrenal h.
conjunctival follicular h.
cutaneous lymphoid h.
cystic h.
cystic glandular h.
desquamated epithelial h.
ductal h.
endometrial h. (EH)
epithelial h.
explosive follicular h.
florid follicular h.
focal cortical h.
focal nodular h. (FNH)
follicular h.
gallium-avid thymic h.
G cell h.
giant lymph node h.
glandular h.
glomerular mesangial h.
hemophagocytic
  histiocytic h.
immunoblastic h.
intimal h.
lymphoid h.
mantle zone h.
medial h.
mixed follicular h.
multicentric angiofollicular
  lymphoid h.
myointimal h.
nodular h.
nodular lymphoid h.
nodular regenerative h.
paracortical h.
plasmacytic h.
polymorphic B-cell h.
reactive h.
reactive follicular h.
reactive lymphoid h.

sclerosing duct h.
sinus h.
Swiss cheese h.
thymic h.
thyroid h.
hyperplastic
  h. achondroplasia
  h. cholecystosis
  h. gastropathy
  h. polyp
hyperpotassemia
hyperprolactinemia
hyperproteinemia
hyperreflexia
  detrusor h.
hypersecretion
  gastric h.
hypersensitivity
  alveolar h.
  delayed h.
  h. lymphadenopathy
  h. pneumonitis
  h. reaction
  tracheobronchial h.
hypersexuality
hypersplenic anemia
hypersplenism
hypertelorism
hypertension
  arterial h.
  benign intracranial h.
  extrahepatic h.
  extrahepatic portal h.
  intracranial h.
  intrahepatic h.
  intrahepatic portal h.
  persistent pulmonary h.
  portal h.
  pregnancy-induced h.
  pulmonary h.
  pulmonary arterial h.
  pulmonary venous h.
  renal allograft-mediated h.
  renovascular h.
  renovascular cause for h.
  suprahepatic h.

NOTES

273

hypertension *(continued)*
    thromboembolic pulmonary
      arterial h.
    venous h.
hypertensive
    h. cardiovascular disease
    h. encephalopathy
    h. intraarterial chemotherapy
Hyper-Tet
hyperthermia
    annular phased array h.
    interstitial h.
    prostatic h.
    h. therapy
    h. treatment
    whole-body h.
hyperthermic
    h. antiblastic perfusion
    h. limb perfusion
hyperthyroidism
hypertonic
    h. glucose
    h. solution
hypertonica
    polycythemia h.
hypertrichosis lanuginosa
hypertrophic
    h. cardiomyopathy
    h. gastritis
    h. olivary degeneration
    h. osteoarthropathy
    h. pulmonary
      osteoarthropathy
    h. pyloric stenosis
    h. subaortic stenosis
hypertrophicans
    osteodermopathia h.
hypertrophy
    asymmetric septal h.
    benign prostatic h.
    Brunner gland h.
    cardiac h.
    compensatory h.
    concentric h.
    focal pyloric h.
    focal renal h.
    interatrial septal h.
    lipomatous h.
    pyloric h.
    septal h.
    septate h.
    symmetric h.

Hypertussis
hyperuricemia
hypervariable
    h. region
    h. sequence
hypervascularity
hyperviscosity syndrome
hypervitaminosis
hypervitaminosis D
hypervolemia
    h. of pregnancy
hypesthesia
    facial h.
hypnoanalgesia
hypnoanesthesia
hypnosis
hypoacousia
hypoalbuminemia
hypoaldosteronism
hypobetalipoproteinemia
hypobilirubinemia
hypocalcemia
    paraneoplastic h.
hypocapnia
hypocarbia
hypocellular acute leukemia
hypocellularity
    bone marrow h.
hypochloremia
hypochlorhydria
hypocholesterolemia
hypochondroplasia
hypochordal arch
hypochromia
hypochromic
    h. anemia
    h. erythrocyte
hypocoagulable
hypocratic fingers
hypocycloidal
hypocythemia
hypocytosis
hypodense
    h. brain lesion
    h. lesion
hypodensity
    nodal h.
    periventricular h.
hypodiploid tumor
hypodiploidy
hypoechogenicity
    false h.

hypoechoic
   h. liver
   h. renal sinus
hypoeosinophilia
hypoferremia
hypofibrinogenemia
hypofluorite
   acyl h.
hypofractionation
hypogammaglobulinemia
   sex-linked h.
   X-linked h.
hypogastric artery
hypogenetic lung syndrome
hypoglossal
   h. canal
   h. fossa
   h. nerve
   h. nerve palsy
   h. palsy
hypoglycemia
hypogonadism
   iatrogenic h.
hypogranular acute promyelocytic
  leukemia
hypogranulocytosis
hypoinflation of the lung
hypointensity
   cortical h.
hypokalemia
hypokinesis
hypolipoproteinemia
hypolobulation
hypomagnesemia
hypometabolism
hyponatremia
   dilutional h.
hypoparathyroidism
hypoperfusion
   cerebral h.
hypoperistalsis syndrome
hypophagia
hypopharyngeal
   h. cancer
   h. tumor
hypopharynx

hypophosphatasia
   congenital lethal h.
hypophosphatemic
   h. osteomalacia
   h. rickets
   h. vitamin D refractory
   rickets
hypophyseal fossa
hypophysectomy
hypophysis
hypophysitis
   lymphoid h.
hypopituitarism
hypoplasia
   bone marrow h.
   cartilage-hair h.
   cerebellar h.
   cerebral white matter h.
   congenital renal h.
   gallbladder h.
   pulmonary h.
   tubular h.
   uterine h.
hypoplastic
   h. heart syndrome
   h. left heart syndrome
   h. penis
   h. right heart syndrome
   h. thumb
hypopotassemia
hypoproteinemia
hypospadias
hyposplenism
hypotelorism
hypotension
   arterial h.
hypothalamic
   h. amenorrhea
   h. blood flow
   h. glioma
hypothalamic-pituitary-adrenal axis
  (HPA)
hypothalamic-pituitary-gonadal
  (HPD)
   h.-p.-g. axis
hypothalamus
hypothenar region

NOTES

hypothermia
    scalp h.
    h. treatment
hypothermic perfusion
hypothesis
    Goldie-Coldman h.
    Korenman estrogen
      window h.
    Norton-Simon h.
    null h.
    Starling h.
    h. testing
    two-hit h.
hypothrombinemia
hypothyroidism
    secondary h.
    tertiary h.
hypotonia
hypouricemia
hypovolemia
hypoxanthine
hypoxemia
hypoxia
    tumor h.
hypoxic
    h. cell cytotoxic agent
    h. cell sensitizer
    h. sensitizer
hypozincemia
HypRho-D
Hyprogest
Hyproval

Hyproxon
Hyrniuk-Bush model
Hyrtl foramen
hysterectomy
    abdominal h.
    extrafascial h.
    modified radical h.
    radical h.
    radical abdominal h.
    radical vaginal h.
    Rutledge classification of
      extended h.
    supracervical h.
    total abdominal h.
    vaginal h.
hysteresis
hystericus
    globus h.
Hysterocath hysterosalpingography
    device
hysterography
hysteromyoma
hysterosalpingo-contrast sonography
hysterosalpingogram (HSG)
hysteroscopy
hysterotomy
hystoincompatibility
Hytrast
Hytrin
Hz
    hertz

I
>I blood group
>I cell disease

I-131
>Albumotope I-131

^{131}I
>iodine-131

^{125}I
>iodine-125

Ia antigen

IAEA
>International Atomic Energy Agency

IAP
>immunosuppressive acidic protein
>IAP tumor marker

iatrogenic
>i. anemia
>i. arteriovenous fistula
>i. disease
>i. hypogonadism
>i. immunosuppression
>i. menopause
>i. TRD

IBC
>iron-binding capacity

IBCA
>isobutyl cyanoacrylate

ibenzmethyzin

ibuprofen

ICA
>immunocytochemical assay
>internal carotid artery

ICAM-1
>intercellular adhesion molecule-1

ICD-O
>International Classification of Diseases for Oncology

ICE
>ifosfamide, carboplatin, etoposide

ice
>dry i.
>i. skater's fracture

iceberg
>i. phenomenon
>i. radiotherapy

ichthyosis
>acquired i.

ICPO protein

ICR
>Institute for Cancer Research

ICRF
>bispiperazinedione

ICRF-159

ICRF-187

ICRP
>International Commission on Radiological Protection

ICRU
>International Commission on Radiation Units and Measurements

icteric

icteroanemia

icterus
>i. neonatorum
>i. praecox

ICV
>intracerebroventricular
>ICV reservoir

IDA
>image display and analysis
>iminodiacetic acid
>IDA scanning

Idamycin

idarubicin

IDC
>invasive ductal carcinoma

IDDM
>insulin-dependent diabetes mellitus

identical twin

IDE particle

idioagglutinin

idioheteroagglutinin

idiopathic
>i. acro-osteolysis
>i. anemia
>i. follicular mucinosis
>i. growth hormone deficiency
>i. hydrocele
>i. hypertrophic subaortic stenosis
>i. hypochromic anemia
>i. interstitial fibrosis
>i. interstitial pneumonitis

idiopathic *(continued)*
  i. intestinal
    pseudoobstruction
  i. megakaryocytic aplasia
  i. plasmacytic
    lymphadenopathy
  i. pulmonary hemosiderosis
  i. thrombocytopenia
  i. thrombocytopenic purpura
    (ITP)
idiotype
  i. antibody
  anti-shared i.
idiotypic antigen
IDMTX
  intermediate-dose methotrexate
idoxuridine (IUDR)
IDX
  4'-iodo-4'-deoxydoxorubicin
IDXrad
IEP
  immunoelectrophoresis
IFA
  immunofluorescence antibody
  incomplete Freund adjuvant
Ifex
  ifosfamide
IFN-α
IFN-α2
IFN-alpha 2
IFN-alpha 2b
IFN-beta
IFN-G
  gamma interferon
IFOS, IFX
  ifosfamide
ifosfamide, iphosphamide (Ifex, IFOS, IFX)
ifosfamide, carboplatin, etoposide (ICE)
ifosfamide, mensa uroprotection, methotrexate, etoposide (IMVP-16)
ifosfamide, Platinol, Adriamycin (IPA)
IFT
  inverse Fourier transform
IFX (*var. of* IFOS)
Ig
  immunoglobulin
  Ig binding
  cytoplasmic Ig
  Ig gene

  platelet-associated Ig (PAIg)
  platelet-directed Ig (PDIg)
IgA
  IgA antibody
  IgA synthesis
IgD
  immunoglobulin D
IgE
  immunoglobulin E
IGF, ILGF
  insulin-like growth factor
IGF-1
  insulin-like growth factor-1
IGF-2
  insulin-like growth factor-2
IGFBP
  insulin-like growth factor-
    binding protein
IgG
  immunoglobulin G
  IgG kappa
IgM
  immunoglobulin M
IgY antibody
II
  Cohn fraction II
  Lynch syndrome II
  Photofrin II
  Renovist II
  Rolloscope II
  Sentinel II
  Stachrom heparin cofactor
    II
  Topo II
    topoisomerase II
  topoisomerase II (Topo II)
III
  antithrombin III (AT III)
  Assera AT III
  Assera-Plate AT III
  Assera protein C
  AT III
    antithrombin III
  Liatest AT III
  Stachrom AT III
  Thrombate III
IL
  interleukin
IL-1
  interleukin-1
IL-2
  interleukin-2

IL-3
   interleukin-3
IL-4
   interleukin-4
IL-5
   interleukin-5
IL-6
   interleukin-6
    rMu IL-6
      murine interleukin-6
IL-7
   interleukin-7
    rMu IL-7
IL-1A
I-labeled B-cell-specific anti-CD20 monoclonal antibody (BIMAb)
IL-1B
    rMu IL-1B
ILE-964
    SDZ ILE-964
ileal
   i. atresia
   i. conduit
   i. loop
   i. loopography
   i. spill
   i. stenosis
ileitis
   backwash i.
   nonsclerosing i.
   regional i.
   terminal i.
   yersinia terminal i.
ileoanal pull-through procedure
ileocecal
   i. cystoplasty
   i. junction
   i. valve
ileocolic artery
ileocolostomy
ileoentectropy
ileofemoral
   i. thrombosis
   i. vein
   i. wing fracture

ileostogram
ileostomy
ileum
   cobblestone i.
   collapsed distal i.
   terminal i.
ileus
   adynamic i.
   cecal i.
   colonic i.
   gallstone i.
   localized i.
   meconium i.
   paralytic i.
   reflex i.
ILGF (*var. of* IGF)
Ilheus virus
ilia (*pl. of* ilium)
   crests of the i.
iliac
   i. artery
   i. artery aneurysm
   i. artery stenosis
   i. crest
   i. fossa abscess
   i. horn
   i. spine
   i. vein
   i. vessel
iliacus
ilii
   osteitis condensans i.
iliocaval thrombus
iliofemoral
   i. artery
   i. thrombosis
ilioinguinal lymph node
ilioneoureterocystotomy
iliopectineal line
iliopsoas
   i. bursa
   i. bursitis
   i. compartment
   i. muscle
   i. tendon

NOTES

iliotibial
    i. band
    i. tract
ilium, pl. **ilia**
    crest of the i.
Ilizarov device
ILL
    intermediate lymphocytic
    lymphoma
ill-defined mass
illicit
    i. drug
    i. sex
Illinois needle
illness comorbidity
illuminator
    Mammo Mask i.
ilmofosine
iludin S
image
    i. acquisition time
    i. amplifier
    i. analysis
    axial i.
    cine magnetic resonance
      function i.
    i. compression
    i. contrast
    contrast-enhanced MR i.
    coronal i.
    i. cytometry
    i. degradation
    degradation of i.
    i. display
    i. display and analysis
      (IDA)
    Doppler i.
    dynamic i.
    flip-angle i.
    flow compensated i.
    flow-on gradient-echo i.
    i. foldover
    i. formation
    ghost i.
    gradient-recalled echo i.
    gray scale i.
    hard-copy i.
    imaginary i.
    in-phase i.
    i. intensifier
    longitudinal i.
    magnitude i.
    i. matrix

    matrix i.
    modulus i.
    i. noise
    opposed-phase i.
    out-of-phase i.
    PC i.
    phase i.
    phase contrast i.
    postexercise i.
    i. postprocessing error
      artifact
    proton density i.
    proton density-weighted i.
    real i.
    real-time echo-planar i.
    i. reconstruction
    i. reconstruction time
    i. recording system
    redistribution i.
    sagittal i.
    second-echo i.
    i. shading
    single-slice gradient-echo i.
    i. spatial resolution
    STIR i.
    stress thallium i.
    striations across i.
    stroke count i.
    subtraction i.
    surface-projection
      rendering i.
    thin-section axial i.
    TR i.
    T1-weighted i.
    T2-weighted i.
    voxel-gradient rendering i.
    zebra stripe i.
ImageMASTER
Imagent
    I. BP
    I. GI
    I. LN
    I. US
image-selected in vivo spectroscopy
imaginary
    i. data
    i. image
    i. mode
    i. number
imaging
    acoustic i.
    anisotropically-rotational
      diffusion i.

anisotropic 3D i.
ARD i.
blood pool i.
bone i.
brain i.
bright field i.
cardiac blood pool i.
i. center information system
i. chain veiling glare
chemical shift i. (CSI)
Chopper-Dixon fat
  suppression i.
cine i.
cine magnetic resonance i.
coded-aperture i.
cold spot i.
color Doppler i.
color-flow Doppler i.
continuous-wave Doppler i.
conventional i.
i. cycle
darkfield i.
3DFT gradient-echo MR i.
diagnostic i.
diffusion i.
digital vascular i.
direct Fourier
  transformation i.
dynamic magnetic
  resonance i.
dynamic volume i.
echo i.
echo-planar i. (EPI)
electrostatic i.
endocrine i.
endometrial chemical
  shift i.
fast i.
fast Fourier i. (FFr)
fat-suppression MR i.
fat/water chemical shift i.
field-echo i.
FLASH magnetic
  resonance i.
flow-sensitive MR i.
Fourier i.
Fourier transform i.

functional i.
gadolinium-enhanced MR i.
gallium i.
gated blood pool i.
gradient-echo i.
gradient-echo MR i.
gradient-to-noise i.
gray scale i.
GRE i.
half-Fourier i. (HFI)
half Nex i.
hepatobiliary i.
high-resolution i.
high-resolution 3DFT MR i.
high-speed i.
hot spot i.
hybrid i.
infarct-avid i.
in-phase i.
interventional i.
iodine fluorescence i.
isotope colloid i.
isotope hepatobiliary i.
isotropic 3D i.
low flip angle gradient-
  echo i.
magnetic resonance i. (MRI)
maxillofacial i.
microwave i.
monoclonal antibody i
MR i.
multiecho i.
multiformatted i.
multiplanar i.
multiple-echo i.
multiple-gated blood pool i.
multiple line scan i.
multiple plane i.
multiple spin echo i.
multislice i.
multislice modified KEW
  direct Fournier i.
musculoskeletal i.
myocardial perfusion i.
myocardial thallium i.
nuclear i.
nuclear cardiovascular i.

NOTES

imaging *(continued)*
    nuclear magnetic resonance i.
    oblique magnetic resonance i.
    opposed-phase i.
    optimum-angle i.
    out-of-phase i.
    paramagnetic enhancement accentuation by chemical shift i.
    perfusion i.
    phase i.
    phase contrast i.
    phase-dependent spectroscopic i.
    phase-offset multiplanar i.
    phase-ordered multiplanar i.
    phase-sensitive gradient-echo MR i.
    photostimulable phosphor digital i.
    planar i.
    planar radionuclide i.
    point i.
    POMP i.
    postoperative i.
    PR i.
    projection-reconstruction i.
    projection tract i.
    proton chemical shift i.
    quantitative i.
    radionuclide i.
    rapid i.
    real-time i.
    real-time color Doppler i.
    reconstructive i.
    reticuloendothelial i.
    rotating frame i.
    selective excitation projection reconstruction i.
    sensitive plane projection reconstruction i.
    sequential first-pass i.
    sequential line i.
    sequential plane i.
    sequential point i.
    short inversion recovery i. (STIR)
    simultaneous volume i.
    single-echo diffusion i.
    single-slice modified KEW direct Fournier i.
    sodium i.
    SPECT i.
    spin-echo i.
    spin-echo magnetic resonance i.
    spin-warp i.
    spoiled gradient-echo i.
    steady-state gradient-echo i.
    i. study
    subsecond FLASH i.
    subtraction i.
    susceptibility i.
    ^{99m}Tc-HMPAO cerebral perfusion SPECT i.
    ^{99m}Tc-HMPAO SPECT i.
    technetium-thallium subtraction i.
    thallium i.
    thallium myocardial scan with SPECT i.
    three-dimensional i.
    three-dimensional fast low-angle shot i.
    three-dimensional Fourier i. (3DFr)
    three-dimensional projection reconstruction i.
    through transfer i.
    transcranial real-time color Doppler i.
    transfer i.
    transverse section i.
    two-dimensional i.
    two-dimensional Fourier i. (2DFr)
    two-dimensional Fourier transformation i.
    velocity i.
    velocity-density i.
    velocity-encoded cine MR i.
    ventilation-perfusion i.
    video i.
    volume i.
    wavelet-encoded magnetic resonance i.

Imatron C-1000 UFCT scanner
imbalance
    electrolyte i.
    i. of phase or gain artifact
IMED
    I. Gemini PC-2 volumetric controller

I. Gemini PC-2 volumetric
pump
I. infusion pump
Imerslund-Graesbeck syndrome
Imerslund syndrome
[131]I-mIB6
monoiodobenzylguanidine
imidazole carboxamide
imidodiphosphonate
5-iminodaunomycin
5-iminodaunorubicin
iminodiacetic acid (IDA)
imipenem
imipramine
immature
i. ovarian teratoma
i. teratoma
immersion technique
immitis
Coccidioides i.
immobilization
immotile cilia syndrome
ImmTher therapy
immune
i. adherence
i. agglutinin
i. antibody
i. clearance
i. complex disease
i. deficiency
i. enhancement
i. function abnormality
i. gamma globulin
i. globulin
i. globulin intravenous
i. hemolytic anemia
i. hydrops
i. interferon
i. marker
i. modulation
i. monitoring technique
i. neutropenia
i. reconstitution
i. response
i. response gene
i. serum (IS)

i. state
i. suppression
i. suppressor (IS)
i. suppressor gene
i. surveillance
i. system
i. system anatomy
i. thrombocytopenic purpura
(ITP)
immune-mediated antileukemia
effect
Immuneron
Immunerora-C
immunifacient
immunity
acquired i.
active i.
adoptive i.
antiviral i.
cell-mediated i. (CMI)
cellular i.
community i.
congenital i.
cross i.
familial i.
genetic i.
herd i.
humoral i.
impaired i.
inherent i.
innate i.
intrauterine i.
native i.
passive transfer of i.
species-specific i.
T-cell-mediated i.
tissue i.
i. transfer
immunization
active i.
passive i.
prophylactic i.
Immuno
Feiba VH I.
immunoadhesin
immunoadjuvant

NOTES

immunoadsorption
   i. column
   i. technique
immunoarchitecture
immunoassay
   enzyme i. (EIA)
   microlatex particle-
    mediated i.
   nephelometric i.
immunoaugmentative therapy
immunobead-binding assay test
immunobiology
immunoblast
immunoblastic
   i. hyperplasia
   i. lymphadenopathy
   i. lymphadenopathy-like
    T-cell lymphoma
   i. lymphoma
   i. sarcoma
immunoblot test
immunoblotting
immunochemical marker
immunochemistry
immunochemotherapy
immunocompetent
   i. cell
   i. lymphocyte
immunocompromised
immunoconjugate
   BR96-DOX i.
   chelate i.
   yttrium-labeled i.
   yttrium-90-labeled anti-B2 i.
immunocytochemical
   i. analysis
   i. assay (ICA)
   i. marker
   i. stain
immunocytochemistry
immunocytoma
   lymphoplasmacytic i.
   lymphoplasmacytoid i.
   plasma cell i.
   polymorphic i.
immunocytometer
immunodeficiency
   cellular i.
   common variable i.
   human i. virus (HIV)
   primary i.
   severe combined i. (SCID)
   i. state

   i. syndrome
   X-linked hyper-IgM i.
immunodepressed
immunodetection
immunodiagnosis in tumor
  immunology
immunodiffusion
   Ouchterony i.
   Oudin i.
immunodominance
immunoelectrophoresis (IEP)
   countercurrent i.
   countercurrent exchanger i.
   crossed i.
   Laurell i.
   rocket i.
   two-dimensional i.
immunofiltration
immunofixation
immunofluorescence
   i. analysis
   i. antibody (IFA)
   i. antibody assay
   indirect i.
   i. technique
Immunogen
   Salk HIV I.
immunogen
immunogenetic
immunogenic determinant
immunogenotypic analysis
immunogenotyping
immunoglobulin (Ig)
   i. A
   i. alpha chain
   B-cell surface i.
   chelated i.
   i. clonality determination
   cytoplasmic i.
   i. D (IgD)
   i. delta chain
   i. E (IgE)
   i. epsilon chain
   i. G (IgG)
   i. G1
   i. gamma chain
   gamma Y i.
   i. gene
   i. gene rearrangement
   i. heavy chain
   heavy-chain i.
   intracellular i.
   intravenous i. (IVIg)

i. kappa chain
i. lambda chain
i. M (IgM)
i. mu chain
i. resilience
secretory i.
i. superfamily
surface i.
surface membrane i.
immunohematopoietic stem cell
immunohistochemical
i. analysis
i. localization
immunohistochemistry
immunohistofluorescence
immunohistologic staining
immunohistology
bone marrow i.
immunoincompetent
immunoisolation
immunologic
i. characterization
i. classification
i. competence
i. enhancement
i. homeostasis
i. memory
i. method of purging
i. paralysis
i. reconstitution
i. suppression
i. surveillance
i. tolerance
i. unresponsiveness
immunology
immunodiagnosis in
tumor i.
transplantation i.
tumor i.
immunolymphoscintigraphy
immunomagnetic
i. bead
i. purging
immunomodulating infection
**immunomodulator (Imreg-1,
Imreg- 2)**
immunopathogenesis

immunoperoxidase
i. stain
immunophenotype
immunophenotypic
i. analysis
i. marker
immunophenotyping
immunophilin
immunophoresis
immunopotentiation
immunoprecipitation
immunoproliferative
i. lesion
i. small intestinal disease
immunoprophylaxis
immunoradioassay (IRA)
immunoradiometric
i. assay (IRMA)
i. assay of antigen activity
immunoreaction
immunoreactive (IR)
immunoregulation
immunoregulatory effector system
immunoresistance
immunorestorative
immunoscintigraphy
immunoselection
immunosorbent
immunostain
immunostaining
Ki-67 i.
immunostimulation
immunosuppression (IS)
iatrogenic i.
immunosuppressive
i. acidic protein (IAP)
i. drug
i. therapy
immunosurveillance
immunotherapy
active nonspecific i.
active specific i.
adjuvant i.
adoptive i.
nonspecific i.
specific i.
tumor i.

NOTES

immunotoxin
CD5-T lymphocyte i.
ST-1 i.
immunotoxin-mediated cytotoxicity
ImmuRAID-AFP
ImmuRAID-CEA
ImmuRAID-hCG
ImmuRAID-LL2
ImmuRAID-MN3
ImmuRAIT-LL2
impacted fracture
impaction
fecal i.
mucoid i.
impaired
i. immunity
i. perfusion
impairment
growth i.
impedance
acoustic i.
diastolic notch i.
i. matching
i. plethysmography (IPG)
imperfecta
dentinogenesis i.
osteogenesis i.
imperforate anus
impingement
posterosuperior glenoid i.
shoulder i.
i. syndrome
implant
carcinomatous i.'s
cesium i.
cochlear i.
collapsed subpectoral i.
ear i.
electrically activated i.
i. fracture
interstitial i.
intracavitary i.
intravitreal i.
mechanically activated i.
metallic otologic i.
ocular i.
otologic i.
penile i.
planar I mesh i.
prosthetic i.
saline i.
silicone i.
subpectoral i.

transperineal i.
transvaginal i.
tumor i.
implantable
i. drug delivery system
i. infusion port
i. infusion pump
i. osmotic pump
i. vascular access device
implantation
i. cyst
radon seed i.
implanted pump
implanter
Wallner interstitial
prostate i.
impotence
arteriogenic i.
vasogenic i.
impression
basilar i.
convolutional i.
extrinsic i.
extrinsic esophageal i.
i. fracture
imprint
tissue i.
impurity
radiochemical i.
radionuclide i.
Imreg-1
immunomodulator
Imreg-2
immunomodulator
Imubind
I. PA1-1 urokinase inhibitor
I. uPA ELISA kit
I. uPAG ELISA kit
urokinase receptor
Imuran
Imuvert
IMVP-16
ifosfamide, mensa uroprotection,
methotrexate, etopside
^{111}In
indium-111
in
i. situ
i. situ assay
i. situ carcinoma of vagina
i. situ hybridization
i. situ vein graft
i. vitro

i. vitro antibody production assay (IVAP)
i. vitro fertilization
i. vitro hybridization
i. vitro transcription assay
i. vivo
i. vivo binding
i. vivo gene transfer
i. vivo labeling
i. vivo stereologic assessment

inactivation
Knudsen hypothesis of tumor suppressor gene i.

inactivator
C1 i.

inactive endometrium

inadequate
i. cranial calcification
i. surgery

inborn error of metabolism

incarcerated hernia

incessant ovulation

incidence
i. rate

incidentaloma

incidental punctate white matter hyperintensity

incisional
i. biopsy
i. hernia

incisor
fascial i.

incisura
i. angularis
i. defect
i. scapulae

incisural epidermoidoma

inclusion
i. cell
i. cyst
cytoplasmic i.
mesothelial cell i.

incognitus
Mycoplasma i.

incoherent motion

income support

incompatibility
ABO i.
Rh i.

incompetence
tricuspid i. (TI)

incompetent
i. cervix
i. ileocecal valve
i. perforators

incomplete
i. band heterotopia
i. fracture
i. Freund adjuvant (IFA)
i. neurofibromatosis
i. obstruction

incomplete neurofibromatosis

incontinence
bladder i.
bowel i.
stress i.

increased
i. isotope uptake
i. markings of emphysema

increta
placenta i.

incubation period

incus, pl. incudes

IND
investigational new drug

indazole
isomer i.

indeterminate cell

indeterminatus
situs i.

index, pl. indices
amniotic fluid i.
ankle-arm i.
ankle-brachial i. (ABI)
bicaudate i.
bifrontal i.
blood-flow i.
Broca i.
cephalic i.
congestion i.
DNA i.
Doppler flow i.
EORTC i.

NOTES

287

index *(continued)*
   free thyroxine i.
   hairy cell i.
   heteroploid i.
   karyopyknotic i.
   Ki-67 i.
   Krebs leukocyte i.
   metacarpal i.
   mitotic i.
   mitotic-karyorrhectic i.
   nuclear contour i.
   penile-brachial i.
   plasma cell labeling i.
   Pourcelot i.
   pulsatility i.
   quantum mottle i.
   red cell i.
   resistive i.
   short-increment sensitivity i.
   Spitzer quality of life i.
   Stuart i.
   therapeutic i.
   tritiated thymidine
     labeling i. (TLI)
   tubular fertility i.
   widened anterior
     meningeal i.
   Wintrobe i.
Index-Cancer
   Functional Living I.-C.
     (FLIC)
Indiana pouch
Indian Club needle
indicator
   prognostic i.
indices (*pl. of* index)
Indiclor
indifferent gonads
indigenous neoplasm
indirect
   i. detection
   i. fluorescent antibody test
   i. hemagglutination
   i. immunofluorescence
   i. laryngoscopy
   i. ultrasound guidance
indistinct liver sign
indium-111 (^{111}In)
   i.-111 antimyosin
     scintigraphy
   i.-111 DTPA
   i.-111 labeling
   i.-111 pentetreotide

indium-111-labeled leukocyte
indium-111-oxime leukocyte
indium-114m
Indocin
indoleamine
indolent
   i. KS
   i. lymphoma
indomethacin
   i. treatment
induced
   i. sputum
   i. sputum test
inducer
   i. T-cell
   i. T-lymphocyte
inductance
induction
   i. chemotherapy
   dorsal i.
   electric i.
   gene i.
   magnetic i.
   neuromuscular system
     electric i.
   ovulation i.
   remission i.
inductive interaction
indwelling catheter
inequality
   limb length i.
   ventilation-perfusion i.
   V/Q i.
inevitable abortion
infancy
   hypercalcemia of i.
infant
   preterm i.
infantile
   i. choriocarcinoma syndrome
   i. cortical hyperostosis
   i. digital fibromatosis
   i. fibrosarcoma
   i. ganglioglioma
   i. hemangioendothelioma
   i. hydrocephalus
   i. hyperostosis
   i. myofibromatosis
   i. polycystic disease
   i. Refsum disease
   i. type polycystic kidney
     disease

infantisepticum
    Corynebacterium i.
infarct
    basal ganglia i.
    bone i.
    lacunar i.
    medullary i.
    myocardial i.
    placental i.
    spinal cord i.
    testicular i.
    watershed i.
infarct-avid imaging
infarction
    acute myocardial i.
    bilateral i.
    bowel i.
    brainstem i.
    cerebral i.
    cortical i.
    dural sinus thrombosis i.
    embolic i.
    hemorrhagic i.
    ischemic i.
    lacunae i.
    lobar renal i.
    medullary i.
    mesenteric i.
    middle cerebral artery i.
    muscle i.
    myocardial i.
    occlusive mesenteric i.
    periventricular
      hemorrhagic i.
    renal i.
    right ventricular i.
    splenic i.
    transcatheter therapeutic i.
    venous i.
infection
    adenovirus i.
    amebic i.
    anaerobic i.
    bacterial i.
    brain i.
    buccal space i.
    congenital i.

cutaneous i.
cutaneous bacterial i.
cutaneous viral i.
cytomegalovirus i.
deep-seated i.
disk space i.
Epstein-Barr i.
fungal i.
gay bowel i.
granulomatous i.
group B streptococcal i.'s
helminthic i.
hepatic fungal i.
herpes simplex i.
herpes simplex virus i.
HIV i.
HIV-1 i.
HIV-2 i.
immunomodulating i.
intraabdominal i.
kala-azar i.
masticator space i.
mycobacterial i.
mycotic i.
neutropenia-related
  bacterial i.
nonopportunistic i.
nosocomial i.
odontogenic i.
opportunistic i. (OI)
parainfluenza virus i.
parasitic i.
pelvic i.
protozoal i.
pulmonary i.
pulmonary bacterial i.
pulmonary fungal i.
pulmonary parenchymal i.
renal fungal i.
respiratory syncytial virus i.
respiratory tract i.
retroperitoneal i.
rickettsial i.
salivary gland i.
shunt i.
spinal i.
subperiosteal i.

NOTES

infection *(continued)*
    temporal space i.
    urinary tract i.
    varicella-zoster i.
    varicella-zoster virus i.
    viral i.
    Walter Reed classification
      for HIV i.
infectious
    i. granuloma
    i. hepatitis
    i. mononucleosis
    i. papilloma virus
    i. process
inferior
    i. accessory fissure
    i. apical aspect of the
      myocardium
    i. colliculus
    i. displacement
    i. mesenteric artery
    i. mesenteric vein
    i. temporal gyrus
    i. triangle sign
    i. vena cava (IVC)
    i. vena cava catheter
    i. vena cava filter
    i. vena cava umbrella filter
    i. venacavography
Inferon
infertility
infestation
    parasitic i.
infiltrate
    alveolar i.
    benign i.
    consolidating i.
    interstitial i.
    Jessner lymphocytic i.
    localized i.
    mottled i.
    patchy i.
    pulmonary i.
    recurrent fleeting lung i.'s
    soft i.
    strandy i.
infiltrating
    i. carcinoma
    i. duct carcinoma
    i. lobular carcinoma
    i. pneumonitis
    i. small cell lobular
      carcinoma

infiltration
    bone i.
    bone marrow i.
    brachial plexus i.
    diffuse fatty i.
    fatty i.
    leukemic i.
    leukocyte i.
    pericapsular fat i.
    pulmonary i. with
      eosinophilia (PIE)
infiltrative disorder
inflammation
    bronchial i.
    esophageal i.
    granulomatous i.
    myocardial i.
    perirectal i.
    retrodiskal
      temporomandibular joint
      pad i.
    spinal i.
inflammatory
    i. aneurysm
    i. aortic aneurysm
    i. bowel disease
    i. breast cancer
    i. breast carcinoma
    i. carcinoma
    i. cholesteatoma
    i. colonic polyp
    i. condition
    i. disease
    i. endometritis
    i. fibrosarcoma
    i. fracture
    i. myofibroblastic tumor
    i. polyp
    i. pseudotumor
    i. response
    i. T-lymphocyte
influenzae
    Haemophilus i.
influenza virus
information
    i. density
    i. system
informed consent
infraclavicular area
infraction
    i. fracture
    Freiberg i.
infraglottic space

infrahilar area
infrahyoid
inframesocolic space
infraorbital groove
infrapatellar
    i. bursa
    i. fat pad
    i. tendon
    i. view
infrapopliteal
    i. angioplasty
    i. transluminal angioplasty
infrapulmonary
infrarenal
infraspinatus
    i. insertion erosion
    i. tendon
infratemporal fossa
infratentorial
    i. syndrome
    i. tumor
infraumbilical omphalocele
Infumed pump
Infumorph 200, 500
infundibula (*pl. of* infundibulum)
infundibular
    i. pulmonary stenosis
    i. stenosis
infundibulopelvic ligament
infundibulum, pl infundibula
    ductus i.
    i. sign
    i. widening
Infusaid pump
infuser
    Baxter i.
    Ohio i.
    Paragon i.
    single-day i.
infusion
    balloon-occluded arterial i.
    i. chemotherapy
    circadian continuous i.
    continuous i.
    epidural i.
    hepatic artery i.
    intraarterial i.

intralymphatic i.
intraportal i.
intravenous i.
local streptokinase i.
multivitamin i. (MVI-12)
neuraxial opioid i.
pediatric multivitamin i.
i. port
portal i.
i. pump
stem cell i.
streptokinase i.
subcutaneous i.
vasopressin i.
ingestion
Ingram-Bachynski classification of hip fractures
inguinal
    i. canal
    i. hernia
    i. lymphadenectomy
    i. lymph node
    i. lymph node metastasis
inguinale
    granuloma i.
    lymphogranuloma i.
    papilloma i.
INH
    isoniazid
inhalation
    hydrocarbon i.
inherent
    i. drug resistance
    i. filter
    i. immunity
inhibiting gene
inhibition
    cyclooxygenase enzyme i.
    leukocyte adherence i.
    leukocyte migration i.
inhibitor
    ACE i.
    alpha 1 proteinase i.
    aromatase i.
    calmodulin i.
    cell growth i.
    cyclooxygenase i.

NOTES

inhibitor *(continued)*
    endogenous GAD i. (EGI)
    Imubind PA1-1 urokinase i.
    lipoxygenase i.
    Merrill-Dow polyamine i.
    mitotic i.
    monamine oxidase i.
     (MAOI)
    nonnucleoside reverse
     transcriptase i.
    plasminogen activator i.
    prostaglandin i.
    protease i.
    reverse transcriptase i.
    serine protease i.
    spindle i.
    tat i.
    topoisomerase i.
    topoisomerase I i.
inhomogeneity
iniencephaly
injection
    bismuth i.
    bolus i.
    contrast i.
    epidural i.
    epidural steroid i.
    extraarachnoid i.
    facet joint i.
    heavy metal i.
    intracavernosal i.
    intracavernous i.
    intramuscular i.
    intrathecal i.
    intratumoral i.
    ipsilateral i.
    percutaneous alcohol i.
    selective i.
    silicone i.
    steroid i.
    subarachnoid i.
    test i.
    trigger point i.
    ultrasonographically-guided i.
injector
    power i.
injury
    acute traumatic aortic i.
     (ATAI)
    aortic i.
    apophyseal i.
    brachial plexus i.
    brachial plexus birth i.

    cervical i.
    clothesline i.
    contrecoup i.
    endothelial i.
    epiphyseal plate i.
    Erb-Duchenne plexus i.
    firearm i.
    glenoid labrum i.
    intraoperative
     gastrointestinal i.
    irradiation i.
    isolated airway i.
    Klumpke brachial plexus i.
    Kulkarni i.
    lateral compartment
     traumatic bony i.
    mechanism of i.
    metatarsal i.
    midtarsal i.
    needle-stick i.
    pericarinal i.
    phrenic nerve i.
    physeal i.
    proximity i.
    radiation i.
    sesamoid i.
    shearing i.
    SLAP i.
    spinal cord i. (SCI)
    stress i.
    superior labral
     anteroposterior i.
    talofibular ligament i.
    tensile i.
    tracheobronchial i. (TBI)
    traumatic aortic i.
    valgus-external rotation i.
    white matter shearing i.
inlet
    thoracic i.
    transaxial thoracic i.
innate immunity
inner
    i. ear
    i. ear atresia
    i. table of the skull
innocent tumor
innominate
    i. artery
    i. artery compression
    syndrome
    i. bone
    i. vein

innovative therapy
inorganic phosphorus (Pi)
inositus
    diabetes i.
In-pentetreotide scintigraphy
in-phase
    i.-p. image
    i.-p. imaging
insertin protein
insertion
    catheter i.
    Huntington rod i.
    subclavian central venous
      catheter i.
    velamentous i.
insertional mutagenesis
inside-out technique
inside-the-needle infusion catheter
insipidus
    diabetes i.
    nephrogenic diabetes i.
inspiration
    degree of i.
    shallow i.
    suspended i.
inspiratory
    i. effort
    i. stridor
    i. view
inspissated
    i. feces
    i. meconium
INSS
    International Neuroblastoma
    Staging System
    INSS stage 1 tumor
instability
    atraumatic, multidirectional,
      bilateral i. (AMBRI)
    dorsal intercalated
      segment i. (DISI)
    volar intercalated segment i.
instillation
    contrast material i.
instillational therapy

Institute
    I. for Cancer Research
      (ICR)
    Dana-Farber Cancer I.
      (DFCI)
    Milan Cancer I.
    National Cancer I. (NCI)
Institut Gustave-Roussy
institutional care
instrument
    alligator-jaw i.
    Kevorkian-Younge cervical
      biopsy i.
    i. output
    Rotex biopsy i.
insufficiency
    adrenal i.
    aortic i.
    i. fracture
    mesenteric vascular i.
    mitral i.
    pulmonary valve i.
    renal i.
    tricuspid i. (TI)
    uteroplacental i.
    vascular i.
    vertebrobasilar i.
insula, pl. insulae
insular
    i. carcinoma
    i. pattern
insulin
    i. clearance
insulin-dependent diabetes mellitus
  (IDDM)
insulin-like
    i.-l. growth factor (IGF,
      ILGF)
    i.-l. growth factor-1 (IGF-1)
    i.-l. growth factor-2 (IGF-2)
    i.-l. growth factor-binding
      protein (IGFBP)
    i.-l. peptide
insulinoma
int-2 proto-oncogene

NOTES

293

intake
    caloric i.
    fluid i.
integral
    i. dose
    i. uniformity
Integra PBS Pageblot test
integrated
    i. optical density (IOD)
    i. optical density histogram
integrin
integumentary barrier
Intelliject pump
intensification
    i. chemotherapy
    dose i.
    frequency i.
    i. regimen
intensification chemotherapy
intensifier
    image i.
intensifying
    i. screen
    i. screen artifact
intensity
    absolute dose i. (ADI)
    dose i. (DI)
    linear degenerative signal i.
    maximum i.
    radiation i.
    SAPA i.
    SATA i.
    signal i.
    spatial average-pulse
      average i.
    spatial average-temporal
      average i.
    spatial peak-temporal
      average i.
    SPTA i.
    temporal average i.
    temporal peak i.
    TP i.
intensive ductal carcinoma
intent
    curative i.
    palliative i.
interaction
    capacitive i.
    dipole-dipole i.
    effector/target cell i.
    electric i.

    inductive i.
    magnetic i.
    mind-body i.
    proton-electron dipole-
      dipole i.
interaorticobronchial diverticulum
interarticularis
    pars i.
interatrial
    i. septal defect
    i. septal hypertrophy
    i. septum
interbody
    i. bone graft
    i. bone plug
    i. fusion
interbronchial diverticulum
intercalated segment
intercalating agent
intercalation
intercalator
    DNA i.
intercarpal ligament
intercavernous sinus
intercellular adhesion molecule-1
  (ICAM-1)
intercervical disk herniation
intercondylar
    i. eminence
    i. femoral fracture
    i. fracture
    i. humeral fracture
    i. notch
    i. tibial fracture
    i. tubercle
intercostal
    i. artery
    i. nerve
    i. space
interdigital neuroma
interdigitating
    i. dendritic cell
    i. dendritic cell sarcoma
interdisciplinary team
interest
    region of i. (ROI)
interface
    bidirectional i.
    bone-air i.
    fat-fluid density i.
    reactive i.
    shear i.

interference
    i. screw
    slice i.
interferon
    i.-α2
    i.-α
    i. alfa
    i. alfa-2a
    i. alfa-2a, recombinant
    i. alfa-2b
    i. alfa-2b, recombinant
    i. alfa-n1
    i. alfa-n3
    alpha i.
    i. alpha
    alpha i.-2A
    alpha i.-2B
    alpha i.-N1
    alpha i.-N3
    i.-β
    i.-β$_2$
    i. beta, recombinant human
    consensus i.
    gamma i. (IFN-G)
    i. gamma-2a
    i. gamma-1b
    human i. (HuIFN)
    human leukocyte i. (HLI)
    immune i
    leukocyte i.
    lymphoblastoid i.
    r-beta-ser i.
    recombinant i.-α
    recombinant alpha i.
    recombinant alpha-26 i.
τ-interferon
interfollicular
    i. mitotic count
    i. pattern
    i. region
intergroup protocol
interhemispheric
    i. cyst
    i. hematoma
    i. subdural hematoma
interlacing

interleaved
    i. acquisition
    i. phase contrast technique
interlesional therapy
interleukin (IL)
    human i.
    murine i.
    recombinant human i.
      (rhIL)
interleukin-1 (IL-1)
    i. beta
    i. receptor antagonist,
      recombinant human
interleukin-2 (IL-2)
    i., liposome-encapsulated
      recombinant
    PEG i.
    polyethylene glycol-
      modified i. (PEG-IL-2)
    i. receptor
    recombinant i. (rIL-2)
interleukin-3 (IL-3)
    iodine-125-labeled i.-3
    murine i.-3
    recombinant human i.-3
interleukin-4 (IL-4)
interleukin-5 (IL-5)
interleukin-6 (IL-6)
    murine i. (rMu IL-6)
interleukin-7 (IL-7)
    murine i.
interleukin-8
interleukin-9
interleukin-10
interleukin-11
interleukin-12
interleukin-3, recombinant human
interleukin-1-alpha,
    i.-a. recombinant human
interleukin-1B
    murine i.
interleukin-1-beta
interleukin-2 PEG (*var. of* PEG-
interleukin-2)
interlobar
    i. artery
    i. fissure

NOTES

interlobular septum
INtermate
Baxter I.
intermedia
massa i.
thalassemia i.
intermediate
i. carcinoma
i. lymphocytic lymphoma
(ILL)
intermediate-dose
i.-d. methotrexate (IDMTX)
i.-d. salvage regimen
intermedius
bronchus i.
nervus i.
vastus i.
intermittent claudication
interna
hyperostosis frontalis i.
internal
i. auditory canal
i. biliary drainage
i. capsule
i. carotid
i. carotid artery (ICA)
i. carotid balloon test
i. double-J catheter
i. fixation fracture
i. hernia
i. iliac
i. jugular vein
i. mammary artery
i. mammary artery
embolization
i. mammary lymph node
i. oblique radiograph
i. radiation therapy
i. rotation view
i. urethrotomy
internal-external
i.-e. catheter
I.-e. Locus of Control Scale
International
I. Atomic Energy Agency
(IAEA)
I. classification of cancer of
cervix
I. Classification of Diseases
for Oncology (ICD-O)
I. Commission on Radiation
Protection
I. Commission on Radiation

Units and Measurements
(ICRU)
I. Commission on
Radiological Protection
(ICRP)
I. Commission on
Radiologic Protection
I. Federation of Gynecology
and Obstetrics (FIGO)
I. Neuroblastoma Staging
System (INSS)
I. System of Units (SI)
I. Union Against Cancer
(UICC)
I. Union Against Cancer-
RO resection (UICC-RO
resection)
I. Workshop on Human
Leukocyte Differentiation
Antigen
internodal tracts
interobserver error
interossei
dorsal i.
palmar i.
plantar i.
interosseous
interperiosteal fracture
interphalangeal joint
interphase cytogenetics
interpolation
interpositi
cavum veli i.
interposition
i. graft
interpretation
intraoperative i.
mirror-image i.
interpulse
i. interval
i. time
interrogation
Doppler i.
intersex
interslice gap
interspace
interspinous
interstice, pl. **interstices**
graft interstices
interstitial
i. antigen-antibody complex
i. brachytherapy
i. calcinosis

i. cell tumor
i. cell tumor of testis
i. cystitis
i. ectopic pregnancy
i. edema
i. emphysema
i. fibrosis
i. hyperthermia
i. implant
i. infiltrate
i. irradiation
i. loculated hematoma
i. lung disease
i. marking
i. nephritis
i. pneumonia
i. pneumonitis
pulmonary i. disease
i. pulmonary edema
pulmonary i. emphysema (PIE)
i. pulmonary fibrosis (IPF)
i. radiotherapy
i. therapy
interstitium
intertrochanteric
i. crest
i. four-part fracture
i. fracture
i. region
interuncal distance
interval
basion-axial i.
basion-dens i.
i. cancer
interpulse i.
progression-free i.
sampling i.
intervention
biliary i.
dietary i.
obstetric i.
i. study
interventional
i. angiography
i. imaging
i. material

i. neuroradiology
i. procedure
i. radiology
interventricular
i. foramen
i. septal defect
i. septum
intervertebral
i. disk
i. foramina
i. osteochondrosis
intervillous thrombosis
intestinal
i. angina
i. atresia
i. bypass procedure
i. carcinoid tumor
i. collateral
i. conduit
i. flora
i. gas pattern
i. lipodystrophy
lipophagic i.
i. lymphangiectasia
i. mesentery
i. obstruction
i. perforation
i. pseudoobstruction
i. pseudoobstruction syndrome
i. tube
intestinalis
pneumatosis i.
pneumatosis cystoides i.
Septata i.
intestine
large i.
papillary adenoma of large i.
small i.
intima
tunica i.
intimal
i. fibroplasia
i. flap
i. hyperplasia
i. tear

NOTES

intopoline
intoxication
psychogenic water i.
intraabdominal
i. arterial hemorrhage
i. calcification
i. hemorrhage
i. infection
i. mass
i. relapse
intraaortic balloon counterpulsation
intraarterial
i. chemotherapy
i. digital subtraction
angiography
i. floxuridine
i. infusion
i. therapy
intraarticular
i. body
i. fracture
i. localized nodular
synovitis
i. proximal tibial fracture
intraaxial neoplasm
intracanalicular
i. irradiation
intracapsular
i. fracture
i. metastasis
intracardiac
i. pressure
i. shunt
intracartilaginous ossification
intracavernosal injection
intracavernous
i. carotid aneurysm
i. injection
intracavitary
i. delivery
i. implant
i. radium
i. therapy
intracellular
i. activation
i. antigen
i. compartment
i. immunoglobulin
i. target
intracellulare
Mycobacterium i.

intracerebral
i. arteriovenous
malformation
i. blood
i. ganglioglioma
i. ganglioma
i. hematoma
i. hemorrhage
i. leukostasis
i. vascular malformation
intracerebroventricular (ICV)
intraconal
i. lesion
i. portion of the eye
intracranial
i. aneurysm
i. arterial aneurysm
i. arteriovenous fistula
i. arteriovenous
malformation
i. calcification
i. circulation
i. cryptococcosis
i. cyst
i. dermoid cyst
i. hematoma
i. hemorrhage
i. hypertension
i. lesion
i. lipoma
i. mass
i. mass lesion
i. MR angiography
i. neoplasm
i. neuroblastoma
i. pneumocephalus
i. pressure
i. tumor
i. vascular abnormality
intractable
i. epilepsy
i. nausea
i. pain
intracystic
i. papillary carcinoma
i. papilloma
intradecidual sign
intraductal
i. breast carcinoma
i. calcification
i. carcinoma
i. mucin-hypersecreting
neoplasm

i. papillary carcinoma
i. papillary neoplasm of the
  pancreas (IPNP)
i. papilloma
i. papillomatosis
i. ultrasonography
intraductal component
  extensive i. c.
intraduodenal choledochal cyst
intradural
  i. epidermoidoma
  i. extramedullary lesion
  i. extramedullary mass
  i. inflammatory disease
intraepidermal carcinoma
intraepithelial
  i. carcinoma
  i. cell
  i. lymphocyte
  i. neoplasia
  i. neoplasia of vagina
  i. neoplasia of vulva
intrahepatic
  i. arterial-portal fistula
  i. bile duct
  i. biliary calculus
  i. biliary cancer
  i. biliary neoplasm
  i. biloma
  i. cholangiocarcinoma
  i. cholestasis
  i. duct
  i. hypertension
  i. pigment stone disease
  i. portacaval shunt
  i. portal hypertension
  i. portosystemic venous
  shunt
  i. radicle
  i. stone
intralesional therapy
intraligamentous myoma
intralobar sequestration
intralobular connective tissue
intraluminal
  i. adenocarcinoma

i. detail
i. diverticulum
i. duodenal diverticulum
i. filling defect
i. flow phenomenon
i. foreign body
i. hemorrhage
i. intubation
i. thrombus
intralymphatic
  i. infusion
  i. radioactivity
  administration
intramammary lymph node
intramedullary
  i. arteriovenous
  malformation
  i. bony disease
  i. compartment neoplasm
  i. demyelination
  i. disease
  i. lesion
  i. nail
  i. rod
  i. tumor biopsy
intramembranous ossification
intrameniscal
  i. cyst
  i. mucoid degeneration
intramural
  i. diverticulosis
  i. esophageal rupture
  i. extramucosal lesion
  i. filling defect
  i. gastric emphysema
  i. hemorrhage
  i. invasion
  i. pseudodiverticulosis
  i. tumor
intramuscular
  i. injection
  i. venous malformation
intranodal myofibroblastoma
in-transit metastasis
intranuclear virion
intraobserver error

NOTES

intraocular
- i. calcification
- i. foreign body
- i. lesion
- i. melanoma
- i. spread

Intra-Op autotransfusion system
intraoperative
- i. angiography
- i. arteriography
- i. cholangiogram
- i. electron beam radiotherapy (IORT)
- i. fracture
- i. gastrointestinal injury
- i. interpretation
- i. radiation
- i. radiotherapy (IORT)
- i. sonography (IOS)
- i. ultrasonography

intraoral cone irradiation
intraorbital
- i. granular cell tumor
- i. lesion

intraosseous
- i. bone lesion
- i. ganglion
- i. keratin cyst
- i. meningioma

intrapancreatic obstruction
intraparenchymal
- i. hematoma
- i. hemorrhage
- i. lymph node
- i. meningioma

intrapericardial portion
intraperitoneal
- i. abscess
- i. air
- i. chemotherapy
- i. drug administration
- i. rupture
- i. thermochemotherapy

intraplacental venous lake
intrapleural chemotherapy
intraportal infusion
intrapulmonary bronchogenic cyst
intrarectal coil
intrarenal
- i. arterial disease
- i. arterial flow

intrascrotal abscess

intrasellar
- i. lesion
- i. mass

Intrasil catheter
intrasinus air-fluid level
intraspinal
- i. administration
- i. enteric cyst

intratemporal fossa
intratesticular
- i. band
- i. cyst

intrathecal
- i. block
- i. chemotherapy
- i. injection
- i. route
- i. therapy

intrathoracic
- i. catheter
- i. cyst
- i. organ involvement
- i. stomach
- i. trachea

intratumoral
- i. fat
- i. injection

intrauterine
- i. contraceptive device (IUD)
- i. gas (IUG)
- i. gestation
- i. growth retardation (IUGR)
- i. immunity
- i. parabiotic syndrome
- i. pregnancy
- i. sonographic diagnosis

intravaginal torsion
intravascular
- i. agent
- i. coil
- i. consumption coagulopathy
- i. filling defect
- i. foreign body
- i. hemolysis
- i. lymphoma
- i. lymphomatosis
- i. metallic fragment embolus
- i. ultrasonography

intravenous (IV)
- i. administration of contrast material

i. alimentation
i. chemotherapy
i. cholangiography
i. cytotoxic drug
i. digital subtraction angiography
i. drug abuse (IVDA)
i. fluid
immune globulin i.
i. immunoglobulin (IVIg)
i. infusion
i. infusion chemotherapy
i. ozone therapy
i. pyelogram (IVP)
i. pyelography
i. urogram (IVU)
i. urography
intraventricular
    i. blood
    i. hemorrhage
    i. hydrocephalus
    i. mass
    i. meningioma
    i. obstructive hydrocephalus
    i. therapy
    i. tumor
intravesical chemotherapy
intravitreal implant
intravoxel
    i. coherent motion
    i. incoherent motion
    i. phase dispersion
intrinsic
    i. asthma
    i. cellular parameter
    i. compression
    i. defect
    i. energy resolution
    i. factor
    i. field uniformity
    i. filling defect
    i. spatial linearity
    i. tyrosine kinase activity
introducer
    Cardak i.
    Check-Flo i.
    Cook i.

Cope-Saddekni i.
Desilets-Hoffman i.
Excalibur i.
Littleford/Spector i.
LPS Peel-away i.
Mylar sheath i.
Nottingham i.
peel-away i.
Razi cannula i.
i. sheath
Tuohy-Borst i.
introduction
    safety wire i.
Intron A (*var. of* interferon alfa-2b)
Intropaque
intubation
    endotracheal i.
    intraluminal i.
    nasogastric i.
    nasotracheal i.
intussusception
    jejunoduodenogastric i.
    jejunogastric i.
    rectal i.
    retrograde jejunoduodenogastric i.
invagination
    basilar i.
invasion
    blood vessel i.
    early stromal i.
    intramural i.
    local i.
    lymphatic vessel i.
    occipital condyle i.
    perineural i.
    serosal i.
    transmural i.
    vascular i.
invasive
    i. cancer
    i. carcinoma
    i. ductal carcinoma (IDC)
    i. lobular carcinoma
    i. mole
    i. pulmonary aspergillosis

NOTES

invasive *(continued)*
  i. squamous cell carcinoma
  i. therapy
  i. thymoma
Inventory
  Brief Symptom I. (BSI)
  State-Trait Anxiety I.
  Zung Depression I.
inverse
  i. comma appearance
  i. follicle
  i. follicle pattern
  i. Fourier transform (IFT)
  i. square law
inversion
  cardiac i.
  chromosome i.
  frequency-selective i.
  magnetic i.
  i. pulse
  i. recovery (IR)
  i. recovery sequence
  i. recovery spin-echo
    sequence (IRSE sequence)
  i. time (TI)
  torcular-lambdoid i.
  i. transfer
inversus
  situs i.
  situs viscus i.
inverted
  i. diverticulum
  i. nipple
  i. papilloma
  i. umbrella defect
inverted-T appearance
inverted-V sign
inverted-Y fracture
investigational
  i. drug
  i. new drug (IND)
Inv group antigen
invisible
  i. light
  i. main pulmonary artery
involucrum
involution
  follicular i.
  HIV-related follicular i.
involved-field
  i.-f. radiation
  i.-f. radiotherapy

involvement
  axillary node i.
  contiguous organ i.
  extramedullary i.
  intrathoracic organ i.
  lymphomatous bone
    marrow i.
  lymph-vascular i. (LVSI)
  metastatic axillary i.
  pagetoid epidermal i.
  supraclavicular node i.
iobenzamic acid
iobutoic acid
iocarmate meglumine
iocarmic acid
iocetamate
IOD
  integrated optical density
iodamic acid
iodamide
iodatol
iodide
  propidium i.
  radioactive i. (RAI)
iodinated
  i. contrast media
  i. tyrosine group
iodination
iodine
  i. allergy
  i. fluorescence imaging
iodine-125 (^{125}I)
iodine-131 (^{131}I)
  i. antiferritin treatment for
    hepatocellular cancer
  i. metaiodobenzylguanidine
  i. OIH
  i. serum albumin
  sodium iodide i.
  i. whole-body scan
iodine-131-6 beta-iodomethyl-19-nor
  cholesterol
iodine-deficiency goiter
iodine-125-labeled
  i.-l. fragment
  i.-l. interleukin-3
iodine-labeled product
iodipamide
  i. ethyl ester
  i. meglumine
  i. methylglucamine
iodixanol
iodized oil

iodoalphionic acid
iodoazomycin arabinoside
iodobenzamide
iodocholesterol
4'-iodo-4'-deoxydoxorubicin (IDX)
iododeoxyuridine (IUDR)
    i. labeling
4-iododexetimide
iododoxorubicin
iodohippurate
iodomethamate
iodophendylate
iodophthalein
iodopyracet
iodovinylestradiol
iodoxamate
iodoxamic acid
iodoxyl
ioglicate
ioglicic acid
ioglucol
ioglucomide
ioglunide
ioglycamic acid
ioglycamide
iogulamide
iohexol
    i. CT ventriculogram
iomide
ion
    i. chamber
    chlorethyl carboniom i.
    heavy i.
ion-bound water
Ionescu-Shiley valve
ionization
ionizing radiation
ionography
iopamidol
iopanoate
iopanoic acid
iopentol
iophendylate
iophenoic acid
iophenoxic acid
ioprocemic acid
iopromide

iopronic acid
iopydol
iopydone
IORT
    intraoperative electron beam
      radiotherapy
    intraoperative radiotherapy
IOS
    intraoperative sonography
iosefamate
iosefamic acid
ioseric acid
iosimide
iosulamide
iosumetic acid
iotasul
ioteric acid
iothalamate
      meglumine i.
iothalamic acid
iotrolan
iotroxamide
iotroxic acid
ioversol
ioxaglate
    i. meglumine
    i. sodium
ioxaglic acid
ioxilan
ioxithalamate
ioxithalamic acid
iozomic acid
IPA
    ifosfamide, Platinol, Adriamycin
    4-hydroxy IPA
IPF
    interstitial pulmonary fibrosis
IPG
    impedance plethysmography
iphosphamide (*var. of* ifosfamide)
IPNP
    intraductal papillary neoplasm of
      the pancreas
ipodate
    i. sodium
ipodic acid
ipomeanol

NOTES

iproplatin
ipsilateral
    i. antegrade arteriography
    i. femoral neck fracture
    i. femoral shaft fracture
    i. injection
    i. lateral ventricle
IR
    immunoreactive
    inversion recovery
IR-192
Ir
    iridium
        Ir gene
^{192}Ir
    iridium-192
^{194}Ir
    iridium-194
IRA
    immunoradioassay
IRCF-187
Iriditope
iridium (Ir)
    i. needle
    i. wire
iridium-192 (^{192}Ir)
iridium-194 (^{194}Ir)
irinotecan
    CPT-11 i.
iris melanoma
IRMA
    immunoradiometric assay
        prolifigen TPA IRMA
iron
    i. binding
    i. deficiency
    i. deficiency anemia
    i. deposition
    ferrous i.
    gadolinium i.
    i. overload
    i. oxide
    i. oxide dextran colloid
    i. stain
    i. storage disease
iron-ascorbate-DTPA
    technetium-99m i.-a.-DTPA
iron-binding
    i.-b. capacity (IBC)
    i.-b. capacity test
iron-dextran particle
irradiation
    abdominal i.

    adjuvant i.
    cardiac i.
    charged-particle i.
    cranial i.
    craniospinal i.
    external beam i.
    external orthovoltage i.
    extracorporeal i.
    fractionated i.
    fractionated external
      beam i.
    gamma i.
    hemibody i.
    hyperfractionated total
      body i.
    i. injury
    interstitial i.
    intracanalicular i.
    intraoral cone i.
    local i.
    low LET external beam i.
    mantle i.
    mediastinal i.
    pelvic i.
    prophylactic i.
    selective i.
    single-fraction total body i.
    surface i.
    i. tolerance
    total body i. (TBI)
    total nodal i.
    UV i.
    whole abdominopelvic i.
      (WAP)
    whole-body i.
    whole-pelvis i.
irreducible fracture
irregular border
irregularity
    avulsive cortical i.
irritable bowel syndrome
irritant
irritation
    chronic i.
    i. fibroma
irrotationally bound water
IRSE sequence
    inversion recovery spin-echo
      sequence
IS
    immune serum
    immune suppressor
    immunosuppression

iscador
ischemia
    cerebral i.
    chemotherapy-induced i.
    focal i.
    focal cerebral i.
    limb i.
    mesenteric i.
    myocardial i.
    nonocclusive mesenteric i.
    organ i.
    radiation-induced i.
    reversible myocardial i.
    stress-induced i.
    testicular i.
ischemic
    i. bowel disease
    i. brainstem
    i. colitis
    i. disease
    i. encephalopathy
    i. heart disease
    i. infarction
    i. necrosis
ischia (*pl. of* ischium)
    transverse diameter
      between i.
ischial
    i. bursitis
    i. spine
    i. tuberosity
ischiopagus
ischium, pl. ischia
ischromatic
isethionate
    pentamidine i.
    piritrexim i.
Is gene
island
    blood i.
    bone i.
    compact i.
    endometrial i.
    fat i.
    Pander i.
    sclerotic bone i.

islet
    i. cell adenoma
    i. cell neoplasm
    i. cell tumor
isoallotypic determinant
isoantibody
isoantigen
isobologram analysis
isobutyl
    i. cyanoacrylate (IBCA)
    dipyridamole technetium-
      99m-2-methoxy i.
isocarboxazid
isochromat
isochromatic
isochromosome
Isocon camera
isocyanate
isocytosis
isodense
    i. subdural hematoma
isodose
    i. curve
    i. line
isoechoic
isoeffect dose
isoenzyme
    creatine kinase-BB i.
      (CK-BB)
    growth-related tumor
      markers ALP i.
    Regan i.
isoenzyme RNase
    ALP i.
isoflurane
isogeneic
    i. antigen
    i. graft
isograft
isohemagglutinin
isoimmunity
isointense
isointensity
Isolar rod
isolated
    i. airway injury
    i. heat perfusion

NOTES

isolated *(continued)*
    i. limb perfusion
    i. tethered cord syndrome
isolation perfusion therapy
isoleucine
isologous neoplasm
isomer indazole
isometric
    i. contractile force ring
    i. transition
isomorphic gliosis
isoniazid (INH)
isonitrile
    dipyridamole technetium-
       99m-2-methoxy isobutyl i.
Isopaque
isopentane
isophil
    i. antibody
    i. antigen
Isopora belli
isoporosis
Isoprinosine
isopropyl pyrrolizine
Isospora
isosporiasis
isosulfan blue
isothiocyanate
    fluorescein i.
Isotope
    i. colloid imaging
    daughter i.
    i. dilution principle
    i. effect
    gamma-emitting i.
    i. hepatobiliary imaging
    labeling of the i.
    low LET i.
    phosphorus i.
    poorly-concentrated i.
    radioactive i.
    rhenium i.
    short-range i.
    strontium i.
    i. uptake
isotretinoin
isotropic
    i. 3D imaging
    i. motion
    i. resolution
    i. tissue
isotropy

isotype
    M-component i.
isotypic determinant
isovaleric acidemia
isovolumetric
    i. contraction
    i. relaxation
isovolumic contraction
Isovue
Isovue M
issue
    vocational i.
isthmus
    aortic i.
    pontine i.
    uterine i.
Itaqui virus
iterative reconstruction
ITP
    idiopathic thrombocytopenic
      purpura
    immune thrombocytopenic
      purpura
      steroid-refractory ITP
itraconzaole
IUD
    intrauterine contraceptive device
IUDR
    idoxuridine
    iododeoxyuridine
IUG
    intrauterine gas
IUGR
    intrauterine growth retardation
IV
    intravenous
    KVO-type IV
Ivalon
    I. embolization
    I. particle
IVAP
    in vitro antibody production
      assay
IVC
    inferior vena cava
IVDA
    intravenous drug abuse
Ivemark syndrome
IVIg
    intravenous immunoglobulin
ivory
    i. phalanx
    i. vertebra

IVP
  intravenous pyelogram
IVU
  intravenous urogram
Ivy bleeding time

IX:Ag
  Asserachrom IX:Ag
  Assera-Plate IX:Ag
Ixodes dammini

NOTES

Jaccoud arthropathy
Jackson
    J. dilator
    J. and Parker classification
      of Hodgkin disease
Jackson-Pratt drain
Jaffe-Campanacci syndrome
Jagziekte disease
jail-bar
    j.-b.'s appearance
    j.-b. chest
    j.-b. rib
Jakob-Creutzfeldt disease
Jaksch
    J. anemia
Jamshidi
    J. adult needle
    J. liver biopsy needle
    J. muscle biopsy needle
    J. needle
Jamshidi-Kormed bone marrow
  biopsy needle
Jansen-type metaphyseal
  chondrodysplasia
Jantene procedure
Japanese
    J. B encephalitis virus
    J. variant
Jarisch-Herxheimer reaction
Jass grading system
jaundice
    neonatal obstructive j.
    obstructive j.
Jaworski body
JC
    JC papovavirus
    JC virus
J chain
Jefferson fracture
Jeffery classification of radial
  fractures
jejunal
    j. diverticulosis
    j. leiomyosarcoma
jejuni
    Campylobacter j.
jejunitis
    ulcerative j.
jejunization

jejunoduodenogastric
    j. intussusception
    retrograde j. intussusception
jejunogastric intussusception
jejunoileal
    j. diverticulum
    j. shunt
jejunum
jelly belly appearance
jennerian
jennerization
Jensen sarcoma
Jerne
    J. plaque assay
    J. theory of antibody
      formation
Jeryl Lynn mumps virus
Jessner lymphocytic infiltrate
jet
    j. lavage
    j. nebulizer
    pressurized fluid j.
    regurgitant j.
    ureteral j.
Jeune
    J. disease
    J. syndrome
Jevity
Jewett
    J. nail
    J. and Whitmore
      classification
Jewett-Strong-Marshall
    J.-S.-M. staging
    J.-S.-M. staging of bladder
      cancer
Job syndrome
Jod-Basedow phenomenon
Joel scanning electron microscope
Johns Hopkins Oncology Center
Johnson & Johnson waterproof
  tape
joining
    j. chain
    j. segment
joint
    acromioclavicular j.
    ankle j.
    atlantoaxial j.
    ball-and-socket j.

joint *(continued)*
    bird-wing j.
    calcaneocuboid j.
    j. capsule
    Charcot j.
    j. chondroma
    Chopart j.
    Clutton painful j.
    coracoclavicular j.
    costotransverse j.
    costovertebral j.
    j. depression fracture
    distal interphalangeal j.
    (DIP)
    j. effusion
    elbow j.
    facet j.
    facet j. injection
    femoropatellar j.
    j. fracture
    hypermobile j.
    interphalangeal j.
    knee j.
    Lisfranc j.
    manubriosternal j.
    metacarpophalangeal j.
    (MCPJ)
    metatarsal j.
    metatarsophalangeal j.
    j. mice
    j. mouse
    neuropathic j.
    patellofemoral j.
    pisotriquetral j.
    proximal interphalangeal j.
    (PIP)
    radioulnar j.
    sacroiliac j.
    scapulothoracic j.
    seagull j.
    shoulder j.
    signal j.
    j. space
    j. space narrowing
    sternoclavicular j.
    sternomanubrial j.
    subtalar j.
    synovial j.
    talocalcaneonavicular j.
    talonavicular j.
    tarsal j.
    temporomandibular j. (TMJ)
    tibiofibular j.
    tibiotalar j.
    transverse tarsal j.
    trapeziometacarpal j.
    uncovertebral j.
    wrist j.
joints of Luschka
Jolly body
Jones
    J. criteria
    J. fracture
Jones-Mote reaction
joule
J-sella
J-shaped stomach
Judet view
Judkins catheter
jugular
    j. bulb anomaly
    j. catheter
    j. compression maneuver
    j. foramen
    j. foramen schwannoma
    j. foramen syndrome
    j. lymph node
    j. node metastatic
    carcinoma
    j. technique
    j. tubercle
    j. vein
    j. vein thrombosis
    j. venous pressure
jugulare
    glomus j.
jugulodigastric node
juice
    cancer j.
junction
    atrioventricular j.
    corticomedullary j.
    costochondral j.
    craniovertebral j.
    EG j.
    esophagogastric j.
    gastroduodenal j.
    gastroesophageal j.
    GE j.
    gray-white j.
    Holliday j.
    ileocecal j.
    rectosigmoid j.
    splenoportal j.
    squamocolumnar j.
    sternochondral j.

temporoparietooccipital j.
ureteropelvic j. (UPJ)
ureterovesical j.
uterovesical j.
junctional
   j. cortical defect
   j. dilatation
   j. epidermolysis bullosa
   j. zone
Junin virus
***jun* proto-oncogene**
Jurkat T-cell line
juvenile
   j. angiofibroma
   j. aponeurotic fibroma
   j. autosomal recessive
     polycystic disease
   j. carcinoma
   j. cell
   j. chronic myelogenous
     leukemia
   j. epiphysitis
   j. fibroadenoma

   j. fibromatosis
   j. hemangiofibroma
   j. hyalin fibromatosis
   j. nephronophthisis
   j. palmoplantar fibromatosis
   j. pilocytic astrocytoma
   j. polyposis
   j. rheumatoid arthritis
   j. xanthogranuloma
juvenilis
   kyphosis dorsalis j.
juxtaarticular
juxtacortical
   j. fracture
   j. osteogenic
   j. osteosarcoma
juxtaductal aortic coarctation
juxtaglomerular tumor
juxtaphrenic peak
juxtaposition
J-wire
   teflonized J-w.

NOTES

311

K

K
- K antigen
- K capture
- K electron
- K shell

³⁹K
- potassium-39

Kabikinase
Kagan staging system
Kager triangle
kala-azar infection
Kaliman atherectomy catheter
kallikrein-inhibiting unit
Kallman syndrome
kangri
- k. burn carcinoma
- k. cancer

kansasii
- *Mycobacterium k.*

kaolin pneumoconiosis
Kaplan-Meier
- K.-M. survival curve
- K.-M. univariant analysis

Kaposi
- K. sarcoma (KS)
- K. varicelliform eruption

kappa
- IgG k.
- k. light chain

Karapandzic flap
Karnofsky
- K. performance score
- K. performance status of chemotherapy
- K. rating scale

Karpas T-cell
Karr method
Karroo syndrome
Kartagener
- K. syndrome
- K. triad

karyolytic
karyometric analysis
karyometry
karyopyknotic index
karyorrhexis
karyotype
Kasabach-Merritt syndrome
Kasai procedure
Kashin-Bek disease

Kast syndrome
Katayama fever
Katzen infusion wire
Kauffmann-White scheme
Kawasaki
- K. disease
- K. syndrome

Kaye tamponade catheter
Kayser-Fleischer ring
Keasby tumor
keep vein open (KVO)
Kegel exercises
Keil
- K. classification of non-Hodgkin lymphoma
- K. tumor cell classification

Kell
- K. antibody
- K. blood group

Kell-Cellano blood group
Kellgren
- K. arthritis
- K. disease

Kemerova virus
Kemohan classification
Kemron
Kensey dynamic angioplasty catheter
Kensey-Nash lithotrite
keratin
- k. ball

keratinizing squamous metaplasia
keratinocyte
- dyskeratotic k.

keratitis
- necrogranulomatous k.

keratoacanthoma
keratoconjunctivitis sicca
keratocyst
- odontogenic k.

keratoma
keratosis
- actinic k.
- seborrheic k.

keratosulfaturia
Kerckring
- K. fold
- K. ossicle

Kerley
- K. A lines

Kerley *(continued)*
  K. B lines
  K. lines
kernel of popcorn appearance
kernicterus
Kernig sign
Kern marker
Kernohan
  K. histiologic grading
    system
  K. notch
ketamine
ketanserin
ketene
  propyl k.
ketoconazole
ketone body
ketoprofen
ketorolac tromethamine
ketosis
3-ketosteroid
Ketostix
Ketron-Goodman syndrome
Kety-Schmidt method
kev, keV
  kiloelectron volt
Kevorkian-Younge cervical biopsy
  instrument
Key-Conwell classification of pelvic
  fractures
Keyes dermatologic punch
keyhole
  k. configuration
  k. limpet hemocyanin
keyhole-shaped craniectomy
KG-1 cell
kHz
  kilohertz
Ki-1
  Ki-1 antigen
  Ki-1 positive lymphoma
Ki-67
  Ki-67 antibody
  Ki-67 immunostaining
  Ki-67 index
  Ki-67 monoclonal antibody
  Ki-67 nuclear antigen
Kidd
  K. antibody
  K. blood group
kidney
  absent k.
  k. adenocarcinoma

  k. adenoma
  k. anomaly
  Ask-Upmark k.
  bilateral large k.
  bilateral small k.
  Brödel-type k.
  cake k.
  k. cancer
  dysgenetic k.
  ectopic k.
  k. failure
  floating k.
  fractured k.
  fused k.
  Hodson-type k.
  horseshoe k.
  lump k.
  medullary sponge k.
  mesonephric k.
  multicystic dysgenetic k.
  multicystic dysplastic k.
  Page k.
  partially-polycystic k.
  pelvic k.
  pole-to-pole length of k.
  Potter type IV k.
  putty k.
  sponge k.
  k. stone
  supernumerary k.
  k. transplant
  unicaliceal k.
  unilateral large smooth k.
  unilateral small k.
  unipapillary k.
kidney-fixing antibody
kidney-shaped distended cecum
kidneys, ureters, bladder (KUB)
kidneys and urinary bladder
  (KUB)
Kiel Pediatric Tumor Registry
Kienböck disease
Kikuchi disease
Kilfoyle classification of condylar
  fractures
kill
  cell k.
  fractional cell k.
  log k.
killed
  k. vaccine
  k. virus
  k. virus vaccine

killer
　　k. cell
　　lymphokine-activated k.
Killian dehiscence
kiloelectron volt (kev, keV)
kilohertz (kHz)
kilovoltage (kV, kv)
　　k. peak (kVp)
　　peak k. (pkV)
Kimmelstiel-Wilson syndrome
Kim-Ray Greenfield caval filter
Kimura disease
Kimura-type choledochal cyst
Kin Air bed
kinase
　　adenylate k. (AK)
　　creatine k. (CK)
　　cytoplasmic protein k.
　　deoxycytidine k.
　　deoxythymidine k.
　　protein k.
　　pyrimidine k.
　　serine k.
　　threonine k.
　　tyrosine k.
　　tyrosine protein k.
kinematics
kinesin protein
kinetic
　　cell k.'s
　　exponential k.'s
　　k. resistance
kinetic-based sequencing
kinetocyte
Kinevac
King-Armstrong unit
kinin
kink
　　k. artifact
　　cervicomedullary k.
kinking
　　aortic k.
kinky-hair syndrome
Kinyoun stain
Ki-ras gene

Kirklin
　　K. meniscal complex
　　K. sign
Kirsten sarcoma virus
kissing
　　k. artifact
　　k. contractions
　　k. cousin sign
　　k. ulcers
kissing-balloon
　　k.-b. angioplasty
　　k.-b. technique
kit
　　CELLFREE Interleukin-2
　　　Receptor k.
　　cold k.
　　Imubind uPA ELISA k.
　　k. ligand
　　Myelo-Nate k.
kit proto-oncogene
Kitzmiller test
Klatskin
　　K. biliary adenocarcinoma
　　K. cholangiocarcinoma
　　K. needle
　　K. tumor
Klebsiella
　　K. oxytoca
　　K. pneumoniae
kleeblatschädel deformity
Kleffner-Landau syndrome
Kleihauer test
Klenow fragment
Klinefelter syndrome
Klippel-Feil syndrome
Klippel-Trenaunay syndrome
Klippel-Trenaunay-Weber-Rubashov
　　syndrome
Klippel-Trenaunay-Weber syndrome
Klonopin
Klumpke
　　K. brachial plexus injury
　　K. paralysis
Km antigen
knee
　　k. fracture

NOTES

knee *(continued)*
  k. joint
  k. joint effusion
knife
  gamma ray k.
knob
  aortic k.
knot
  false k.
  true k.
knuckle
  k. sign
Knudsen hypothesis of tumor suppressor gene inactivation
Koate-HP, -HS, -HT
Kobak needle
Kobert test
Koch
  K. phenomenon
  K. postulate
Kocher
  K. fracture
  K. maneuver
Kock pouch
Koenen tumor
KoGENate
Köhler disease
Kohn pore
koilocytotic cell
Kolmer test
Kommerell diverticulum
Kontrast U
Konȳne 80
Konȳne-HT
Kopan
  K. breast lesion localization hookwire
  K. needle
Korenman estrogen window hypothesis
Korin fever
Kormed liver biopsy needle
Körner septum
Kostmann syndrome
Kovalevsky canal
Kowarsky test
Kr
  krypton
Krabbe disease
K-ras proto-oncogene

Krebs leukocyte index
Krishan procedure for DNA analysis by flow cytometry
Kronlein orbitotomy
Krukenberg tumor
krusei
  Candida k.
Kruskal-Wallis nonparametric analysis of variance
krypton (Kr)
  k. laser
krypton-81
krypton-81m
KS
  Kaposi sarcoma
  indolent KS
K-space
KUB
  kidneys, ureters, bladder
  kidneys and urinary bladder
Kugelberg-Welander disease
Kugel collateral
Kulchitsky cell
Kulkarni injury
Kumba virus
Kümmel disease
Kun colocolpopoiesis
Kupffer
  K. cell
  K. cell sarcoma
Kussmaul sign
kV, kv
  kilovoltage
Kveim
  K. antigen
  K. test
KVO
  keep vein open
KVO-type IV
kVp
  kilovoltage peak
kwashiorkor
Kwik Board IV and arterial line stabilizer
Kynacyte
kyphoscoliosis
kyphosis
  k. dorsalis juvenilis
Kytril

L1210
L1210 leukemia
murine leukemia L1210
L-696,229
L-697,661
L-735,524
L26 antigen
LA
leuprolide acetate
Labbé vein
labeled
l. leukocyte scan
l. thyroxine
labeling
l. abnormality
antibody l.
indium-111 l.
iododeoxyuridine l.
l. of the isotope
technetium-99m antibody l.
in vivo l.
labialis
herpes l.
labia majora
lability
genetic l.
Laboratories
Venereal Disease
Research L. (VDRL)
laboratory
l. finding
l. marker
l. study
labral-capsular
l.-c. complex
shoulder l.-c. complex
La Bross spot test
labrum
glenoid l.
labrum-ligament complex (LLC)
labyrinth, labyrinthus
labyrinthine
l. disease
l. fistula
labyrinthitis ossificans
labyrinthus (*var. of* labyrinth)
lace-like appearance
laceration
bladder l.
parenchymal l.

lacerum
foramen l.
lac operon
lacrimal
l. artery
l. canaliculi
l. gland
l. mass
l. nerve
l. recess
l. sac
β-lactam
lactamase
lactate
l. proton
Ringer l.
lactated Ringer solution
lactating
l. adenoma
l. breast
lactation
lactescent blood
lactic
l. acidosis
l. dehydrogenase (LDH)
lactiferous duct
Lactobacillus
L. casei
L. casei factor
L. lactis Dorner factor
lactoferrin
lactogen
human placental l. (hPL)
lacto-N-fucopentose III
lacuna, lacune, pl. **lacunae**
lacunaire
état l.
lacunar
l. cell
l. infarct
l. skull
lacune (*var. of* lacuna)
LAD
left anterior descending
ladakamycin
Ladd bands
ladder effect
ladderlike pattern
Ladendorff test
L.A.E. 20

Laënnec cirrhosis
Laetrile
laeve
    chorion l.
LaGrange classification of humeral
  supracondylar fractures
lag screw
Laimer
    triangle of L.
LAK cell
lake
    intraplacental venous l.
    maternal l.
    venous l.
laked blood
Laki-Lorand factor
Lallemand body
Lallemand-Trousseau body
LAM-1
    leukocyte adhesion molecule-1
lambda
    l. light chain
lambdoid
    l. suture
    l. synostosis
lambdoidal suture
lamblia
    Giardia l.
lambliasis
lamella
    basal l.
lamellar periosteal reaction
lamina
    l. dura
    external elastic l.
    l. papyracea
    l. propria
    vertebral l.
laminar
    l. air flow
    l. flow
    l. fracture
laminated gallstone
laminectomy
laminin receptor
laminogram
laminography
laminotomy
lamivudine
Lamprene
Lancefield classification
lanceolate deformity
Lancereaux diabetes

Landau diamagnetism
Landschutz tumor
Landzert fossa
Langat virus
Langerhans
    L. cell
    L. cell histiocytosis
Langer-Saldino disease
Langhans giant cell
Lansing virus
lanthanide metal
lanthanides
lanthanum
lanuginosa
    hypertrichosis l.
Lanz line
LAO
  left anterior oblique
laparoscopic
    l. abdominal tumor
    diagnosis laparoscopic
    abdominal tumor diagnosis
    l. cholecystectomy
laparoscopy
laparotomy
    staging l.
lap-belt ecchymosis
Laplace law
lap seatbelt fracture
Laredo-Bard needle
large
    l. agranular lymphocyte
    l. bowel
    l. cell carcinoma
    l. cell immunoblastic
    lymphoma
    l. cell lung cancer
    l. cell lymphoma
    l. cell undifferentiated
    carcinoma
    l. clothing artifact
    l. column of Bertin
    l. granular lymphocyte
    l. granular lymphocyte
    antigen
    l. granular lymphocytic
    (LGL)
    l. granular lymphocytic
    leukemia
    l. intestine
    l. intestine neoplasm
    l. loop excision
    l. loop excision of

transformation zone
(LLETZ)
l. noncleaved cell lymphoma
l. noncleaved follicular
center cell
l. plaque parapsoriasis
l. septum of Bertin
large-bore catheter
large-core technique
large-for-gestational age (LGA)
Lariam
Larmor
L. equation
L. frequency
L. precession
Larsen-Johannson disease
laryngeal
l. cancer
l. cartilage
l. forceps
l. granuloma
l. neoplasm
l. nerve
l. papillomatosis
l. skeleton
l. stridor
laryngectomy
supraglottic l.
vertical partial l.
laryngitis
viral spasmodic l.
laryngography
laryngomalacia
laryngopyocele
laryngoscopy
indirect l.
laryngotracheitis
laryngotracheobronchitis
larynx
laser
argon l.
l. balloon
l. beam
l. biliary lithotripsy
endoscopic l.
l. energy
l. energy absorption

Excimer dye l.
helium-cadmium l.
krypton l.
Nd:YAG l.
neodymium:yttrium-
aluminum-garnet laser
neodymium:yttrium-
aluminum-garnet l.
(Nd:YAG laser)
l. recanalization
smart l.
l. system
TEC-2100 postioning l.
l. therapy
laser-assisted balloon angioplasty
Lasix
Lassa fever virus
late antigen
latency
molecular l.
latent
l. carcinoma
l. iron-binding capacity
(LIBC)
l. membrane protein-1
(LMP-1)
latent carcinoma
late-onset dwarfism
lateral
l. aberrant thyroid
carcinoma
l. compartment traumatic
bony injury
l. condylar humeral fracture
l. decubitus radiograph
l. decubitus view
l. extension view
l. flexion view
l. geniculate body
l. lemniscus tract
l. malleolar fracture
l. mass
l. meningocele
l. oblique radiograph
l. oblique view
l. pharyngeal wall
l. projection

NOTES

lateral *(continued)*
    l. radiograph
    l. recess
    l. recess stenosis
    l. rectus muscle
    l. resolution
    l. root
    l. skull radiograph
    l. spinothalamic tract
    l. subluxation
    l. sulcus
    l. tibial plateau fracture
    l. ventricle
lateralis
    sinus l.
lateromedial oblique view
latex
    l. agglutination
    l. balloon
    l. condom
    l. dam
    D-Di l.
    Spli-Prest l.
Latino virus
latissimus dorsi
latitude
    l. film
LATS
    long-acting thyroid stimulator
lattice
    l. theory
laudanum
Laue x-ray crystallography
Lauge-Hansen classification of ankle fractures
Laugier fracture
Laurell
    L. immunoelectrophoresis
    L. technique
Laurence-Moon-Biedl syndrome
Lauren classification
lavage
    antral l.
    bronchoalveolar l. (BAL)
    gastric l.
    jet l.
    peritoneal l.
law
    Behring l.
    Curie l.
    Dulong and Petit l.
    Faraday l.
    Fick l.
    Gibbs-Donnan l.

    inverse square l.
    Laplace l.
    Le Borgne l.
    Lenz l.
    Poiseuille l.
    Wolff l.
lawn plate
Law view
layer
    basalis l.
    boundary l.
    half-life l.
    half-value l. (HVL)
    tenth-value l.
layered gallstone
lazaroid
lazy leukocyte syndrome
LBL
    lymphoblastic lymphoma
L-buthionine sulfoximine
L-CF
    leucovorin-citrovorum factor
L-chain myeloma
lck
    lck oncogene
    lck proto-oncogene
LD
    lethal dose
    LD antigen
LDH
    lactic dehydrogenase
LDL
    low-density lipoprotein
LDR
    low-dose rate
    LDR intracavitary radiation therapy
LE
    lupus erythematosus
    LE factor
    LE prep
Le
    Lewis
    Le blood group antigen
    Le Borgne law
Le Fort
    Le Fort fibular fracture
    Le Fort fracture
    Le Fort mandibular fracture
    Le Fort procedure
    Le Fort-Wagstaffe fracture
lead
    bipolar l.

l. line
pacemaker l.
l. pipe colon
l. pipe fracture
l. poisoning
precordial l.
l. shield
leaf of the diaphragm
leafless tree appearance
leaflet
bridging l.
heart valve l.
valve l.
League of Nations staging
leak
calibrated l.
transient chyle l.
urine l.
leakage
bile l.
silicone implant l.
leaky gene
leatherbottle stomach
lecithin
egg l.
Leclercq test
lectin
l. agglutination
l. cell adhesion molecule
Ulex europaeus I l.
lectin-binding site
Lederer anemia
Lee
L. needle
L. & Westcott needle
leeching
LEEP
loop electrosurgical excision
procedure
LEEP conization
Lee-White clotting time
Le Fort fracture
left
l. anterior descending
(LAD)
l. anterior descending artery
l. anterior oblique (LAO)

l. anterior oblique view
l. atrioventricular groove
artery
l. circumflex artery
l. common carotid artery
l. coronary artery
l. heart catheterization
l. heart syndrome
l. lateral decubitus film
l. parietal syndrome
l. pulmonary artery
l. ventricle
l. ventricular aneurysm
l. ventricular configuration
l. ventricular ejection
fraction
l. ventricular failure
l. ventricular function
l. ventricular gated blood
pool scan
l. ventricular inflow tract
obstruction
l. ventricular outflow tract
l. ventricular outflow tract
obstruction
l. ventriculography
left-sidedness
bilateral l.-s.
left-side-down position
left-to-right shunt
Legg-Calvé-Perthes disease
Legionella
L. pneumophila
legionella
l. pneumonia
legionellosis
Legionnaire's disease
Leiner disease
leiomyoblastoma
leiomyofibroma
leiomyoma
l. cutis
epithelioid l.
parasitic l.
pedunculated l.
uterine l.
vascular l.

NOTES

leiomyomatosis
    l. peritonealis disseminata
leiomyomatous
    l. hamartoma
    l. tumor
leiomyosarcoma
    esophageal l.
    gastric l.
    jejunal l.
    retroperitoneal l.
    uterine l.
Leishman chrome cell
Leishman-Donovan body
Leishmania
    L. tropica
leishmaniasis
L electron
lemniscus, pl. lemnisci
    medial l.
lemon sign
length
    crown-rump l. (CRL)
    femoral l. (FL)
    fetal femoral l.
    focal l.
    humeral l.
    limb l.
    pulse l.
    renal l. measurement
Lennert
    L. classification for
      follicular lymphoma
    L. lymphoma
    L. pattern
lens
    acoustic l.
    catadioptric l.
lenticulostriate
    l. arteries
    l. vessel
lentiform nucleus
lentigo maligna
lentil
    l. agglutination binding
    l. lectin affinity
      chromatography
Lentinan
lentivirus
    bovine l.
Lenz law
leontiasis ossea
Leon virus

Lepore
    hemoglobin L.
    L. trait
    L. virus
lepra
    l. cell
    l. reaction
leprae
    Mycobacterium l.
lepromin
Lepron Depot
leprosy
leptocyte
leptocytosis
    hereditary l.
leptomeningeal
    l. anastomosis
    l. cancer
    l. carcinoma
    l. carcinomatosis
    l. cyst
    l. enhancement
    l. failure
    l. lymphoma
    l. metastasis
    l. space
leptomeninges
leptomeningitis
leptomeningoencephalitis
leptomyelolipoma
leptospirosis
Leriche syndrome
Leri-Layani-Weill syndrome
Leri pleonosteosis
lesbian
Lesch-Nyhan syndrome
Leser-Trélat sign
lesion
    admixture l.
    angiocentric
      immunoproliferative l.
      (AIL)
    angiocentric
      lymphoproliferative l.
    annular constricting l.
    aortic valve l.
    apple core l.
    atherosclerotic l.
    axillary skin l.
    Bankart l.
    barrel-shaped l.
    benign l.
    benign bone l.

benign lymphoepithelial l.
benign lymphoproliferative l.
benign vascular l.
blastic l.
bone l.
bone marrow l.
brain l.
breast l.
bubbly bone l.
bull's-eye l.
carpet l.
cavitary lung l.
cavitary small bowel l.
centrilobular l.
cochlear l.
coin l.
constricting l.
cutaneous l.
destructive bone l.
diffuse ulcerative l.
discrete l.
dorsal route entry zone l.
enhancing l.
enhancing brain l.
eosinophilic
  fibrohistiocytic l.
epididymis l.
epidural extramedullary l.
erythrodermatous l.
expansile l.
expansile unilocular well-
  demarcated bone l.
extracranial mass l.
extrahepatic l.
extratesticular l.
fibrohistiocytic l.
fibrous bone l.
fibrous polypoid l.
focal parenchymal brain l.
focal splenic l.
genetic l.
Ghon l.
Gill l.
glomerular l.
high-intensity l.
hyperdense l.
hyperdense brain l.

hyperintense l.
hyperintense brain l.
hyperpigmented l.
hypodense l.
hypodense brain l.
immunoproliferative l.
intraconal l.
intracranial l.
intracranial mass l.
intradural extramedullary l.
intramedullary l.
intramural extramucosal l.
intraocular l.
intraorbital l.
intraosseous bone l.
intrasellar l.
low-attenuation l.
lucent l.
lucent lung l.
lumbar spine l.
lung l.
lymphoepithelial l.
lymphoproliferative l.
lytic l.
macroscopic l.
mass l.
mesencephalic low density l.
mesenchymal l.
metastatic l.
mixed fat-water density l.
mixed sclerotic and lytic
  bone l.
mucocutaneous l.
mucosal l.
multifocal enhancing l.
multilocular cystic l.
needle localization of
  breast l.
neurovascular l.
nodular l.
nodule-in-nodule l.
nonmeningiomatous
  malignant l.
nonperforative l.
nucleus ambiguus l.
occult l.
ocular l.

NOTES

lesion *(continued)*
    ocular adnexal l.
    optic nerve l.
    orbital l.
    osteoblastic l.
    osteochondral l.
    osteolytic l.
    osteosclerotic l.
    ostial l.
    paraorbital l.
    patch l.
    perforative l.
    perisellar vascular l.
    photon-deficient bone l.
    pigmented l.
    polypoid l.
    prechiasmal optic nerve l.
    presacral cystic l.
    radiodense l.
    reactive lymphoid l.
    reverse Hill-Sachs l.
    rim-enhancing l.
    ring l.
    saddle l.
    satellite l.
    sclerosing l.
    sclerotic l.
    sessile l.
    sinonasal l.
    sinusoidal l.
    skeletal l.
    skin l.
    skip l.
    SLAP l.
    space-occupying l.
    spiculated l.
    spleen l.
    squamous intraepithelial l.
    stellate l.
    stellate border breast l.
    stenotic l.
    suprasellar l.
    suprasellar low-density l.
    trabeculated bone l.
    unilocular cystic l.
    visceral l.
    Waldeyer ring l.
    well-circumscribed l.
lesser
    l. curvature of the stomach
    l. multangular bone
    l. omentum
    l. petrosal

    l. sac
    l. sac hernia
    l. trochanter
    l. trochanteric fracture
LET
    linear energy transfer
lethal
    l. bone dysplasia
    l. dose (LD)
    l. dwarfism
    l. gene
    l. midline granuloma
    l. musculoskeletal dysplasia
letrazuril
Letterer-Siwe disease
lettering artifact
Leu-8 antigen
leucine
    l. aminopeptidase
    l. radical
    l. zipper
leucoerythroblastic reaction
Leucomax
leucovorin
    calcium l.
    l. calcium
    l. rescue
    l. rescue factor
leucovorin-citrovorum factor (L-CF)
leucovorin, Oncovin, methotrexate, Adriamycin, cyclophosphamide (LOMAC)
Leu-Dox
    N-1-leucyldoxorubicin
leukapheresis
leukemia
    acute l.
    acute basophilic l. (ABL)
    acute eosinophilic l.
    acute erythroblastic l.
    acute granulocytic l.
    acute lymphoblastic l. (ALL)
    acute lymphocytic l. (ALL)
    acute lymphoid l.
    acute megakaryoblastic l.
    acute megakaryocytic l.
    acute mixed lineage l.
    acute monoblastic l.
    acute monocytic l.
    acute myeloblastic l.
    acute myelocytic l. (AML)
    acute myelogenous l. (AML)
    acute myeloid l. (AML)

acute myelomonocytic l.
acute nonlymphoblastic l.
  (ANLL)
acute nonlymphocytic l.
  (ANLL)
acute nonlymphoid l.
acute progranulocytic l.
acute promyelocytic l.
  (APL)
adult T-cell l. (ATL)
aleukemic l.
aleukocythemic l.
basophilic l.
basophilocytic l.
B-cell acute lymphoblastic l.
B-cell acute lymphocytic l.
B-cell chronic lymphocytic l.
Binet staging system for
  chronic lymphocytic l.
blast cell l.
BN acute myelocytic l.
  (BNML)
Burkitt l.
child lymphoblastic l.
chronic l.
chronic granulocytic l.
chronic lymphocytic l.
  (CLL)
chronic lymphoid l.
chronic monocytic l.
chronic myelocytic l. (CML)
chronic myelogenous l.
  (CML)
chronic myeloid l. (CML)
chronic myelomonocytic l.
  (CMML)
chronic neutrophilic l.
compound l.
l. cutis
embryonal l.
eosinophilic l.
l. eradication
feline l.
granular acute
  lymphoblastic l.
granulocytic l.
Gross l.

hairy cell l. (HCL)
hand-mirror cell l.
hemoblastic l.
hemocytoblastic l.
hypergranular acute
  promyelocytic l.
hypocellular acute l.
hypogranular acute
  promyelocytic l.
l. inhibitory factor (LIF)
juvenile chronic
  myelogenous l.
L1210 l.
large granular lymphocytic l.
leukemic l.
leukopenic l.
LGL l.
lineage switch l.
lymphatic l.
lymphoblastic l.
lymphocytic l.
lymphoid l.
mast cell l.
mature cell l.
megakaryocytic l.
meningeal l.
metachronous l.
microgranular acute
  promyelocytic l.
micromyeloblastic l.
mixed l.
mixed cell l.
monocytic l.
myeloblastic l.
myelocytic l.
myelogenic l.
myeloid l.
myelomonocytic l.
Naegeli-type of monocytic l.
neutrophilic l.
non-B cell l.
non-T cell l.
null cell acute
  lymphocytic l.
null cell lymphoblastic l.
oral hairy l.
plasma cell l.

NOTES

leukemia *(continued)*
    polymorphocytic l.
    postthymic l.
    postthymic T-cell l.
    pre-B acute lymphoblastic l.
    precursor B acute
      lymphoblastic l.
    preplasmacytic l.
    pre-T acute lymphocytic l.
    prolymphocytic l. (PLL)
    promyelocytic l.
    Rauscher l.
    Rieder cell l.
    Schilling type of
      monocytic l.
    l. screen
    splenic l.
    stem cell l.
    subleukemic l.
    T-cell acute lymphoblastic l.
    T-cell prolymphocytic l.
    testicular l.
    thrombocytic l.
    thymic l.
    l. transcript
leukemic
    l. blast progenitor
    l. cell
    l. clone
    l. infiltration
    l. leukemia
    l. reticuloendotheliosis
leukemogenesis
leukemogenic potential
leukemoid
Leukeran
Leukine
leukoagglutinin
leukocidin
    Neisser-Wechsberg l.
    Panton-Valentine l.
leukocoria (*var. of* leukokoria)
leukocyte
    l. acid phosphatase stain
    l. adherence inhibition
    l. adhesion deficiency
    l. adhesion molecule-1
      (LAM-1)
    l. alkaline phosphatase
    l. common antigen
    l. diapedesis
    l. filter

    gallium-67-labeled l.'s
    hyaline l.
    indium-111-labeled l.
    indium-111-oxime l.
    l. infiltration
    l. interferon
    l. migration inhibition
    l. transfusion
leukocythemia
leukocytic
    l. crystal
    l. sarcoma
leukocytoclastic vasculitis
leukocytoma
leukocytopenia
leukocytopoiesis
leukocytosis
    lymphocytic l.
leukodepletion
leukodystrophy
    globoid cell l.
    metachromatic l.
leukoencephalopathy
    disseminated necrotizing l.
    periventricular l.
    progressive multifocal l.
    radiation-induced l.
    spongiform l.
leukoerythroblastic anemia
leukoerythroblastosis
leukoglobulin
leukokinin
leukokoria, leukocoria
leukolymphosarcoma
leukomalacia
    periventricular l.
leukopenia
    autoimmune l.
    hairy l.
leukopenic leukemia
leukopheresis
leukoplakia
    hairy l.
leuko-poor
    l.-p. blood component
    l.-p. red blood cells
leukorrhea
leukosarcoma
leukosarcomatosis
leukosialin
leukostasis
    intracerebral l.

Leukotrap
L. RC system
L. red cell storage system
leukotrienes
leucovorin (LV)
leucovorin-modulated 5-FU
Leu monoclonal antibody
leupeptin
leuprolide
l. acetate (LA)
leuprorelin acetate
leurocristine
Leustatin
LEV
levamisole
levamisole (LEV)
levator
l. ani
l. palpebrae
l. palpebrae superioris
l. palpebrae superiosus
l. scapulae
l. veli palatini
LeVeen shunt
level
air-fluid l.
aldosterone l.
amylase l.
attenuation l.
base-plus-fog l.
complement 3, 4 l.
creatinine l.
energy l.
fat-fluid l.
fluid l.
fluid-fluid l.
intrasinus air-fluid l.
peak-dose l.
prodrug l.
serum phenytoin l.
significance l.
supraventricular l.
level-dependent
blood oxygenation l.-d.
(BOLD)
Levin tube
levocardia

Levo-Dromoran
Levolist
levorphanol
levosulpiride
levothyroxine
Levy, Rowntree, and Marriott
method
Lewis (Le)
L. A antigen
L. antibody
L. and Benedict method
L. blood group
L. blood group antigen
Lewissohn method
Leyden
hemophilia B L.
Leydig
L. cell
L. cell adenoma
L. cell tumor
LFA-1
LFA-2
LFA-3
LFT
liver function test
Lf unit
LGA
large-for-gestational age
LGL
large granular lymphocytic
LGL leukemia
LH
luteinizing hormone
L&H
L&H cell
L&H nodular pattern
L&H type
LH-RF agonist
LHRH
luteinizing hormone-releasing
hormone
LHRH analog
Liacopoulos phenomenon
Liang and Pardee method
liarozole fumarate
Liatest AT III
Liatest protein S

NOTES

LIBC
  latent iron-binding capacity
liblomycin
Libman-Sacks endocarditis
library
  DNA l.
  gene l.
Librium
lichen myxedematosus
lichenoid
  l. drug eruption
  l. graft-versus-host disease
lichenoides
  pityriasis l.
Lichtenstein-Jaffe disease
Lichtheim plaque
lid droop
lidocaine
  l. hydrochloride
  viscous l.
lidofenin
  technetium-99m l.
Liebow
  usual interstitial pneumonia
  of L.
lienis
  sustentaculum l.
LIF
  leukemia inhibitory factor
LIFE
  lung imaging fluorescent
  endoscopy
life
  l. event
  quality of l.
  l. style
  l. table survival
LifePort infusion set
Li-Fraumeni cancer syndrome
ligament
  anterior cruciate l.
  arcuate l.
  broad l.
  calcaneofibular l.
  coccygeal l.
  collateral l.
  conoid l.
  Cooper l.
  Cooper suspensory l.
  coracoacromial l.
  coracoclavicular l.
  coracohumeral l.
  coronary l.

  deltoid l.
  dentate l.
  falciform l.
  glenohumeral l.
  hepatoduodenal l.
  humeral avulsion of the
  glenohumeral l.
  l. of Humphry
  infundibulopelvic l.
  intercarpal l.
  lunatotriquetral l.
  median cruciate l.
  meniscofemoral l.
  periodontal l.
  petroclinoid l.
  phrenicocolic l.
  popliteal l.
  posterior longitudinal l.
  rhomboid l.
  round l.
  sacrotuberous l.
  splenorenal l.
  talofibular l.
  trapezoid l.
  l. of Treitz
  triangular l.
  uterosacral l.
  vesicosacral l.
  Wrisberg l.
ligamenta flava
ligamentous calcification
ligamentum
  l. arteriosum
  l. flavum
  l. flavum thickening
  l. nuchae
  l. patellae
  l. teres
  l. venosum fissure
ligand
  l. agent
  l. blotting
  kit l.
ligase
ligation
  hepatic artery l.
light
  bili l.
  l. bulb appearance
  l. chain isotype suppression
  l. collection system
  invisible l.
lighter-than-bile contrast agent

Lightwood syndrome
Lillehei-Kaster valve
Lillie hematoxylin
lily-pad sign
limb
l. abnormality
l. bud
l. ischemia
l. length
l. length inequality
l. perfusion
l. reduction
l. reduction abnormality
l. reduction anomaly
limb-body wall complex
Limberg flap
limb-girdle muscular dystrophy
limb-lengthening
l.-l. procedure
limb-sparing surgery
limbus vertebra
limit
eye exposure l.
Nyquist l.
limitation
beam l.
l. of motion
limited examination
limited-slice
l.-s. computed tomography
limited-stage disease
limulus anti-DPS factor
limy bile
LINAC
linear accelerator
Lincoln log vertebra
Lindau tumor
line
air-fluid l.
aneuploid cell l.
anterior junction l.
azygoesophageal l.
Beau l.'s
Blummenstat l.
cell l.
CEM/HIV-1 cell l.
central venous pressure l.

Chamberlain l.
Chaussier l.
clinoparietal l.
clivus torcula l.
Conradi l.
Crampton l.
curved radiolucent l.
epiphyseal l.
fat l.
fat-density l.
Fleischner l.
l. focus principle
fracture l.
Fränkel white l.
gallbladder-vena cava l.
gaussian l.
gluteal l.
Granger l.
growth arrest l.
Gubler l.
Hampton l.
Harris l.'s
Hickman l.
His l.
human AML cell l.
humeral l.
iliopectineal l.
l. integral concept
isodose l.
Jurkat T-cell l.
Kerley l.'s
Kerley A l.'s
Kerley B l.'s
Lanz l.
lead l.
Looser l.'s
lorentzian l.
Mach l.
McGregor l.
McKee l.
McRae l.
Meyer l.
mouse germ l.
Muercke l.
Nelaton l.
Ohngren l.
l. pairs

NOTES

line *(continued)*
paraspinal l.
PICC l.
pleural l.
posterior junction l.
properitoneal fat l.
psoas l.
radiocapitellar l.
radiolucent crescent l.
Reid base l.
l. of Retzius
septal l.
l. shape
Shenton l.
spectral l.
l. spread function
subclavian l.
suture l.
tram l.
transverse lucent
  metaphyseal l.'s
trough l.
Twining l.
Ullmann l.
Wackenheim l.
water density l.
Wegner l.
l. width
Z l.
Zahn l.
zero l.
linea
l. alba
l. semilunaris
lineage
chromaffin l.
l. fidelity
ganglionic l.
l. heterogeneity
macrophage l.
mixed l.
l. promiscuity
l. restriction
schwannian l.
l. switch
l. switch leukemia
lineage-associated
l.-a. antigen
l.-a. gene
linear
l. accelerator (LINAC)
l. amplifier
l. array

l. array transducer
l. degenerative signal
  intensity
l. energy transfer (LET)
l. fracture
l. gradient
l. pharmacokinetic model
l. phosphates
l. polarization
l. prediction with singular
  value decomposition
l. radiopacities
l. tomography
linearity
absolute l.
differential l.
gradient l.
intrinsic spatial l.
linearly-polarized coil
Linell-Ljungberg classification
lingual
l. artery
l. nerve
l. thyroid
l. tonsils
lingula
lingular
l. division of the left lung
l. pneumonia
lining
mucosal l.
linitis
l. plastica
l. plastica carcinoma
linkage
l. analysis
chemical l.
l. disequilibrium
thiourea l.
Linomide
Linsman water test
Linson electronic cell counter
Linton procedure
Lintro-Scan
Lioresal
liothyronine sodium
lip
l. cancer
cleft l.
hilar l.
lipemia
l. retinalis

lipid
>blood l.
>l. cell neoplasm
>l. cholecystitis
>l. content of storage fats
>l. cyst
>egg lecithin l.
>l. emulsion
>l. fraction relaxation rate
>l. granulomatosis
>l. pheresis
>l. storage disease

lipid-associated sialic acid
lipid-coated virus
lipid-containing
>l.-c. vesicle

lipidema
lipid-lowering
>l.-l. therapy

Lipiodol
Lipisorb dressing
lipoblastoma
lipoblastomatosis
lipocalcinogranulomatosis
lipodystrophy
>intestinal l.
>mesenteric l.

lipofibroadenoma
lipofibroma
lipogenic tumor
lipogranuloma
lipogranulomatosis
>disseminated l.

lipohemarthrosis
Lipo-Hepin
lipoid
>l. granuloma
>l. granulomatosis
>l. pneumonia

lipoleiomyoma
lipoma
>l. arborescens
>intracranial l.
>l. macrodystrophia
>pericallosal l.
>l. sarcomatodes
>l. sarcomatosum

lipomatosa
>macrodystrophia l.

lipomatosis
>central sinus l.
>epidural l.
>mediastinal l.
>multiple symmetrical l.
>pelvic l.
>peripelvic l.
>renal sinus l.

lipomatous hypertrophy
lipomyelomeningocele
lipomyeloschisis
liponecrosis
>l. macrocystica calcificans
>l. microcystica calcificans

lipophagia granulomatosis
lipophagic
>l. granuloma
>l. intestinal

lipophilic dye
lipoplethoric diabetes
lipopolysaccharide
lipoprotein
>high-density l. (HDL)
>low-density l. (LDL)

lipoproteinemia
lipoproteinosis
liposarcoma
>myxoid l.
>myxomatous l.
>pleomorphic l.
>retroperitoneal l.
>l. of uterus

liposclerotic mesenteritis
liposomal
>l. daunorubicin
>l. preparation

liposome
>dactinomycin-loaded l.

lipotropin
lipoxygenase
>l. enzyme
>l. inhibitor

Lippes loop
lipping
Lipschutz body

NOTES

331

liquefaciens
    Enterobacter l.
    Moraxella l.
    Serratia l.
liquefaction
liquid
    l. extraction
    l. nitrogen
    Polycose l.
    Sustacal l.
Liquipake
Lisch nodule
Lisfranc
    L. amputation
    L. fracture
    L. joint
lissencephaly
listeria
    Cryptosporidium l.
    l. encephalitis
Listeria monocytogenes
listeriosis
lithiasis
lithium-7
lithium carbonate
lithotripsy
    biliary l.
    candela l.
    electrohydraulic l. (EHL)
    extracorporeal shock-wave l.
      (ESWL)
    laser biliary l.
    rotational contact l.
    shock-wave l.
    ultrasonic l.
lithotripter
    Dornier HM3 l.
    Dornier HM4 l.
    Siemens Lithostar l.
    Wolf Piezolith 2200 l.
lithotrite
    Kensey-Nash l.
Littleford/Spector introducer
Little Leaguer's elbow
littoral cell
liver
    l. abscess
    l. agenesis
    l. biopsy
    l. cancer
    l. cell adenoma
    l. cell carcinoma
    fatty l.
    l. fluke
    l. function test (LFT)
    hypoechoic l.
    l. mass
    l. metastasis
    l. scan
    l. transplant
liver-lung scan
live virus vaccine
living
    activities of daily l. (ADL)
Livingstone-Wheeler regimen
LLC
    labrum-ligament complex
LLETZ
    large loop excision of
    transformation zone
L-leucovorin
Lloyd-Roberts open reduction of Monteggia fracture
L-lysine
L-17M
LMP-1
    latent membrane protein-1
LMR
    localized magnetic resonance
LMWH
    low molecular weight heparin
    Hepanorm L.
L-myc-1,2 proto-oncogene
L-myc oncogene
LN
    Imagent LN
load
    viral l.
loading
    coil l.
    contrast l.
    l. dose
    fracture callus l.
lobar
    l. bronchi
    l. dysmorphism
    l. emphysema
    l. holoprosencephaly
    l. nephronia
    l. pneumonia
    l. renal infarction
lobation
    fetal l.
    persistent cortical l.
lobe
    accessory l.

azygos l.
caudate l.
frontal l.
hepatic l.
hot caudate l.
occipital l.
parietal l.
prominent pyramidal l.
pyriform l.
Riedel l.
spigelian l.
succenturiate l.
temporal l.
lobectomy
sleeve l.
Lobstein disease
lobular
l. calcification
l. carcinoma
l. carcinoma in situ
l. microcalcification
l. neoplasia
l. pneumonia
lobulated
lobulation
fetal l.
lobule
fat l.
local
l. anesthesia
l. anesthetic
l. coil
l. excision
l. invasion
l. irradiation
l. recurrence
l. streptokinase infusion
l. surgery
localization
cellular l.
immunohistochemical l.
needle l.
needle-hookwire l.
pelvis for IUD l.
percutaneous l.
radiotherapy l.
l. technique

localized
l. ileus
l. infiltrate
l. magnetic resonance
(LMR)
l. mastocytoma
l. shimming
localizing
l. probe
l. sign
locally advanced cancer
loci (*pl. of* locus)
lock
field l.
heparin l., hep lock
locked nuclear magnetization
LOCM
low-osmolar contrast medium
locoregional
l. disease
l. failure
l. field radiotherapy
loculated
l. effusion
l. hydropneumothorax
l. pleural fluid
loculation of fluid
loculus
locus, pl. loci
ATPase l.
cut l.
HGPT l.
Lodine
Loevit cell
Löffler
L. eosinophilia
L. fibroplastic endocarditis
L. pneumonia
L. syndrome
Löfgren syndrome
L-ofloxacin
log
l. amplifier
cell kill l.
l. effect
l. kill

NOTES

log-kill
> l.-k. model

LOH at 16q

lollipop
> l. follicle
> l. tree appearance

LOMAC
> leucovorin, Oncovin,
> methotrexate, Adriamycin,
> cyclophosphamide

Lometrexol

Lomotil

lomustine (CCNU)

Lone Star fever

long
> l. axis view
> l. bone
> l. oblique fracture
> l. segmental diaphyseal
> uptake bone scintigraphy
> l. terminal repeat

long-acting
> l.-a. thyroid stimulator
> (LATS)
> l.-a. thyroid stimulator
> protector

long-chain fatty acid

Longdwel needle

longitudinal
> l. acoustic wave
> l. fasciculus
> l. fissure
> l. image
> l. magnetization
> l. recovery time
> l. relaxation
> l. relaxation time
> l. relaxivity (R1)
> l. scan

long-term
> l.-t. storage
> l.-t. survivor
> l.-t., U-loop nephrostomy
> catheter

longus
> l. colli muscle
> extensor carpi radialis l.
> extensor digitorum l.
> extensor hallucis l.
> extensor pollicis l.

lonidamine

loop
> l. of bowel

l. catheter
conductive l.
Cope l.
l. distribution
duodenal l.
efferent l.
l. electrosurgical excision
procedure (LEEP)
flow volume l.
l. of Henle
ileal l.
Lippes l.
sentinel l.
l. snare
V2 l.
V3 l.
Waltman l.

looped Silastic Universal stent

loopography
> ileal l.

loose
> l. body
> l. fracture
> l. intraarticular body

Looser
> L. lines
> L. zone

lophosphamide

LORAD StereoGuide

lorazepam

lordosis

lordotic
> l. curve
> l. view

lorentzian
> l. curve
> l. field mapping
> l. line

Lorenzo oil

lorry driver's fracture

Lortab

losoxantrone HCl

loss
> cochlear hearing l.
> coincidence l.
> dielectric l.
> hair l.
> high-velocity signal l.
> retrocochlear hearing l.
> signal l.
> time-of-flight signal l.
> volume l.
> weight l.

Lossen rule
Lostorfer corpuscle
Louis angle
Louis-Bar syndrome
lovastatin
low
  l. anterior resection
  l. back syndrome
  l. bandwidth
  l. columnar cell
  l. flip angle gradient-echo
    imaging
  l. frequency blood group
  l. LET external beam
    irradiation
  l. LET isotope
  l. molecular weight heparin
    (LMWH)
low-attenuation
  l.-a. lesion
  l.-a. mass
low-density
  l.-d. lipoprotein (LDL)
  l.-d. mass
low-dose
  l.-d. chemotherapy
  l.-d. heparin
  l.-d. rate (LDR)
low-energy fracture
lower
  l. basilar aneurysm
  l. esophageal sphincter
  l. extremity
  l. lobe pneumonia
  l. motor neuron
lowered tumor antigenicity
low-grade
  l.-g. B-cell lymphoma
  l.-g. lymphoma
low-lying placenta
low-molecular keratin stain
low-osmolar
  l.-o. contrast material
  l.-o. contrast medium
    (LOCM)

low-pass
  l.-p. filter
  l.-p. filtering
low-power field (lpf)
low-pressure hydrocephalus
low-profile angioplasty balloon
low-residue diet
Lowsley lobar anatomy
low-speed rotational angioplasty
loxoribine
LP
  lumbar puncture
  lymphomatous polyposis
LPAM, L-PAM
lpf
  low-power field
L-phase variant
L-phenylalanine mustard (L-PAM)
L-phenylalanine mustard,
  vinblastine (PAVe)
LPS Peel-away introducer
L/TFZ-Thymomodulin
L-transposition
L-tryptophan
^{197}Lu
  lutetium-177
lucency
  sandlike l.
lucent
  l. lesion
  l. lung lesion
Lucey-Driscoll syndrome
Luciani-Wenckebach phenomenon
Lucké adenocarcinoma
lückenschädel
Lucke virus
Luer-Lok adapter
lues
luetic
  l. aortitis
  l. diaphysitis
Lugano classification for testicular
  tumor
Lugol
  L. dye esophagoscopy
  L. solution

NOTES

Lukes

L. and Butler classification
of Hodgkin disease

L. and Collins classification
of non-Hodgkin lymphoma

lumbar

l. artery
l. canal
l. disk
l. diskectomy
l. hernia
l. myelogram
l. nerve root
l. nerve root blockade
l. plexus
l. puncture (LP)
l. root avulsion
l. spine
l. spine burst fracture
l. spine fracture
l. spine lesion
l. spine stenosis
l. synovial cyst
l. vertebra

lumbosacral

l. agenesis
l. canal
l. spine

lumbrical

lumen, pl. lumina

l. diameter
double l.
false l.
gastric l.
tracheal l.

luminal

l. caliber
l. narrowing
l. plug

luminance

lumpectomy

lump kidney

lunate

l. dislocation
l. tilt

lunate-shaped trachea

lunatomalacia

lunatotriquetral ligament

Lund-Amplatz retrievable filter

Lunderquist

L. catheter
L. wire
L. wire guide

**Lunderquist-Ring torque control
wire**

lung

l. abscess
air-filled l.
l. apices
l. biopsy
bird-fancier's l.
l. block
bullous l. disease
l. cancer
L. Cancer Symptom Scale
l. capacity
l. carcinoma
l. cavity
coin lesion of l.
collapsed l.
l. compliance
consolidated l.
l. density
diffuse l. disease
farmer's l.
l. field
l. fissure
folded l.
l. function testing
horseshoe l.
hypoinflation of the l.
l. imaging fluorescent
endoscopy (LIFE)
l. lesion
lingular division of the
left l.
malt worker's l.
mushroom worker's l.
l. nodularity
l. nodule
l. parenchyma
l. perfusion
pigeon breeder's l.
respirator l.
l. reticulations
rheumatoid l.
right l.
l. shielding
shunt to the l.
silo-filler's l.
l. transplant
l. tumor
unilateral hyperlucent l.
l. volume
l. window
l. zone

Lunyo virus
Luprolide
Lupron
    L. Depot
lupus
    l. erythematosus (LE)
    l. pneumonitis
Luque rod
Luria-Delbruck
    L.-D. fluctuation test
    L.-D. model
Luschka
    foramen of L.
    joints of L.
lusitaniae
    Candida *l.*
lusoria
    arteria l.
luteal cyst
luteinized
    l. thecoma of ovary
    l. unruptured follicle
luteinizing
    l. hormone (LH)
    l. hormone-releasing agonist
    l. hormone-releasing
    hormone (LHRH)
Lutembacher syndrome
lutetium-177 (^{197}Lu)
Lutheran
    L. antibody
    L. blood group
LuVax
luxatio erecta
Lux culture dish
luxury perfusion
LV
    leucovorin
    LV + 5-FU
LVSI
    lymph-vascular involvement
lwoffi
    Acinetobacter *l.*
LY186641
LY188011
Ly antigen
Lyb antigen

Lyell syndrome
lye stricture
lyl-1 oncogene activation
Lyl B-cell
Lym-1 monoclonal antibody
Lyme
    L. arthritis
    L. borreliosis
    L. disease
lympangiomyomatosis
lymph
    l. node
    l. node drainage
    l. node fibrosis
    l. node histology
    l. node metastasis
    l. node station
lymphadenectomy
    bilateral l.
    inguinal l.
    Meigs pelvic l.
    paraaortic l.
    pelvic l.
    retroperitoneal l.
lymphadenitis
    dermatopathic l.
    histiocytic necrotizing l.
    mesenteric l.
    postvaccinial l.
    regional granulomatous l.
lymphadenoma cell
lymphadenopathy
    angioblastic l.
    angioimmunoblastic l.
    axillary l.
    benign l.
    dermatopathic l.
    hypersensitivity l.
    idiopathic plasmacytic l.
    immunoblastic l.
    massive l.
    mediastinal l.
    mesenteric l.
    peripancreatic l.
    persistent generalized l.
    plasmacytic l.
    reactive l.

NOTES

lymphadenopathy *(continued)*
    retroperitoneal l.
    secondary axillary l.
    superficial l.
    l. syndrome
    toxoplasmosis l.
lymphadenopathy-associated virus
lymphangiectasia
    congenital l.
    generalized l.
    intestinal l.
    pulmonary l.
lymphangiography effect
lymphangiography-related
lymphangioleiomyomatosis
lymphangioma
    cavernous l.
    cystic l.
    pancreatic cystic l.
    retroperitoneal l.
    simple capillary l.
lymphangiomatosis
lymphangiomyomatosis
lymphangiosarcoma
lymphangitic carcinomatosis
lymphangitis
    l. carcinomatosa
lymphangitis carcinomatosa
lymphapheresis
lymphatic
    l. canal
    l. carcinomatosis
    l. drainage
    l. drainage of genitalia
    l. leukemia
    l. malformation
    l. metastasis
    paracervical l.
    l. permeation
    l. sarcoma
    l. spread
    l. system
    l. tracking
    l. vessel invasion
lymphatica
    pseudopolyposis l.
lymphaticum
    angioma l.
Lymphazurin
lymphedema
    postmastectomy l.
lymph-mode
    curvature l.-m.

lymphoblast
    l. mutation assay
lymphoblastic
    l. leukemia
    l. lymphoma (LBL)
    l. lymphoma-leukemia
lymphoblastoid interferon
lymphoblastoma
lymphocele
lymphocyst
lymphocytapheresis
lymphocyte
    l. activator
    amplifier T-l.
    B-l.
    clonal B-l.
    l. count
    cytotoxic T-l.
    l. depletion
    l. function antigen
    l. gene rearrangement
    hand-mirror l.
    helper T-l.
    immunocompetent l.
    inducer T-l.
    inflammatory T-l.
    intraepithelial l.
    large agranular l.
    large granular l.
    l. migration
    l. mitogenic factor
    monocytoid B-l.
    natural killer l.
    peripheral blood l.
    plasmacytoid l.
    l. proliferation
    l. proliferation assay
    l. recombinase
    small l.
    T-l.
    thymic l.
    tumor-infiltrating l.
    villous l.
lymphocyte-activating factor
lymphocyte-defined
lymphocyte-depleted
lymphocyte-depletion Hodgkin disease
lymphocyte-predominant Hodgkin disease
lymphocyte-stimulating hormone

lymphocytic
l. angiitis and
granulomatosis
l. bronchitis
l. choriomeningitis
l. and histiocytic nodular
Hodgkin disease
l. interstitial pneumonia
l. interstitial pneumonitis
large granular l. (LGL)
l. leukemia
l. leukocytosis
l. lymphoma
l. thyroiditis
well-differentiated l.
lymphocytoma
lymphocytopenia
lymphocytopoiesis
lymphocytosis
lymphoepithelial
l. cyst
l. lesion
l. parotid tumor
l. tumor
lymphoepithelioid cell lymphoma
lymphoepithelioma
salivary gland l.
lymphogranuloma
l. benignum
l. inguinale
l. malignum
Schaumann l.
venereal l.
l. venereum
l. venereum antigen
l. venereum virus
lymphogranulomatosis
lymphogranulomatosis X
lymphography
lymphohistiocytic variant
lymphohistiocytosis
familial hemophagocytic l.
hemophagocytic l.
lymphoid
l. cell
l. hemoblast of Pappenheim
l. hyperplasia

l. hypophysitis
l. inflammatory
pseudotumor
l. interstitial pneumonia
l. interstitial pneumonitis
l. leukemia
l. marker
l. organ
l. precursor cell
l. proliferation
l. stem cell
l. tissue
lymphokine
lymphokine-activated
l.-a. killer
l.-a. killer cell
lymphoma
acute lymphoblastic l.
adult T-cell l.
African Burkitt l.
AIDS-related l.
anaplastic large cell l.
(ALCL)
anaplastic large cell
Ki-1- positive l.
angiocentric T-cell l.
angioimmunoblastic
lymphadenopathy-like
T- cell l.
angioimmunoblastic
lymphadenopathy with
dysproteinemia-like
T- cell l.
angiotropic large cell l.
B-cell l.
Bennett classification of l.
Berard classification for
follicular l.
biclonal follicular l.
Burkitt l.
B-zone small lymphocytic l.
(BZSLL)
centracytic l.
central nervous system l.
centroblastic l.
centrocytic l.
cerebral l.

NOTES

lymphoma *(continued)*
    colorectal l.
    cutaneous l.
    cutaneous angiocentric
      T-cell l.
    cutaneous B-cell l.
    cutaneous T-cell l.
    diffuse l.
    diffuse aggressive l.
    diffuse intermediate
      lymphocytic l.
    diffuse large cell l. (DLCL)
    diffuse lymphocytic l.
    diffuse mixed small and
      large cell l.
    diffuse small cell
      lymphocytic l.
    diffuse small cleaved cell l.
    endemic Burkitt l.
    enteropathy-associated l.
    enteropathy-associated
      T-cell l.
    erythrophagocytic
      T-gamma l.
    extranodal l.
    extranodal follicular l.
    follicular l.
    gastric l.
    gastrointestinal l.
    gluten enteropathy-associated
      T-cell l.
    hepatosplenic l.
    high-grade B-cell l.
    histiocytic l.
    Hodgkin l.
    immunoblastic l.
    immunoblastic
      lymphadenopathy-like
      T-cell l.
    indolent l.
    intermediate lymphocytic l.
      (ILL)
    intravascular l.
    Keil classification of non-
      Hodgkin l.
    Ki-1 positive l.
    large cell l.
    large cell immunoblastic l.
    large noncleaved cell l.
    Lennert l.
    Lennert classification for
      follicular l.
    leptomeningeal l.

    low-grade l.
    low-grade B-cell l.
    lymphoblastic l. (LBL)
    lymphocytic l.
    lymphoepithelioid cell l.
    lymphoplasmacytic l.
    lymphoplasmacytoid l.
    malignant l.
    mantle cell l.
    mantle zone l.
    mediastinal l.
    mediastinal B-cell l.
    mediastinal large B-cell l.
    Mediterranean l.
    mesencephalic cerebral l.
    mesenteric l.
    metastatic l.
    metastatic testicular l.
    mixed small cleaved and
      large cell l.
    mixed small and large
      cell l.
    monocytoid B-cell l.
    monomorphic l.
    multiclonal follicular l.
    multilobated T-cell l.
    nodular l.
    nodular histiocytic l.
    nodular poorly-differentiated
      lymphocytic l. (NPDL)
    non-Hodgkin l. (NHL)
    North American Burkitt l.
    null cell l.
    l. of ocular adnexa
    ocular adnexal l.
    ovarian l.
    l. of ovary
    peripheral l.
    peripheral T-cell l.
    perirenal l.
    peritoneal l.
    plasmablastic l.
    plasmacytoid lymphocytic l.
    pleomorphic T-cell l.
    polymorphic B-cell l.
    postthymic T-cell l.
    precursor B-cell l.
    primary l.
    primary central nervous
      system l.
    primary CNS l.
    primary mediastinal B-cell l.
    primary refractory Burkitt l.

pseudo-T-cell l.
pulmonary l.
pyothorax-associated
  pleural l.
Rappaport classification
  of l.
recurrent l.
renal l.
retroperitoneal l.
l. screen
sinonasal l.
skeletal l.
small cleaved cell l.
small lymphocytic l.
small non-cleaved cell l.
spinal epidural l.
splenic B-cell l.
sporadic Burkitt l.
systemic l.
T-cell l.
T-cell lymphoblastic l.
T-cell-rich B-cell l.
T-gamma l.
thyroid l.
true histiocytic l.
T-zone l.
U-cell l.
uterine corpus l.
Waldeyer ring l.
working formulation of non-
  Hodgkin l.
lymphomagenesis
lymphoma-leukemia
  lymphoblastic l.-l.
lymphomasonography
  primary l.
lymphomatoid
  l. granulomatosis
  l. panniculitis
  l. papulosis
lymphomatosis
  intravascular l.
lymphomatosum
  cystadenoma l.
  papillary cystadenoma l.
lymphomatous
  l. bone marrow involvement

l. lymph node
l. polyposis (LP)
l. type
lymphomyeloma
lymphopenia
lymphophagocytosis
lymphoplasmacytic
  l. immunocytoma
  l. lymphoma
lymphoplasmacytoid
  l. immunocytoma
  l. lymphoma
lymphopoiesis
lymphoproliferation
  posttransplantation l.
lymphoproliferative
  l. disorder
  l. lesion
  l. syndrome
lymphoprotease
lymphoreticular
  l. cell
lymphosarcoma
lymphosarcomatosis
lymphoscintigraphy
lymphotoxic antibody
lymphotoxin
  l. antitumor activity
  tumor necrosis factor-β-l.
lymph-vascular involvement (LVSI)
Lynbya majuscula
Lynch
  L. syndrome
  L. syndrome II
Lyon phenomenon
lyophilization
lyophilized
  l. acemannin
  l. recombinant interferon
    formulation
lysin
lysis
  blade-of-grass l.
  candle flame l.
  clot l.
  complement l.

NOTES

lysis *(continued)*
    complement-mediated l.
    follicle l.
Lysodren
lysosomal storage disease
lysosome
lysozyme
lyssa body

lyt-10
    lyt-10 oncogene activation
    lyt-10 proto-oncogene
lyt-1 **proto-oncogene**
Lyt antigen
lytic
    l. lesion

M2
    vincristine, carmustine,
      cyclophosphamide, melphalan,
      prednisone
M344
      M344 antibody
      M344 antigen
99m
      CEA-Tc 99m
      technetium-99m, 99mTc
        (^{99m}Tc)
MAA
    macroaggregated albumin
    technetium-99m
      macroaggregated albumin
Maass double-helix stent
MAb
    monoclonal antibody
      PM-81 MAb
MAC
    methotrexate, actinomycin D,
      chlorambucil
    Mycobacterium avium complex
Mac-1 antigen
Macaca nemestrina
MACC
    methotrexate, ara-C,
      cyclophosphamide, CCNU
MacConkey agar
maceration
Mach
      M. band
      M. band effect
      M. line
Machado-Guerreiro test
Machado test
machine
      cobalt megavoltage m.
      focused, segmented,
        ultrasound m. (FSUM)
      megavoltage m.
Machupo virus
MAC III
    methotrexate, actinomycin D,
      cyclophosphamide
Macleod syndrome
MACOB
    methotrexate, Adriamycin
      (doxorubicin),

      cyclophosphamide, Oncovin
      (vincristine), bleomycin
MACOB with leucovorin
    methotrexate, Adriamycin,
      cyclophosphamide, Oncovin,
      prednisone, bleomycin, with
      leucovorin
MACOP-B
    methotrexate-leucovorin,
      Adriamycin,
      cyclophosphamide, Oncovin,
      prednisone, bleomycin
macrencephaly, macrenephalia
macroadenoma
    pituitary m.
macroaggregated albumin (MAA)
macrobiotic
macrocalcification
macrocephaly, macrocephalia
macrocirculation
macrocyst
    adrenocortical m.
macrocystic
      m. adenoma
      m. cystadenoma
      m. encephalomalacia
      m. neoplasm
      m. pilocytic cerebellar
        astrocytoma
macrocythemia
macrocytic anemia
macrocytosis
Macrodantin pneumonia
macrodystrophia
    lipoma m.
    m. lipomatosa
macrofollicular adenoma
$\alpha_2$2-macroglobulin
macroglobulinemia
    Waldenström m.
macroglossia
macrolide
Macrolin
macromolecular
      m. complex
      m. conjugate
      m. hydration effect
      m. nonlipid compound
      m. polar compound
      m. tumbling

macromolecule
macronodular
    m. cirrhosis
    m. lung disease
macronutrient
macrophage
    alveolar m.
    armed m.
    m. chemotactic factor
    colony-forming unit
      granulocyte, erythrocyte,
      megakaryocyte, m.
      (CFU- GEMM)
    m. colony-stimulating factor
      (M-CSF)
    fixed m.
    free m.
    m. growth factor
    Hansemann m.
    m. lineage
    m. lineage antigen
    peritoneal m.
    m. variant
macrophage-activating factor
macrophage-inhibition factor
macrophagocyte
macrophthalmos
macroscopic
    m. lesion
    m. magnetic moment
    m. magnetization vector
macrosomia
Macrotec
MACS
    Multicenter AIDS Cohort Study
macule
    varicella m.
maculopathy
Madayag needle
MADDOC
    mechlorethamine, Adriamycin,
      dacarbazine, DDP, Oncovin,
      cyclophosphamide
      MADDOC chemotherapy
Madelung deformity
maduromycosis
Maertel regimen
Maffucci
    M. disease
    M. syndrome
mafosfamide
MAG3
    Technescan MAG3

Magendie foramen
Maggi biopsy needle
magic
    m. angle
    m. angle effect
"magic angle" artifact
Magic catheter
Magill Pain Questionnaire
magna
    cisterna m.
    coxa m.
    mega cisterna m.
Magnacal
Magnes biomagnetometer system
magnesemia
magnesium
    m. chloride
    m. citrate
magnet
    hybrid m.
    permanent m.
    resistive m.
    superconducting m.
magnetic
    m. anisotropy
    m. bead
    m. bolus tracking
    m. dipole
    m. dipole-dipole coupling
    m. dipole moment
    m. domain
    m. field
    m. field gradient
    m. field perturbation
    m. flux
    m. flux density
    m. induction
    m. interaction
    m. inversion
    m. material
    m. microsphere
    m. moment
    m. radiation exposure
    m. resonance (MR)
    m. resonance angiography
      (MRA)
    m. resonance imaging
      (MRI)
    m. resonance spectroscopy
      (MRS)
    m. resonance venography
    m. shielding

spin-echo m. resonance
imaging
m. susceptibility
m. susceptibility artifact
m. tape storage
magnetically responsive microsphere
magnetism
nuclear m.
magnetite (Fe$_3$O$_4$)
m. in tumor targeting
magnetization
equilibrium m.
locked nuclear m.
longitudinal m.
net transverse m.
m. precession angle
rephased transverse m.
residual m.
rest m.
spatial modulation of m.
m. transfer
m. transfer technique
transverse m.
magnetogyric ratio
magnetohydrodynamic effect
magneton
Bohr m.
magnetopharmaceutical
magnetophosphene
magnetotherapy
Magnevist
magnification
m. angiography
electronic m.
m. mammography
spot m.
m. view
Magniter-AMT-1
magnitude
m. image
m. reconstruction
magnitude preparation-rapid
acquisition gradient echo
(MP-RAGE)
MAID
mesna, Adriamycin, ifosfamide,
dacarbazine

mesna, Adriamycin, interleukin-
3, dacarbazine
MAIDS
murine-acquired
immunodeficiency syndrome
main
m. magnetic field
inhomogeneity artifact
m. pancreatic duct (MPD)
m. papillary duct (MPD)
m. pulmonary artery
mainline granulomatosis
mainstem bronchus
Maisonneuve
M. fibular fracture
M. fracture
Majewski disease
Majocchi granuloma
major
m. fissure
m. gene
globus m.
m. histocompatibility
antigens
m. histocompatibility
complex
m. histocompatibility
complex antigen
rhomboid m.
thalassemia m.
majuscula
Lynbya m.
MAK-6
monoclonal anticytokeratin
MAK-6 cocktail
Makar stricture
Makonde virus
malabsorption
paraneoplastic m.
m. syndrome
maladie de Roger
malaise
malakoplakia
renal parenchymal m.
malalignment
malar
m. bone

NOTES

malar *(continued)*
m. eminence
m. fracture
malaria
malarial rosette
Malassezia furfur
maldescended testis
maldevelopment
pubic bone m.
male
m. breast
m. pseudohermaphroditism
m. sexual dysfunction
m. Turner syndrome
maleate
DABIS m.
thiethylperazine m.
Malecot
M. biliary drainage catheter
M. catheter
M. stent
malformation
anorectal m.
Arnold-Chiari m.
arteriovenous m. (AVM)
capillary m.
cardiovascular m.
central nervous system m.
cerebral m.
cerebral arteriovenous m.
cerebral vascular m.
cerebrovascular m.
Chiari I m.
Chiari II m.
congenital m.
congenital heart m.
congenital vascular m.
cystic adenomatoid m.
Dandy-Walker m.
DeMyer system of
cerebral m.
extremity m.
fetal cystic adenomatoid m.
frontal arteriovenous m.
frontoparietal
arteriovenous m.
galenic venous m.
intracerebral
arteriovenous m.
intracerebral vascular m.
intracranial arteriovenous m.
intramedullary
arteriovenous m.

intramuscular venous m.
lymphatic m.
mixed venous-lymphatic m.
Mondini m.
neural axis vascular m.
occult vascular m.
pulmonary m.
pulmonary arterial m.
pulmonary arteriovenous m.
spinal vascular m.
telencephalic m.
vascular m.
vein of Galen m.
venous m.
malfunction
Malgaigne
M. fracture
M. pelvic fracture
maligna
lentigo m.
malignancy
extrapelvic m.
gastrointestinal m.
gynecologic m.
hematologic m.
hypercalcemia of m.
meningeal m.
mimicker of m.
occult primary m. (OPM)
pelvic m.
secondary m.
T-cell m.
uroepithelial m.
urogenital m.
vulvar m.
malignant
m. angioendotheliomatosis
m. breast cancer
m. calcification
m. carcinoid syndrome
m. cell
m. down
m. effusion
m. fibrous histiocytoma
m. gastric ulcer
m. glioma
m. granuloma
m. hepatoma
m. histiocytoma
m. histiocytosis
m. lentigo melanoma
m. lymphoma

m. lymphoproliferative
disorder
m. mastocytosis
m. melanoma
m. melanoma in situ
m. mesothelioma
m. mixed müllerian tumor
m. mixed tumor
m. myoepithelioma
m. nephrosclerosis
m. otitis
m. ovarian teratoma
m. ovarian tumor
m. reticulosis
m. small round cell tumor
m. teratoma
m. tumor
m. tumor of cervix
malignum
adenoma m.
lymphogranuloma m.
Malin syndrome
mallei (*pl. of* malleus)
malleolar fracture
malleolus, pl. **malleoli**
mallet fracture
malleus, pl. **mallei**
Mallory-Weiss
M.-W. esophageal tear
M. W. syndrome
malmoense
Mycobacterium m.
malnutrition
malondialdehyde
malpighian
m. body
m. corpuscle
malpositioned testis
malrotation
midgut m.
renal m.
MALT
MALT function
maltophilia
Pseudomonas m.
Xanthomonas m.
malt worker's lung

malunited fracture
mamillothalamic fasciculus
Mamm-Aire HF
mammalian cell
mammary
m. artery
m. duct
m. dysplasia
m. gland
m. proliferative disease
m. serum antigen (MSA)
m. tissue
mammillary system
mammography
magnification m.
orthogonal projection m.
screening m.
spot compression
magnification m.
x-ray m.
Mammo-lock needle
Mammo-Lume
Mammo Mask illuminator
Mammomat
mammoplasia
mammoplasty
augmentation m.
postreduction m.
reduction m.
Mammorex
Mammospot
Mammotest unit
mammotome
Biopsys m.
Mammotrax
mAMSA, m-AMSA
amsacrine
management
data m.
pain m.
Manan needle
**Manchester system for radium
therapy**
Mancini plate
mandible
mandibular
m. condyle

NOTES

mandibular *(continued)*
    m. disorder
    m. division
    m. foramen
    m. fossa
    m. ramus
mandibularis
    torus m.
mandibulectomy
mandibulofacial dysostosis
maneuver
    Adson m.
    Hampton m.
    jugular compression m.
    Kocher m.
    pull m.
    push m.
    Valsalva m.
manganese
    m. acetate
    m. chloride
    m. citrate
    m. sulfate
manganese-BOPTA
manganese tetrasodium-meso-tetra (Mn-TPPS$_4$)
manganese tetrasodium-meso-tetra (40-sulfonatophenyl) porphine
Mangevist
Mani cerebral catheter
manifestation
    cardiopulmonary m.
    ocular m.
    oral m.
manipulation
    bile duct m.
    guidewire m.
mannitol
mannosyl
Mann-Whitney U test
manometry
Mantel-Cox test
M antigen
mantle
    m. cell
    m. cell lymphoma
    cerebral m.
    m. irradiation
    m. radiotherapy
    m. zone
    m. zone hyperplasia
    m. zone lymphoma
    m. zone nodule
    m. zone pattern
Mantou method
manual differential
manubriosternal
    m. joint
manubrium, pl. manubria
MAO
    monoamine oxidase
MAOI
    monamine oxidase inhibitor
Maolate
map
    cancer m.
    chromosome m.
    genetic linkage m.
maple bark disease
mapping
    brain m.
    digital road m.
    gene m.
    lorentzian field m.
    phase m.
    phase difference m.
    phase-velocity m.
    road m.
    susceptibility m.
    two-dimensional m.
    velocity m.
marantic endocarditis
marasmus
marble bone disease
marbling
Marburg virus
Marcaine
marcellomycin
marcescens
    Serratia m.
March
    M. disease
    M. fracture
Marchand cell
Marchiafava-Bignami disease
Marchiafava-Micheli disease
Marek herpesvirus disease
Marfan syndrome
margin
    anal m.
    m. of apposition
    costal m.
    disk m.
    enhancing ventricular m.'s
    overhanging m.

periarticular m.
psoas m.
marginal
    m. artery of Drummond
    m. erosion
    m. fracture
    m. sclerosis
    m. spurring
    m. ulceration
    m. zone cell
    m. zone pattern
Marie-Strumpell disease
marihuana, marijuana
Marinol
Marituba virus
marker
    AFP tumor m.
    alkaline phosphatase
      isoenzyme tumor m.
    B-hCG tumor m.
    biochemical m.
    CA 15-3 breast cancer
      tumor m.
    CA 549 breast cancer
      tumor m.
    CA M26 tumor m.
    CA M29 tumor m.
    CA 125 ovarian tumor m.
    CASA tumor m.
    CA 125-11 tumor m.
    CA 19-9 tumor m.
    CA 195 tumor m.
    CA 27.29 tumor m.
    CA 50 tumor m.
    CA 72-4 tumor m.
    CD5 m.
    CEA tumor m.
    cell-lineage m.
    CK-BB tumor m.
    clonal m.
    CYFRA 21-1 tumor m.
    erythroid m.
    FT tumor m.
    genetic m.
    granulocytic m.
    6-HIAA tumor m.
    HSAP tumor m.

hyaluronan m.
IAP tumor m.
immune m.
immunochemical m.
immunocytochemical m.
immunophenotypic m.
Kern m.
laboratory m.
lymphoid m.
MCA tumor m.
M-CSF serum m.
megakaryocytic m.
membrane m.
metallic m.
monocytic m.
MSA tumor m.
myeloid m.
neuron-specific enolase
  tumor m.
nipple m.
NSE lung cancer tumor m.
NSE tumor m.
OVX1 serum m.
PAP tumor m.
proliferation m.
PSA prostate cancer
  tumor m.
PSA tumor m.
radiopaque m.
Rnase tumor m.
SCC tumor m.
serologic m.
serum tumor m.
sialic acid tumor m.
sitz m.
surrogate m.
TPA tumor m.
tumor m.
marking
    confluence of vascular m.
    convolutional m.
    digital m.'s
    genetic m.
    interstitial m.
    sutural m.
Markov process
Marlex mesh

NOTES

marneffei
  Penicillium m.
Maroteaux-Lamy syndrome
marrow
  m. ablation
  bone m.
  calvarial m.
  m. cell
  facial m.
  fatty m.
  m. graft rejection
  hematopoietic m.
  myelophthisis m.
  nonpurged m.
  pediatric fatty m.
  m. progenitor
  purged m.
  red m.
  shunting of tracer to the
    bone m.
  m. toxic drug
marrow-ablative chemoradiation
masculinization
masfin gene
mask
  Aquaplast m.
masked virus
masking
  unsharp m.
Mason-Pfizer monkey virus
***mas* proto-oncogene**
mass
  abdominal m.
  abdominopelvic m.
  adnexal m.
  adrenal m.
  adrenal cystic m.
  anterior mediastinal m.
  atomic m.
  benign m.
  bleeder in tumor m.
  brain m.
  calcified renal m.
  cardiophrenic angle m.
  circumscribed m.
  complex chest m.
  congenital nasal m.
  conglomerate m.
  cystic adrenal m.
  cystic chest m.
  cystic pelvic m.
  m. defect
  dense brain m.

dominant m.
dumbbell m.
m. effect
exophytic gut m.
extracardiac m.
extrauterine pelvic m.
extravascular m.
fallopian tube m.
groin m.
hilar m.
ill-defined m.
intraabdominal m.
intracranial m.
intradural extramedullary m.
intrasellar m.
intraventricular m.
lacrimal m.
lateral m.
m. lesion
liver m.
low-attenuation m.
low-density m.
mediastinal m.
mediastinal high-
  attenuation m.
mesenteric m.
mixed-density m.
multiloculated renal m.
myocardial m.
noncalcified nodular m.
nonopaque intraluminal m.
ovarian m.
parasellar m.
pediatric m.
pelvic m.
perivascular m.
pleural m.
posterior mediastinal m.
presacral m.
pulmonary m.
pulsatile m.
renal m.
retrobulbar m.
solitary pulmonary m.
m. spectrophotometer (MS)
m. spectrophotometric
  detector
stellate m.
suprasellar m.
thymic m.
tooth m.
tubal m.
tumor m.

umbilical m.
uncinate process m.
uterine m.
well-defined m.
Massachusetts General Teflon catheter
massa intermedia
masseter muscle
massive
  m. lymphadenopathy
  m. osteolysis
Masson
  M. pseudoangiosarcoma
  M. trichrome stain
MAST
  motion artifact suppression technique
  MAST suit
  MAST technique
mast
  m. cell
  m. cell disease
  m. cell-enhancing activity
  m. cell growth factor
  m. cell leukemia
  m. cell nevus
  m. cell sarcoma
Mastadenovirus
mastectomy
  extended radical m.
  modified radical m.
  radical m.
  subcutaneous m.
  total m.
mastication muscle
masticator space infection
mastitis
  cystic m.
  m. fibrosa cystica
  fibrous m.
  granulomatous m.
  plasma cell m.
  puerperal m.
mastocytoma
  localized m.
mastocytosis
  malignant m.

mastoid
  m. antrum
  m. complex
  m. emissary vein
  m. foramen
  m. lymph node
mastoidectomy
mastoiditis
mastoplasia (*var. of* mazoplasia)
masturbation
Masugi nephritis
MAT
  multiple agent therapy
matched
  m. lymphocyte transfusion
  m. related donor
  m. unrelated donor (MUD)
matching
  impedance m.
mater
  dura m.
  pia m.
material
  amorphous extracellular m.
  anthracotic m.
  autologous m.
  ballistic m.
  byproduct m.
  coffee-grounds m.
  columnization of contrast m.
  contrast m.
  dental m.
  fecal m.
  ferromagnetic m.
  flow of contrast m.
  hand-instilled contrast m.
  interventional m.
  intravenous administration of contrast m.
  low-osmolar contrast m.
  magnetic m.
  nonionic contrast m.
  semisolid fecal m.
  silicotic m.
  vicarious excretion of contrast m.

NOTES

maternal
    m. gonad
    m. lake
    m. serum alpha-fetoprotein
      (MSAFP)
mathematical modeling technique
Mathews classification of
  olecranon fractures
matrix, pl. matrices
    acquisition m.
    data m.
    display m.
    extracellular m.
    image m.
    m. image
    m. metalloproteinase
    protein m.
    m. protein
    reduced-acquisition m.
      (RAM)
matter
    cytotoxic edema of the
      gray m.
    heterotopic gray m.
    particulate m.
    periventricular white m.
Matuhasi-Ogata phenomenon
Matulane
maturation
    m. arrest
mature
    m. cell leukemia
    m. cystic teratoma
    m. ovarian teratoma
maturity
    cytologic m.
Maurer dot
maxilla, pl. maxillae
maxillary
    m. antrum
    m. artery
    m. division
    m. sinus
    m. sinus radiograph
maxillofacial
    m. fracture
    m. imaging
maximal
    m. drug concentration
      (C_{max})
    m. midexpiratory flow rate
    m. permissible dose

maximum
    m. entropy processing
    m. intensity
    m. permissible body burden
    m. permissible concentration
    m. permissible dose
    m. tolerated dose (MTD)
maximum-intensity projection
Max protein
Maxwell pair
Mayaro virus
Mayer-Rokitansky-Küster-Hauser
  syndrome
Mayer view
May-Hegglin anomaly
Mazabraud syndrome
Mazicon
mazoplasia, mastoplasia
Mazzariello-Caprini forceps
M-BACOD
    high-dose methotrexate,
      bleomycin, Adriamycin,
      cyclophosphamide, Oncovin,
      dexamethasone
    methotrexate-leucovorin,
      bleomycin, Adriamycin,
      cyclophosphamide, Oncovin,
      dexamethasone
m-BACOD
    moderate-dose methotrexate,
      bleomycin, Adriamycin,
      cyclophosphamide, Oncovin,
      dexamethasone
M-BACOS
    methotrexate, bleomycin,
      Adriamycin,
      cyclophosphamide, Oncovin,
      Solu-Medrol
MBC
    methotrexate, bleomycin,
      cisplatin
MBD
    methotrexate, bleomycin, DDP
MBP
    modified Bagshawe protocol
MC
    mitoxantrone, cytarabine
MC-540
    merocyanine 540
MCA tumor marker
MCBP
    melphalan, cyclophosphamide,
      BCNU, prednisone

MCC gene
McCoy culture medium
McCune-Albright syndrome
McDonough sarcoma virus
McFarlane skin flap
McGahan drainage catheter
McGregor line
McIndoe-Hayes construction
McIndoe vaginal creation
McKee line
McKrae herpes simplex virus
McKusick-Kaufman syndrome
McLeod phenotype
M-component
    M.-c. isotype
MCP
    metacarpophalangeal
MCPJ
    metacarpophalangeal joint
McRae line
M-CSF
    macrophage colony-stimulating
    factor
       M-CSF serum marker
MCTD
    mixed connective tissue disease
MCT oil
MCV
    mean corpuscular volume
    melanoma whole-cell vaccine
MDA
    M. D. Anderson
M. D. Anderson (MDA)
    M. D. A. Cancer Center
    M. D. A. cancer staging
    M. D. A. grading system
MDLO
    metoclopramide,
    dexamethasone, lorazepam,
    ondansetron
MDMS
    methylene dimethane sulfonate
MDR
    multidrug resistance
mdr-1
    mdr-1 gene
    mdr-1 oncogene

mdr gene
MDR-TB
    multidrug-resistant tuberculosis
MDS
    myelodysplastic syndrome
meal
    barium m.
mean
    m. corpuscular hemoglobin
    m. corpuscular volume
    (MCV)
    m. transit time
measles
    m. pneumonia
    m. vaccine
measurement
    ankle-brachial pressure m.
    blood flow m.
    1D phase m.
    2D phase m.
    end-diastolic velocity m.
    fetal m.
    fetal foot-length m.
    fetal long bone m.
    flow cytometric DNA m.
    multicolor
    immunofluorescence m.
    peak-and-trough drug m.
    phase-sensitive flow m.
    pulse-echo distance m.
    renal length m.
    temperature distribution m.
    time-of-flight flow m.
    time-velocity m.
    transcutaneous oxygen
    pressure m. (tcPO$_2$)
    trough drug m.
    true conjugate m.
    xenon CT m.
meatus, pl. meatus
    nasal m.
mebendazole
mebrofenin
MeCCNU
    methyl-CCNU
    methyl-1-[2-chloroethyl]-3-
    cyclhexyl-1-nitrosurea

NOTES

mechanical
- m. bowel obstruction
- m. sector scanner
- m. thrombectomy
- m. ventilation

mechanically activated implant

mechanism
- autocrine m.
- cellular cytotoxic m.
- contrecoup m.
- heat transfer m.
- homing m.
- host defense m.
- host response m.
- m. of injury
- osseous pinch m.
- paracrine m.
- pathogenetic m.
- resistance m.
- thermoregulatory m.
- tumorigenic m.
- watershed m.

mechlorethamine
- m. hydrochloride

mechlorethamine, Adriamycin, dacarbazine, DDP, Oncovin, cyclophosphamide (MADDOC)

mechlorethamine, Oncovin, procarbazine, prednisone (MOPP)

mechlorethamine, Oncovin, procarbazine, prednisone, Adriamycin, bleomycin, vinblastine (MOPP/ABV)

mechlorethamine, Oncovin (vincristine), procarbazine, prednisone (MOPP)

mechlorethamine, vinblastine, procarbazine, prednisone (MVPP)

mechlorethamine, vincristine, vinblastine, procarbazine, prednisone (MVVPP)

Mecholyl test

Meckel
- M. cave
- M. diverticulum
- M. syndrome

Meckel-Gruber syndrome

meclofenamate sodium

meclofenamic acid

Meclomen

meclopromide

meconium
- m. aspiration
- m. aspiration syndrome
- m. ileus
- m. ileus equivalent
- inspissated m.
- m. peristalsis
- m. peritonitis
- m. plug syndrome
- m. pseudocyst

MED
- minimum effective dose
- multiple epiphyseal dysplasia

media (*pl. of* medium)
- contrast m.
- iodinated contrast m.
- otitis m.
- tunica m.
- water-soluble contrast m.

medial, medialis
- m. angle
- m. dissection
- m. epicondyle
- m. fibroplasia
- m. geniculate body
- m. hyperplasia
- m. lemniscus
- m. longitudinal fasciculus
- m. oblique view

median
- m. cruciate ligament
- multiples of the m.
- m. nerve
- m. septum
- m. sternotomy
- m. survival time (MST)

mediastinal
- m. abscess
- m. adenoma
- m. adenopathy
- m. B-cell lymphoma
- m. biopsy
- m. bronchogenic cyst
- m. cyst
- m. dorsal enteric cyst
- m. emphysema
- m. fat
- m. fibrosis
- m. germ cell tumor
- m. hemorrhage
- m. high-attenuation mass
- m. irradiation
- m. large B-cell lymphoma

m. lipomatosis
m. lymphadenopathy
m. lymph node
m. lymphoma
m. mass
m. neoplasm
m. pseudomass
m. retraction
m. seroma
m. shift
m. tube
m. vein
m. viscera
m. widening
m. window
mediastinitis
fibrosing m.
sclerosing m.
mediastinoscopy
mediastinum
m. testis
mediator
m. cell
chemical m.
mediator-related symptom
medical
m. internal radiation dose
m. internal radiation
dosimetry (MIRD)
m. therapy
medication
concomitant m.
medicine
allopathic m.
alternative m.
Ayurvedic m.
holistic m.
nuclear m.
**Medilase angioscope-laser delivery
system**
Medinvent
M. stent
M. vascular stent
mediolateral view
Mediport infusion access device
Medisperse

Mediterranean
M. anemia
M. fever
M. Kaposi sarcoma (MEKS)
M. lymphoma
medium, pl. media
m. chain triglycerides
contrast m.
diatrizoate meglumine
radiopaque m.
HAT m.
high-osmolar contrast m.
(HOCM)
hot contrast m.
low-osmolar contrast m.
(LOCM)
McCoy culture m.
radiochromic dosimetry m.
Thayer-Martin culture m.
medium-energy collimator
medius
scalenus m.
Medix MF-5500X
Medrol
M. Dosepak
medronate
technetium-99m m.
medroxyprogesterone
m. acetate (MPA)
Medtronic infusion pump
Medtronic-Wiktor stent
medulla
hyperechoic renal m.
m. oblongata
renal m.
medullaris
conus m.
medullary
m. artery
m. calcification
m. carcinoma
m. cystic disease
m. infarct
m. infarction
m. nephrocalcinosis
m. pyramid
m. rod

NOTES

medullary *(continued)*
    m. sarcoma
    m. sponge
    m. sponge kidney
    m. thyroid carcinoma
medulloblastoma
    m. metastasis
medusa
    caput m.
Medx camera
mefenamic acid
megacalices
    congenital m.
megacalicosis
Megace
    M. oral suspension
mega cisterna magna
megacolon
    aganglionic m.
    toxic m.
megacystic microcolon
megacystis-microcolon-intestinal
  hypoperistalsis syndrome
megaduodenum
megaesophagus
MegaFlo infusion set
megahertz (MHz)
megakaryoblast
megakaryocyte
    m. colony-forming unit
    m. colony-stimulating factor
      (MEG-CSF)
    m. progenitor
megakaryocytic
    m. leukemia
    m. marker
megakaryocytopoiesis
megaloblast
megaloblastic anemia
megalocytosis
megaloencephaly
megaloureter, megaureter
    congenital primary m.
    primary m.'s
megavitamin therapy
megavolt (MeV)
megavoltage
    m. machine
    m. radiation
MEG-CSF
  megakaryocyte colony-
    stimulating factor

megestrol
    m. acetate
meglumine
    diatrizoate m.
    m. diatrizoate
    iocarmate m.
    iodipamide m.
    m. iothalamate
    ioxaglate m.
Meigs
    M. pelvic lymphadenectomy
    M. syndrome
Meigs-Okabayashi procedure
Meigs-Salmon syndrome
Meissner plexus
MEKS
    Mediterranean Kaposi sarcoma
MEL
    melphalan
Melacine
    M. regimen
melanin
melanocarcinoma
melanocyte
melanocytoma
    meningeal m.
melanocytosis
    meningeal m.
melanoma
    acral lentiginous m.
    amelanotic m.
    anorectal m.
    balloon-cell m.
    benign juvenile m.
    Bombriski m.
    Breslow thickness in
      malignant m.
    m. cell lysate vaccine
    choroidal m.
    ciliary body m.
    Clark staging system for
      malignant m.
    Cloudman m.
    cutaneous m.
    desmoplastic m.
    halo m.
    Harding-Passey m. (HPM)
    intraocular m.
    iris m.
    malignant m.
    malignant lentigo m.
    melanotic m.
    metastatic m.

minimal deviation m.
nodular m.
regional m.
spitzoid malignant m.
subungual m.
superficial spreading m.
uveal m.
vulvar m.
m. whole-cell vaccine
(MCV)
melanoma-associated antigens
melanomatosis
melanosis
m. coli
neurocutaneous m.
melanosome
melanotic
m. carcinoma
m. melanoma
m. neuroectodermal tumor
melatonin
meleagridis
Cryptosporidium m.
melena
melenic stool
melioidosis
mellitus
diabetes m.
insulin-dependent
diabetes m. (IDDM)
non-insulin-dependent
diabetes m. (NIDDM)
Melnick-Needles syndrome
melorheostosis
melphalan (MEL)
m. hydrochloride
melphalan, cyclophosphamide,
BCNU, prednisone (MCBP)
melphalan, prednisolone (MP)
melting sign
MelVax
membranacea
placenta m.
membranaceum
caput m.
membrane
amniotic m.

basement m.
glomerular basement m.
(GBM)
hourglass m.
m. marker
mucous m.
plasma m.
rolling m.
Shrapnell m.
surface m.
synovial m.
tympanic m.
membranous
m. obstruction of inferior
vena cava
m. stenosis
Memorial Sloan-Kettering Cancer
Center
memory
m. cell
immunologic m.
m. phenomenon
thermal shape m.
MEN
multiple endocrine neoplasia
menadione
Mendelson syndrome
Menest
Ménétrier disease
Menghini
M. biopsy technique
M. needle
Mengo virus
Ménière disease
meningeal
m. artery
m. artery groove
m. carcinoma
m. carcinomatosis
m. cell tumor
m. fibrosis
m. leukemia
m. malignancy
m. melanocytoma
m. melanocytosis
m. sarcoma
meninges (*pl. of* meninx)

NOTES

meningioangiomatosis
meningioma
    cerebellopontine angle m.
    clivus m.
    cystic intraparenchymal m.
    falx m.
    globular m.
    intraosseous m.
    intraparenchymal m.
    intraventricular m.
    meningothelial m.
    multicentric m.
    olfactory groove m.
    optic nerve sheath m.
    optic sheath m.
    parasagittal m.
    periauricular m.
    perioptic m.
    posterior fossa m.
    m. of posterior fossa
    sphenoid ridge m.
    spinal m.
    suprasellar m.
    temporal m.
    tentorial m.
    tuberculum sellae m.
meningioma-en-plaque
meningiomatosis
meningitidis
    Neisseria m.
meningitis
    AIDS-related
      lymphomatous m.
    aseptic m.
    bacterial m.
    carcinomatous m.
    cryptococcal m.
    epidural m.
    granulomatous m.
    Haemophilus influenzae m.
    neoplastic m.
    pseudomonas m.
    purulent m.
    salmonella m.
meningocele
    cervical m.
    lateral m.
    occipital m.
    sacral m.
    traumatic m.
meningococcal
    m. vaccine
meningococcemia

meningoencephalitis
    spirochetal m.
meningoencephalocele
meningohypophyseal artery
meningomyelocele
meningothelial meningioma
meninx, pl. meninges
meniscal ossicle
menisci (*pl. of* meniscus)
meniscofemoral ligament
meniscotibial separation
meniscocapsular
    m. attachment
    m. separation
meniscus, pl. menisci
    m. sign
Menkes syndrome
menogaril
menopausal
    m. gonadotropin
    m. symptom
menopause
    iatrogenic m.
    premature m.
menorrhagia
menotropin
menstrual
    m. age
    m. cycle
    m. function
menstrualis
    herpes m.
mensuration
    fetal m.
Mentor prostatic biopsy needle
MEP
    mitomycin C, etoposide, Platinol
meperidine
    m. hydrochloride
Mephyton
Mepron
meptazinol
merbarone
2-mercaptoethanesulfonate
mercaptopurine
6-mercaptopurine (6-MP)
Mercator projection
Mercedes-Benz sign
Merchant view
Mercier urethral dilator
mercury artifact
Meritene
Merkel cell tumor

mermaid syndrome
merocyanine 540 (MC-540)
Merrill-Dow polyamine inhibitor
mertiatide
    technetium-99m m.
mesencephalic
    m. cerebral lymphoma
    m. low density lesion
    m. vein
mesencephalitis
mesencephalon
mesenchymal
    m. chondrosarcoma
    m. hamartoma
    m. lesion
    m. neoplasm
    m. sex cord stromal tumor
    m. stromal cell
    m. tumor
mesenchyme
    nonspecific m.
mesenchymoma
    atrial m.
mesenteric
    m. adenitis
    m. adenopathy
    m. artery
    m. border
    m. calcification
    collateral m. circulation
    m. cyst
    m. infarction
    m. ischemia
    m. lipodystrophy
    m. lymphadenitis
    m. lymphadenopathy
    m. lymph node
    m. lymphoma
    m. mass
    m. panniculitis
    superior m.
    m. vascular insufficiency
    m. vein
    m. vessel
mesentericoparietal fossa
mesenteritis
    fibrosing m.

liposclerotic m.
    retractile m.
    sclerosing m.
mesenteroaxial volvulus
mesentery
    intestinal m.
mesh
    Marlex m.
    Prolene m.
    tantalum m.
    tubular wire m.
mesial temporal sclerosis
mesna
mesna, Adriamycin, ifosfamide,
    dacarbazine (MAID)
mesna, Adriamycin, interleukin-3,
    dacarbazine (MAID)
Mesnex
mesoappendix
mesoatrial shunt
mesoblastic nephroma
mesocardia
mesocaval shunt
mesocolon
    sigmoid m.
    transverse m.
mesodermal
    m. dysplasia
    m. sarcoma
mesomelia
mesomelic
    m. dwarfism
    m. dysplasia
mesometanephric carcinoma
meson
    negative π-m.
mesonephric
    m. adenocarcinoma
    m. carcinoma
    m. duct
    m. kidney
mesonephroi (pl. of mesonephros)
mesonephroid tumor
mesonephroma
mesonephros, pl. mesonephroi
mesothelial
    m. cell

NOTES

mesothelial *(continued)*
  m. cell inclusion
  m. cyst
  m. tissue
mesothelioma
  asbestos-related m.
  biphasic malignant m.
  epithelioid malignant m.
  malignant m.
  peritoneal m.
  pleural m.
  sarcomatoid malignant m.
messenger RNA (mRNA)
Mestinon
mestranol
mesylate
  atevirdine m.
  crisnatol m.
  deazaguanine m.
met
  met gene
  met proto-oncogene
meta-analysis
meta-azidopyrimethamine ethanesulfonate
metabolic
  m. acidosis
  m. bone disease
  m. bone disorder
  m. bone series
  m. complication
  m. disease
  m. emergency
metabolism
  arachidonic acid m.
  glucose m.
  hepatic m.
  inborn error of m.
  m. in intraperitoneal chemotherapy
  myocardial m.
  prostaglandin endoperoxide m.
metabolite
metacarpal
  m. bone
  m. fracture
  m. index
  m. sign
metacarpophalangeal (MCP)
  m. joint (MCPJ)
metacarpus
metachromatic leukodystrophy

metachronous
  m. carcinoma
  m. leukemia
metaclopramide
metadiaphyseal
metadiaphysis
metaiodobenzylguanidine
  iodine-131 m.
metal
  m. biopsy guidance attachment
  m. chelate complex
  m. dilator
  lanthanide m.
  radioactive m.
  transition m.
metallic
  m. artifact
  m. clip
  m. foreign body
  m. fragment
  m. fragment embolization
  m. marker
  m. needle
  m. otologic implant
  m. pointer
  m. rod fixation
  m. staple
  m. suture
  m. track of bullet
metalloporphyrin
metalloproteinase
  matrix m.
metalloproteinase-like, disintegrin-like, cysteine-rich protein
metalloproteinase-proteolytic enzyme
metallothionein
metamyelocyte
metanephric blastema
metanephros
metaphyseal, metaphysial
  m. bands
  m. chondrodysplasia
  m. dysostosis
  m. dysplasia
  m. fracture
  Schmid-like m. chondrodysplasia
metaphysis, pl. metaphyses
  frayed metaphyses
metaplasia
  agnogenic myeloid m.
  keratinizing squamous m.

myeloid m.
postpolycythemic
  myeloid m.
squamous m.
metaplastic carcinoma
metastasis, pl. metastases
adnexal m.
adrenal m.
aortic node m.
axillary node m.
blastic m.
bone m.
bony m.
brain m.
breast m.
calcified m.
calcified liver m.
calcifying m.
cavitating m.
celiac lymph node m.
cerebral m.
clivus m.
cystic m.
distant m.
drop m.
echopenic liver m.
extracapsular m.
extrathoracic m.
floxuridine in hepatic
  metastases
hematogenous m.
hepatic m.
hernia m.
inguinal lymph node m.
intracapsular m.
in-transit m.
leptomeningeal m.
liver m.
lymphatic m.
lymph node m.
medulloblastoma m.
necrotic m.
nodal m.
orbital m.
osseous m.
osteoblastic m.
ovarian cancer m.

paracardiac m.
parasellar m.
parenchymal brain m.
peritoneal m.
placental m.
pulmonary m.
skeletal m.
skip m.
sphenoid sinus m.
stomach cancer m.
testicular m.
tumor node m. (TNM)
uterine sarcoma m.
Virchow m.
metastasize
metastatic
  m. adenocarcinoma
  m. adenopathy
  m. axillary involvement
  m. breast cancer
  m. calcification
  m. carcinoid syndrome
  m. carcinoma
  m. cascade
  m. contamination
  m. lesion
  m. lymph node tumor
  m. lymphoma
  m. melanoma
  m. testicular lymphoma
  m. tumor
Metastron
metatarsal
  m. bone
  m. fracture
  m. injury
  m. joint
  m. synostosis
metatarsophalangeal
  m. joint
  m. joint arthritis
metatarsus adductus
metatrophic
  m. dwarfism
  m. dysplasia
metatypical carcinoma
metaxalone

NOTES

**Metchnikoff cellular immunity
theory**
metencephalon
meteorism
methacholine
methadone
methanol
 m. extraction residue of
  bacillus Calmette-Guérin
  vaccine
 m. freezing method
methemoglobin
methemoglobinemia
methiodal
methionine
methocarbamol
method
 AMeX m.
 antibody linkage m.
 Autenrieth and Funk m.
 B_0-gradient m.
 Clark-Collip m.
 Clausen m.
 Cockroft m.
 Cope m.
 Dixon m.
 Dixon fat suppression m.
 Epstein m.
 Fahraeus m.
 fibrin plate m.
 Fick m.
 Fisk and Subbarow m.
 Folin m.
 Folin and Wu m.
 freehand m.
 gradient m.
 gradient-echo m.
 gradient-reversal fat
  suppression m.
 Greenwald and Lewman m.
 Hagedorn and Jansen m.
 Hammerschlag m.
 Hawkins m.
 histochemical m.
 Hoechst dye m.
 Karr m.
 Kety-Schmidt m.
 Levy, Rowntree, and
  Marriott m.

 Lewis and Benedict m.
 Lewissohn m.
 Liang and Pardee m.
 Mantou m.
 methanol freezing m.
 Meyerding m.
 Nikiforoff m.
 Oliver-Rosalki m.
 Paris m.
 Pfiffner and Myers m.
 Sahli m.
 Shaffer-Hartmann m.
 single-stick m.
 Stammer m.
 three-dimensional-FATS m.
 Tilden m.
 triangulation m.
 trocar drainage m.
 two-dye m.
 Welcker m.
 Westergren m.
 Wintrobe and Landsberg m.
 Wroblewski m.
 x-line m.
methodology
 assay m.
methohexital
Methosarb
methotrexate, amethopterin (MTX)
 high-dose m. (HDMTX)
 intermediate-dose m.
  (IDMTX)
**methotrexate, actinomycin D,
chlorambucil (MAC)**
**methotrexate, actinomycin D,
cyclophosphamide (MAC III)**
**methotrexate, Adriamycin,
cyclophosphamide, Oncovin,
prednisone, bleomycin, with
leucovorin (MACOB with
leucovorin)**
**methotrexate, Adriamycin
(doxorubicin), cyclophosphamide,
Oncovin (vincristine), bleomycin
(MACOB)**
**methotrexate, ara-C,
cyclophosphamide, CCNU
(MACC)**
methotrexate, bleomycin,

Adriamycin, cyclophosphamide,
Oncovin, Solu-Medrol (M-
BACOS)
methotrexate, bleomycin, cisplatin
(MBC)
methotrexate, bleomycin, DDP
(MBD)
methotrexate-leucovorin,
Adriamycin, cyclophosphamide,
Oncovin, prednisone, bleomycin
(MACOP-B)
methotrexate-leucovorin, bleomycin,
Adriamycin, cyclophosphamide,
Oncovin, dexamethasone (M-
BACOD)
methotrexate, vinblastine,
Adriamycin, cisplatin (MVAC)
methotrimeprazine
methoxsalen
methoxyflurane
methoxyphenylisocyanate
methydiphosphonate bone scan
methyl
    m. benzoate
    m. CCNU
    m. guanine
    m. methacrylate
methyl-2-carbomethoxy-3-phenyl
  tropane
methyl-ABV
methylacetylenic putrescine
methyl-CCNU (MeCCNU)
methylcellulose
methyl-1-[2-chloroethyl]-3-cyclhexyl-
  1-nitrosurea (MeCCNU)
methylene
    m. dimethane sulfonate
    (MDMS)
    m. diphosphonate
methyl-GAG
methylglucamine
    iodipamide m.
methylglyoxal bisguanylhydrazone
methylhydrazine
    procarbazine m.
methylmalonic acidemia

methylmercaptopurine
    m. riboside
methyl nitrosurea
methylphenidate
methylprednisolone
    m. acetate
    m. sodium succinate
N-methylspiroperidol
methyl-*tert*-butyl ether
methyl testosterone
methyltyrosine
methylxanthine
methysergide
metoclopramide
metoclopramide, dexamethasone,
  lorazepam, ondansetron (MDLO)
metolazone
metopic suture
metrizamide
metrizoate
    sodium m.
metrizoic acid
metrofibroma
metronidazole
metroplasty
metrorrhagia
MeV
    megavolt
Mewissen infusion catheter
Mexate
Mexican
    M. hat erythrocyte
    M. hat sign
mexiletine
Meyer
    M. dysplasia
    M. line
    supratubercular ridge of M.
Meyer-Betz disease
Meyerding method
Meyers-McKeever classification of
  tibial fractures
mezlocillin
MF-5500X
    Medix MF-5500X

NOTES

M1G8
    monoclonal antibody M1G8
MHA-TPA
    microhemagglutination assay-
        Treponema pallidum assay
MHz
    megahertz
mica pneumoconiosis
mice
    joint m.
Michaelis
    M. buffer
    M. complex
    rhomboid of M.
Michaelis-Gutmann body
Michel anomaly
michellamine B
Mick afterloading needle
Mickey Mouse ears pelvis
miconazole
micrencephaly
microabscess
    Pautrier m.
microadenoma
    pituitary m.
microangiopathic anemia
microangiopathy
    mineralizing m.
    thrombotic m.
microbial flora
microbiology
microcalcification
    ductal m.
    lobular m.
microCase
Micro-Cast collimator
microcatheter
microcephaly
    cytomegalovirus with m.
microcirculation
microcoil
    Hilal m.
microcolon
    megacystic m.
microculture tetrazolium dye assay
microcyst
    milk-of-calcium m.
microcystic
    m. adenoma
    m. degeneration
    m. encephalomalacia
    m. lumbar spine

    m. pilocytic cerebellar
        astrocytoma
microcystica
microcytosis
microcytotoxicity assay
microelectrophoresis
microembolization
    ferromagnetic m.
microembolus
microencapsulation assay
microenvironment
    bone marrow m.
    hematopoietic m.
microfibrillar collagen
microfluorometry
microfollicular adenoma
microgastria
microglandular adenosis
microglial cell
microglioma
β_2-microglobulin
micrognathia
microgranular acute promyelocytic
    leukemia
microhemagglutination
    m. assay-Treponema
        pallidum assay (MHA-
        TPA)
microhomology
microinvasive
    m. carcinoma
    m. carcinoma classification
microlatex particle-mediated
    immunoassay
micro liquid extraction
microlithiasis
    alveolar m.
micromegakaryocyte
micromelia
    bowed m.
    extreme m.
micromelic
    m. dwarfism
    m. dysplasia
micrometastasis, pl. micrometastases
Micro-Mist nebulizer
micromyeloblastic leukemia
micronest
    endocrine cell m.
micronodular
    m. cirrhosis
    m. lung disease
micronutrient

microorganism
Micropaque
microphage
microphthalmus
Micropore tape
microprolactinoma
microscope
    Joel scanning electron m.
    Rheinberg m.
microscopically normal tissue
microscopy
    cryoelectrom m.
    darkfield m.
    electron m.
microsequencing
microsomal hydroxylation
microspectrofluorometry
microsphere
    acrylic m.
    degradable starch m.
    ferromagnetic m.
    gelatin-encapsulated
      nitrogen m.
    magnetic m.
    magnetically responsive m.
    paramagnetic m.
    Silastic m.
    silicone m.
    stainless steel m.
    starch m.
    superparamagnetic m.
    therapeutic m.
Microsporida
microsporidiosis
Microsporum canis
microti
    Babesia m.
Microtrast
microvascular disease
microvillus
microwave
    m. fixation
    m. imaging
microwell
MIC tube
midazolam
midbrain

midcarpal dislocation
midclavicular
    m. planes
midcoronal plane
Middeldorph tumor
middle
    m. cerebral artery
    m. cerebral artery infarction
    m. cranial fossa
    m. ear
    m. ear neoplasm
    m. fossa syndrome
    m. meningeal
    m. meningeal artery groove
Middlebrook
    M. agar
    M. broth
Middlebrook-Dubos
    hemagglutination test
midfoot fracture
midfrontal
    m. plane
    m. plane coronal section
midgut
    m. malrotation
    m. volvulus
midhumeral line
midline
    m. cystic structure
    m. granuloma
    m. malignant reticulosis
    m. shift
midobenzoyl-N-hydroxysuccinimide
  ester
midsagittal plane
midshaft fracture
midtarsal injury
midthalamic plane
midthoracic spine
Miescher granulomatosis
mifepristone (RU 486)
migraine
migrans
    erythema m.
    necrolytic erythema m.
    visceral larva m.
migrant pattern

NOTES

migration
    cell m.
    cellular m.
    embolus m.
    m. inhibitory factor
    lymphocyte m.
    neuronal m.
    neutrophil m.
    phagocyte m.
Mikity-Wilson syndrome
Mikulicz
    M. disease
    M. syndrome
Milan Cancer Institute
Milch classification of humeral
  fractures
Miliaria 538
miliary
    m. nodule
    m. pattern
    m. pulmonary tuberculosis
    m. tuberculosis
militate against
milk
    m. of calcium
    m. factor
    m. fat globule protein
milk-alkali syndrome
milkmaid's elbow dislocation
milkman's
    m. fracture
    m. pseudofracture
    m. syndrome
milk-of-calcium
    m.-o.-c. bile
    m.-o.-c. microcyst
Miller
    M. Behavioral Style Scale
    M. stent
Miller-Abbott tube
Miller-Duker syndrome
million
    parts per m. (ppm)
Millipore filter
miltefosine
Milwaukee
    M. brace
    M. shoulder syndrome
mimicker of malignancy
mind-body interaction
mineral
    clay m.
    m. oil aspiration

mineralization
mineralizing microangiopathy
mineralocorticoid secretion
miner's anemia
miniature uterine cavity
miniaturized mitral valve
Mini-Balloon system
minicalyx
minicholecystostomy
    surgical-radiologic m.
minicoil
minification
minimal
    m. deviation melanoma
    m. differentiation
    m. port diameter (MPD)
    m. residual disease (MRD)
minimum effective dose (MED)
mining
    uranium m.
minipilon fracture
minisatellite DNA
Minnesota tube
minor
    m. fissure
    rhomboid m.
    teres m.
Minot-Murphy diet
minute
    double m.
miosis
miotic
mirabile
    rete m.
MIRD
    medical internal radiation
    dosimetry
Mirizzi syndrome
mirror
    beam-splitting m.
mirror-image
    m.-i. artifact
    m.-i. interpretation
    m.-i. reflection
mismapping
    phase m.
mismatch
    ventilation-perfusion m.
mismatched related donor
misonidazole
misoprostol
mispair
misplaced thoracentesis

misregistration
- m. artifact
- chemical shift m.
- oblique flow m.

missed
- m. abortion
- m. testicular torsion

missense mutation
missile effect
missing pulse steady-state free precession sequence
mistletoe
- European m.

MIT-C
- mitomycin C

Mithracin
mithramycin
mitis
- *Streptococcus m.*

mitochondrial
- m. antibody
- m. encephalomyopathy

mitogen
- pokeweed m.

mitogenic factor
mitoguazone
mitolactol
mitomycin
- m. cardiotoxicity
- m. C, etoposide, Platinol (MEP)

mitomycin C (MIT-C)
mitomycin, vinblastine, Platinol (MVP)
mitonafide
mitoquidone
mitosis
- quantal m.

mitotane
mitotic
- m. figure
- m. index
- m. inhibitor

mitotic-karyorrhectic index

mitotoxicity
mitoxantrone, mitozantrone (DHAD)
- m. hydrochloride

mitoxantrone, cytarabine (MC)
mitral
- m. annulus calcification
- m. component
- m. insufficiency
- m. regurgitation
- m. regurgitation artifact
- m. stenosis
- m. valve
- m. valve prolapse
- m. valve stenosis

Mitsuda antigen
Mix D
mixed
- m. cell leukemia
- m. cellularity Hodgkin disease
- m. cellularity type
- m. chimerism
- m. connective tissue disease (MCTD)
- m. fat-water density lesion
- m. follicular hyperplasia
- m. germ cell tumor
- m. gonadal dysgenesis
- m. leukemia
- m. lineage
- m. mesodermal sarcoma
- m. mesodermal tumor
- m. müllerian sarcoma
- m. opioid agonist-antagonist
- m. ovarian mesodermal sarcoma
- m. pattern
- m. rheumatoid and degenerative arthritis
- m. sclerotic and lytic bone lesion
- m. small cleaved and large cell lymphoma
- m. small and large cell lymphoma
- m. tumor

NOTES

mixed *(continued)*
    m. tumor of salivary gland
    m. tumor of skin
    m. type carcinoma
    m. venous-lymphatic
      malformation
mixed-density mass
mixture
    barium m.
MK-217 (biphosphonate)
MK-906 (tinasteride)
M-mode echocardiography
MN blood group
MNSs blood group
Mn-TPPS$_4$
    manganese tetrasodium-meso-
      tetra
MO1 antigen
Moberg-Gedda fracture
mobile
    cecum m.
    m. magnetic resonance
    m. radiography
mobility shift assay
mobilization
    stem cell m.
Mobin-Uddin
    M.-U. filter
    M.-U. umbrella filter
Mobitz heart block
modality
mode
    amplitude m.
    brightness m.
    continuous m.
    dispersion m.
    m. I additivity
    m. II additivity
    imaginary m.
    motion m.
    pulsed m.
    stimulated-echo
      acquisition m. (STEAM)
model
    Cox proportional
      hazards m.
    Dayhoff m.
    M. Forty
    Goldie-Coldman m.
    hematopoietic-inductive
      microenvironment m.
    Hyrniuk-Bush m.
    linear pharmacokinetic m.

    log-kill m.
    Luria-Delbruck m.
    multiresolution tree m.
    multistage Markov m.
    primate m.
    Skipper-Schabel m.
    m. system
    till birth and death m.
    Trentin hematopoietic-
      inductive
      microenvironment m.
    Zimmerman-Brittin
      exchange m.
modeling
modeling-derivation
moderate-dose methotrexate,
   bleomycin, Adriamycin,
   cyclophosphamide, Oncovin,
   dexamethasone (m-BACOD)
modification
    fiber tip m.
    glutathione m.
    Gunderson-Sosin m.
    posttranslation m.
    Rosch m.
    thiol m.
modified
    m. Bagshawe protocol
      (MBP)
    m. radical hysterectomy
    m. radical mastectomy
    m. Simpson rule
modifier
    biological response m.
      (BRM)
    response m.
modifying gene
modulation
    amplitude m.
    antigenic m.
    biochemical m.
    immune m.
    m. potential
    specific m.
    m. transfer function
modulator
    combined m.'s
module
    diode m.
modulus
    bulk m.
    m. image
Mohs micrographic surgery

moiety
  arginine-glycine-aspartic
    acid m.
  glucopyranoside m.
moiré pattern
Moi-Stir
  M.-S. oral spray
  M.-S. swabstick
molar
  m. pregnancy
  m. tooth fracture
mole
  amniography in
    hydatidiform m.
  Breus m.
  complete m.
  hydatidiform m.
  invasive m.
  partial m.
molecular
  m. approach
  m. cell biology
  m. cloning
  m. diffusion
  m. epidemiology
  m. genetic analysis
  m. genetics
  m. genetic technique
  m. hybridization study
  m. latency
  m. study
  m. technique
  m. weight
  m. weight dependence of
    relaxation
molecule
  accessory adhesion m.
  adhesion m.
  cell adhesion m.
  homing m.
  lectin cell adhesion m.
  neural cell adhesion m.
molecule-1
  intercellular adhesion m.-1
    (ICAM-1)
  leukocyte adhesion m.-1
    (LAM-1)

molgramostim
Moll
  adenocarcinoma of M.
molle
  fibroma m.
  papilloma m.
molluscum
  m. contagiosum
  fibroma m.
  m. fibrosum
Molnar disk
Moloney test
Molulsky dye reduction test
molybdenum
  m. target
  m. target tube
moment
  macroscopic magnetic m.
  magnetic m.
  magnetic dipole m.
  nuclear magnetic m.
  quadripole m.
  zeroth m.
momentum
  angular m.
**monamine oxidase inhibitor
  (MAOI)**
Mönckeberg
  M. calcification
  M. sclerosis
Mondini
  M. anomaly
  M. malformation
Mondor disease
mongolism
mongoloid features
moniliasis
moniliid
monitor
  dosimetristradiation
    beam m.
  patient dose m.
monitoring
  m. electrode
  physiologic m.

NOTES

monitoring *(continued)*
    m. technique
    therapeutic drug m.
monoamine oxidase (MAO)
monoblast
    m. predominance
monocellular suspension
monochorionic
    m. diamniotic twin
      pregnancy
    m. monoamniotic twin
      pregnancy
    m. twin
monochorionic-monoamniotic twin
monochromatism, monochromasy
Monoclate
Monoclate P
monoclonal
    m. antibody (MAb)
    m. antibody B72.3
    m. antibody-defined antigen
    m. antibody imaging
    m. antibody M1G8
    m. antibody PC10
    m. antibody therapy
    m. anticytokeratin (MAK-6)
    m. band
    m. gammopathy
    m. gammopathy of
      undetermined significance
    m. origin
    m. spike
monoclonality
monocrotaline
monocular blindness
monocyte
    m. colony-stimulating factor
    m. lineage antigen
    m. presenting
    m. tissue factor
monocyte-macrophage progenitor
monocytic
    m. leukemia
    m. marker
    m. sarcoma
monocytogene
    heat-killed Listeria m.'s
    Listeria m.'s
monocytoid
    m. B-cell
    m. B-cell lymphoma
    m. B-lymphocyte
monocytopenia

monocytosis
Mono-Diff test
monogamous
monohistiocyte
monoiodobenzylguanidine
    (^{131}I- mIB6)
monokine
monoligand nitrosurea
monomalleolar fracture
monomorphic
    m. adenoma
    m. lymphoma
mononeuritis multiplex
mononuclear
    m. cell
    m. phagocyte
mononucleosis
    infectious m.
monooctanoin
monooleate
    polyethylene sorbitan m.
monophasic
Monophen
monophosphate
    adenosine m.
    deoxyadenosine m. (dAMP)
    fludarabine m. (FAMP)
Monopty needle
monosomy
    m. 5q-syndrome
    m. 7 syndrome
monosomy X
Monospot test
monostotic
    m. fibrous dysplasia
monoventricle
monovular twin transfusion
Monox-IX
monozygotic twin
Monro
    foramen of M.
Monsel solution
Monte Carlo simulation
Monteggia fracture
Montercaux fracture
Montgomery glands
moon sign
Moore fracture
Mooser cell
MOPP
    mechlorethamine, Oncovin,
      procarbazine, prednisone
    mechlorethamine, Oncovin

(vincristine), procarbazine,
prednisone
MOPP/ABV
mechlorethamine, Oncovin,
procarbazine, prednisone,
Adriamycin, bleomycin,
vinblastine
Moranyl
Moraxella
M. *bovis*
M. *catarrhalis*
M. liquefaciens
morbidity
m. rate
morbilliform rash
Morbillivirus
Morgagni
M. hernia
M. hydatid
sinus of M.
M. syndrome
tubercle of M.
Morison pouch
morphea
m. form basal cell
carcinoma
morphine
m. sulfate (MS)
morphogen
morphogenetic protein
morpholino
m. anthracycline
morphologic
m. classification
m. growth
m. pattern
morphologically normal
morphology
m. system CAS-200
Morquio syndrome
mortality
m. rate
mortise
ankle m.
m. radiograph
m. view
Morton neuroma

morula
morular cell
mosaic pattern
Moser balloon
Mose technique
mos **proto-oncogene**
Mosse syndrome
Mossuril virus
Mostofi histologic typing
moth-eaten
m.-e. appearance
m.-e. bone destruction
m.-e. calyx
mother cell
mother-in-law phenomenon
motif
protein m.
motilin
motility
antroduodenal m.
m. disorder
m. of Golden
motion
m. artifact
m. artifact suppression
technique (MAST)
m. blur
brownian m.
m. compensation gradient
pulse
incoherent m.
intravoxel coherent m.
intravoxel incoherent m.
isotropic m.
limitation of m.
m. mode
paradoxical m.
patient m.
perturbed water m.
random m.
regional wall m.
respiratory m.
rotational m.
stationary zero-order m.
translational m.
m. unsharpness
within-view m.

NOTES

motional
> m. averaging
> m. narrowing

motion-induced phase shift

Motofen

motor
> m. area
> m. deficit
> m. nucleus

Mott
> M. body
> M. cell

mottle
> quantum m.

mottled
> m. appearance
> m. infiltrate

mottling
> m. pattern

Mouchet fracture

moulage sign

Mounier-Kuhn
> M.-K. disease
> M.-K. syndrome

mountain anemia

mouse
> m. bed sign
> m. cancer
> cancer-free white m.
> Carworth Farm m.
> m. erythrocyte receptor
> m. germ line
> Harvard m.
> joint m.
> m. leukemia virus
> m. mammary tumor factor
> m. mammary tumor virus
> New Zealand black m.
> m. parotid tumor virus
> transgenic m.
> Webster strain m.

mouth
> floor of m.

mouthwash
> biotene m.
> swish and swallow m.

movement
> m. artifact
> fetal m. (FM)
> fetal breathing m. (FBM)
> systolic anterior m.

moving boundary electrophoresis

moyamoya disease

MP
> melphalan, prednisolone

6-MP
> 6-mercaptopurine

MPA
> medroxyprogesterone acetate

MPD
> main pancreatic duct
> main papillary duct
> minimal port diameter
> multiplanar display

MPGR
> multiple planar gradient-recalled
> MPGR technique

MP-RAGE
> magnitude preparation-rapid
> acquisition gradient echo
> MP-RAGE technique

MR
> magnetic resonance
> MR angiography
> MR imaging

MRA
> magnetic resonance angiography

MRD
> minimal residual disease

MRI
> magnetic resonance imaging
> cine MRI
> pulse MRI

mRNA
> messenger RNA

MRS
> magnetic resonance spectroscopy
> slice point MRS

MS
> mass spectrophotometer
> morphine sulfate
> MS Contin

MSA
> mammary serum antigen
> muscle-specific actin
> MSA tumor marker

MSAFP
> maternal serum alpha-
> fetoprotein

MST
> median survival time

MTD
> maximum tolerated dose

MTN blot

MTX
> methotrexate

MU
  M. filter
Mucha-Habermann disease
mucicarmine stain
mucinosa
  alopecia m.
mucinosis
  erythrodermic follicular m.
  follicular m.
  idiopathic follicular m.
  papular m.
mucinous
  m. adenocarcinoma of ovary
  m. carcinoma
  m. cystadenocarcinoma
  m. cystadenoma
  m. cystadenoma of ovary
  m. tumor
mucin-producing
  m.-p. adenocarcinoma
  m.-p. carcinoma
mucleated erythrocyte
mucocele
  breast m.
  frontal sinus m.
  frontoethmoidal m.
  orbital m.
mucocutaneous
  m. lesion
  m. pigmentation
  m. reaction
mucoepidermoid
  m. carcinoma
  m. tumor
mucoid
  m. adenocarcinoma
  m. impaction
mucoid adenocarcinoma
mucolipidosis, pl. **mucolipidoses**
mucomycosis
mucopolypeptide
mucopolysaccharidosis,
  pl. **mucopolysaccharidoses**
mucopyocele
Mucor

mucormycosis
  rhinocerebral m.
mucosa
  buccal m.
  endocervical m.
  gingival m.
  m. muscularis
  oral m.
  polypoid m.
  prolapsed antral m.
  prolapsed gastric m.
mucosa-associated
  m.-a. lymphoid tissue
mucosal
  m. barrier
  m. destruction
  m. fold
  m. gland
  m. lesion
  m. lining
  m. neuroma syndrome
  m. pattern
  m. relief radiography
  m. stripe sign
  m. thickening
  m. toxicity
  m. ulceration
mucositis
  oral m.
  oropharyngeal m.
  radiation m.
mucous
  m. bronchogram
  m. colitis
  m. cystadenocarcinoma
  m. membrane
  m. plug
  m. plug syndrome
  m. pseudomass
mucoviscidosis
mucus (noun)
mucus stretchability
MUD
  matched unrelated donor
  MUD transplant
Muercke line

NOTES

MUGA
multiple gated acquisition
MUGA scan
mu heavy-chain disease
Mukherjee-Sivaya view
mule-spinner's cancer
Müller
M. duct body
M. empyema
M. empyema catheter
M. test
müllerian
m. adenosarcoma
m. duct
m. duct anomaly
m. duct cyst
m. duct formation and
fusion
m. sarcoma of uterus
m. structure
m. tumor
multangular
m. bone
m. ridge fracture
multiagent chemotherapy
**Multicenter AIDS Cohort Study
(MACS)**
multicentric
m. angiofollicular lymphoid
hyperplasia
m. carcinoma
m. Castleman disease
m. germinoma
m. glioblastoma
m. meningioma
m. osteosarcoma
multicentricity
multiclonal follicular lymphoma
multiclonality
multicolony-stimulating factor
multicolor
m. data analysis
m. immunofluorescence
measurement
Multicrystal camera
multicystic
m. dysgenetic kidney
m. dysplasia
m. dysplastic kidney
multidrug resistance (MDR)
multidrug-resistant
m.-r. phenotype
m.-r. tuberculosis (MDR-TB)

multiecho
m. imaging
preinversion m. (PRIME)
multifactorial
multifiber catheter
multifocal
m. anaplastic astrocytoma
m. brain tumor
m. enhancing lesion
m. subperitoneal sclerosis
multifocality
multiformat camera
multiformatted imaging
multiforme
erythema m.
glioblastoma m. (GBM)
granuloma m.
multileaf collimating system
multilineage origin
multilobated
m. nucleus
m. T-cell lymphoma
multilocular
m. cyst
m. cystic lesion
m. cystic nephroma
m. renal cyst
multilocularis
Echinococcus m.
multiloculated renal mass
multilog effect
multimerization
multimodality therapy
multinodular goiter
multipartite patella
multiplanar
m. display (MPD)
m. gradient-recalled echo
m. gradient refocused
m. gradient refocused
sequence
m. imaging
phase-ordered m. (POMP)
m. reformations
multiple
m. agent therapy (MAT)
m. basal cell neuromas
syndrome
m. core biopsy
m. cyst
m. drug resistance
m. enchondromatosis

m. endocrine neoplasia (MEN)
m. endocrine neoplasia syndrome
m. endocrine neoplasia, type 1
m. endocrine neoplasia, type 2
m. epiphyseal dysplasia (MED)
m. fetuses
m. gaited acquisition scan (MUGA scan)
m. gated acquisition (MUGA)
m. gestation
m. gland disease
m. hamartoma syndrome
m. idiopathic hemorrhagic
m. line scan imaging
m. lymphomatous polyposis
m.'s of the median
m. myeloma
m. myeloma staging
m. myelomatosis
m. plane imaging
m. pulmonary calcification
m. quantum experiment
m. sclerosis
m. sensitive point
m. spin echo imaging
m. stones
m. symmetrical lipomatosis
m. thyroid cyst
multiple-drug resistance gene
multiple-echo imaging
multiple-gated blood pool imaging
multiple planar gradient-recalled (MPGR)
multiple-sidehole infusion catheter
multiplex
dysplasia epiphysealis m.
mononeuritis m.
myeloma m.
myelomatosis m.
multiplexing
multiploid tumor

multiploidy
Multi-Pro biopsy needle
multipurpose catheter
multiray fracture
multiresolution tree model
multiseptated gallbladder
multislice
m. flow-related enhancement
m. imaging
m. modified KEW direct Fournier imaging
multistage Markov model
multisweep
high-resolution m.
multisystem organ failure
multitargeted chemotherapy
multivariant
m. analysis
m. regressional analysis
multivitamin infusion (MVI-12)
multizone transmit-receive focus
mummified cell
mumps
m. skin test antigen
m. virus
mural
m. fibrosing alveolitis
m. nodule
m. thickening
m. thrombus
muramidase
muramyl-tripeptide
mu receptor
murine
m. colony-forming unit
m. granulocyte-macrophage colony-stimulating growth factor
m. interleukin
m. interleukin-3
m. interleukin-6 (rMu IL-6)
m. interleukin-7
m. interleukin-1B
m. leukemia L1210
m. leukemia P388
m. monoclonal antibody

NOTES

murine *(continued)*
    m. protein
    m. sarcoma virus
murine-acquired immunodeficiency syndrome (MAIDS)
muris
    Cryptosporidium m.
murmur
    Austin Flint m.
    heart m.
muromonab-CD3 *(var. of* anti-CD3)
Murphy sign
Murray Valley encephalitis virus
Murri disease
muscarinic receptor
muscle
    abductor m.
    accessory m.
    m. actin
    anconeus m.
    autologous m.
    ciliary m.
    dartos m.
    m. of deglutition
    detrusor m.
    external oblique m.
    extraocular m.
    genioglossus m.
    m. hemoglobin
    hyoglossus m.
    iliopsoas m.
    m. infarction
    lateral rectus m.
    longus colli m.
    masseter m.
    mastication m.
    mylohyoid m.
    palatal m.
    papillary m.
    paraspinal m.
    Passavant m.
    pectoralis m.
    pharyngeal m.
    psoas m.
    pterygoid m.
    pupillary constrictor m.
    pyloric m.
    quadriceps m.
    rectus m.
    rotator cuff m.
    m. sarcoma

    serratus anterior m.
    smooth m.
    m. spindle
    sternocleidomastoid m.
    sternohyoid m.
    sternothyroid m.
    strap m.
    striated m.
    styloglossus m.
    stylohyoid m.
    temporalis m.
    tensor veli palatini m.
    transversus abdominis m.
muscle-specific actin (MSA)
muscular
    m. dystrophy
    m. slip
muscularis
    mucosa m.
    m. propria
musculoaponeurotic structure
musculocutaneous
    rectus abdominis m. flap
musculoskeletal
    m. imaging
    m. radiography
    m. system
    m. tumor
musculus uvula
mushroom
    m. appearance
    m. catheter
    shiitake m.
    m. sign
    m. worker's lung
mustache sign
mustard
    nitrogen m. (HN_2, NM)
    M. operation
    phenylalanine m.
    L-phenylalanine m. (L-PAM)
    phosphoramide m.
    M. procedure
    spirohydantoin m.
    uracil m.
Mustargen
mustine
mutagen
mutagenesis
    insertional m.
mutagenicity
Mutamycin

mutant
> m. cell
> m. gene

mutation
> dominant lethal m.
> genetic m.
> missense m.
> point m.
> somatic m.
> transcriptional m.
> wimp m.

mutational dysostosis
mutogenicity
MVAC
> methotrexate, vinblastine, Adriamycin, cisplatin

MVI-12
> multivitamin infusion

MVI pediatric
MVP
> mitomycin, vinblastine, Platinol

MVPP
> mechlorethamine, vinblastine, procarbazine, prednisone

MVVPP
> mechlorethamine, vincristine, vinblastine, procarbazine, prednisone

myalgia
myasthenia gravis
myasthenic syndrome
myb
> *myb* protein
> *myb* proto-oncogene

myc
> *myc* oncogene
> *myc* protein

mycalamide A
Mycelex troche
mycetoma
mycobacteria
mycobacterial infection
Mycobacterium
> *M. avium*
> *M. avium* complex (MAC)
> *M. avium-intracellulare*

> *M. avium-intracellulare* enteritis
> *M. bovis*
> *M. fortuitum*
> *M. genavense*
> *M. gordonae*
> *M. haemophilum*
> *M. intracellulare*
> *M. kansasii*
> *M. leprae*
> *M. malmoense*
> *M. scrofulaceum*
> *M. tuberculosis*
> *M. ulcerans*
> *M. xenopi*

Mycobutin
Mycoplasma
> *M. fermentans pneumoniae*
> *M. incognitus*
> *M. pneumoniae*

mycoplasma
> m. pneumonia

mycoplasmal
Mycosel agar
mycosis
> m. fungoides
> m. fungoides/Sézary syndrome

mycotic
> m. aneurysm
> m. aortic aneurysm
> m. infection
> m. stomatitis

Mycotoruloides
myelencephalon
myelin
> m. base protein
> m. pallor

myelination
> nerve fiber m.
> optic pathway m.

myelinoclastic disorder
myelinolysis
> central pontine m. (CPM)
> pontine m.

NOTES

myelitis
    radiation m.
    transverse m.
myeloablation
myeloablative
myeloblast
myeloblastic leukemia
myeloblastoma
myelocele
myelocystocele
myelocyte
    eosinophilic m.
myelocytic leukemia
myelocytoma
myelocytomatosis
myelodysplasia
myelodysplastic syndrome (MDS)
myelofibrosis
    acute m.
myelogenesis
myelogenic
    m. leukemia
    m. sarcoma
myelogenous leukemia
myelogram
    cervical m.
    lumbar m.
myelography
    extraarachnoid m.
myeloid
    m. associated antigen
    m. blood element
    m. cell
    m. depletion
    m. disease
    m. engraftment
    m. growth factor
    m. leukemia
    m. lineage antigen
    m. marker
    m. metaplasia
    m. precursor cell
    m. progenitor
    m. sarcoma
myeloid/erythroid ratio
myelolipoma
    adrenal m.
myeloma
    amyloidosis of multiple m.
    Bence Jones m.
    CALLA-positive m.
    m. cell
    endothelial m.

    giant cell m.
    L-chain m.
    multiple m.
    m. multiplex
    nonsecreting m.
    nonsecretory m.
    plasma cell m.
    m. protein
    smoldering multiple m.
    solitary m.
myelomalacia
    cystic m.
myelomatosis
    multiple m.
    m. multiplex
myelomeningocele repair
myelomonocyte
myelomonocytic
    m. antigen
    m. leukemia
Myelo-Nate
    M.-N. kit
    M.-N. needle
    M.-N. set
myelopathic anemia
myelopathy
    carcinomatous m.
    cystic m.
    necrotizing m.
    paracarcinomatous m.
    posttraumatic cystic m.
    subacute necrotizing m.
myeloperoxidase
    m. stain
myelophthisic
    m. anemia
myelophthisis marrow
myelopoiesis
myeloproliferative
    m. disorder
    m. syndrome
myelosarcoma
myelosarcomatosis
myeloschisis
myelosclerosis
myelosis
    chronic megakaryocytic m.
    erythremic m.
myelosuppression
    m. chemotherapy
    dose-limiting m.
myelotomy
myelotoxic drug

myelotoxicity
myl
>   *myl* oncogene
>   *myl* proto-oncogene

Mylar sheath introducer
myleogenous
Myleran
mylohyoid muscle
myoablative therapy
myoblast
myoblastoma
>   granular cell m.

myocardial
>   m. blood flow
>   m. cell
>   m. contractility
>   m. deposition disease
>   m. fibrosis
>   m. function
>   m. function assessment
>   m. hypertrophy
>   m. infarct
>   m. infarction
>   m. inflammation
>   m. ischemia
>   m. mass
>   m. metabolism
>   m. perfusion
>   m. perfusion imaging
>   m. pulsation
>   m. tagging
>   m. thallium imaging
>   m. toxicity
>   m. twist
>   m. wall

myocardiopathy
myocarditis
myocardium
>   inferior apical aspect of
>   the m.
>   ventricular m.

myoclonus
myocutaneous flap
myocytoma
MyoD gene
Myodil
myoD protein

myoepithelial sialoadenitis
myoepithelioma
>   malignant m.

myofascial
>   m. pain
>   m. pain dysfunction
>   syndrome

myofibrillar dropout
myofibroblastic tumor
myofibroblastoma
>   intranodal m.

myofibrohistiocytic proliferation
myofibroma
myofibromatosis
>   infantile m.

myogenesis
myoglobin
myoglobinuria
myoglobulinuria
myointimal hyperplasia
myoma
>   intraligamentous m.
>   uterine m.

myomalacia
myomatous polyp
myomectomy
myometrium
myopathy
>   carcinomatous m.
>   steroid m.

myopia
Myoplex
myosarcoma
Myoscint
myosin
myosis
>   endolymphatic stromal m.

myositis
>   m. ossificans
>   m. ossificans progressiva

myotonic disorder
myotube
myxedema
myxedematosus
>   lichen m.

myxochondrofibrosarcoma
myxofibroma

NOTES

myxofibrosarcoma
myxoglobulosis
myxoid
    m. liposarcoma
    m. malignant fibrous
      histiocytoma
myxoma
    atrial m.
    m. sarcomatosum

myxomatodes
    carcinoma m.
    fibroma m.
myxomatous liposarcoma
myxopapillary ependymoma
myxosarcoma
myxovirus

N$_{aqs}$
>number of planar acquisitions
>per phase-encoding step

N1-alkyl-2-iodo-lyseric acid diethylamide

N-2 fluorenylacetamide

N901 blocked ricin

^{24}Na
>sodium-24

^{23}Na
>sodium-23

NAA
>*N*-acetylaspartate

nabilone

nabothian cyst

N-acetylation polymorphism

N-acetylcysteine

N-acetyl-L-cysteine

N-acetyltransferase

Naclerio
>V-sign of N.

nadir
>n. count

NADPH-dependent oxidase

Naegeli-type of monocytic leukemia

nafidimide

Nageotte cell

NAG vibrio

nail
>n. hyperpigmentation
>intramedullary n.
>Jewett n.
>Rush intramedullary n.
>Smith-Petersen n.
>Zickel n.

nail-patella syndrome

nail-plate device

naked-facet sign

Na-K exchange pump

nalbuphine
>n. hydrochloride

Nalfon

naloxone

naltrexone

nana
>*Hymenolepis n.*

nanogram

nanoparticle

napkin-ring
>n.-r. carcinoma
>n.-r. trachea

Napoleon hat sign

Naprosyn

naproxen

Narcan

naris, pl. nares

narrow chest

narrowing
>arteriolar n.
>colonic n.
>concentric n.
>degenerative n.
>disk space n.
>duodenal n.
>eccentric n.
>esophageal n.
>gastric n.
>glottic n.
>joint space n.
>luminal n.
>motional n.
>nasopharyngeal n.
>oropharyngeal n.
>rectal n.
>retropharyngeal n.
>stomach n.
>subglottic n.
>supraglottic n.
>vallecular n.

nasal
>n. bridge
>n. cavity
>n. cavity cancer
>n. conchae
>n. cycle
>n. meatus
>n. septum
>n. spine
>n. turbinate
>n. vestibule cancer

nasobiliary catheter

nasociliary nerve

nasofrontal duct

nasogastric (NG)
>n. intubation
>n. tube

nasojejunal feeding tube

nasolacrimal duct

nasoorbital fracture
nasopalatal fissure
nasopharyngeal
n. blastomycosis
n. cancer
n. carcinoma
n. hematoma
n. mucus retention cyst
n. narrowing
n. squamous cell carcinoma
nasopharynx
nasotracheal intubation
National
N. Association of Tumor Registrars (NATR)
N. Biomedical Tracer Facility (NBTF)
N. Cancer Institute (NCI)
N. Coalition for Cancer Survivorship (NCCS)
N. Collaborative Diethylstilbestrol Adenosis Project (DESAD)
N. Council on Radiation Protection and Measurements (NCRP)
N. Marrow Donor Program
N. Prostatic Cancer Project criteria
N. Research Council (NRC)
N. Surgical Adjuvant Breast and Bowel Project
N. Surgical Adjuvant Breast Project
native
n. aorta
n. ʟ-asparaginase
n. immunity
n. vessel
NATR
National Association of Tumor Registrars
natural
n. antibody
n. history
n. killer cell
n. killer cell antigen
n. killer lymphocyte
n. selection theory
Naumoff disease
nausea
intractable n.

Navane
Navelbine
navicula
bipartite n.
carpal n.
navicular
n. bone
n. fracture
n. view
navicularis
fossa n.
naviculocapitate fracture
NBTF
National Biomedical Tracer Facility
NCCS
National Coalition for Cancer Survivorship
NCI
National Cancer Institute
NCRP
National Council on Radiation Protection and Measurements
Nd:YAG
neodymium:yttrium-aluminum-garnet
Nd:YAG laser
near
n. drowning
n. field
Nearly Me breast form
nebulizer
DeVilbiss n.
Emerson-Segal Medimizer demand n.
Fisons n.
hand-held n.
Hudson n.
jet n.
Micro-Mist n.
PulmoMate n.
Raindrop n.
Respirguard n.
Schuco n.
Selrodo n.
ultrasonic n.
NebuPent
neck
n. coil
n. fracture
potato tumor of n.
webbed n.

necrobiotic
n. nodule
n. xanthogranuloma
necrobiotic xanthogranuloma
necrogranulomatous
n. keratitis
necrolysis
epidermal n.
toxic epidermal n.
necrolytic
n. erythema migrans
n. migratory erythema
necrosis
acute tubular n.
aseptic n.
avascular n.
coagulative n.
cortical n.
cystic medial n.
dirty n.
fat n.
hepatic n.
ischemic n.
papillary n.
postsurgical fat n.
posttraumatic fat n.
radiation n.
renal cortical n.
renal papillary n.
renal tubular n.
soft-tissue n.
stellate cell n.
subcapsular hepatic n.
traumatic fat n.
tubular n.
vascular n.
necrotic
n. cell death
n. core
n. metastasis
n. pseudocyst
necrotizing
n. angiitis
n. enterocolitis
n. fasciitis
n. myelopathy
n. pancreatitis

n. papillitis
n. stomatitis
n. ulcerative gingivitis
NED-SD
no evidence of disease-stationary
disease
needle
Abrams biopsy n.
abscission n.
Accucore II biopsy n.
Ackermann n.
Adson-Murphy n.
Agnew tattooing n.
Amplatz angiography n.
Amplatz TLA n.
Amsler n.
aspiration n.
atraumatic n.
Baltaxe-Mitty-Pollack n.
Bauer Temno biopsy n.
B-D bone marrow biopsy n.
beveled-tip n.
biopsy n.
n. biopsy
Buerger prostatic n.
butterfly n.
cesium n.
Charles vacuuming n.
Chiba n.
Colapinto n.
communal n.
Conrad-Crosby bone marrow
biopsy n.
Cook endomyocardial n.
Cope biopsy n.
Cournand arteriography n.
Cournand-Grino
angiography n.
Craig n.
Deschamps n.
diamond-tip n.
discission n.
Dos Santos n.
E-Z-EM n.
E-Z-EM cut biopsy n.
Ferris bone marrow
aspiration n.

NOTES

383

needle *(continued)*
flexible biopsy n.
Franklin-Silverman biopsy n.
Franseen n.
French spring-eye n.
full-intensity n.
Greene n.
guaiac n.
Hagedorn n.
half-intensity n.
Hawkins n.
Hawkins-Akins n.
Hawkins breast lesion
  localization n.
Hawkins one-stick n.
Homerlok n.
Homer Mammalok n.
Huber n.
Illinois n.
Indian Club n.
iridium n.
Jamshidi n.
Jamshidi adult n.
Jamshidi-Kormed bone
  marrow biopsy n.
Jamshidi liver biopsy n.
Jamshidi muscle biopsy n.
Klatskin n.
Kobak n.
Kopan n.
Kormed liver biopsy n.
Laredo-Bard n.
Lee n.
Lee & Westcott n.
n. localization
n. localization of breast
  lesion
Longdwel n.
Madayag n.
Maggi biopsy n.
Mammo-lock n.
Manan n.
Menghini n.
Mentor prostatic biopsy n.
metallic n.
Mick afterloading n.
Monopty n.
Multi-Pro biopsy n.
Myelo-Nate n.
nonsheathed n.
OSTYCUT bone biopsy n.
PercuGuide n.
percutaneous n.

Pharmaseal n.
pleural biopsy n.
ProBloc insulated regional
  block n.
n. pyelography
226 Ra n.
Ring drainage catheter n.
Rosenthal aspiration n.
Rotex n.
Rutner biopsy n.
scalp vein n.
Seldinger n.
sheathed n.
skinny n.
small bore n.
small caliber n.
spinal n.
Sprotte n.
subdural n.
Sure-Cut n.
Teflon-coated n.
Terry-Mayo n.
tie-on n.
TLA n.
Tocantins bone marrow
  biopsy n.
n. track
transaxillary n.
translumbar aortography n.
Travenol biopsy n.
trocar n.
Tru-Cut biopsy n.
Tru-Cut liver biopsy n.
Tuohy aortography n.
Turkel n.
Turner n.
Tworek bone marrow-
  aspirating n.
Vacutainer n.
Veenema-Gusberg prostatic
  biopsy n.
Veress n.
Vim-Silverman n.
n. visualization
Westcott n.
Zavala lung biopsy n.
needle-hookwire localization
needle-stick injury
Neel temperature
Neer classification
Neer-Horowitz classification of
  humeral fractures

nef
n. gene
n. protein
negative
E rosette n.
guaiac n.
n. π-meson
n. predictive value
Rh n.
n. selection procedure
tumor receptor protein n.
negatron
Negri body
Neill-Mooser body
Neisser granule
Neisseria
N. gonorrhoeae
N. meningitidis
neisserial
Neisser-Wechsberg leukocidin
Nelaton line
Nelson
N. syndrome
N. tumor
nematode
nemestrina
Macaca n.
neoadjuvant
n. chemotherapy
n. therapy
neoantigen
neocarzinostatin
Neocholex
neocytosis
neodymium:YAG laser therapy
neodymium:yttrium-aluminum-garnet (Nd:YAG)
n.-y.-a.-g. laser (Nd:YAG laser)
neoformans
Cryptococcus n.
neogalactosyl albumin
neoglycoalbumin
neoglycoprotein
neointima formation
Neo-Iopax

neonatal
n. ascites
n. cardiac failure
n. hepatitis
n. intracranial hemorrhage
n. intraventricular hemorrhage
n. lung disease
n. obstructive jaundice
n. pneumonia
n. wet lung disease
neonatorum
hemophilia n.
icterus n.
neoplasia
anal intraepithelial n. (AIN)
B-cell n.
cervical intraepithelial n. (CIN)
endocrine n.
endometrial intraepithelial n. (EIN)
gestational trophoblastic n.
Hürthle cell n.
intraepithelial n.
lobular n.
multiple endocrine n. (MEN)
ovarian intraepithelial n.
vulvar intraepithelial n.
neoplasm, pl. neoplasia
adrenocortical n.
alpha islet cell n.
B-cell n.
bone n.
borderline malignant epithelial n.
borderline malignant epithelial ovarian n.
bronchopulmonary n.
cavitating n.
cervical intraepithelial n.
choroid plexus n.
connective tissue n.
cranial nerve n.
cutaneous n.
cystic n.

NOTES

385

neoplasm *(continued)*
  ductectatic mucinous
    cystic n.
  epithelial n.
  esophageal n.
  external ear n.
  fibrillary astrocytic n.
  germ cell n.
  gestational trophoblastic n.
  hepatic n.
  hernia n.
  histiocytic n.
  histoid n.
  indigenous n.
  intraaxial n.
  intracranial n.
  intraductal mucin-
    hypersecreting n.
  intrahepatic biliary n.
  intramedullary
    compartment n.
  islet cell n.
  isologous n.
  large intestine n.
  laryngeal n.
  lipid cell n.
  macrocystic n.
  mediastinal n.
  mesenchymal n.
  middle ear n.
  neuroendocrine n.
  neuroepithelial n.
  osteocartilaginous
    parasellar n.
  ovarian n.
  ovarian lipid cell n.
  ovarian malignant
    epithelial n.
  papillary cystic n.
  pearly n.
  plasma cell n.
  primary n.
  skeletal n.
  n. staging
  supratentorial n.
  T-cell n.
  thoracic spinal n.
  thymic n.
  transitional cell n.
  trochlear nerve n.
  vaginal intraepithelial n.
    (VAIN)
  vulvar intraepithelial n.

neoplastic
  n. arachnoiditis
  n. calcification
  n. cell
  n. clone
  n. follicle
  n. fracture
  n. meningitis
  n. polyp
  n. proliferating
    angioendotheliomatosis
  n. state
neoplasticum
  Gongylonema n.
neopterin
Neosar
neovascularization
neovasculature
  tumor n.
nepheline pneumoconiosis
nephelometric immunoassay
nephrectomy
nephritis
  acute diffuse bacterial n.
  acute focal bacterial n.
  acute interstitial n.
  bacterial n.
  diffuse bacterial n.
  focal bacterial n.
  glomerular n.
  hereditary n.
  hereditary chronic n.
  Heymann n.
  interstitial n.
  Masugi n.
  nephrocalcinosis n.
  radiation n.
  salt-losing n.
nephroblastoma
  cystic n.
  cystic partially-
    differentiated n.
  polycystic n.
nephroblastomatosis
nephrocalcinosis
  cortical n.
  medullary n.
  n. nephritis
  renal cortical n.
nephrogenic
  n. adenoma
  n. diabetes insipidus

nephrogram
cortical rim n.
obstructive n.
shell n.
striated n.
sunburst n.
Swiss cheese n.
nephrolithiasis
nephrolithotomy
nephroma
congenital mesoblastic n.
cystic n.
mesoblastic n.
multilocular cystic n.
nephromalacia
nephronia
lobar n.
nephronophthisis
juvenile n.
nephronophthisis
nephropathic cystinosis
nephropathy
analgesic n.
obstructive n.
reflux n.
urate n.
uric acid n.
nephrosclerosis
malignant n.
nephroscope
Alken-Marberger n.
flexible n.
percutaneous n.
rigid n.
Wickham-Miller n.
nephroscopic fulguration
nephroscopy
percutaneous n.
nephrosis
nephrostolithotomy
caliceal n.
nephrostomy
n. catheter
circle wire n.
n. dilator
n. drainage

percutaneous n.
n. puncture
nephrotic syndrome
nephrotomograms
nephrotoxicity
cisplatin n.
nephroureteral stent
nephrourology
nerve
abducent n.
accessory n.
acoustic n.
n. block
n. cell tumor
cochlear n.
cranial n.
facial n.
femoral n.
n. fiber myelination
frontal n.
glossopharyngeal n.
hypoglossal n.
intercostal n.
lacrimal n.
laryngeal n.
lingual n.
median n.
nasociliary n.
oculomotor n.
ophthalmic n.
optic n.
peripheral n.
peroneal n.
recurrent laryngeal n.
n. root sheath
n. root sleeve
sacral n.
n. sheath tumor
spinal n.
trigeminal n.
trochlear n.
nervosa
anorexia n.
nervous
n. system
nervus intermedius
nesidioblastoma

NOTES

nest
    cancer n.
    solid cell n.
    von Brunn cell n.'s
nested primer
net transverse magnetization
network theory
Neufeld reaction
Neumann cell
Neupogen
neural
    n. arch
    n. axis vascular
      malformation
    n. canal
    n. cell adhesion molecule
    cervical n. foramen
    n. foramen
    n. foramen remodeling
    n. foramina
    n. tissue
    n. tube
    n. tube defect (NTD)
    n. tumor
neuraminidase
neuraxial opioid infusion
neuraxonal dystrophy
neurenteric cyst
neurilemoma
neurinoma
    acoustic n.
neuritis
    herpetic n.
    optic n.
    VIII nerve n.
    VIII nerve herpetic n.
neuroablation
neuroablative technique
neuroadenolysis
neuroangiography
neuroarthropathy
neuroaugmentation
neuroblastoma
    Evans stages of n.
    hemorrhagic n.
    intracranial n.
    olfactory n.
neurocardiology
neurocutaneous
    n. disorder
    n. melanosis
    n. syndrome
neurocysticercosis

neurocytoma
neurodiagnostic evaluation
neuroectoderm
neuroectodermal
    n. dysplasia
    n. tumor
neuroendocrine
    n. cancer
    n. cells
    n. neoplasm
    n. tumor
neuroepithelial
    n. neoplasm
    n. tumor
neuroepithelioma
    primitive n.
neurofibroma
    aryepiglottic fold n.
    facial n.
    plexiform n.
    storiform n.
neurofibromatosis
    abortive n.
    incomplete n.
    segmental n.
    von Recklinghausen n.
neurofibrosarcoma
neurogastrointestinal peptide
neurogenic
    n. bladder
    n. bladder dysfunction
    n. fracture
    n. tumor
neuroglial
    n. cell
    n. tumor
neuroimaging
    functional n.
    three-dimensional n.
neuroimmunology
neuroleptic agent
Neurolite
neurologic
    n. adverse effect
    n. assessment
    n. deficit
    n. paraneoplastic syndrome
neurologist
neurolytic
    n. block
    n. nerve block
neuroma
    acoustic n.

digital n.
facial n.
interdigital n.
Morton n.
postamputation n.
trigeminal n.
neuromatosa
elephantiasis n.
neuromuscular
n. dysfunction
n. function
n. system electric induction
neuromyopathy
carcinomatous n.
neuron
lower motor n.
upper motor n.
neuronal
n. cell origin tumor
n. migration
n. proliferation
neuron-specific
n.-s. enolase
n.-s. enolase tumor marker
neuropathic
n. arthropathy
n. fracture
n. joint
n. pain
neuropathicum
papilloma n.
neuropathology
neuropathy
acute n.
chemotherapy-induced
peripheral n.
compression n.
cranial n.
paraneoplastic sensory n.
peripheral n.
postherpetic n.
vinca-related n.
neuropore
neuroradiologist
neuroradiology
interventional n.
pediatric n.

neuroreceptor
neurosarcoma
neurosonography
Neurostat Mark II cryoanalgesia system
neurostimulating procedure
neurosurgery
ablative n.
neurosurgical approach
neurosyphilis
neuroticum
papilloma n.
neurotoxicity
neurotransmitter
neurovascular
n. bundle
n. lesion
neurulation
neutral endopeptidase
neutralization
cisplatin n.
NeuTrexin
neutrino
neutron
n. activation analysis
n. capture therapy
fast n.
n. radiation
neutropenia
febrile n.
high-grade n.
immune n.
neutropenia-related bacterial infection
neutropenic fever
neutrophil
n. alkaline phosphatase
n. chemotactic factor
n. count
n. engraftment
n. lobe count
n. migration
n. migration-inhibition factor
polymorphonuclear n.
n. pooling
n. reserve

NOTES

neutrophil-activating peptide
neutrophilia
neutrophilic
>n. cell
>n. eccrine hidradenitis
>n. leukemia

neutropoiesis
nevi (*pl. of* nevus)
nevirapine
nevoid basal cell carcinoma
nevus, pl. nevi
>Becker n.
>benign n.
>blue n.
>dysplastic n.
>ectopic n.
>n. flammeus
>giant melanocytic n.
>mast cell n.
>port wine n.
>Spitz n.
>n. vasculosus
>n. verrucosus
>verrucous n.
>n. of vulva

new
>n. tuberculin

newborn
>focal atelectasis of the n.
>respiratory distress
>syndrome of n. (RDS)
>transient respiratory distress
>of n.
>transient tachypnea of n.
>(TTN)

Newcastle disease
Newman classification of radial
neck and head fractures
Newvicon camera tube
New Zealand black mouse
Nezelof syndrome
***N*-formyl-1-methionyl-1-leucyl-1-**
phenylalamine (FMLP)
NG
>nasogastric
>NG tube

N(H)
>hydrogen density
>N(H) weighted

NHL
>non-Hodgkin lymphoma

nicardiosis
nicardipine

niche
Nichols radioimmunoassay
nick translation
nicotinamide
>n. adenine dinucleotide
>n. adenine dinucleotide
>phosphate

nicotine
>n. dependence

NIDDM
>non-insulin-dependent diabetes
>mellitus

Niemann-Pick disease
Nievergelt syndrome
niger
>*Aspergillus n.*

nightstick fracture
night sweats
nigra
>substantia n.

nigricans
>acanthosis n.

niguldipine
Nikiforoff method
nilutamide
nimustine (ACNU)
nine-mile fever
niobium/titanium superconductor
Niopam
Nipent
Nippe test
nipple
>adenoma of n.
>aortic n.
>n. aspiration cytology
>deep to the n.
>n. discharge
>inverted n.
>n. marker
>out-of-profile n.
>Paget disease of n.
>n. retraction
>n. shadow

nipple-areolar
>n.-a. complex
>n.-a. reconstruction

Nissen
>N. fundoplication
>N. fundoplication procedure

Nitinol
>N. filter
>N. goose-neck snare
>N. hydrophilic-coated wire

N. inferior vena cava filter
N. stent
nitrate
    gallium n.
    vinblastine, ifosfamide,
      gallium n. (VIG)
nitric oxide hemoglobin
nitriloacetic acid
nitrite
    amyl n.
    butyl n.
nitroalkane
nitroblue tetrazolium
nitrofurantoin
nitrogen
    blood urea n. (BUN)
    liquid n.
    n. mustard (HN_2, NM)
nitrogen-14
nitrogen-15
nitrogen-phosphorus detector
nitroglycerin
nitroimidazole
    n. compound
nitrosomethylurea
nitrosurea
    monoligand n.
nitrous oxide
nitroxide-stable free radical
Nizoral
N-1-leucyldoxorubicin (Leu-Dox)
NM
    nitrogen mustard
nm23 gene
N-methylglucamine
N-methylhydrazine
NMR
    nuclear magnetic resonance
    continuous-wave NMR
    CW NMR
    surface-coil NMR
***N-myc-1,2* proto-oncogene**
N-myc copy number
no
    n. evidence of disease-
      stationary disease (NED-
      SD)
    n. frequency wrap
Nocardia
    N. asteroides
nocardia osteomyelitis
nocardiosis
    granulomatous n.
nociceptive
nodal
    n. disease
    n. hypodensity
    n. metastasis
    n. sampling
node
    aortic lymph n.
    atrioventricular n.
    AV n.
    axillary lymph n.
    azygos lymph n.
    Bouchard n.
    cartilaginous n.
    cervical lymph n.
    diaphragmatic lymph n.
    facial lymph n.
    first echelon lymph n.
    Ghon n.
    Heberden n.
    Henson n.
    ilioinguinal lymph n.
    inguinal lymph n.
    internal mammary lymph n.
    intramammary lymph n.
    intraparenchymal lymph n.
    jugular lymph n.
    jugulodigastric n.
    lymph n.
    lymphomatous lymph n.
    mastoid lymph n.
    mediastinal lymph n.
    mesenteric lymph n.
    occipital lymph n.
    paraaortic lymph n.
    parotid lymph n.
    pelvic lymph n.
    periaortic lymph n.
    popliteal n.

NOTES

node *(continued)*
retrocrural n.
retropharyngeal lymph n.
SA n.
Schmorl n.
second echelon lymph n.
sentinel n.
shotty n.
sinoatrial n. (SA)
Sister Mary Joseph n.
spinal accessory lymph n.
subcarinal lymph n.
supraclavicular lymph n.
supratrochlear n.
Virchow n.
node-negative
n.-n. cancer
n.-n. patient
nodosa
periarteritis n.
polyarteritis n.
salpingitis isthmica n.
nodosum
erythema n.
polyarteritis n.
nodular
n. disorder
n. enhancement
n. fasciitis
n. histiocytic lymphoma
n. hyperplasia
n. lesion
n. lymphoid hyperplasia
n. lymphoma
n. melanoma
n. pattern
n. poorly-differentiated
lymphocytic lymphoma
(NPDL)
n. regenerative hyperplasia
n. sclerosing
n. sclerosing Hodgkin
disease
n. sclerosis
n. thyroid disease
nodularity
lung n.
nodule
cavitating lung n.
cerebral n.
cold n.
discordant thyroid n.
echogenic n.

fatty dysplastic regenerative
hepatic n.
Gamna-Gandy n.
hot thyroid n.
Lisch n.
lung n.
mantle zone n.
miliary n.
mural n.
necrobiotic n.
prostatic hyperplastic n.
pulmonary n.
regenerating n.
rheumatoid n.
Rokitansky n.
Scheuermann n.
siderotic n.
solitary pulmonary n.
subcutaneous n.
thyroid n.
nodule-in-nodule lesion
Noguchi test
noise
acoustic n.
image n.
quantum n.
random n.
n. spike artifact
statistical n.
structured n.
systematic n.
thermal n.
total image n.
white n.
Nolvadex
nomenclature
FIGO n.
nominal standard dose (NSD)
nonaccidental trauma
nonalkylating agent
nonaneurysmal perimesencephalic
subarachnoid hemorrhage
nonangiogenic cell
non-A, non-B hepatitis
nonatherosclerotic disease
non-B
n.-B. cell leukemia
nonbacterial
n. endocarditis
n. gastric emphysema
noncalcified
n. nodular mass
n. ocular process

noncardiogenic
    n. pulmonary edema
noncausal association
nonchromaffin paraganglioma
noncleaved
noncommunicating hydrocephalus
noncontiguous fracture
nonconvoluted type
nondisplaced fracture
nondysgerminoma
nonencapsulated sclerosing tumor
nonepithelial tumor
nonferromagnetic MR-compatible
  frame
nongestational choriocarcinoma
nonhematopoietic
    n. element
    n. growth factor
    n. stem cell
non-Hodgkin lymphoma (NHL)
nonhomogeneous
nonideal pulse
nonimmune
    n. hydrops
    n. hydrops fetalis
noninfiltrating lobular carcinoma
non-insulin-dependent diabetes
  mellitus (NIDDM)
noninvasive
    n. aspergillosis
    n. diagnosis
    n. procedure
nonionic
    n. contrast material
nonionizing radiation
nonislet cell carcinoma
nonlactating breast
nonlethal
    n. dwarfism
    n. dysplasia
nonlinear
    n. least squares regression
      analysis
    n. sampling
nonlymphocytic
nonmeningiomatous malignant
  lesion

nonmyelosuppressive
    n. agent
    n. toxicity
nonneoplastic disease
nonnucleated
nonnucleoside reverse transcriptase
  inhibitor
nonobstructive hydrocephalus
nonocclusive mesenteric ischemia
nonopaque
    n. calculus
    n. intraluminal mass
    n. stone
nonopioid analgesic
nonopportunistic infection
nonossifying fibroma
nonosteogenic fibroma
nonoverlapping toxicity concept
nonoxynol-9
nonpalpable abnormality
nonparametric
nonperforative lesion
nonphyseal fracture
nonplanar slice
nonpurged marrow
non-rhabdo soft tissue sarcoma
non-rib-bearing vertebrae
nonrotation
nonrotational burst fracture
nonsaturable drug
nonsclerosing
    n. ileitis
    n. tumor
nonsecreting myeloma
nonsecretory myeloma
nonselective pulse
nonseminomatous
    n. germ cell tumor
    n. tumor
nonsense codon
nonsheathed needle
non-small cell lung cancer
nonspecific
    n. esterase
    n. esterase stain
    n. immunotherapy
    n. mesenchyme

NOTES

nonspecific *(continued)*
    n. reaction
    n. staining
nonsquamous carcinoma
nonsteroidal anti-inflammatory drug
  (NSAID)
nonstress test (NST)
nonstructural gene
nonsuppurative
    n. ascending cholangitis
    n. destructive cholangitis
nonsyncytium-inducing
nonsystemic
non-T cell leukemia
non-T, non-B acute lymphocytic
  leukemia of childhood
nontropical sprue
nonuniform excitation
nonunion
    bony n.
    fracture n.
nonunited fracture
nonvisualization
Noonan syndrome
norethynodrel
norfloxacin
normal
    n. gestation
    n. hematopoietic cell
    morphologically n.
    n. perfusion pressure
      breakthrough
    n. planar MR anatomy
    n. pressure hydrocephalus
    (NPH)
    n. tissue
    n. variant
normalization
    assay n.
normal-pressure hydrocephalus
normoblast
    basophilic n.
    orthochromic n.
    polychromatophilic n.
normochromic
    n. anemia
    n. erythrocyte
normocytic anemia
Normocytin
normocytosis
normotensive
normovolemia
Norport pump

Norpramin
Norrie disease
Norris corpuscle
North
    N. American blastomycosis
    N. American Burkitt
    lymphoma
Northern
    N. blot
    N. blot analysis
    N. blot test
    N. hybridization
Norton-Simon hypothesis
nortriptyline
Norwalk agent
Norwood procedure
nosocomial
    n. anemia
    n. infection
    n. pneumonia
notch
    apical n.
    dicrotic n.
    fibular n.
    intercondylar n.
    Kernohan n.
    n. protein
    semilunar n.
    septal n.
    sigmoid n.
    n. sign
    sternal n.
    trochlear n.
notching
    rib n.
notochord
notochordal process
no-touch technique
Nottingham introducer
Novantrone
novo
    de n.
novobiocin
Novopaque
NovoSeven
nozzle effect
NPDL
    nodular poorly-differentiated
    lymphocytic lymphoma
NPH
    normal pressure hydrocephalus
_N_-phosphonoacetyl-L-aspartic acid
  (PALA)

NR antigen
N-ras
    N-r. oncogene
    N-r. proto-oncogene
NRC
  National Research Council
  Nuclear Regulatory Commission
N-region
NSABP protocol
NSABT protocol B23
NSAID
  nonsteroidal anti-inflammatory
    drug
NSC-102816
NSD
  nominal standard dose
NSE
    NSE lung cancer tumor
     marker
    NSE tumor marker
NSI variant of HIV
NST
  nonstress test
N-**succinamidylproprionate (SPDP)**
Ntaya virus
NTD
  neural tube defect
NTP
  nucleoside triphosphate
Nubain
nubbin sign
nuchae
  ligamentum n.
nuchal
    n. cyst
    n. cyst syndrome
    n. skin thickening
    n. thickening
nuclear
    n. abnormality
    n. angiography
    n. antigen
    n. bubbling artifact
    n. cardiovascular imaging
    n. cell
    n. contour index
    n. convolution

    n. DNA
    n. factor
    n. fragmentation
    n. grade
    n. imaging
    n. magnetic moment
    n. magnetic resonance
     (NMR)
    n. magnetic resonance
     imaging
    n. magnetic resonance
     tomography
    n. magnetism
    n. medicine
    n. membrane abnormality
    n. organizing region
    n. Overhauser effect
    n. polarization
    n. proliferation antigen
    n. protein
    n. signal
    n. spin
    n. spin quantum number
nuclear/cytoplasmic ratio
**Nuclear Regulatory Commission
(NRC)**
nucleated
    n. cell count
    n. red blood cell
nuclei (*pl. of* nucleus)
nucleic
    n. acid
    n. acid hybridization
nucleolar organizing region
nucleon
nucleoside
    n. analog
    n. phosphonate
    n. triphosphate (NTP)
nucleotidase
    5' n.
nucleotide
    tricyclic n.
Nucletron simulator
nucleus, pl. nuclei
    n. ambiguus lesion
    basal n.

NOTES

nucleus *(continued)*
    caudate n.
    dentate n.
    Edinger-Westphal n.
    head of the caudate n.
    lentiform n.
    motor n.
    multilobated n.
    n. pulposus
    n. pulposus herniation
    quadripolar n.
    sensory n.
    sixth n.
nuclide
Nu-Derm foam island dressing
Nu Gauze dressing
null
    n. cell
    n. cell acute lymphocytic
      leukemia
    n. cell adenoma
    n. cell lymphoblastic
      leukemia
    n. cell lymphoma
    n. hypothesis
    n. point
nulling
    gradient moment n. (GMN)
nulliparous patient
    adolescent n. p.
    postmenopausal n. p.
nullizygosity
number
    average gradient n.
    n. of excitations
    imaginary n.
    N-myc copy n.
    nuclear spin quantum n.
    Reynolds n.
    spin n.
    spin quantum n.
number of excitations
number of planar acquisitions per phase-encoding step (N_{aqs})

numerary renal anomaly
nummular pneumonia
Numorphan
nurse cell
nursemaid's elbow
nurse-patient ratio
nutation
nutcracker fracture
Nutren with fiber
nutrient
    n. artery
    n. artery growth
    n. canal
    n. foramen
nutrition
    enteral n.
    glutamine-supplemented total
      parenteral n.
    parenteral n.
    total enteral n. (TEN)
    total parenteral n. (TPN)
nutritional
    n. assessment
    n. disorder
    n. prevention
    n. status
    n. support
    n. therapy
Nutritionals
    Bio-Defense N.
NX
    regional lymph nodes cannot be
    addressed
Nydrazid
Nyegaard
Nyquist
    N. criterion
    N. frequency
    N. limit
    N. sampling theorem
    N. theorem
nystatin
Nystatin-LF I.V.

Oakley-Fulthorpe technique
Oak Ridge National Laboratory
  (ORNL)
O antigen
oat
    o. cell
    o. cell carcinoma
    o. cell lung cancer
OBD
    optimum biologic dose
obesity
    o. in endometrial sarcoma
objective symptoms
object-plane blur
obligate chain terminator
oblique
    o. coronal plane
    o. fissure
    o. flow misregistration
    o. fracture
    left anterior o. (LAO)
    o. magnetic resonance
     imaging
    o. projection
    o. radiograph
    right anterior o. (RAO)
    right posterior o. (RPO)
    o. sagittal sequence
    o. slice
    superior o.
    o. view
obliquity
obliterans
    atherosclerosis o.
    bronchiolitis o.
    endarteritis o.
    thromboangiitis o.
obliteration
    subdeltoid fat plane o.
oblongata
    medulla o.
O'Brien classification of radial
  fractures
obstetric
    o. intervention
    o. sonography
    o. ultrasonography
obstetrics
obstipation

obstruction
    airway o.
    aqueductal o.
    arachnoid villi o.
    biliary tract o.
    biliary tree o.
    bladder outlet o.
    bowel o.
    bronchial o.
    catheter o.
    colonic o.
    congenital duodenal o.
    distal common bile duct o.
    duodenal o.
    duodenal-gastric outlet o.
    extrahepatic o.
    extrahepatic binary o.
    fetal renal o.
    gastric outlet o.
    gastrointestinal o.
    gastrointestinal tract o.
    incomplete o.
    intestinal o.
    intrapancreatic o.
    left ventricular inflow
     tract o.
    left ventricular outflow
     tract o.
    mechanical bowel o.
    partial small bowel o.
    pelvic venous o.
    renal o.
    segmental biliary o.
    small bowel o.
    strangulated o.
    superior vena cava o.
    suprapancreatic o.
    thrombotic o.
    tubal o.
    ureteral o.
    ureteropelvic junction o.
    ureterovesical junction o.
    urinary o.
    venous o.
    ventricular o.
obstructive
    o. calculus
    o. cardiomyopathy
    chronic o. pulmonary
     disease (COPD)

obstructive *(continued)*
> chronic o. uropathy
> o. colorectal cancer
> o. disease
> o. emphysema
> o. hydrocephalus
> o. jaundice
> o. lung disease
> o. nephrogram
> o. nephropathy
> o. pancreatitis
> o. pulmonary disease
> o. uropathy

obtundation
obturator
> o. avulsion fracture
> o. canal
> o. externus
> o. fascia
> o. foramen
> o. internus
> o. line

OC-125
occipital
> o. artery
> o. bone
> o. cephalocele
> o. condyle fracture
> o. condyle invasion
> o. horn
> o. lobe
> o. lymph node
> o. meningocele
> o. sinus

occipitoatlantoaxial anomaly
occipitofrontal fasciculus
occipitomental projection
occipitoparietal region
occiput
occlusal film
occlusion
> angiographic o.
> arterial o.
> balloon o.
> balloon test o.
> carotid o.
> carotid artery o.
> cerebral sinovenous o.
> coronary o.
> diathermic vascular o.
> dural sinus o.
> fresh thrombotic o.
> percutaneous thermal o.

> plastic stent o.
> subclavian vein o.
> o. therapy
> thermal o.
> thrombotic o.
> transcatheter o.
> tubal o.
> ureteral o.
> venous o.
> vertebrobasilar o.

occlusive
> o. cerebrovascular disease
> o. mesenteric infarction
> o. vascular disease

occult
> o. blood
> o. blood in stool
> o. blood testing
> o. cancer
> o. carcinoma
> o. carcinoma of the thyroid
> o. clonal B-cell population
> o. fracture
> o. lesion
> o. papillary carcinoma
> o. primary malignancy (OPM)
> o. primary tumor of testis
> o. residual herniated disk
> o. tumor cell
> o. vascular malformation

occulta
> spina bifida o.

Occupational Safety and Health Administration (OSHA)
OCG
> oral cholecystography

ochronosis
OctreoScan
octreotide
> o. scan

ocular
> o. adnexa
> o. adnexal inflammatory pseudotumor
> o. adnexal lesion
> o. adnexal lymphoid proliferation
> o. adnexal lymphoma
> o. herpes
> o. implant
> o. lesion
> o. manifestation

o. radiation therapy (ORT)
o. rhabdomyosarcoma
o. toxicity
o. toxoplasmosis
oculomotor nerve
oculoplethysmography
OD
optical density
odd-echo dephasing
Oddi
sphincter of O.
odontogenic
calcifying epithelial o.
o. cyst
o. fibroma
o. infection
o. keratocyst
o. pain
o. tumor
odontoid
o. condyle fracture
o. fracture
odontoideum
os o.
odontoid process
odontoma
odynophagia
Office of Health Technology
Assessment (OHTA)
offset
chemical shift spatial o.
quarter-detector o.
o. RF spin echo
ofloxacin
Ogawa model for hematopoiesis
Ogden classification of epiphyseal
fractures
Ogilvie syndrome
O-glycanase enzyme
O-glycosylation
Ohio infuser
4-OHIPA
4-hydroxyifosfamide
Ohngren line
OHS
ovarian hyperstimulation
syndrome

OHTA
Office of Health Technology
Assessment
OI
opportunistic infection
OIH
orthoiodohippurate
iodine-131 OIH
oil
brominized o.
o. cyst
o. emulsion
ethiodized o.
iodized o.
Lorenzo o.
MCT o.
rapeseed o.
o. tumor
oily granuloma
ointment
Chloresium o.
collagenase o.
Elase o.
Panafil o.
Santyl o.
Travase o.
OK-432
okadaic acid
OKB7 monoclonal antibody
OKT3 anti-CD3 monoclonal
antibody
Olbert
O. balloon catheter
O. dilator
olecranon
o. bursa
o. fossa
o. fracture
o. process
oleic acid
oleogranuloma
olfactory
o. bulb
o. groove meningioma
o. neuroblastoma
o. tract
oligemia

NOTES

oligoastrocytoma
    recurrent vermian o.
oligodendrocyte
oligodendroglioma
    bifrontal o.
    subependymal o.
oligodendrogliomas
oligodeoxynucleotide
oligohydramnios
oligomeganephronia
oligomer
oligomerization
oligometastasis
oligonucleotide
    antisense o.
oligoribonucleotide
oligosaccharide
oligospermia
oliguria
olivary degeneration
Oliver-Rosalki method
olivopontocerebellar atrophy
Ollier disease
olycystic ovarian disease
Olympus GF-UM2, GF-UM3
    echoendoscope
omega-sella
Omenn syndrome
omenta (*pl. of omentum*)
omental
    o. bursa
    o. cake
    o. cyst
omentectomy
omentum, pl. omenta
Ommaya reservoir
Omnipaque
Omniscan
omovertebral bone
omphalocele
    infraumbilical o.
omphalomesenteric
    o. cyst
    o. duct
    o. remnant
omphalopagus
Oncaspar
onchocerciasis
ONCOCIN information system
oncocytic hepatocellular tumor
oncocytoma

oncofetal
    o. antigen
    o. protein
oncogene
    gene
    abl o.
    o. activation
    bcl-1 o.
    bcl-2 o.
    bcl-3 o.
    B-lym o.
    can o.
    c-ets o.
    c-fms o.
    c-fos o.
    c-myb o.
    c-myc o.
    dek o.
    E2A o.
    erb B o.
    fms o.
    HER-2/neu o.
    HOX11 o.
    H-ras o.
    lck o.
    L-myc o.
    mdr-1 o.
    myc o.
    myl o.
    N-ras o.
    p53 o.
    PBX1 o.
    RARα o.
    ras o.
    Rb1 o.
    rel o.
    rhombotin-2/Ttg-1 o.
    rhombotin/Ttg-1 o.
    rhombotin/Ttg-2 o.
    R-ras o.
    tal o.
    tal-1 o.
    tan-1 o.
    tcl-1 o.
    tcl-2 o.
    tcl-3 o.
    tcl-4 o.
    viral o.
oncogenic
    o. agent
    o. rickets
Oncoject
oncologic emergency

oncologist
    radiation o.
oncology
    American Society of
      Preventive O. (ASPO)
    American Society for
      Therapeutic Radiology
      and O. (ASTRO)
    International Classification
      of Diseases for O.
      (ICD-O)
    O. Nursing Society (ONS)
    radiation o.
    Society of Gynecologic O.
      (SGO)
    Society of Surgical O.
      (SSO)
    surgical o.
oncolysate
    vaccinia melanoma o.
      (VMO)
Oncolysin B
oncoplastic carcinoma
oncoprotein
OncoRad
    O. for bladder
    O. OV103
    O. PR
OncoScint
    O. CR103
    O. CR372
    O. CR/OV
    O. OV103
    O. PR
    O. scan
oncosis
Oncotech assay
OncoTrac
Oncovin
Oncovirinae
ondansetron
    metoclopramide,
      dexamethasone,
      lorazepam, o. (MDLO)
Ondrox
one-dimensional phase encoding

on-end
    seen o.-e.
one-part fracture
one-session removal
one-sided image reconstruction
one-tail test
onion
    o. skin appearance
    o. skin periosteal reaction
ONS
    Oncology Nursing Society
onycholysis
onychomycosis
onychoosteodysplasia
    familial o.
oocyte
    o. retrieval
    transvesical o. retrieval
oogenesis
oophorectomy
    prophylactic o.
oophoropexy
oophorus
    cumulus o.
oozing
    venous o.
opacification
    collecting system o.
    contrast o.
opacity
OPAL knowledge-entry system
opaque
    o. stone
open
    keep vein o. (KVO)
    o. reduction and internal
      fixation (ORIF)
open-book fracture
open-break fracture
open-ended guidewire
opening
    aortic o.
    caval o.
    esophageal o.
open-mouth view
operation
    Amussat o.

NOTES

operation *(continued)*
    biliary-enteric anastomosis o.
    Duhamel o.
    Emmet o.
    Mustard o.
    pulsed-mode o.
    second-look o.
    Whipple o.
    Williams copulating
      pouch o.
operative cholangiogram
operator
    o. exposure
    o. gene
operculofrontal artery
operculum, pl. **opercula**
operon
    lac o.
OPG
    ophthalmoplethysmography
ophthalmic
    o. artery
    o. division
    o. nerve
    o. vein
ophthalmicus
    herpes zoster o.
ophthalmopathy
ophthalmoplegia
ophthalmoplethysmography (OPG)
opiate receptor
opioid
    o. agonist
    o. analgesic
    o. antagonist
    o. receptor
    rectal o.
OPM
    occult primary malignancy
opponens
    o. digiti minimi
    o. pollicis
opportunistic infection (OI)
opposed-phase
    o.-p. image
    o.-p. imaging
opposite of FISP
Op-Site
    O.-S. dressing
    O.-S. TFD
opsoclonus
opsomyoclonus syndrome
opsonization

opsonizing antibody
optic
    o. canal
    o. chiasm
    o. complex tumor
    o. drusen
    o. foramen
    o. glioma
    o. nerve
    o. nerve glioma
    o. nerve lesion
    o. nerve sheath meningioma
    o. neuritis
    o. pathway myelination
    o. radiation
    o. sheath meningioma
optical
    o. density (OD)
    o. fiber
    o. flare
    o. system
optimization
optimum-angle imaging
optimum biologic dose (OBD)
Optiray
Orabilex
Oragrafin
oral
    o. bile desaturating agent
    o. cancer
    o. candidiasis
    o. cavity
    o. cavity tumor
    o. cephalocele
    o. cholecystogram
    o. cholecystography (OCG)
    o. complication
    o. copulation
    o. cryotherapy
    o. hairy leukemia
    o. hygiene
    o. hyperpigmentation
    o. magnetic particle
    o. manifestation
    o. mucosa
    o. mucositis
    o. thrush
    o. ulcer
Oramorph
    O. SR
orange
    acridine o.
OraQuick test

OraSure test
Ora-Swab
Ora-Testryl
Oravue
orbit
    floor of the o.
orbital
    o. abscess
    o. apex syndrome
    o. canal
    o. cavity
    o. emphysema
    o. exenteration
    o. fissure
    o. floor fracture
    o. fracture
    o. granulocytic sarcoma
    hybridized o.
    o. lesion
    o. metastasis
    o. mucocele
    o. pseudotumor
    o. rhabdomyosarcoma
    o. rim
    o. varix
    o. varix ophthalmic vein
    o. wall
orbitopathy
    thyroid o.
orbitotomy
    Kronlein o.
orchiectomy
    radical o.
orchitis
ordered phase encoding
Oreton
organ
    o. ablation
    erythroid o.
    o. failure
    o. ischemia
    lymphoid o.
    secondary retroperitoneal o.
    target o.
    o. toxicity
    o. transplant
    o. volume

organelle
    cytoplasmic o.
    sphere o.
organic
    o. erectile dysfunction
    o. free radical
organification defect
organism
    Gram-negative o.
    Gram-positive o.
    pleuropneumonia-like o.
Organization
    World Health O. (WHO)
organization
    preferred provider o.
organizing interstitial pneumonia
organoaxial
    o. rotation
    o. volvulus
organogenesis
organoid tumor
organ-restricted lymphoid subset
organ-specific antigen
organs of Zuckerkandl
orgasmic problem
Oriental
    O. cholangiohepatitis
    O. cholangitis
    O. lung fluke
orientation
    angle of o.
ORIF
    open reduction and internal
    fixation
orifice
origin
    anomalous o.
    cell of o.
    cellular o.
    monoclonal o.
    multilineage o.
    o. of the renal artery
Ormond disease
Ornidyl
ornithine decarboxylase
ORNL
    Oak Ridge National Laboratory

NOTES

orofacial carcinoma
orofacial-digital syndrome
oropharyngeal
    o. cancer
    o. dysfunction
    o. emptying
    o. mucositis
    o. narrowing
oropharynx
    boost to the o.
orphan
    enteric cytopathogenic
      bovine o.
    enteric cytopathogenic
      human o.
    enteric cytopathogenic
      monkey o.
ORT
    ocular radiation therapy
Orthicon camera
orthochromatic erythroblast
orthochromic
    o. erythrocyte
    o. normoblast
Orthoclone OKT3 monoclonal
  antibody
orthodeoxia
orthogonal
    o. projection mammography
orthoiodohippurate (OIH)
Ortho-mune antibody
orthopaedic, orthopedic
orthopanogram
orthotopic ureterocele
orthovoltage radiation
Orthozyme-CD5+
Ortolani test
Orudis
os
    o. calcis
    cervical o.
    external o.
    o. fabella
    o. odontoideum
    o. peroneum
    o. styloidium
    o. trigonum
Osbil
oscillating gradient
oscilloscope
Osgood-Schlatter disease

OSHA
    Occupational Safety and Health
    Administration
Osler syndrome
osmium-194
Osmolite
    O. HN
osmotherapy
osmotic fragility test
ossea
    leontiasis o.
osseocartilaginous
    o. arch
osseoligamentous
    o. arch
    o. ring
osseous, osteal
    o. abnormality
    o. dysplasia
    o. metastasis
    o. pinch mechanism
    o. structure
    o. union
ossicle
    accessory o.
    Kerckring o.
    meniscal o.
ossificans
    labyrinthitis o.
    myositis o.
ossification
    o. of cartilaginous structure
    o. centers
    diaphyseal o.
    ectopic o.
    endochondral o.
    heterotopic o.
    intracartilaginous o.
    intramembranous o.
    paravertebral o.
    soft tissue o.
    vertebral arch ligament o.
ossifying
    o. epiphysis
    o. fibroma
Ossirene
ossium
    fibrogenesis imperfecta o.
    fragilitas o.
Ostalloy 202 alloy
osteal (*var. of* osseous)
    o. stenosis

osteitis
o. condensans ilii
condensing o.
o. deformans
o. fibrosa
o. fibrosa cystica
o. pubis
osteoarthritis
early o.
erosive o.
premature o.
osteoarthropathy
hypertrophic o.
hypertrophic pulmonary o.
pulmonary o.
osteoblast
osteoblastic
o. lesion
o. metastasis
o. osteosarcoma
osteoblastoma
osteocarcinoma
osteocartilaginous
o. exostosis
o. parasellar neoplasm
o. tumor
osteochondral
o. fracture
o. lesion
o. loose body
o. slice fracture
osteochondritis
o. dissecans
osteochondrodysplasia
osteochondrodystrophy
osteochondroma
solitary o.
osteochondromatosis
bursal o.
synovial o.
tenosynovial o.
osteochondroplastica
tracheobronchopathia o.
tracheopathia o.
osteochondrosarcoma

osteochondrosis
intervertebral o.
spinal o.
osteoclast-activating factor
osteoclastic
osteoclastoma
o. giant cell tumor
osteocystoma
osteocyte
osteocytoma
osteodermopathia hypertrophicans
osteodiastasis
osteodystrophy
Albright hereditary o.
congenital renal o.
renal o.
osteofibroma
osteofibrous dysplasia
osteogenesis
o. imperfecta
o. imperfecta tarda
osteogenesis imperfecta
osteogenic
o. fibroma
juxtacortical o.
o. sarcoma
telangiectatic o.
osteohypertrophic nevus flammeus
osteoid
o. osteoma
o. seam
o. stroma
osteoclysis
essential o.
massive o.
osteolytic lesion
osteoma
cancellous o.
choroidal o.
fibrous o.
osteoid o.
osteomalacia
famine o.
hypophosphatemic o.
osteomeatal unit
osteomyelitis
bacterial o.

NOTES

osteomyelitis *(continued)*
    BCG o.
    hematogenous o.
    nocardia o.
    recurrent multifocal o.
    sacral o.
osteomyelofibrosis
osteonecrosis
    dysbaric o.
    spontaneous o.
osteoonychodysostosis
osteopathia condensans disseminata
osteopenia
osteopetrosis
    cranial o.
osteophyte
    anterior o.
    bridging o.
    o. formation
    posterior o.
osteophytic spurring
osteopoikilosis
osteoporosis
    o. circumscripta
    posttraumatic o.
    regional migratory o.
osteoradiologist
osteoradiology
osteoradionecrosis
osteosarcoma
    o. antigen-associated
      monoclonal antibody
    chondroblastic o.
    epithelioid o.
    extraosseous o.
    extraskeletal o.
    extremity o.
    fibroblastic o.
    juxtacortical o.
    multicentric o.
    osteoblastic o.
    parosteal o.
    periosteal o.
    small cell o.
    surface o.
osteosarcomatosis
osteosclerosis
    diffuse o.
    subchondral o.
    o. vertebral sarcoidosis
osteosclerotic lesion
osteotomy
ostia (*pl. of* ostium)

ostial lesion
ostiomeatal complex
ostium, pl. ostia
    o. primum
    o. primum atrial septal
      defect
    o. secundum
    o. secundum atrial septal
      defect
ostomy
OSTYCUT bone biopsy needle
Otic
    Cortisporin O.
otic
    o. capsule
    o. ganglion
otitis
    o. externa
    malignant o.
    o. media
otologic implant
otorrhea
otosclerosis
    cochlear o.
    stapedial o.
ototoxicity
Otto pelvis
Ouchterony immunodiffusion
Oudin immunodiffusion
out
    silhouetted o.
outer table of the skull
outlet
    thoracic o.
out-of-phase
    o.-o.-p. image
    o.-o.-p. imaging
out-of-profile nipple
out-of-slice artifact
outpatient biopsy
output
    cardiac o.
    instrument o.
OV103
    OncoRad O.
    OncoScint O.
ovalbumin
ovale
    foramen o.
    patent foramen o. (PFOB)
oval window
ovarian
    o. ablation

o. abscess
o. artery
o. cancer
o. cancer metastasis
o. carcinoid tumor
o. carcinoma
o. choriocarcinoma
o. cycle
o. cyst
o. cystadenocarcinoma
o. cystadenoma
o. cystectomy
o. cystic teratoma
o. dysgenesis
o. dysgerminoma
o. edema
o. edometrioid carcinoma
o. embryonal teratoma
o. failure
o. fibroma
o. follicle
o. fossa
o. function
o. gonadoblastoma
o. granulosa-stromal cell tumor
o. granulosa-theca cell tumor
o. hilar cell tumor
o. hyperstimulation syndrome (OHS)
o. intraepithelial neoplasia
o. lipid cell neoplasm
o. lymphoma
o. malignant epithelial neoplasm
o. mass
o. neoplasm
o. pediatric dysgerminoma
o. proliferative cystadenoma
o. remnant syndrome
o. torsion
o. tubular adenoma
o. tumor
o. vein
o. vein syndrome

ovarii
struma o.
ovary
hilar cell tumor of o.
luteinized thecoma of o.
lymphoma of o.
mucinous adenocarcinoma of o.
mucinous cystadenoma of o.
palpable postmenopausal o.
postmenopausal o.
sclerocystic o.
stromal carcinoid of o.
teratoblastoma of o.
teratocarcinoma of o.
thecoma of o.
transposition of o.
undifferentiated carcinoma of o.
overcirculation
pulmonary o.
o. vascularity
overdevelopment
bone o.
overdistention
overexpressed receptor
overexpression
p53 protein o.
overframing
horizontal o.
overgrowth
epiphyseal o.
overhanging margin
Overhauser
O. effect
O. technique
overhead film
overlapping
overload
fluid o.
iron o.
overlying
o. bowel content
o. bowel gas
o. bowel shadows

NOTES

overriding
    o. aorta
    o. of fracture fragments
oversampling
over-the-guidewire dilator
over-the-needle infusion catheter
ovoid
    afterloading tandem and o.'s
ovulation
    incessant o.
    o. induction
ovulatory failure
ovum
    blighted o.
OVX1 serum marker
owl's eye inclusion body
Owren-Koller buffer
oxaliplatin
oxalosis
    primary o.
oxantrazole
oxazaphosphorine alkylating agent
oxazepam
oxidase
    monoamine o. (MAO)
    NADPH-dependent o.
oxidation
    hemoglobin o.
    o. state
oxide
    crystalline iron o.
    iron o.
    nitrous o.
    superparamagnetic agent
    iron o.
    zinc o.
oxidized
    o. cellulose
    o. hemoglobin
oxidronate
    technetium-99m o.

oxime
    hexamethylpropyleneamine o. (HMPAO)
oximeter
    Critikon o.
oximetry
    pulse o.
ox red blood cell
Oxycel
oxycephaly
oxycodone
oxygen
    o. delivery
    o. demand
    o. enhancement ratio
    o. extraction rate
    o. free radical
    hyperbaric o.
    o. reduction product
    o. therapy
oxygen-15
oxygen-17
oxygenated hemoglobin
oxygenation
    cell o.
    extracorporeal membrane o. (ECMO)
    tissue o.
    tumor o.
oxygenator
    extracorporeal membrane o. (ECMO)
oxygen-free water
oxyhemoglobin
oxymorphone
oxyphilic adenoma
oxytoca
    Klebsiella o.
oxytocin
Oz antigen

P-170
　P-glycoprotein
P24
　　P24 antigen
　　P24 antigen capture assay
　　P24 antigen test
P388
　　murine leukemia P388
P450
　　cytochrome P450
P50
P53
　　P53 oncogene
　　P53 protein
　　P53 protein overexpression
³²P
　phosphorus-32
P170 protein
P185 protein
***p40* T-cell growth factor**
PA
　　posteroanterior
　　PA chest film
　　PA projection
　　Stachrom PA
PAC
　　premature atrial contraction
PAC-1
　　Platinol, Adriamycin,
　　　cyclophosphamide
pacchionian
　　p. bodies
　　p. depression
　　p. granulations
PACE
　　Platinol, Adriamycin,
　　　cyclophosphamide, etopside
Pace assay
pacemaker
　　bipolar p.
　　p. lead
　　p. wire
pachydermoperiostosis
pachygyria
pachymeningitis
Pacific yew
packed
　　p. beads
　　p. erythrocytes
　　p. red blood cells

packing for bleeding
paclitaxel
PACS
　　picture archival communication
　　system
pad
　　branch p.
　　p. effect
　　epicardial fat p.
　　pericardial fat p.
　　Sat p.
　　p. sign
padding
　　antral p.
Page
　　P. grade (2/2, 3/3) for
　　　breast tumor
　　P. kidney
Pageblot system
Paget
　　P. carcinoma
　　P. disease
　　P. disease of nipple
pagetic
pagetoid
　　p. epidermal involvement
　　p. reticulosis
PAI
　　Stachrom PAI
PAI-1
　　Asserachrom PAI-1
PAI-3
　　Stachrom PAI-3
PAIg
　　platelet-associated Ig
pain
　　abdominal p.
　　acute flank p.
　　bone p.
　　p. cocktail
　　deafferentation p.
　　existential p.
　　flank p.
　　intractable p.
　　p. management
　　myofascial p.
　　neuropathic p.
　　odontogenic p.
　　phantom limb p.
　　pleuritic p.

pain *(continued)*
   radicular p.
   referred p.
   spiritual p.
painless thyroiditis
pair
   base p.
   HIV-1 specific primer p.
   line p.'s
   Maxwell p.
   p. production
paired inferior vena cava
Pais fracture
PALA
   N-phosphonoacetyl-L-aspartic
   acid
palatal muscle
palate
   cleft p.
palatine
   p. foramen
   p. suture
palatoglossus
palatopharyngeus
Palestrant/Simon filter
palilalia
palindrome
Pall
   P. ELD-96 Set Saver filter
   P. filter
   P. filter PL100KL/50K
   P. filter RC50KL
   P. leukocyte removal filter
   P. transfusion filter
palliation
palliative
   p. care
   p. chemotherapy
   p. esophagostomy
   p. gastrostomy
   p. intent
   p. surgery
   p. therapy
pallidum
   direct fluorescent antibody
   staining for *Treponema p.*
   (DFA-TP)
   Treponema p.
pallidus
   globus p.
pallor
   myelin p.

palmar
   p. angulation
   p. displacement
   p. fasciitis
   p. fibromatosis
   p. interossei
   p. surface
palmaris
   p. brevis
   p. longus
palmatae
   plicae p.
Palmaz balloon expandable stent
Palmaz-Schatz biliary stent
palmitate
   retinyl p.
palmoplantar
   p. erythrodysesthesia
   syndrome
palpable postmenopausal ovary
palpation
palpatory T stage prostate cancer
palpebra, pl. **palpebrae**
   levator palpebrae
palsy
   Bell p.
   cerebral p.
   Erb p.
   Erb-Duchenne p.
   hypoglossal p.
   hypoglossal nerve p.
   progressive supranuclear p.
   VI cranial nerve p.
   waiter's tip p.
L-PAM
   L-phenylalanine mustard
pamidronate
   p. disodium
p-aminobenzoic acid
pampiniform plexus
pan
   p. B-cell antigen
   p. T-cell antibody
   p. T-cell antigen
panacinar emphysema
Panafil ointment
Panax ginseng
pan-B antibody
panbronchiolitis
   diffuse p.
pancake appearance
Pancoast tumor

pancreas
annular p.
body of the p.
p. divisum
ectopic p.
fatty p.
head of the p.
intraductal papillary
neoplasm of the p. (IPNP)
pancreatic
p. abscess
p. adenocarcinoma
p. allograft
p. ascites
p. biopsy
p. calcification
p. cancer
p. carcinoma
p. cholera
p. cyst
p. cystic fibrosis
p. cystic lymphangioma
p. deivisum
p. disease
p. duct
p. duct dilatation
p. fluid collection
p. head
p. islet cell tumor
p. oncofetal antigen
p. polypeptide
p. pseudocyst
p. pseudocyst drainage
p. transplant
pancreaticoblastoma
pancreaticoduodenal artery
pancreaticoduodenectomy
pancreatitis
acute p.
chronic p.
diffuse p.
edematous p.
focal p.
hemorrhagic p.
hereditary p.
necrotizing p.
obstructive p.

phlegmonous p.
suppurative p.
tropical p.
pancreatography
percutaneous p.
pancreozymin
Pancretec
P. pump
P. 2000 pump
pan-cultured
pancuronium bromide
pan-cytokeratin antibody
pancytopenia
panda appearance
pandemic
Pander island
Pandora pneumonitis
panel
antibody p.
panencephalitis
sclerosing p.
subacute sclerosing p.
Paneth cell
panhematopoietic cell antigen
panhypopituitarism
panic
homosexual p.
panimmunity
Panje voice button
panlobular emphysema
panmyelopathy
panmyelosis
Panner disease
panni (pl. of pannus)
panniculitis
fasciitis p.
lymphomatoid p.
mesenteric p.
systemic nodular p.
panniculus
panning
p. dish
pannus, pl. panni
p. formation
synovial p.
Panomat infusion pump

NOTES

411

panoramic
    p. radiograph
    p. surface projection
Panorex view
pansinusitis
pan-T antigen assay
Panton-Valentine leukocidin
Pantopaque
    P. cisternography
PAP
    peroxidase-antiperoxidase
    prostatic acid phosphatase
    PAP tumor marker
Pap
    Papanicolaou
    Pap smear
Papanicolaou (Pap)
    P. smear
    P. test
Papavasiliou classification of olecranon fractures
papaverine
paper radioimmunosorbent test (PRIST)
papilla, pl. papillae
    circumvallate p.
    p. of columnar epithelium
    columnar epithelium p.
    duodenal p.
    smudged p.
    p. of Vater
    p. of Vater enlargement
papillary
    p. adenocarcinoma
    p. adenoma of large intestine
    p. blush
    p. carcinoma
    p. cystadenoma lymphomatosum
    p. cystic adenoma
    p. cystic neoplasm
    p. epididymal cystadenoma
    p. muscle
    p. muscle rupture
    p. necrosis
    p. projection
    p. serous carcinoma
    p. stenosis
    p. thyroid carcinoma
    p. tumor
papilledema

papillitis
    necrotizing p.
papillocarcinoma
papillogram
papilloma
    p. acuminatum
    basal cell p.
    p. caniculum
    canine oral p.
    choroid plexus p.
    p. diffusum
    ductal p.
    p. durum
    fibroepithelial p.
    hard p.
    Hopmann p.
    p. inguinale
    intracystic p.
    intraductal p.
    inverted p.
    p. molle
    p. neuropathicum
    p. neuroticum
    penile squamous p.
    soft p.
    squamous cell p.
    transitional cell p.
    p. venereum
    villous p.
    zymotic p.
papillomatosis
    intraductal p.
    laryngeal p.
    tracheobronchial p.
Papillomavirus
papillomavirus
    human p. (HPV)
Papillon-Lefevre syndrome
papillotomy
papovavirus
    JC p.
Pappenheim
    lymphoid hemoblast of P.
Pappenheimer body
PAPS
    primary antiphospholipid antibody syndrome
papular
    p. mucinosis
    p. rash
papule
    Gottron p.
    varicella p.

papulonodule
erythematous p.
papulosis
bowenoid p.
lymphomatoid p.
papyracea
lamina p.
PAR
plain abdominal radiography
paraaortic
p. hematoma
p. lymphadenectomy
p. lymph node
p. node sampling
parabiotic syndrome
parabolic velocity profile
paracarcinomatous myelopathy
paracardiac
p. metastasis
p. tumor
paracentesis
paracentral artery
paracervical lymphatic
paracetamol
paracoccidioidal granuloma
paracoccidioidomycosis
paracolic gutter
paracortical hyperplasia
paracrine
p. mechanism
paradigm
Halsted p.
paradoxical
p. cerebral embolism
p. enhancement
p. middle turbinate
p. motion
paradoxicum
carcinoma p.
paradoxus
pulsus p.
paraduodenal
p. fossa
p. hernia
paraesophageal hernia
paraffin
p. block embedding

p. cancer
p. tissue section
p. tumor
paraffinoma
paraformaldehyde
paraganglioma
nonchromaffin p.
Paragon
P. ambulatory pump
P. immunofixation
electrophoresis
P. infuser
paragonimiasis, paragonimosis
parahiatal hernia
paraimmunoblastic variant
parainfluenza
p. virus
p. virus infection
para-iodobenzoyl conjugate
**para-isopropyliminodiacetic acid
(PIPIDA)**
paralaryngeal space
parallax view
parallel
p. channel sign
p. data acquisition coil
p. line equal spacing bar
pattern
p. plate dialyzer
paralysis
antigenic p.
diaphragmatic p.
Erb p.
Erb-Duchenne p.
Erb-Duchenne-Klumpke p.
facial p.
hernia p.
immunologic p.
Klumpke p.
phrenic nerve p.
residual p.
vocal cord p.
paralytic ileus
paramagnetic
p. artifact
p. contrast
p. contrast agent

NOTES

413

paramagnetic *(continued)*
    p. contrast enhancement
    p. enhancement accentuation
    p. enhancement accentuation
      by chemical shift imaging
    p. iron species
    p. microsphere
    p. shift relaxation
paramagnetism
    apparent p.
    collective p.
paramedian
parameningeal rhabdomyosarcoma
parameniscal cyst
paramesonephric duct cyst
parameter
    cell-cycle p.
    extrinsic cellular p.
    growth p.'s
    intrinsic cellular p.
    timing p.'s
parametrectomy
    radical p.
parametric
parametrium, pl. **parametria**
paranasal
    p. sinus
    p. sinus cancer
    p. sinusitis
paraneoplasia
paraneoplastic
    p. acrokeratosis
    p. anemia
    p. anorexia
    p. basophilia
    p. cachexia
    p. dermatomyositis
    p. ectopic ACTH
      production
    p. encephalomyelitis
    p. endocarditis
    p. eosinophilia
    p. erythema
    p. erythrocytosis
    p. granulocytosis
    p. hepatopathy
    p. hypercalcemia
    p. hypercoagulability
    p. hypocalcemia
    p. malabsorption
    p. polymyositis
    p. sensory neuropathy

    p. syndrome
    p. thrombocytosis
paraorbital
    p. lesion
paraosteoarthropathy
paraovarian cyst
paraparesis
    tropical spastic p.
    X-linked spastic p.
parapelvic cyst
parapharyngeal
    p. abscess
    p. space
    p. space cyst
Paraplatin
paraplegia
parapneumonic effusion
paraproteinemia
parapsilosis
    Candida p.
parapsoriasis
    large plaque p.
Paraquat poisoning
pararectal fossa
pararenal space
parasagittal meningioma
parasellar
    p. dermoid tumor
    p. mass
    p. metastasis
parasitic
    p. fibroid
    p. granuloma
    p. infection
    p. infestation
    p. leiomyoma
paraspinal
    p. abscess
    p. calcification
    p. line
    p. muscle
parasternal scanning
parasympathetic fibers
paratesticular
    p. rhabdomyosarcoma
    p. tumor
parathormone
parathymus gland
parathyroid
    p. adenoma
    p. biopsy
    p. carcinoma
    ectopic p.

p. gland
p. gland enlargement
p. hormone (PTH)
p. hormone-related protein
(PTHrP)
p. scintigraphy
p. tumor
p. tumor ablation
p. vein
paratracheal
p. adenopathy
p. tissue stripe
paratrooper's fracture
paratubal serous cyst
paraumbilical vein
paraurethral cyst
paravaginal soft tissue
paravertebral
p. ossification
p. scanning
paravesical fossa
parenchyma
brain p.
breast p.
cerebral p.
glandular p.
hepatic p.
lung p.
renal p.
parenchymal
p. blastoma
p. brain metastasis
p. breast pattern
p. cysticercosis
p. hematoma
p. laceration
parent drug
parenteral
p. chemotherapy
p. nutrition
p. therapy
Parenti-Fraccaro disease
parent-infant traumatic stress
syndrome
parietal
p. bone
p. boss

p. convexity
p. eminence
p. foramen
p. lobe
p. peritoneum
p. pleura
p. pleural scarring
parietooccipital area
Parinaud
P. phenomenon
P. syndrome
Paris
P. method
P. method for radium
therapy
parity bit
Park
transverse lines of P.
Parke corner sign
Parkes-Weber syndrome
Parkinson disease
Parodi-Irgens sarcoma virus
paromomycin
paroöphoron
parosteal
p. osteosarcoma
p. sarcoma
parotid
p. abscess
p. duct
p. gland
p. gland sialography
p. lymph node
p. tumor
parotitis
epidemic p.
parous patient
parovarian cyst
paroxysmal
p. auricular tachycardia
(PAT)
p. nocturnal hemoglobinuria
(PNH)
p. supraventricular
tachycardia
parplatin

NOTES

415

parrot
> p.'s beak labral tear
> p.'s beak tear
> frontal bossing of P.
> P. pseudopalsy

pars, pl. **partes**
> p. defect
> p. infravaginalis gubernaculi
> p. interarticularis
> p. interarticularis fracture
> pedicles and p.

partial
> p. anomalous pulmonary
>   venous return
> p. complex seizure
> p. duplication
> p. Fourier technique
> p. mole
> p. saturation
> p. shunt
> p. small bowel obstruction
> p. thromboplastin time
>   (PTT)
> p. volume effect

partially-implantable catheter
partially-polycystic kidney
partial saturation spin-echo (PSSE)
particle
> p. accelerator
> alpha p.
> p. beam radiation therapy
> Dane p.'s
> heavy charged p.
> IDE p.
> iron-dextran p.
> Ivalon p.
> oral magnetic p.
> submicron magnetic p.
> Zimmerman elementary p.

particulate
> p. air filtration system
> p. embolization
> p. matter

parts per million (ppm)
parturition
Parvovirus
parvovirus
> human p. (HPV)

parvum
> *Corynebacterium p.*
> *Cryptosporidium p.*

PAS
> periodic acid-Schiff
>   PAS stain

Paschen body
P.A.S. Port catheter
passage
> adiabatic fast p. (AFP)

Passavant muscle
passive
> p. atelectasis
> p. congestive failure
> p. diffusion
> p. immunization
> p. shield
> p. shielding
> p. shimming
> p. smoking
> p. transfer of immunity

Passovoy factor
Pasteur Institute bacillus Calmette-Guérin vaccine
PAT
> paroxysmal auricular tachycardia
> percutaneous aspiration
>   thromboembolectomy

patch
> p. angioplasty
> ash leaf p.
> blood p.
> Carrel p.
> fentangle p.
> GORE-TEX p.
> p. graft
> p. lesion
> Peyer p.
> pigskin p.
> salmon p.
> sclerotic calvarial p.
> Shagreen rough skin p.
> transdermal medication p.

patchy
> p. area of density
> p. area of pneumonia
> p. infiltrate

Pate clip
patella
> p. alta
> p. baja
> bipartite p.
> high-lying p.
> squared p.

patellae
> chondromalacia p.

patellar
>p. button
>p. fracture
>p. sleeve fracture
>p. tendon

patellectomy
patellofemoral
>p. disorder
>p. joint

patency
patent
>p. ductus arteriosus (PDA)
>p. foramen ovale (PFOB)

Paterson-Brown-Kelly syndrome
Paterson-Kelly syndrome
pathogen
pathogenesis
pathogenetic mechanism
pathognomonic
pathologic, pathological
>p. cell death
>p. feature
>p. fracture

pathologist
>Cancer Committee of
>College of American P.'s

pathology
>Armed Forces Institute
>of P. (AFIP)
>focal p.
>surgical p.

pathophysiology
pathway
>catabolic p.
>c-fos-dependent p.
>c-fos-independent p.
>Embden-Meyerhof p.
>enzymatic p.
>folate uptake p.

patient
>p. advocate
>Artma Virtual P.
>p. care
>chemotherapy-responsive p.
>cured p.
>p. dose monitor
>febrile p.

>Fontan p.
>gynecologic cancer p.
>high-risk p.
>p. motion
>node-negative p.
>parous p.
>premenopausal p.
>receptor-negative p.
>terminally ill p.
>p. volume

patient-controlled analgesia (PCA)
pattern
>acinar p.
>airspace-filling p.
>airway p.
>alveolar p.
>atypical vessel
> colposcopic p.
>band p.
>beam p.
>beast stromal p.
>bony trabecular p.
>bronchovascular p.
>bull's-eye p.
>butterfly p.
>canalicular
> immunostaining p.
>centrum semiovale p.
>circadian p.
>coiled-spring p.
>corkscrew p.
>cribriform p.
>degenerative nuclear p.
>diffuse p.
>dissemination p.
>divergent spiculated p.
>echodense p.
>echolucent p.
>fibrous nodular p.
>flow p.
>follicular p.
>four-quadrant bar p.
>gas p.
>germinal center p.
>ground-glass p.
>gyriform p.
>haustral p.

NOTES

pattern *(continued)*
    hepatic echo p.
    high-velocity flow p.
    honeycomb p.
    insular p.
    interfollicular p.
    intestinal gas p.
    inverse follicle p.
    ladderlike p.
    Lennert p.
    L&H nodular p.
    mantle zone p.
    marginal zone p.
    migrant p.
    miliary p.
    mixed p.
    Moiré p.
    morphologic p.
    mosaic p.
    mottling p.
    mucosal p.
    nodular p.
    parallel line equal spacing
     bar p.
    parenchymal breast p.
    PLES bar p.
    postembolization
     angiographic p.
    prominent ductal p.
    pseudofollicular growth p.
    pseudomantle zone p.
    pulmonary vascular p.
    p. recognition
    reticulonodular p.
    rosary bead p.
    rugal p.
    sheetlike growth p.
    shish kebab p.
    sinus p.
    slice-of-sausage p.
    snowflake p.
    spectral p.
    spoiler gradient p.'s
    spoke wheel p.
    p. of spread
    starry sky p.
    storiform-pleomorphic p.
    sunburst p.
    Tabar p.
    transducer beam p.
    tubular gas p.
    urticaria p.
patulous

pauciostotic
paucity
Paul-Bunnell-Davidsohn test
Pauling theory of antibody
    formation
Pautrier microabscess
Pauwels fracture
PAVe
    L-phenylalanine mustard,
     vinblastine
Pavlik harness
paxillin protein
Paxipam
P blood group
PBX1
    PBX1 oncogene
    PBX1 proto-oncogene
PC10
    PC10 antigen
    monoclonal antibody PC10
PC-1 antigen
PCA
    patient-controlled analgesia
    PCA antigen
PCA-1 antigen
PCB
    procarbazine
P-cell stimulating factor
PCH-paroxysmal cold
    hemoglobineria
PC image
PCIS
    postcardiac injury syndrome
PCOD
    polycystic ovarian disease
PCP
    phencyclidine
    Pneumocystis carinii pneumonia
PCV protocol
PCZ
    procarbazine
PDA
    patent ductus arteriosus
PDIg
    platelet-directed Ig
PDQ information system
PDTA
    propanoldiaminotetraacetic acid
PE
    Platinol (cisplatin), etoposide
PEACH approach
peak
    p. area

Bragg p.
juxtaphrenic p.
p. kilovoltage (pkV)
kilovoltage p. (kVp)
photon p.
p. shape
spread Bragg p.
temporal p.
p. velocity
peak-and-trough drug measurement
peak-dose level
pearl
p. necklace gallbladder
p. tumor
pearl-and-string sign
pearly
p. neoplasm
p. tumor
peau
p. d'orange
p. d'orange appearance
p. d'orange skin
p. d'orange skin thickening
PEB
Platinol, etoposide, bleomycin
pectineus, pectineal
pectoral girdle
pectoralis
p. minor
p. muscle
pectoris
angina p.
pectus
p. carinatum deformity
p. excavatum deformity
pedes (*pl. of* pes)
pediatric
p. fatty marrow
p. fibroxanthoma
p. hemangioma
p. mass
p. multivitamin infusion
MVI p.
p. neuroradiology
p. radiology
p. solid tumor

pedicle
p. fracture
p.'s and pars
vascular p.
pedicolaminar fracture-dislocation
peduncle
cerebral p.
pedunculated
p. leiomyoma
peel-away
p.-a. banana catheter
p.-a. catheter
p.-a. introducer
p.-a. sheath
PEG
percutaneous endoscopic
gastrostomy
polyethylene glycol
PEG interleukin-2
PEG tube
peg
p. cell
cerebellar p.
PEG-ADA
polyethylene glycol-modified
adenosine deaminase
pegademase bovine
PEG-L-asparaginase
Pegasys workstation
PEG-IL-2
polyethylene glycol-modified
interleukin-2
PEG-interleukin-2, interleukin-2
PEG
PEG-intron A
PEG-L-ASP
polyethylene glycol-conjugated L-
asparaginase
pegnology
PEI
Platinol (cisplatin), etoposide,
ifosfamide
PEIT
percutaneous ethanol injection
therapy
PEIT therapy
Pel-Ebstein fever

NOTES

Pelger-Huet
>P.-H. anomaly
>P.-H. cell

peliosis
>p. hepatis
>p. hepatitis

Pelizaeus-Merzbacher disease
Pelkan spur
Pellegrini-Stieda disease
pellet artifact
pellucidum
>cavum septum p.
>septum p.

pelvic
>p. abscess
>p. arteriogram
>p. artery
>p. aspiration biopsy
>p. biopsy
>p. brim
>p. exenteration
>p. exostosis
>p. fibrolipomatosis
>p. fracture
>p. girdle
>p. infection
>p. inflammatory disease (PID)
>p. inlet
>p. irradiation
>p. kidney
>p. lipomatosis
>p. lymphadenectomy
>p. lymph node
>p. lymph node dissection (PLND)
>p. malignancy
>p. malignancy in pregnancy
>p. mass
>p. outlet
>p. recurrence
>p. rest
>p. ring fracture
>p. sonography
>p. steal
>p. steal test
>p. straddle fracture
>p. vascular trauma
>p. vein thrombosis
>p. venous obstruction
>p. venous stenosis
>p. wall

pelvimetry
>radiographic p.

pelvis
>android p.
>bifid renal p.
>brim of the p.
>champagne glass p.
>extrarenal renal p.
>false p.
>goblet-shaped p.
>p. for IUD localization
>Mickey Mouse ears p.
>Otto p.
>renal p.
>shielding of the abdomen and p.
>wineglass p.

pelvocalyceal system
pemphigoid
Pena Shokeir syndrome
pencil-in-cup deformity
penciling
>p. of the distal clavicle
>p. of terminal tufts

Pendred syndrome
penetrating
>p. aortic ulcer
>p. fracture
>p. TRD

penetration
>bowel wall p.
>rectal p.

penicillamine
penicillin
Penicillium marneffei
penile
>p. artery
>p. fibromatosis
>p. implant
>p. plaque
>p. prosthesis
>p. sonography
>p. squamous papilloma
>p. urethra
>p. urethra diverticulum
>p. vein
>p. vessel

penile-brachial index
penis
>hypoplastic p.

peniscopy
Penrose drain
pentacene

pentagastrin
pentalogy
    p. of Cantrell
    p. of Fallot
Pentam
pentamethylmelamine
pentamidine
    aerosolized p.
    p. isethionate
pentazocine
pentetide
    satumomab p.
pentetreotide
    indium-111 p.
pentobarbital
pentosan polysulfate
pentostatin
pentoxifylline (PTX)
pentretreotide scan
penumbra, pl. penumbrae
pepleomycin
Pepper
    P. syndrome
    P. tumor
pepsinogen C
Peptamen
peptic
    p. esophagitis
    p. ulcer
    p. ulcer disease
peptichemio
peptide
    atrial natriuretic p.
    chemotactic p.
    fusion p.
    gastrin-releasing p.
    insulin-like p.
    neurogastrointestinal p.
    neutrophil-activating p.
    p. T
    vasoactive intestinal p.
    (VIP)
perchlorate
    potassium p.
    p. washout test
Percocet
Percoll

percreta
    placenta p.
Percuflex antegrade stent
PercuGuide needle
percussion
    p. and postural drainage
    (PPD)
percutaneous
    p. alcohol injection
    p. aspiration
    thromboembolectomy
    (PAT)
    p. atherectomy
    p. biliary drainage
    p. biopsy
    p. catheter drainage
    p. cecostomy
    p. cholangiography
    p. cholecystectomy
    p. cholecystostomy
    p. dilatation of biliary duct
    p. drainage
    p. endofluoroscopy
    p. endoscopic gastrostomy
    (PEG)
    p. endoscopic gastrostomy
    tube
    p. endoscopy
    p. enterostomy
    p. ethanol ablation
    p. ethanol ablation of
    tumor
    p. ethanol injection therapy
    (PEIT)
    p. fetal tissue sampling
    p. fine-needle aspiration
    (PFNA)
    p. fine-needle aspiration
    biopsy (PFNAB)
    p. gastroenterostomy
    p. gastrostomy
    p. liver biopsy
    p. localization
    p. low-stress angioplasty
    p. microwave coagulation
    therapy
    p. needle

NOTES

percutaneous *(continued)*
    p. needle biopsy
    p. needle puncture
    p. nephroscope
    p. nephroscopy
    p. nephrostomy
    p. nephrostomy catheter
    p. pancreatography
    p. placement
    p. portocaval anastomosis
    p. thermal occlusion
    p. transcatheter therapy
    p. transhepatic biliary drainage (PTBD)
    p. transhepatic biliary procedure
    p. transhepatic catheter
    p. transhepatic cholangiography
    p. transhepatic drainage
    p. transhepatic sclerosis
    p. transluminal angioplasty (PTA)
    p. transluminal coronary angioplasty (PTCA)
    p. tumor ablation
    p. umbilical blood sampling (PUBS)
    p. venoablation
perfloxacin
perflubron
perfluorochemical
perfluorooctyl bromide
perforated
    p. appendicitis
    p. hollow viscus
    p. ulcer
perforating
    p. colorectal cancer
    p. vein
perforation
    colon p.
    colonic p.
    esophageal p.
    gallbladder p.
    intestinal p.
    ureteral p.
    vascular p.
perforative lesion
perforator
    incompetent p.'s
performance status

perfringens
    Clostridium p.
perfused twin
perfusion
    brain p.
    capillary p.
    continuous hyperthermic peritoneal p. (CHPP)
    p. defect
    first-pass cardiac p.
    hyperthermic antiblastic p.
    hyperthermic limb p.
    hypothermic p.
    p. imaging
    impaired p.
    isolated heat p.
    isolated limb p.
    limb p.
    lung p.
    p. lung scan
    luxury p.
    p. measurement technique
    myocardial p.
    regional vascular p.
    p. therapy
    unilateral lung p.
    ventilation-p. (V/Q)
Pergamid
pergolide
Pergonal
periampullary carcinoma
perianal area
periaortic
    p. lymph node
    p. mediastinal hematoma
periaortitis
periapical
    p. cemental dysplasia
    p. granuloma
periarteriolar lymphoid sheath
periarteritis nodosa
periarticular
    p. fluid collection
    p. fracture
    p. margin
periauricular meningioma
peribronchial
    p. cuffing
pericaliceal cyst
pericallosal
    p. artery
    p. lipoma
    p. vein

pericapsular fat infiltration
pericardial
    p. cyst
    p. defect
    p. disease
    p. effusion
    p. fat pad
    p. fluid
    p. hematoma
    p. knock sound
    p. sac
pericardiectomy
pericardiocentesis
pericardiotomy syndrome
pericarditis
    chemotherapy-induced p.
    constrictive p.
    radiation-induced p.
pericardium
pericarinal injury
pericaval
pericholecystic
    p. abscess
    p. fluid
    p. fluid collection
perichondrium
pericranii
    sinus p.
pericyst
peridontal space
peridiaphragmatic hematoma
peridiploid
peridiverticulitis
periductal
    p. calcification
    p. fibrosis
perigastric fat
perigraft
    p. fluid
    p. hematoma
perihepatic space
perilobular connective tissue
perilunar dislocation
perilunate dislocation
perimedial fibroplasia
perimembranous ventricular septal
  defect

perimenopause
    premature p.
perimesencephalic cistern
perimetry testing
perinatal
    p. anoxia
    p. asphyxia
    p. mortality rate
perinea (pl. of perineum)
perineoplasty
perinephric
    p. abscess
    p. abscess drainage
    p. fluid collection
    p. hematoma
    p. hemorrhage
    p. space hemorrhage
perineum, pl. perinea
perineural
    p. fibrosis
    p. invasion
    p. sacral cyst
    p. tumor spread
period
    embryonic p.
    fetal p.
    G_O p.
    incubation p.
    phase encoding p.
    postbiopsy p.
    straight line recovery p.
    window p.
periodic
    p. acid-Schiff (PAS)
    p. acid-Schiff reaction
    p. acid-Schiff stain
    p. acid staining
periodontal
    p. disease
    p. ligament
perioptic meningioma
periorbital
    p. directional Doppler
    ultrasonography
    p. Doppler
    p. edema

NOTES

periosteal
  p. artery
  p. desmoid
  p. dysplasia
  p. elevation
  p. new bone formation
  p. osteosarcoma
  p. reaction
  p. resorption
  p. sarcoma
periosteum
periostitis
peripancreatic lymphadenopathy
peripelvic
  p. cyst
  p. fat proliferation
  p. lipomatosis
peripheral
  p. arterial disease
  p. balloon angioplasty
  p. blood
  p. blood lymphocyte
  p. blood mononuclear cells
  p. blood progenitor cells
  p. blood stem cell
  p. blood stem cell
    autografting
  p. blood stem cell
    transplant
  p. carcinoma
  p. chondrosarcoma
  p. gating
  p. lymphoid cell
  p. lymphoma
  p. nerve
  p. nerve block
  p. nervous system
  p. neuroectodermal tumor
  p. neurologic adverse effect
  p. neuropathy
  p. ossifying fibroma
  p. pseudoaneurysm
  p. pulmonary artery stenosis
  p. stem cell
  p. stem cell transplant
  p. T-cell lymphoma
  p. vascular disease
  p. vasculature
  p. vessel
periphery
periprosthetic fracture
perirectal
  p. cellulitis

  p. disease
  p. inflammation
perirenal
  p. abscess
  p. hematoma
  p. lymphoma
  p. space
  p. venous collaterals
perisellar vascular lesion
peristalsis
  esophageal p.
  hyperactive p.
  meconium p.
  ureteral p.
  yo-yo p.
peristaltic
  p. activity
  p. wave
peritendinitis
peritendinous calcification
peritetraploid
perithelial cell
perithyroid vein
peritoneal
  p. carcinomatosis
  p. cavity
  p. cavity fluid
  p. cytology
  p. dialysis
  p. dissemination
  p. fluid
  p. inclusion cyst
  p. lavage
  p. lymphoma
  p. macrophage
  p. mesothelioma
  p. metastasis
  p. reflection
  p. space
  p. spill
peritonei
  carcinomatosis p.
  pseudomyxoma p.
peritoneography
**peritoneopericardial diaphragmatic
  hernia**
peritoneoplasty
peritoneoscopy
peritoneovenous shunting
peritoneum
  p. desmoid tumor
  parietal p.
  visceral p.

peritonitis
  meconium p.
  tuberculous p.
peritrochanteric fracture
peritrophoblastic flow
peritubular vascular structure
periungual fibroma
periureteral disease
periureteric venous ring
periurethral gland
perivalvular pseudoaneurysm
perivascular
  p. fibrosis
  p. mass
  p. pseudorosette
  p. space
periventricular
  p. border
  p. calcification
  p. hemorrhagic infarction
  p. hypodensity
  p. leukoencephalopathy
  p. leukomalacia
  p. plaque
  p. white matter
perivillous fibrin deposition
periwinkle alkaloid
Perls stain
Perma-Cath
permanent magnet
permeability
permeation
  lymphatic p.
permeative neuroectodermal tumor
pernicious anemia
peroneal
  p. artery
  p. brevis tendon
  common p. artery
  p. longus tendon
  p. nerve
  p. retinaculum
  p. vein
peroneum
  os p.
peroneus
  p. longus

p. longus muscle avulsion
  p. tertius
Perox-A-Mint
peroxicam
peroxidase
  horseradish p.
  platelet p.
peroxidase-antiperoxidase (PAP)
peroxide
  hydrogen p.
  zinc p.
perphanazine
Per-Q-Cath catheter
Persantine
persistent
  p. common atrioventricular
    canal
  p. cortical lobation
  p. fetal circulation
  p. generalized
    lymphadenopathy
  p. hyperparathyroidism
  p. hyperplastic primary
    vitreous
  p. left inferior vena cava
  p. left superior vena cava
  p. ostium atrioventriculare
    commune
  p. primitive trigeminal
    artery
  p. pulmonary hypertension
  p. truncus arteriosus
personal ionization chamber
personality disorder
pertechnate
  technetium p.
pertechnetate
  p. sodium
  technetium-99m p.
Pertofrane
Pertscan 99m
perturbation
  magnetic field p.
perturbed water motion
pertussis
  Bordetella p.
pes, pl. pedes

NOTES

pes *(continued)*
p. anserinus
p. anserinus bursitis
p. cavus
p. planus
pessary
p. cell
pestis
Yersinia p.
PET
positron emission tomography
PET scan
petechia, pl. **petechiae**
petechial hemorrhage
petroclinoid ligament
petrosal
p. foramen
p. sinus
p. vein
petrositis
apical p.
petrous
p. apex
p. bone
p. pyramid
p. ridge
Peutz-Jeghers syndrome
Peyer patch
Peyronie disease
PF
protection factor
PF4
Asserachrom PF4
PFE
Platinol (cisplatin), 5-FU,
etoposide
Pfeifer
P. dynamic angioplasty
catheter
P. milling catheter
Pfeiffer
P. disease
P. syndrome
Pfiffner and Myers method
Pfister-Schwartz stone basket
PFL
Platinol, 5-fluorouracil,
leucovorin
PFNA
percutaneous fine-needle
aspiration

PFNAB
percutaneous fine-needle
aspiration biopsy
PFOB
patent foramen ovale
PFS
progression-free survival
PGA
polyglandular autoimmune
syndrome
PGE
prostaglandin E
PGF
prostaglandin F
P-glycoprotein (P-170, P-gp)
P-gp
P-glycoprotein
PGSE
pulsed-gradient spin-echo
PGY1 **gene**
PGY3 **gene**
phacoma (*var. of* phakoma)
phacomatosis (*var. of*
phakomatosis)
phage
phagocyte
p. migration
mononuclear p.
polymorphonuclear p.
phagocytic
p. cell
p. defense
phagocytopoiesis
phagocytosis
granulocyte p.
phakoma, phacoma
phakomatosis, phacomatosis
phalangeal
p. diaphyseal fracture
p. fracture
phalanx, pl. **phalanges**
drumstick phalanges
hourglass phalanges
ivory p.
rectangular phalanges
phallectomy
phantom
Alderson
anthropomorphic p.'s
p. dosimetry
Hine-Duley p.
p. limb pain
reference p.

p. study
p. tumor
velocity-evaluation p.
wax p.
pharmacoangiography
pharmacodynamic-pharmacokinetic relationship
pharmacodynamics
pharmacokinetic
pharmacokinetic-pharmacodynamic relationship
pharmacologic
   p. aid
   p. maintenance erection flow
   p. method of purging
pharmacology
   cellular p.
Pharmaseal needle
Pharmorubicin
pharyngeal
   p. abscess
   p. artery
   p. herpes
   p. muscle
   p. plexus
   p. recess
   p. wall cancer
   p. wall carcinoma
pharyngobasilar fascia
pharyngoesophagogram
pharynx
   postcricoid p.
phase
   accelerated p.
   accumulative p.
   p. angle
   arterial p.
   blastic p.
   p. cancellation intensity artifact
   cellular p.
   chronic p.
   p. coherence
   p. contrast
   p. contrast angiography
   p. contrast image

p. contrast imaging
p. cycling
p. difference mapping
p. discontinuity artifact
p. encoding
p. filtering
G-p.
p. gain
p. II autologous vaccination
p. image
p. imaging
p. I, phase II, phase III protocol
M-p.
p. mapping
p. mismapping
S-p.
p. shift
p. shift artifact
spent p.
synthesis p.
washin p.
washout p.
zero p.
phase-angle display redundancy
phased
   p. array
   p. array scanner
   p. array transducer
phase-dependent spectroscopic imaging
phase-encoding
   p.-e. artifact
   p.-e. direction
   p.-e. gradient
   p.-e. period
phase-offset multiplanar (POMP)
   p.-o. m. imaging
phase-ordered
   p.-o. multiplanar (POMP)
   p.-o. multiplanar imaging
phase-preserving reconstruction
phase-sensitive
   p.-s. detector
   p.-s. flow measurement
   p.-s. gradient-echo MR imaging

NOTES

phase-velocity mapping
phasicity
Phemister triad
phencyclidine (PCP)
Phenergan
phenethylamine
phenobutiodyl
phenol
phenomenon, pl. phenomena
   autoimmune p.
   Berry-Dedrick p.
   Bordet-Gengou p.
   Danysz p.
   dawn p.
   Denys-Leclef p.
   Doppler p.
   Dubin-Johnson p.
   embolic p.
   entry p.
   first-set p.
   flare p.
   flip-flop p.
   flow p.
   fogging p.
   gene-silencing p.
   Gengou p.
   Gibbs p.
   Gilbert p.
   Hamburger p.
   Hektoen p.
   hematocrit p.
   Hurst p.
   iceberg p.
   intraluminal flow p.
   Jod-Basedow p.
   Koch p.
   Liacopoulos p.
   Luciani-Wenckebach p.
   Lyon p.
   Matuhasi-Ogata p.
   memory p.
   mother-in-law p.
   Parinaud p.
   prozone p.
   Raynaud p.
   recall p.
   resonance p.
   Simonsen p.
   spin-phase p.
   stalactite p.
   Theobald Smith p.
   truncation p.
   Twort-d'Herelle p.

   vacuum p.
   vacuum disk p.
   Will Rogers p.
   window-period p.
phenothiazine
phenotype
   Bombay p.
   Cellano p.
   debrisoquine metabolic p.
   McLeod p.
   multidrug-resistant p.
   T-cell p.
phenotypic escape
phenoxybenzamine
phentetiothalein
phentolamine
phenylalanine
   p. mustard
phenylephrine
phenylhydrazine anemia
phenylketonuria
phenyloxazolone
phenylzine sulfate
phenytoin
phenytoin-induced pseudolymphoma
   syndrome
pheochromocytoma
pheresis
   lipid p.
Philadelphia
   P. chromosome
   P. chromosome-negative
   P. chromosome-positive
Philippine dengue
phlebitis
phlebography
phlebolith
phlebolith-like calcification
phlebomyomatosis
phlegmon
phlegmonous
   p. gastritis
   p. pancreatitis
phocomelia, phocomely
phonation
phonoangiography
phorbol ester
phosgene
phosphatase
   acid p.
   alkaline p.
   alkaline phosphatase-anti-
    alkaline p.

heat-stable alkaline p.
HSAP p.
leukocyte alkaline p.
neutrophil alkaline p.
placental alkaline p.
prostatic acid p. (PAP)
tartrate-resistant acid p.
phosphate
    chromic p.
    chromium p.
    condensed p.'s
    p. diabetes
    etoposide p.
    fludarabine p.
    linear p.'s
    nicotinamide adenine
      dinucleotide p.
    p. reaction
    sodium p.
    triciribine p.
phosphatidylinositol
phosphocreatine
phosphodiester
phosphoethanolamine
phosphokinase
    creatine p. (CPK)
phospholipase cyl-1 expression
phospholipidosis
phospholipoproteinosis
phosphomonoester (PME)
phosphonate
    nucleoside p.
    tetraazacyclododecanete-
      traacetic tetramethylene p.
      (DOTP)
phosphonoformic acid
phosphor
    photostimulable p.
    photostimulable p. digital
      imaging
    p. plate
phosphoramide mustard
phosphorus
    inorganic p. (Pi)
    p. isotope
    p. trihydrazide complex
phosphorus-32 (^{32}P)

phosphorus-31 spectroscopy
phosphorylase
    purine nucleoside p. (PNP)
phosphorylation
    tyrosine p.
phosphotope oral solution
photo
    p. cell
    p. transformation
photoactivation
photoaffinity
photobleaching
photochemotherapy
    topical p.
photocoagulation
photodensitometry
photodermatitis
photodiode
photodisintegration
photodynamic therapy
photoelectric
    p. absorption
    p. emission
    p. system
photoexcitation
Photofrin
    P. II
photolysis
    flash p.
photometer
    HemoCue p.
photomicrograph
    cystic hyperplasia p.
photon
    annihilation p.'s
    p. peak
photon-deficient bone lesion
photopeak
photopenia
photopenic
photoplethysmography (PPG)
photoprotein
    aequorin p.
photoradiation
photosensitivity dermatitis
photosensitization

NOTES

photostimulable
    p. phosphor
    p. phosphor digital imaging
phototherapy
    HpD p.
phototimer
phototreatment
phrenic
    p. ampulla
    p. artery
    p. nerve injury
    p. nerve paralysis
phrenicocolic ligament
phrenoesophageal
phrygian
    p. cap
    p. cap deformity
phrynoderma
phthisis
    p. bulbi
phycobiliprotein
phycoerythrin
phycomycosis
phyllodes, phylloides
    cystosarcoma p.
    p. tumor
physaliferous cell
physeal
    p. bar
    p. fracture
    p. injury
physical
    p. examination
    p. half-life
    p. handicap
    p. restoration
    p. restraining
physics
    Doppler p.
    radiation p.
physiologic
    p. cell death
    p. monitoring
    p. staging
physis
phytate colloid
phytobezoar
phytohemagglutinin
    p. antigen
Pi
    inorganic phosphorus
pia mater

PICA
    posterior-inferior
    communicating artery
pica artifact
PICC line
picibanil
Pick
    P. disease
    P. tubular adenoma
picket fence appearance
pickettii
    Pseudomonas p.
picometer (pm)
picture
    p. archival communication
    system (PACS)
    p. frame appearance
    p. frame vertebra
PID
    pelvic inflammatory disease
PIE
    pulmonary infiltration with
    eosinophilia
    pulmonary interstitial
    emphysema
    PIE disorder
Piedmont fracture
Pierre Robin syndrome
piezoelectric
    p. effect
    p. generator
    p. transducer
pigeon-breast deformity
pigeon breeder's lung
pigment
    p. change
    p. stone
    p. stone disease
pigmentation
    flagellate p.
    mucocutaneous p.
pigmented
    p. dermatofibrosarcoma
    p. lesion
    p. villonodular synovitis
pigmentosa
    urticaria p.
pigmentosum
    xeroderma p.
pigskin patch
pigtail catheter
pilaris
    pityriasis rubra p.

pilar tumor of scalp
pillar
    faucial p.
pillion fracture
pillow fracture
pilocystic astrocytoma
piloid astrocytoma
pilon
    p. ankle fracture
    p. fracture
pilosity
pim-1 proto-oncogene
pin
    Hagie p.
    Smith-Petersen p.
    track of p.
Pindborg tumor
pindolol
pineal
    p. body
    p. cyst
    p. dysgerminoma
    p. germ cell tumor
    p. gland
    p. gland tumor
    p. parenchymal tumor
    p. region
    p. region tumor
    p. teratocarcinoma
    p. teratoma
    p. tumor
pinealcytoma
pinealoblastoma, pineoblastoma
pinealoma
    ectopic p.
pine cone extract
pineoblastoma
pineoblastoma (*var. of*
  pinealoblastoma)
pineocytoma
ping-pong
    p.-p. ball deformity
    p.-p. fracture
    p.-p. volume
pinhole camera
pink tetralogy
Pinnacle

pinning
    hip p.
Pinocchio cell
pinocytosis
pinocytotic vacuole
P32 intraperitoneal treatment
pion
PIP
    proximal interphalangeal joint
piperacillin
piperazinedione
piperazine estrone sulfate
pipe-smoker's cancer
pipestem ureter
pipetting
PIPIDA
    para-isopropyliminodiacetic acid
    technetium-99m
Pipkin classification of femoral
  fractures
pipobroman
pirarubicin
piriform
    p. recess
    p. sinus
piriformis
piritrexhim
piritrexim
    p. isethionate
piroxantrone (PXT)
pisiform
    p. fracture
pisotriquetral joint
piston-like reflux
pit
    herniation p.
pitch-worker's cancer
Pitressin
Pittsburgh pneumonia agent
pituicytoma
pituitary
    p. adenoma
    p. apoplexy
    p. dwarfism
    p. fossa
    p. gland
    p. macroadenoma

NOTES

pituitary *(continued)*
    p. microadenoma
    p. region
    p. stone
    p. tumor
pityriasis
    p. lichenoides
    p. lichenoides chronica
    p. lichenoides et
      varioliformis acuta
      (PLEVA)
    p. rubra pilaris
Pityrosporum
pixel
PIXY321
Pixykine
pkV
    peak kilovoltage
placement
    percutaneous p.
    transpapillary p.
placenta
    p. abruptio
    p. accreta
    battledore p.
    circummarginate p.
    circumvallate p.
    p. edema
    extrachorial p.
    p. extrachorialis
    p. increta
    low-lying p.
    p. membranacea
    p. percreta
    p. previa
placentae
    abruptio p.
placental
    p. abruption
    p. alkaline phosphatase
    p. cyst
    p. infarct
    p. metastasis
    p. septal cyst
    p. septum
    p. transfer
placentation
placode
plafond
    p. fracture
    tibial p.
plagiocephaly

plain
    p. abdominal radiography
      (PAR)
    p. film
    p. radiograph
    p. radiography
plan
    accrual p.
    comprehensive care p.
    posterior transaxial scan p.
plana
    vertebra p.
planar
    echo p.
    p. imaging
    p. I mesh implant
    p. radionuclide imaging
Planck constant
plane
    axial p.
    coronal p.
    fascial p.
    fat p.
    midcoronal p.
    midfrontal p.
    midsagittal p.
    midthalamic p.
    oblique coronal p.
    sagittal p.
    scan p.
    sensitive p.
    subcostal p.
    thalamic p.
    transaxial p.
    transaxial scan p.
    transtubercular p.
    transverse p.
planimetry
planning
    discharge p.
    Prowess treatment p.
plant
    p. alkaloid
    p. remedy
plantar, plantaris
    p. arch
    p. aspect
    p. compartmental anatomy
    p. fasciitis
    p. fibromatosis
    p. interossei
    p. spur
    p. surface

planum sphenoidale
planus
    pes p.
plaque
    atheromatous p.
    atherosclerotic p.
    carotid artery p.
    Hollenhorst p.'s
    Lichtheim p.
    penile p.
    periventricular p.
    pleural p.
plaque-forming cell
Plasbumin
plasma
    p. cell
    p. cell antigen
    p. cell dyscrasia
    p. cell granuloma
    p. cell immunocytoma
    p. cell interstitial
      pneumonitis
    p. cell labeling index
    p. cell leukemia
    p. cell mastitis
    p. cell myeloma
    p. cell neoplasm
    citrated p.
    p. clot
    cyroprecipitate-depleted p.
    p. depletion
    expanded p.
    p. expander
    p. fraction
    fresh frozen p.
    p. membrane
    p. membrane blebbing
    platelet-free p.
    pooled p.
    p. protein fraction
    p. tetranectin
plasmablast
plasmablastic lymphoma
plasmacytic
    p. hyperplasia

    p. lymphadenopathy
    p. sarcomatosis
plasmacytoid
    p. differentiation
    p. lymphocyte
    p. lymphocytic lymphoma
    p. transformation
    p. variant
plasmacytoma, plasmocytoma
    anaplastic p.
    extramedullary p.
    extramedullary leukemic p.
    p. growth factor
    solitary p.
plasmacytosis
Plasmalyte
Plasmanate
plasmapheresis through a Prosorba
plasmin
plasminogen
    p. activator inhibitor
    Stachrom p.
plasmocytoma (*var. of*
  plasmacytoma)
plaster cast
plastic
    p. block embedding
    p. bowing fracture
    p. section
    p. stent occlusion
plastica
    linitis p.
plate
    blood agar p.
    Casper p.
    chorionic p.
    compression p.
    cribriform p.
    D-Di p.
    epiphyseal growth p.
    Fresnel zone p.
    growth p. complex
    lawn p.
    Mancini p.
    phosphor p.
    pterygoid p.

NOTES

plate *(continued)*
    quadrigeminal p.
    quadrilateral p.
    Sabourad p.
    selenium p.
    septal cartilage p.
    Spli-Prest p.
plateau
    tibial p.
platelet
    adhesive p.
    p. agglutination
    p. aggregation
    p. aggregation alteration
    p. clumping
    p. concentrate
    p. count
    hemolysis, elevated liver
      enzymes, low p.'s
    p. neutralization procedure
      (PNP)
    p. peroxidase
    p. refractoriness
    single-donor p.'s
    p. suspension
      immunofluorescence test
      (PSIFT)
    p. transfusion
platelet-activating factor
platelet-associated Ig (PAIg)
platelet-derived
    p.-d. autoantibody
    p.-d. growth factor
    p.-d. growth factor-AA
    p.-d. growth factor-BB
platelet-directed Ig (PDIg)
platelet factor 4
platelet-free plasma
plateletpheresis
platelet-poor blood
platelet-rich blood
plate-like atelectasis
platform
    positioning p.
platinating agent
Platinol
Platinol, Adriamycin,
  cyclophosphamide (PAC-1)
Platinol, Adriamycin,
  cyclophosphamide, etopside
  (PACE)
Platinol-AQ
Platinol (cisplatin), etoposide (PE)

Platinol (cisplatin), etoposide,
  ifosfamide (PEI)
Platinol (cisplatin), 5-FU,
  etoposide (PFE)
Platinol, etoposide, bleomycin
  (PEB)
Platinol, 5-fluorouracil, leucovorin
  (PFL)
Platinol, vinblastine, bleomycin
  (PVB)
Platinol, vinblastine, bleomycin
  (PVB)
platinum
    cis-dichlorotranshydroxybis-
      isoprophylamine p.
    p. coil
    rhodamine p.
platinum-based regimen
platinum-liposome
platybasia
platypelloid
platyspondyly generalisata
pleiotropic
    p. cytokine
    p. gene
pleomorphic
    p. adenoma
    p. liposarcoma
    p. rhabdomyosarcoma
    p. T-cell lymphoma
    p. type
    p. xanthoastrocytoma
pleonosteosis
    Leri p.
PLES bar p.
plesiotherapy
plethora
plethysmography
    impedance p. (IPG)
pleura, pl. **pleurae**
    parietal p.
    visceral p.
pleural
    p. aspergillosis
    p. biopsy
    p. biopsy needle
    p. calcification
    p. cavity
    p. cyst
    p. disease
    p. effusion
    p. fluid
    p. fluid aspiration

p. fluid collection
p. line
p. mass
p. mesothelioma
p. plaque
p. reaction
p. space
p. stripe
subpulmonic p. space
p. tail sign
pleural-based
pleural-fluid hyaluronic acid
pleurectomy
pleurisy
pleuritic pain
pleuropericardial
p. adhesion
p. cyst
pleuroperitoneal shunting
pleuropneumonia-like organism
pleuropulmonary blastoma
pleuroscopy
PLEVA
pityriasis lichenoides et
varioliformis acuta
plexiform neurofibroma
Plexiglas radiographic ruler
plexogenic pulmonary arteriopathy
plexus
Batson p.
brachial p.
celiac p.
cervical p.
choroid p.
glomus of choroid p.
lumbar p.
Meissner p.
pampiniform p.
prostatic venous p.
sacral p.
tympanic p.
plica, pl. **plicae**
plicae circulares
plicamycin
PL100KL/50K
Pall filter PL100KL/50K

PLL
prolymphocytic leukemia
PLND
pelvic lymph node dissection
ploidy
DNA p.
p. status
tumor p.
plop
tumor p.
plot
Sips p.
Wu-Kabat p.
plug
bone p.
dermoid p.
echogenic p.
finger-in-the-glove mucous p.
finger-like mucous p.
p. flow
interbody bone p.
luminal p.
mucous p.
toothpaste shadows
mucous p.
plumbism
plumbline view
Plumicon camera tube
Plummer disease
Plummer-Vinson syndrome
plunging ranula
**pluripotential immunoproliferative
syndrome**
pluripotent stem cell
Plus
DPS P.
PM
prednimustine
PM-81
PM-81 MAb
PM-81 monoclonal antibody
pm
picometer
PME
phosphomonoester

NOTES

435

pML
posterior mitral valve leaflet
anterior tracking of pML
PMMA
polymethylmethacrylate
PMN-elastase
pneumatic reduction
pneumatization
pneumatized
pneumatocele
postinfectious p.
traumatic p.
pneumatocyst
pneumatosis
p. coli
p. cystoides intestinalis
epidural p.
gastric p.
p. intestinalis
p. sphenoidale
pneumaturia
pneumobilia
pneumocephalus
intracranial p.
pneumococcal
p. pneumonia
p. vaccine
pneumococcitis
Pneumococcus
pneumocolon
pneumoconiosis, pl. pneumoconioses
aluminum p.
barium p.
bauxite p.
carbon p.
coal worker's p.
complicated p.
fiberglass p.
Fuller earth p.
kaolin p.
mica p.
nepheline p.
sericite p.
silicate p.
sillimanite p.
talc p.
tungsten carbide p.
zeolite p.
Pneumocystis
P. carinii
P. carinii pneumonia (PCP)
Pneumocystis-related vasculitis

pneumocystosis
cutaneous p.
pneumohemothorax
pneumohydrothorax
pneumomediastinum
spontaneous p.
traumatic p.
pneumonectomy
p. chest
pneumonia
adenovirus p.
alveolar p.
aspiration p.
atypical measles p.
Bacillus anthracis p.
bilateral lower lobe p.
bronchiolitis obliterans-
organizing p.
caseous p.
cavitating p.
cholesterol p.
chronic eosinophilic p.
community-acquired p.
concomitant p.
cytomegalovirus p.
desquamative interstitial p.
endogenous lipid p.
eosinophilic p.
extensive bilateral p.
golden p.
Gram-negative p.
Haemophilus influenzae p.
herpesvirus p.
interstitial p.
legionella p.
lingular p.
lipoid p.
lobar p.
lobular p.
Löffler p.
lower lobe p.
lymphocytic interstitial p.
lymphoid interstitial p.
Macrodantin p.
measles p.
mycoplasma p.
neonatal p.
nosocomial p.
nummular p.
organizing interstitial p.
patchy area of p.
pneumococcal p.

Pneumocystis carinii p.
(PCP)
postobstructive p.
primary atypical p.
proteus p.
pseudomonas p.
Pseudomonas aeruginosa p.
*Pseudomonas
pseudomallei* p.
recurrent p.
round p.
segmental p.
staphylococcal p.
streptococcal p.
usual interstitial p.
varicella-zoster p.
viral p.
pneumoniae
Diplococcus p.
Klebsiella p.
Mycoplasma p.
Mycoplasma fermentans p.
Streptococcus p.
pneumonitis
bacterial p.
chemical p.
cytomegalovirus
interstitial p.
hypersensitivity p.
idiopathic interstitial p.
infiltrating p.
interstitial p.
lupus p.
lymphocytic interstitial p.
lymphoid interstitial p.
Pandora p.
plasma cell interstitial p.
radiation p.
unusual interstitial p.
usual interstitial p.
pneumopathy
cobalt p.
Pneumopent
pneumopericardium
pneumoperitoneum
pneumophila
Legionella p.

pneumoretroperitoneum
pneumosinus dilatans
pneumothorax, pl. pneumothoraces
catamenial p.
spontaneous p.
tension p.
traumatic p.
PNH
paroxysmal nocturnal
hemoglobinuria
PNH prep alloimmunization
PNP
platelet neutralization procedure
purine nucleoside phosphorylase
POACH
prednisone, Oncovin
(vincristine), ara-C
(cytarabine),
cyclophosphamide,
hydroxydaunomycin
pocket
p. chamber
p. shot
pocketing of barium
podophyllotoxin
POEMS
polyneuropathy, organomegaly,
endocrine abnormalities, M-
protein, skin changes
polyneuropathy, organomegaly,
endocrinopathy, monoclonal
gammopathy, and skin
hyperpigmentation
POEMS syndrome
Pohl test
poikilocytosis
poikiloderma
point
bleeding p.
bounce p.
Cannon p.
choroid p.
colliculocentral p.
copular p.
p. imaging
multiple sensitive p.
p. mutation

NOTES

point *(continued)*
    null p.
    pressure p.
    p. scanning
    sensitive p.
    p. spread function
    sylvian p.
    time p.'s
    0 time p.'s
pointer
    metallic p.
point-resolved spectroscopy
Poiseuille law
poisoning
    arsenic p.
    carbon monoxide p.
    lead p.
    Paraquat p.
    radiation p.
pokeweed mitogen
Poland
    P. classification of
      epiphyseal fractures
    P. syndrome
polar anemia
polar-bound water
polarization
    dynamic nuclear p. (DNP)
    fluorescence p.
    linear p.
    nuclear p.
Polaroid film
pole-to-pole length of kidney
pol gene
policy
    standardized care p.
poliomyelitis
pollen antigen
pollicis
    adductor p.
    extensor p. brevis
    extensor p. longus
    flexor p. brevis
    flexor p. longus
    opponens p.
***pol* protein**
polyacrylamide bead
polyadenopathy
    angiofollicular and
      plasmacytic p.
polyarteritis
    p. nodosa
    p. nodosum

polyarthropathy
polychondritis
    relapsing p.
polychromasia
polychromatic cell
polychromatophilic
    p. erythroblast
    p. normoblast
polychromic erythrocyte
polyclonal
    p. antibody
    p. CD3 antibody
polyclonality
Polycose
    P. liquid
polycystic
    p. kidney disease
    p. nephroblastoma
    p. ovarian disease (PCOD)
    p. renal disease
polycythemia
    p. hypertonica
    p. rubra vera
    spurious p.
    p. vera
polydactyly
polyembryoma
polyester
    sucrose p. (SPE)
polyestradiol
polyethylene
    p. balloon catheter
    p. catheter
    p. double-pigtail stent
    p. glycol (PEG)
    p. glycol-conjugated
      L-asparaginase (PEG-L-ASP)
    p. glycol-modified adenosine
      deaminase (PEG-ADA)
    p. glycol-modified *E. coli*
      ASN-ase
    p. glycol-modified
      interleukin-2 (PEG-IL-2)
    p. sorbitan monooleate
    p. tubing
    p. ureteral stent
polyglandular autoimmune
  syndrome (PGA)
polyglutamylation
polyhydramnios
polylactic acid
poly-L-lysine slide
polylobulated cell

polylysine
polylysine-DOTA
polylysine-Gd-DOTA
polylysine-Gd-DTPA
polymastia
polymerase
    p. chain reaction
    p. chain reaction assay
    DNA p.
    reverse transcriptase p.
    Taq p.
polymer fume fever
polymerizing tissue adhesive
polymethylmethacrylate (PMMA)
polymicrogyria
polymorphic
    p. B-cell hyperplasia
    p. B-cell lymphoma
    p. immunocytoma
    p. reticulosis
polymorphism
    genetic p.
    N-acetylation p.
    restriction fragment
      length p.
polymorphocytic leukemia
polymorphonuclear
    p. neutrophil
    p. phagocyte
polymyalgia rheumatica
polymyositis
    paraneoplastic p.
polyneuropathy
    Déjérine-Sottas
      hypertrophic p.
    distal predominantly
      sensory p.
polyneuropathy, organomegaly,
    endocrine abnormalities, M-
    protein, skin changes (POEMS)
polyneuropathy, organomegaly,
    endocrinopathy, monoclonal
    gammopathy, and skin
    hyperpigmentation (POEMS)
polynucleotide
Polyomavirus
polyostotic fibrous dysplasia

polyp
    adenomatous p.
    adenomatous colonic p.
    antral p.
    antrochoanal p.
    carpet p.
    choanal p.
    cholesterol p.
    colonic p.
    colorectal p.
    endometrial p.
    epithelial p.
    epithelial colonic p.
    fibroepithelial p.
    fibroid p.
    gastric p.
    hamartomatous p.
    hyperplastic p.
    inflammatory p.
    inflammatory colonic p.
    myomatous p.
    neoplastic p.
    regenerative p.
    retention p.
    sessile p.
    vascular fibrous p.
    villous p.
polypectomy
    colonoscopic p.
polypeptide
    pancreatic p.
polyphosphate
polyploidization
polypoid
    p. adenoma
    p. fibroma
    p. lesion
    p. mucosa
polyposis
    adenomatous p. syndrome
    familial adenomatous p.
    (FAP)
    familial multiple p.
    familial p. syndrome
    juvenile p.
    lymphomatous p. (LP)

NOTES

polyposis *(continued)*
    multiple lymphomatous p.
    p. syndrome
polyradiculoneuropathy
polyradiculopathy
polyreactive antibody
polyribosome
polysaccharide
    p. antigen
    p. vaccine
polysplenia syndrome
polystotic
polysucrose
polysulfate
    pentosan p.
polytetrafluoroethylene (PTFE)
    expanded p. (E-PTFE)
    p. graft
    p. shunt
polythelia
polyvinyl
    p. alcohol
    p. alcohol foam
    p. chloride balloon catheter
POMP
    phase-offset multiplanar
    phase-ordered multiplanar
    POMP imaging
Pompe
    P. disease
    P. syndrome
Ponomar transjugular clot-trapper device
pons, pl. pontes
Ponstel
ponticulus posticus
pontine
    p. angle tumor
    p. cistern
    p. glioma
    p. hydatid cyst
    p. isthmus
    p. myelinolysis
    p. syndrome
pontis
    basis p.
    brachium p.
pontomesencephalic vein
pool
    blood p.
    gene p.
    stem cell p.
pooled plasma

pooling
    neutrophil p.
poorly-concentrated isotope
poorly-differentiated
    p.-d. infiltrating duct carcinoma
    p.-d. lymphocytic
popcorn
    p. like calcification
    p. Reed-Sternberg cell
popcornlike appearance
popliteal
    p. artery
    p. artery aneurysm
    p. artery trifurcation
    p. cyst
    p. fossa
    p. ligament
    p. node
    p. space
    p. tendon
    p. vein
popliteus bursa
Poppel sign
population
    occult clonal B-cell p.
    predominating p.
population-based registry
porcelain gallbladder
porcine
    p. gallbladder
    p. xenograft
pore
    Kohn p.
    skin p.
porencephalic cyst
porencephaly
    true p.
porfiromycin
porphyria
    p. cutanea tarda
port
    Celsite implanted p.
    implantable infusion p.
    infusion p.
    subcutaneous implanted injection p.
    p. wine nevus
    p. wine stain
portable
    p. chest film
    p. infusion pump

p. radiography
p. view
Port-A-Cath
P.-A.-C. catheter
portacaval shunt
portagram
ᵀ-p.
porta hepatis
portal
p. flow
p. hypertension
p. infusion
p. space
p. triad
p. vein
p. vein aneurysm
p. vein system
p. vein thrombosis
p. venography
p. venous gas
p. venous system
portion
Fc p.
intrapericardial p.
supraclinoid p.
portio vaginalis
Portland
hemoglobin P.
portography
portohepatic
portohepatic venous shunt
portopulmonary venous anastomosis
portosplenic thrombosis
portosystemic
p. anastomosis
p. collateral
p. collateral circulation
p. collateral vessel
p. gradient
p. shunt
Posada fracture
position
cardiac p.
catheter p.
p. encoding

Feist-Mankin p.
Fick p.
Fowler p.
Fuchs p.
left-side-down p.
prone p.
reclining p.
right-side-down p.
semiupright p.
supine p.
upright p.
positioning platform
positive
p. predictive value
Rh p.
p. selection
TRAP p.
positron
p. emission tomography (PET)
p. scintillation camera
postamputation neuroma
postangioplasty
p. intimal flap
p. restenosis
postaugmentation
postbiopsy
p. change
p. period
p. renal AV fistula
p. skin thickening
postbulbar
p. ulcer
p. ulceration
postcardiac injury syndrome (PCIS)
postcentral gyrus
postcholecystectomy syndrome
postcoital test
postcricoid
p. defect
p. pharyngeal cancer
p. pharynx
postductal aortic coarctation
Postel destructive coxarthropathy

NOTES

postembolization
   p. angiographic pattern
   p. syndrome
posterior
   p. arch fracture
   p. cardinal vein
   p. cerebral artery
   p. cervical space
   p. circulation
   p. communicating artery
   p. communicating artery
    aneurysm
   p. descending artery
   p. drawer sign
   p. element fracture
   p. fossa
   p. fossa circulation
   p. fossa meningioma
   p. fossa tumor
   p. iliac crest
   p. inferior cerebellar artery
   p. junction line
   p. longitudinal ligament
   p. mediastinal mass
   p. mitral valve leaflet
    (pML)
   p. osteophyte
   p. pituitary fossa
   p. pituitary gland ectopia
   p. proctotomy
   p. ring fracture
   p. scalloping
   p. tibial artery
   tibialis p.
   p. tibial tendon
   p. transaxial scan plan
   p. urethral valve
   p. urethrovesical angle
   p. wall fracture
posterior-inferior
   p.-i. cerebellar artery
    aneurysm
   p.-i. communicating artery
    (PICA)
posteroanterior (PA)
   p. projection
posterooblique view
posterosuperior glenoid
  impingement
postevacuation film
postexercise image
postganglionic sympathetic fibers

postherpetic neuropathy
postictal
posticus
   ponticulus p.
postinfectious
   p. encephalomyelitis
   p. pneumatocele
postinflammatory
   p. adenopathy
   p. renal atrophy
   p. scarring
postirradiation
   p. fracture
   p. sarcoma
   p. study
postlumpectomy
   p. skin thickening
postmastectomy lymphedema
postmaturity syndrome
postmenopausal
   p. adnexal cyst
   p. endometrium
   p. estrogen therapy
   p. nulliparous patient
   p. ovary
   p. uterine atrophy
   p. woman
postmenopause
postmicturitional adrenergic attack
postmortem
postmyocardial infarction syndrome
postobstructive
   p. pneumonia
   p. renal atrophy
postoperative
   p. bladder dysfunction
   p. chemotherapy
   p. complication
   p. fracture
   p. imaging
   p. pelvic radiation
   p. sepsis
   p. seroma
postpericardiotomy syndrome
postphlebitic syndrome
postpolio syndrome
postpolycythemia
postpolycythemic myeloid
  metaplasia
postprimary pulmonary tuberculosis
postradiation therapy
postradical neck dissection

postreduction
p. mammoplasty
p. view
postrenal failure
postrubella syndrome
poststenotic dilatation
postsurgical fat necrosis
postterm pregnancy
posttherapy change
postthoracotomy change
postthymic
p. leukemia
p. T-cell leukemia
p. T-cell lymphoma
posttranslation modification
posttransplantation
p. lymphoproliferation
p. lymphoproliferative
disorder
posttraumatic
p. chondrolysis
p. cystic myelopathy
p. fat necrosis
p. hemorrhage
p. hydrocephalus
p. intradiploic
pseudomeningocele
p. osteoporosis
p. spinal cord cyst
p. subcapsular hepatic fluid
collection
postulate
Koch p.
postural reduction
postvaccinial lymphadenitis
postvasectomy change in
epididymis
postvoiding film
postvoid residual
potassium
p. bromide
p. perchlorate
p. space
potassium-39 (^{39}K)
potato tumor of neck
potency

potential
brainstem auditory-
evoked p.'s
leukemogenic p.
modulation p.
proliferating p.
somatosensory-evoked p.
tumoricidal p.
zeta p.
potentially lethal x-ray damage
repair
potentiator
Pott
P. ankle fracture
P. disease
P. fracture
P. puffy tumor
P. shunt
Potter
P. classification
P. dysplasia
P. syndrome
P. type IV kidney
Potter-Bucky diaphragm
pouch
arachnoid retrocerebellar p.
p. of Douglas
gastric p.
Hartmann p.
Indiana p.
Kock p.
Morison p.
Rathke p.
rectouterine p.
rectovaginal p.
rectovesical p.
uterovesical p.
Zenker p.
Pourcelot index
povidone
Powassan virus
powder
Gelfoam p.
p. pseudocalcification
shark p.
tantalum p.

NOTES

443

power
- p. gain
- p. injector
- p. ratio
- resolving p.

PPD
- percussion and postural drainage
- PPD test

PPG
- photoplethysmography

ppm
- parts per million

P30 protein

PR
- PR imaging
- OncoRad PR
- OncoScint PR

Pr
- Pr antigen

PRAD-1 gene expression

praecox
- icterus p.

Praestholm

Prausnitz-Kustner antibody

prazosin

PRE agent

pre-B acute lymphoblastic leukemia

pre-B-cell growth factor

precancerous
- p. change
- p. condition
- p. disease

precentral
- p. artery
- p. gyrus

precentroblast

precession
- p. angle
- fast imaging with steady-state free p. (FISP)
- free p.
- Larmor p.
- steady-state free p.

precessional frequency

prechiasmal optic nerve lesion

precipitin

preclinical study

precocious puberty

precordial lead

precordium

pre-criblé
- état p.-c.

precuneus

precursor
- p. B acute lymphoblastic leukemia
- p. B-cell
- p. B-cell lymphoma
- bone marrow myeloid p. (BMMP)
- p. cell tumor
- erythroid p.
- hematopoietic p.
- p. T-cell

PRED
- prednisone

predental space

predictive
- p. value of negative test
- p. value of positive test
- p. value of test

predisposing condition

prediverticular
- p. change
- p. disease

prednimustine (PM)

prednisolone
- melphalan, p. (MP)

prednisone (PRED)

prednisone, methotrexate-leucovorin, Adriamycin, cyclophosphamide, etoposide (ProMACE)

prednisone, methotrexate-leucovorin, Adriamycin, cyclophosphamide, etoposide, cytarabine, bleomycin, Oncovin, methotrexate (ProMACE-CytaBOM)

prednisone, Oncovin (vincristine), ara-C (cytarabine), cyclophosphamide, hydroxydaunomycin (POACH)

predominance
- monoblast p.

predominating population

preeclampsia

preemphasis

preepiglottic
- p. soft tissue
- p. space

preexposure prophylaxis

preferential
- p. B-cell panhematopoietic antigen
- p. T-cell panhematopoietic antigen

preferred provider organization

prefrontal artery
pregnancy
anembryonic p.
diamniotic p.
dichorionic diamniotic
twin p.
ectopic p.
hypervolemia of p.
interstitial ectopic p.
intrauterine p.
molar p.
monochorionic diamniotic
twin p.
monochorionic
monoamniotic twin p.
pelvic malignancy in p.
postterm p.
prevalence ectopic p.
selective reduction of p.
sextuplet p.
p. test
tubal p.
p. tumor
twin p.
twin ectopic p.
p. wastage
pregnancy-induced hypertension
preintegration complex
**preinvasive disease of cervix,
vagina, and vulva**
preinversion multiecho (PRIME)
Prekallikrein
Stachrom P.
preleukemia
preload
premalignant condition
premammillary artery
Premarin
premasseteric
p. space
p. space abscess
premature
p. atrial contraction (PAC)
p. menopause
p. osteoarthritis
p. perimenopause
p. placental senescence

p. thelarche
p. ventricular contraction
(PVC)
prematurity
retinopathy of p.
premedication
premenopausal patient
prenatal testing
preneoplastic
preoperative chemotherapy
prep
LE p.
preparation
bowel p.
buffy coat p.
crush p.
cytocentrifuge p.
Debrun latex balloon p.
p. error
flow cytometry sample p.
liposomal p.
prepatellar
p. bursa
p. bursitis
preplacental hemorrhage
preplasma cell
preplasmacytic leukemia
prepontine
p. cistern
p. white epidermoidoma
prepped and draped
prepubertal development of breast
prepyloric ulcer
prerenal failure
presacral
p. anomaly
p. cystic lesion
p. mass
p. space
presaturation
fat p.
p. pulse
spatial p.
p. technique
presbyesophagus
presentation
aleukemic p.

NOTES

presentation *(continued)*
    antigen p.
    breech p.
    brow p.
presenting
    monocyte p.
preservation
    breast p.
presinusoidal
pressor unit
pressure
    acoustic p.
    p. amplitude
    blood p.
    p. half-time
    intracardiac p.
    intracranial p.
    jugular venous p.
    p. point
    shock wave p.
pressurized fluid jet
prestenotic dilatation
presurgical chemotherapy
pre-T acute lymphocytic leukemia
preterm
    p. delivery
    p. infant
pretherapy baseline
prethymic
prethymocyte
pretibial dimple
pretreatment
    p. assessment
    p. evaluation
prevalence
    p. ectopic pregnancy
    p. rate
prevention
    American Stop Smoking Intervention Study for Cancer P. (ASSIST)
    hormonal p.
    nutritional p.
prevertebral
    p. soft tissue
    p. width
previa
    placenta p.
    vasa p.
priapism
prilocaine
primaquine

primary
    p. amenorrhea
    p. antiphospholipid antibody syndrome (PAPS)
    p. aspergillosis
    p. atypical pneumonia
    p. biliary cirrhosis
    p. cancer
    p. carcinoma
    p. central nervous system
    p. central nervous system lymphoma
    p. chemotherapy
    p. cholangitis
    p. CNS lymphoma
    p. healing after radiation therapy
    p. hepatocellular carcinoma
    p. hyperparathyroidism
    p. immunodeficiency
    p. implanted tumor
    p. lymphoma
    p. lymphomasonography
    p. mediastinal B-cell lymphoma
    p. megaureter
    p. neoplasm
    p. oxalosis
    p. pulmonary tuberculosis
    p. radiation
    p. refractory Burkitt lymphoma
    p. sclerosing
    p. sclerosing cholangitis
    p. systemic amyloidosis
    unknown p.
    p. yolk sac
primate model
PRIME
    preinversion multiecho PRIME pulse sequence
primed lymphocyte typing
primer
    nested p.
priming effect
primitive
    p. acoustic (otic) artery
    p. gut
    p. hypoglossal artery
    p. neuroectodermal tumor
    p. neuroepithelial tumor
    p. neuroepithelioma
    p. stem cell

p. streak
p. yolk sac
primordial
p. cyst
p. germ cell
primum
ostium p.
septum p.
principle
antianemia p.
Bernoulli p.
Fick p.
Fuchs p.
Haber toxicologic p.
Huygens p.
isotope dilution p.
line focus p.
submicron magnetic p.
tracer p.
transforming p.
print-through
Prinzmetal angina
Priodax
prion
Priscoline
PRIST
paper radioimmunosorbent test
private antigen
probability
conditional p.
probe
bcr/abl DNA p.
biotinylated HPV DNA p.
genetic p.
hot-tip p.
hybrid p.
hybridization p.
localizing p.
relaxation p.
sapphire tip p.
shift p.
special p.
TEE p.
UBCR p.
probenecid
Probit analysis

problem
colostomy-related p.
orgasmic p.
sexual p.
ProBloc insulated regional block needle
proboscis
Probst
bundles of P.
procainamide
procarbazine (PCB, PCZ)
p. hydrochloride
p. methylhydrazine
procarcinogen
procedure
Bankart p.
Blalock-Hanlon p.
Boari flap p.
Bricker p.
bypass p.
catheter-directed
interventional p.
Chamberlain p.
Cleveland p.
Darrach p.
endoscopic p.
Fontan p.
gastric bypass p.
gastric pull-through p.
Giemsa trypsin banding p.
Gill p.
Hancock p.
Hedley p.
heparinization p.
ileoanal pull-through p.
interventional p.
intestinal bypass p.
Jantene p.
Kasai p.
Le Fort p.
limb-lengthening p.
Linton p.
loop electrosurgical
excision p. (LEEP)
Meigs-Okabayashi p.
Mustard p.
negative selection p.

NOTES

procedure *(continued)*
    neurostimulating p.
    Nissen fundoplication p.
    noninvasive p.
    Norwood p.
    percutaneous transhepatic
      biliary p.
    platelet neutralization p.
      (PNP)
    psoas-hitch p.
    Rashkind p.
    Rastelli p.
    revascularization p.
    Roux-en-Y p.
    Senning p.
    Soave p.
    spatial localization p.
    Swenson pull-through p.
    two-step p.
    Waldhausen p.
    Waterhouse transpubic p.
    Whipple p.
    York-Mason p.
process
    acromion p.
    alveolar p.
    articular p.
    clinoid p.
    convolution p.
    coracoid p.
    coronoid p.
    cystic p.
    ensiform p.
    freezing p.
    granulomatous p.
    infectious p.
    Markov p.
    noncalcified ocular p.
    notochordal p.
    olecranon p.
    pterygoid p.
    radial styloid p.
    space-occupying p.
    spinous p.
    styloid p.
    temporal p.
    transverse p.
    uncinate p.
    xiphoid p.
processing
    maximum entropy p.

processor
    array p.
    fast array p.
processus vaginalis
prochlorperazine
procoagulant
procollagen
Procrit
proctitis
    herpetic p.
Proctofoam-HC
proctoperineoplasty
proctoscopic examination
proctoscopy
proctosigmoidoscopy
proctotomy
    posterior p.
Procysteine
procysteine
Pro-Depo
prodrug level
product
    c-erbB-2 gene p.
    envelope gene p.
    fibrin degradation p.
      (FbDP)
    fibrinogen split p.'s
    fibrin split p.'s
    gene p. (gp)
    iodine-labeled p.
    oxygen reduction p.
    pyrolysis p.
    respiratory burst p.
    stem cell p.
    α-1 thymosin p.
    tumor-cell p.
production
    ectopic parathormone p.
    pair p.
    paraneoplastic ectopic
      ACTH p.
proerythroblast
profile
    biophysical p.
    coagulation p.
    flow p.
    P. of Mood States
    projection p.
    vector p.
    velocity p.
profilogram
profluens
    hydrops tubae p.

profunda
 colitis cystica p.
 p. femoris artery
profundus
 flexor digitorum p.
profusion
progenitalis
 herpes p.
progenitor
 p. cell
 p. cell antigen
 erythroid p.
 hematopoietic p.
 leukemic blast p.
 marrow p.
 megakaryocyte p.
 monocyte-macrophage p.
 myeloid p.
Progens
progeny
 radon p.
progeria
 adult p.
Progestasert
progestational agent
progesterone
 p. receptor
progestin
 p. receptor
prognostic
 p. factor
 p. indicator
prognosticator
Prograf
program
 Cancer Surveillance P.
  (CSP)
 conditioning p.
 National Marrow Donor P.
 Sedlachek p.
 Solid Tumor Autologous
  Marrow Transplant P.
  (STAMP)
 stripping p.
programmed cell death
programmer
 pulse p.

progression
 terminal p.
 tumor p.
progression-free
 p.-f. interval
 p.-f. survival (PFS)
progressiva
 chronica et p.
 encephalopathia
  subcorticalis p.
 fibrodysplasia ossificans p.
 myositis ossificans p.
 rhinitis gangrenosa p.
progressive
 p. diaphyseal dysplasia
 p. disease
 p. massive fibrosis
 p. multifocal
  leukoencephalopathy
 p. primary tuberculosis
 p. saturation
 p. spin saturation
 p. supranuclear palsy
 p. systemic sclerosis
progressively transformed germinal center
ProHance
Project
 National Collaborative
  Diethylstilbestrol
  Adenosis P. (DESAD)
 National Surgical Adjuvant
  Breast P.
 National Surgical Adjuvant
  Breast and Bowel P.
projectile vomiting
projection
 anteroposterior p.
 AP p.
 apical lordotic p.
 back p.
 bony p.
 cross-table lateral p.
 Didiee p.
 divergent ray p.
 fan beam p.
 p. fiber damage

NOTES

projection *(continued)*
    filtered back p.
    frog-leg lateral p.
    Granger p.
    half-axial p.
    Hermodsson tangential p.
    lateral p.
    maximum-intensity p.
    Mercator p.
    oblique p.
    occipitomental p.
    PA p.
    panoramic surface p.
    papillary p.
    posteroanterior p.
    p. profile
    Rhese p.
    submental vertex p.
    submentovertical p.
    surface p.
    p. tract imaging
    Waters p.
projection-reconstruction
    p.-r. imaging
    p.-r. technique
projector
    cine p.
Prokine
prolactin
    p. elevation
prolactinoma
prolactin-producing adenoma
prolapse
    gastroduodenal mucosal p.
    gastrojejunal mucosal p.
    mitral valve p.
prolapsed
    p. antral mucosa
    p. gastric mucosa
Prolastin
Prolene mesh
Proleukin
proliferating
    p. cell nuclear antigen
    p. potential
proliferation
    p. antigen
    p. area
    benign p.
    B-lymphocyte p.
    cell p.
    extranodal p.
    histiocytic p.

    lymphocyte p.
    lymphoid p.
    p. marker
    myofibrohistiocytic p.
    neuronal p.
    ocular adnexal lymphoid p.
    peripelvic fat p.
    small lymphoid cell p.
    stem cell p.
    systemic polyclonal
      immunoblastic p.
proliferation-associated antigen
proliferative
    p. disorder
    p. stage
prolifigen TPA IRMA
prolymphoblastic
prolymphocyte
prolymphocytic
    p. leukemia (PLL)
    p. transformation
prolymphocytoid
    p. transformation
    p. variant
ProMACE
    prednisone, methotrexate-
    leucovorin, Adriamycin,
    cyclophosphamide, etoposide
ProMACE-CytaBOM
    prednisone, methotrexate-
    leucovorin, Adriamycin,
    cyclophosphamide, etoposide,
    cytarabine, bleomycin,
    Oncovin, methotrexate
Promega Cell Titer 96 cell
    proliferation assay
promegakaryocyte
promethazine
prominent
    p. ductal pattern
    p. ductal vascular structure
    p. pyramidal lobe
promiscuity
    lineage p.
ProMod
promonocyte
promoter
    p. element
    gene p.
    p. trap
promyelocyte
promyelocytic leukemia
pronation

pronation-abduction fracture
pronation-eversion fracture
pronator
  p. fat pad sign
  p. quadratus
  p. teres
pronephron
  rudimentary p.
pronephros, pl. **pronephroi**
prone position
proneural gene
pronormoblast
Propac
propagation speed artifact
propanoldiaminotetraacetic acid (PDTA)
properidine
properitoneal
  p. fat
  p. fat line
prophylactic
  p. antibiotic
  p. antibody
  p. chemotherapy
  p. immunization
  p. irradiation
  p. oophorectomy
  p. therapy
prophylaxis
  antibiotic p.
  hemorrhagic cystitis p.
  preexposure p.
propidium iodide
propionate
  dromostanolone p.
  testosterone p.
propionibacterium acne
propirimine
propofol
proportion
  aneurysmal p.'s
proportional ratio
propoxyphene
propranolol
propria
  lamina p.
  muscularis p.

proprioception nerve fiber
proptosis
propyliodone
propyl ketene
Proscar
prosencephalon
Prosorba
  P. column
  P. column platelet
    replenisher
  plasmapheresis through a P.
prostacyclin
prostaglandin
  p. E (PGE)
  p. E₁
  p. endoperoxide metabolism
  p. F (PGF)
  p. inhibitor
  p. synthesis
prostanoic acid
prostate
  p. cancer
  p. capsule
  p. gland
  transurethral incision of
    the p. (TUIP)
prostatectomy
  radical retropubic p.
prostate-specific antigen (PSA)
prostatic
  p. acid phosphatase (PAP)
  p. adenoma
  p. cancer
  p. carcinoma
  p. cyst
  p. hyperplastic nodule
  p. hyperthermia
  p. portion of the urethra
  p. stent
  p. transition zone
  p. urethra
  p. urethroplasty
  p. venous plexus
prostatism
prostatitis
  granulomatous p.
prostatodynia

NOTES

prosthesis
    aortic bifurcation p.
    Austin Moore hip p.
    ball-and-socket p.
    hip p.
    penile p.
    self-expanding
      endovascular p.
prosthetic
    p. device
    p. implant
    p. replacement
    p. valve
Prostigmin
protamine
proteamaculans
    Serratia p.
protease
    CD26 p.
    p. inhibitor
protection
    p. factor (PF)
    radiation p.
    regions of p.
    S1 nuclease p.
protective environment
protector
    long-acting thyroid
      stimulator p.
protein
    actin p.
    alpha-actinin p.
    B-cell epitope p.
    bcl-2 p.
    Bence Jones p.
    p. binding
    p. C
    caldesmon p.
    p. C anticoagulant system
    catenin-a p.
    CD4 p.
    c-erbB-2 oncogene, p.
    clathrin p.
    c-myc p.
    C-reactive p.
    cross-reactive p. (CRP)
    cyclin D p.
    delta p.
    drug resistance p.
    dynein p.
    p. electrophoresis
    Epstein-Barr early region p.
      (EBER protein)

erb A p.
p. factor
focal adhesion kinase p.
foculin p.
G p.
gag p.
glial acidic p.
glial fibrillary acidic p.
Golgi-specific p.
GTP-binding p.
heat shock p.
Hektoen, Kretschmer, and
  Welker p.
HIV envelope p.
ICPO p.
immunosuppressive acidic p.
  (IAP)
insertin p.
insulin-like growth factor-
  binding p. (IGFBP)
p. kinase
kinesin p.
matrix p.
p. matrix
Max p.
metalloproteinase-like,
  disintegrin-like, cysteine-
  rich p.
milk fat globule p.
morphogenetic p.
p. motif
murine p.
myb p.
myc p.
myelin base p.
myeloma p.
myoD p.
nef p.
notch p.
nuclear p.
oncofetal p.
P170 p.
P185 p.
P30 p.
p53 p.
parathyroid hormone-
  related p. (PTHrP)
paxillin p.
pol p.
pS2 p.
radixin p.
recombinant fusion p.
rev p.

Rex p.
p. S
S100 p.
shuttle p.
synapsin Ia p.
talin p.
Tat p.
tat p.
Tax p.
tensin p.
tenuin p.
trimeric p.
tublin p.
vif p.
vinculin p.
viral envelope p.
vpr p.
ZEBRA p.
zyxin p.
protein-1
latent membrane p. (LMP-1)
proteinase
aspartic p.
cysteine p.
serine p.
protein-binding abnormality
protein-losing enteropathy
proteinosis
alveolar p.
pulmonary alveolar p.
proteinuria
Bence Jones p.
Tamm-Horsfall p.
Protenate
proteoglycan binding
proteoglycans
proteolytic enzyme
proteus
p. pneumonia
p. syndrome
prothombinemia
prothrombin time (PT)
prothymocyte
protocol
ABOV p.
BR96-DOX p.

BUDR p.
CHAD p.
intergroup p.
modified Bagshawe p. (MBP)
NSABP p.
PCV p.
phase I, phase II, phase III p.
Spigos p.
T-2 p.
Thaw p.
Vokes chemotherapy p.
protocol-specified dose
protogram
transhepatic p.
proton
p. chemical shift imaging
p. density
p. density image
p. density-weighted image
lactate p.
p. magnetic resonance
p. magnetic resonance signal
p. nuclear magnetic resonance spectroscopy
p. nuclear magnetic resonance spectrum
p. relaxation
p. relaxation enhancement
p. spectroscopy
p. spin-lattice relaxation time
proton-electron dipole-dipole interaction
proton-proton magnetization exchange
proto-oncogene
abl p.-o.
bcl-2 p.-o.
c-abl p.-o.
can p.-o.
c-cis p.-o.
c-fms p.-o.
c-myb p.-o.
dek p.-o.
E2A p.-o.

NOTES

proto-oncogene *(continued)*
    erb A p.-o.
    erb B p.-o.
    ets-1 p.-o.
    ets-2 p.-o.
    fes p.-o.
    fgr p.-o.
    fos p.-o.
    G p.-o.
    gip2 p.-o.
    gsp p.-o.
    hck p.-o.
    HOX11 p.-o.
    H-ras p.-o.
    hst (K-fgf) p.-o.
    int-2 p.-o.
    jun p.-o.
    kit p.-o.
    K-ras p.-o.
    lck p.-o.
    L-myc-1,2 p.-o.
    lyt-1 p.-o.
    lyt-10 p.-o.
    mas p.-o.
    met p.-o.
    mos p.-o.
    myb p.-o.
    myl p.-o.
    N-myc-1,2 p.-o.
    N-ras p.-o.
    PBX1 p.-o.
    pim-1 p.-o.
    raf-1 p.-o.
    RARα p.-o.
    ras p.-o.
    rel p.-o.
    ret p.-o.
    rhombotin-2/Ttg-1 p.-o.
    rhombotin/Ttg-1 p.-o.
    ros p.-o.
    sea p.-o.
    ski p.-o.
    src p.-o.
    tal-1 p.-o.
    tan-1 p.-o.
    trk p.-o.
    yes p.-o.
protoplasmic astrocytoma
protozoal infection
protracted exposure sensitization
protrusio acetabuli

protrusion
    acetabular p.
    disk p.
protuberans
    dermatofibrosarcoma p.
prourokinase
Provera
Provider 6000 ambulatory dual channel infusion pump
provirus
provocation
    secretin p.
provocative testing
Prowazek body
Prowazek-Greeff body
Prower factor
Prowess treatment planning
proxetil
    cefpodoxime p.
proximal
    p. femoral fracture
    p. femur
    p. fibula
    p. humeral fracture
    p. interphalangeal joint (PIP)
    p. loop syndrome
    p. tibia
    p. tibial fracture
    p. tibial metaphyseal fracture
    p. tubular adenoma
proximity injury
prozone phenomenon
prune belly syndrome
pruned-tree appearance
pruritus
    vulvar p.
Prussak space
Prussian
    P. blue
    P. blue reaction
pS2 protein
PSA
    prostate-specific antigen
    PSA prostate cancer tumor marker
    PSA slope
    PSA tumor marker
    PSA velocity
PSA-immunoperoxidase
psammocarcinoma
psammoma body

psammomatoid ossifying fibroma
psathyrosis
Pseudallescheria boydii
pseudarthrosis, pseudoarthrosis
pseudoacardia
pseudoachondroplasia
pseudoagglutination
pseudoanemia
pseudoaneurysm
    hepatic artery p.
    peripheral p.
    perivalvular p.
    splenic artery p.
pseudoangiosarcoma
    Masson p.
pseudoarthritis
pseudoarthrosis (*var. of*
    pseudarthrosis)
pseudoarticulation
pseudoascites
pseudobiopsy technique
pseudo-blind loop syndrome
pseudocalcification
    powder p.
pseudocalculus
pseudocarcinoma
pseudocarcinomatous
pseudoclonality
    T-cell p.
pseudocoarctation
pseudocryptorchidism
pseudocyst
    meconium p.
    necrotic p.
    pancreatic p.
    subarticular p.
pseudodiffusion
pseudodiploidy
pseudodiverticulosis
    esophageal intramural p.
    intramural p.
pseudodiverticulum
    retrograde ureteral p.
pseudofollicle
pseudofollicular
    p. growth pattern
    p. proliferation center

pseudofracture
    p. artifact
    milkman's p.
pseudogating
    diastolic p.
pseudogene segment
pseudogestational sac
pseudoglioma
pseudogout
pseudogynecomastia
pseudohermaphroditism
    female p.
    male p.
pseudo-Hodgkin disease
pseudohypoparathyroidism
pseudo-Kaposi syndrome
pseudokidney sign
pseudoleukemia
pseudolymphoma
    p. syndrome
pseudomantle zone pattern
pseudomass
    mucous p.
pseudomembranous
    p. candidiasis
    p. colitis
pseudomeningocele
    posttraumatic intradiploic p.
Pseudomonas
    P. aeruginosa
    P. aeruginosa pneumonia
    P. fluorescens
    P. hyperimmune globulin
    P. maltophilia
    P. pickettii
    P. pseudomallei pneumonia
    P. stutzeri
pseudomonas
    p. meningitis
    p. pneumonia
Pseudomonas exotoxin
pseudomucinous cystadenocarcinoma
pseudomyxoma peritonei
pseudoneoplasm
pseudoneuroma

NOTES

pseudoobstruction
  chronic idiopathic
    intestinal p.
  idiopathic intestinal p.
pseudoobstruction
  intestinal p.
pseudoomphalocele
pseudopalsy
  Parrot p.
pseudopancreatitis
pseudo-Pelger-Huet change
pseudoperoxidase
pseudopod formation
pseudopodia
pseudopolyp
pseudopolyposis lymphatica
pseudoporencephaly
pseudoprecocious
pseudo-pseudohypoparathyroidism
pseudopyogenic granuloma
pseudorosette
  perivascular p.
pseudorosettes
pseudosacculation
pseudosarcoma
pseudosarcomatous fasciitis
pseudostricture
pseudo-T-cell lymphoma
pseudothickening
pseudotruncus arteriosus
pseudotumor
  atelectatic asbestos p.
  p. cerebri
  inflammatory p.
  lymphoid inflammatory p.
  ocular adnexal
    inflammatory p.
  orbital p.
  p. sign
  vermian p.
  xanthomatous p.
pseudoureterocele
pseudoxanthoma elasticum
PSIFT
  platelet suspension
    immunofluorescence test
psittaci
  Chlamydia p.
psittacosis
psoas
  p. line
  p. major
  p. margin

  p. muscle
  p. shadow
  p. stripe
psoas-hitch procedure
psoralen
psoralen and ultraviolet A (PUVA)
psoriasis
psoriatic arthritis
^{31}P spectroscopy
PSSE
  partial saturation spin-echo
    PSSE technique
psychiatric comorbidity
psychogenic water intoxication
psychoimmunoneurology
psychological
  p. approach
  p. factor
  p. support
psychometrics
psychomimetic drug
psychoneuroimmunology
psychosis
  AIDS p.
psychosocial aspect
PT
  prothrombin time
PTA
  percutaneous transluminal
    angioplasty
PTBD
  percutaneous transhepatic biliary
    drainage
PTCA
  percutaneous transluminal
    coronary angioplasty
pteronyssimus
  Dermatophagoides p.
pterygium colli
pterygoid
  anal p.
  p. artery
  p. canal
  p. fossa
  p. muscle
  p. plate
  p. process
pterygopalatine
  p. fossa
  p. ganglion
PTFE
  polytetrafluoroethylene

PTH
  parathyroid hormone
PTHrP
  parathyroid hormone-related
  protein
ptosis
ptotic
PTT
  partial thromboplastin time
PTX
  pentoxifylline
pubertal development
puberty
  precocious p.
pubic
    p. arch
    p. bone maldevelopment
    p. crest
    p. rami
    p. ramis
    p. ramus
    p. tubercle
pubis
    osteitis p.
    symphysis p.
public antigen
PUBS
  percutaneous umbilical blood
  sampling
PUCK film changer
pudenda
  ulcerating granuloma of p.
pudendal
pudendi
  granuloma p.
puerperal mastitis
puff-of-smoke vessels
pullback
    p. atherectomy catheter
    p. pressure gradient
pull maneuver
PulmoMate nebulizer
pulmonale
    cor p.
pulmonary
    p. adenopathy
    p. adverse effect

p. agenesis
p. alveolar proteinosis
p. angiography
p. angioma
p. aplasia
p. arterial hypertension
p. arterial malformation
p. arteriography
p. arteriovenous aneurysm
p. arteriovenous fistula
p. arteriovenous
  malformation
p. arteriovenous shunt
p. artery
p. artery aneurysm
p. artery hemorrhage
p. asbestosis
p. atresia
p. bacterial infection
p. blood flow
chronic obstructive p.
  disease (COPD)
p. circulation
p. complication
p. consolidation
p. contusion
p. cyst
diffuse p. alveolar
  hemorrhage
p. disorder
p. dysmaturity
p. edema
p. embolectomy
p. emboli
p. embolic disease
p. embolism
p. emphysema
p. endocrine cell
p. fibrosis
p. function test
p. fungal infection
p. hemosiderosis
p. hyalinizing granuloma
p. hypertension
p. hypoplasia
p. infection
p. infiltrate

NOTES

pulmonary *(continued)*
    p. infiltration with
      eosinophilia (PIE)
    p. interstitial disease
    p. interstitial emphysema
      (PIE)
    p. lymphangiectasia
    p. lymphoid disorder
    p. lymphoma
    p. mainline granulomatosis
    p. malformation
    p. mass
    p. metastasis
    p. nodule
    noncardiogenic p. edema
    p. osteoarthropathy
    p. outflow tract
    p. overcirculation
    p. parenchymal infection
    p. resection
    p. sequelae
    p. sequestration
    p. sling
    p. sulcus
    p. telangiectasia
    p. thromboembolic disease
    p. thromboembolism
    p. toxicity
    p. trunk
    p. tuberculosis
    p. tumor
    p. valve
    p. valve insufficiency
    p. valve stenosis
    p. varix
    p. vascular congestion
    p. vascularity
    p. vascular pattern
    p. vasculature
    p. vein
    p. venolobar syndrome
    p. venoocclusive disease
    p. venous congestion
    p. venous hypertension
    p. venous return
    p. vessel
pulmonic
    p. click
    p. stenosis
pulp
    red p.
    white p.

pulposus
    herniated nucleus p. (HNP)
    nucleus p.
pulsatile mass
pulsatility
    arterial p.
    p. index
pulsating exophthalmos
pulsation
    myocardial p.
pulse
    binomial p.
    bounding peripheral p.
    p. chlorambucil
    depth p.
    p. design
    detection p.
    dorsalis pedis p.
    p. fashion pulse spray
    femoral p.
    p. flip angle
    frequency-selective p.
    gradient p.
    hard p.
    p. height analyzer
    inversion p.
    p. length
    motion compensation
      gradient p.
    p. MRI
    nonideal p.
    nonselective p.
    p. oximetry
    presaturation p.
    p. programmer
    radiofrequency p.
    p. repetition frequency
    p. repetition time
    saturation p.
    selective p.
    sequence p.
    p. sequence
    p. shape
    shaped p.
    soft p.
    spoiler p.
    tailored p.
    twin-peaked p.
    twister p.
    p. VAC
    velocity-compensating
      gradient p.
    water-hammer p.

pulsed
    p. Doppler
    p. Doppler waveforms
    p. mode
    p. wave
pulsed-field gel electrophoresis
pulsed-gradient spin-echo (PGSE)
pulsed-gradient spin-echo technique
pulsed-mode operation
pulse-echo distance measurement
pulse-timing diagram
pulsion diverticulum
pulsus
    p. paradoxus
    p. parvus et tardus
pump
    aortic balloon p.
    Autosyringe p.
    CADD-PLUS p.
    CADD-TPN p.
    Cobe double blood p.
    Cormed p.
    Deltec-Pharmacia CADD p.
    Disetronic infuser syringe p.
    Graseby p.
    Hakim valve and p.
    IMED Gemini PC-2
     volumetric p.
    IMED infusion p.
    implantable infusion p.
    implantable osmotic p.
    implanted p.
    Infumed p.
    Infusaid p.
    infusion p.
    Intelliject p.
    Medtronic infusion p.
    Na-K exchange p.
    Norport p.
    Pancretec p.
    Pancretec 2000 p.
    Panomat infusion p.
    Paragon ambulatory p.
    portable infusion p.
    Provider 6000 ambulatory
     dual channel infusion p.
    Sartorius breast p.

    Travenol Infusor p.
    p. twin
    Verifuse ambulatory
     infusion p.
punch
    p. biopsy
    Keyes dermatologic p.
punched-out
    p.-o. appearance
    p.-o. area
    p.-o. bony defect
punch-through
puncta (*var. of* punctum)
punctata
    chondrodysplasia p.
    rhizomelic
     chondrodysplasia p.
punctate
    p. calcification
    p. white matter
     hyperintensity
punctation
punctum, puncta
puncture
    antegrade p.
    cisternal p.
    direct needle p.
    lumbar p. (LP)
    nephrostomy p.
    percutaneous needle p.
    retrograde nephrostomy p.
    spinal p.
    p. transducer
    ultrasound-guided
     nephrostomy p.
pupil
    Argyll-Robertson p.
pupillae
    sphincter p.
pupillary
    p. constrictor muscle
    p. dilatation
Purdue Pegboard Test
pure red cell aplasia
purged marrow
purging
    bone marrow p.

NOTES

purging *(continued)*
    immunologic method of p.
    immunomagnetic p.
    pharmacologic method of p.
purified protein derivative
purine
    p. analog
    p. antimetabolite
    p. nucleoside phosphorylase
      (PNP)
Purinethol
Purkinje fibers
purple mutation system
purpura
    autoimmune
      thrombocytopenic p.
      (AITP)
    Henoch-Schonlein p.
    idiopathic
      thrombocytopenic p. (ITP)
    immune
      thrombocytopenic p. (ITP)
Purtillo syndrome
purulent
    p. meningitis
    p. synovitis
pus
    frank p.
push maneuver
putamen
putrescine
    methylacetylenic p.
putty kidney
PUVA
    psoralen and ultraviolet A
    PUVA radiation
PVB
    Platinol, vinblastine, bleomycin
    PVB study
PVC
    premature ventricular
      contraction
PXT
    piroxantrone
pyarthroses
pyarthrosis, pl. **pyarthroses**
pycnodysostosis
pyelitis
    p. cystica
pyelocaliectasis
pyelocalyceal, pyelocaliceal
    p. system
pyelogenic cyst

pyelogram
    antegrade p.
    intravenous p. (IVP)
pyelography
    intravenous p.
    needle p.
    retrograde p.
pyelolymphatic backflow
pyelolysis
pyelonephritis
    atrophic p.
    emphysematous p.
    p. in exenteration
    suppurative p.
    xanthogranulomatous p.
pyeloplasty
pyelorenal backflow
pyelotubular backflow
pyeloureteritis cystica
pyeloureterostomy
pyelovenous backflow
pygopagus
pyknodysostosis
pyknosis
pyknotic
    p. body
Pyle disease
pylori
    Campylobacter p.
    Helicobacter p.
pylori (*pl. of* pylorus)
pyloric
    p. antrum
    p. canal
    p. hypertrophy
    p. muscle
    p. sphincter
    p. stenosis
    p. stricture
    p. teat
pyloroplasty
pylorospasm
pylorus, pl. **pylori**
pyocele
pyoderma granulosa
pyogenes
    Streptococcus p.
pyogenic
    p. abscess
    p. cholangitis
    p. granuloma
pyogenic granuloma

pyogenicum
   granuloma p.
pyometra
pyomyositis
pyonephrosis
pyopneumothorax
pyorrhea
pyosalpinx
pyothorax
pyothorax-associated pleural
   lymphoma
pyoureter ectopic ureterocele
pyramid
   petrous p.
   renal p.
   renal medullary p.
pyramidal
   p. fracture
   p. system
   p. tract
pyrazinamide
pyrazine diazohydroxide
pyrazoloacridine
pyretic therapy
pyribenzamine
pyridinone
pyridoxilated stroma-free
   hemoglobin

Pyridoxine
pyridoxine-responsive anemia
4-pyridylsulfide
pyriform
   p. lobe
   p. sinus
   p. sinus cancer
pyriformis
pyrilamine
pyrimethamine
pyrimidine
   p. antagonist
   halogenated p.
   p. kinase
Pyrolite
pyrolysis product
pyronin Y
pyrophosphate
   technetium-99m p.
   technetium stannous p.
pyrrolizidine alkaloid
pyrrolizine
   isopropyl p.
pyuria
   sterile p.

NOTES

Q
> Q factor
> Q fever

16q
> LOH at 16q

QA antigen

QC-PCR
> quantitative competitive polymerase chain reaction

QLQ-C30
> Quality of Life Questionnaire-C30

Q-PCR
> quantitative polymerase chain reaction

Q-prep system

Q-switching

Q-TWiST
> time without symptoms or toxicity

quadrant

quadrantectomy

quadratic
> q. dependence
> q. phase gain

quadrature
> q. coil
> q. detection
> q. detector
> q. excitation
> q. phase detector artifact

quadratus
> q. femoris
> q. lumborum
> q. plantae

quadriceps
> q. femoris
> q. femoris tendon reflex test
> q. muscle
> q. tendon
> q. tendon tear

quadrigeminal
> q. cistern
> q. plate
> q. vein

quadrilateral plate

quadriplegia

quadriplegic

quadripolar
> q. nucleus
> q. signal broadening

quadripole
> q. broadening
> q. moment

qualitative clot retraction

quality
> q. control
> q. factor
> q. of life
> Q. of Life Questionnaire-C30 (QLQ-C30)
> spectral q.

quantal mitosis

quanti-Pirquet test

quantitative
> q. amniotic fluid volume
> q. competitive polymerase chain reaction (QC-PCR)
> q. computed tomography
> q. evaluation
> q. imaging
> q. polymerase chain reaction (Q-PCR)
> q. risk assessment

quantization error

quantum
> q. detection efficiency
> q. energy
> q. mottle
> q. mottle index
> q. noise
> q. sink

quarter-detector offset

quasispecies

quellung reaction

quenching

Quercitin

questionnaire
> European Organization for Research and Treatment of Cancer Core Quality of Life Q.-C30 (EORTC QLQ-C30)
> Magill Pain Q.
> Quality of Life Q.-C30 (QLQ-C30)

Queyrat erythroplasia

Quick test

quiescent fraction
quinacrine
Quinamm
quinazoline
Quinby classification of pelvic
   fractures

quinine sulfate
quinolone
quintana
   Rochalimaea q.
Quinton central venous catheter
quinuclidinyl ester

R

R
  roentgen
R1
  longitudinal relaxivity
R2
  transverse relaxivity
R-75251
R85,246
RA
  RA latex fixation test
Ra
  radium
²²⁶Ra
  radium-226
  ²²⁶Ra needle
Raaf catheter
RAB
  remote afterloading
    brachytherapy
rabbit
  r. antirat ferritin
  r. ears strands
  r. fibroma
  r. fibroma virus
rabies immune globulin
Rabkin Nitinol coil stent
racemose cyst
racemosum
  angioma venosum r.
rachitic rosary
Raclopride
rad
  radiation absorbed dose
radial
  r. aplasia
  r. artery
  r. fracture
  r. head fracture
  r. neck fracture
  r. scar
  r. styloid fracture
  r. styloid process
radian
radiata
  corona r.
radiation
  r. absorbed dose (rad)
  alpha r.
  characteristic r.
  r. chimera

r. cystitis
r. dose
r. effect
electromagnetic r.
r. enhancement
r. exposure
external beam r.
r. fibrosis
gamma r.
r. hepatitis
high linear energy
  transfer r.
r. injury
r. intensity
intraoperative r.
involved-field r.
ionizing r.
megavoltage r.
r. mucositis
r. myelitis
r. necrosis
r. nephritis
neutron r.
nonionizing r.
r. oncologist
r. oncology
optic r.
orthovoltage r.
r. physics
r. pneumonitis
r. poisoning
postoperative pelvic r.
primary r.
r. protection
PUVA r.
radiofrequency r.
r. response
r. risk
scatter r.
secondary r.
r. sensitivity testing
r. sensitizer
solar r.
superficial r.
supervoltage r.
r. therapy (RT, XRT)
tissue tolerance to r.
total lymphoid r. (TLI)
ultraviolet r.
r. weighting factor

radiation-induced
r.-i. ischemia
r.-i. leukoencephalopathy
r.-i. pericarditis
r.-i. peripheral nerve tumor
r.-i. pulmonary toxicity
radical
r. abdominal hysterectomy
r. axillary dissection
r. cystectomy
free r.
r. hysterectomy
leucine r.
r. mastectomy
r. neck dissection
nitroxide-stable free r.
r. orchiectomy
organic free r.
oxygen free r.
r. parametrectomy
r. retropubic prostatectomy
stable free r.
r. surgery
r. vaginal hysterectomy
r. vulvectomy
radices (*pl. of* radix)
radicle
biliary r.
intrahepatic r.
radicular
r. artery
r. cyst
r. pain
radiculopathy
Radinyl
radioactive
r. colloid
r. gold
r. half-life
r. iodide (RAI)
r. iodine (RAI)
r. isotope
r. metal
r. radon
r. tracer
radioaerosol
radioassay
radiobiologic
r. equivalent (RBE)
r. study
radiobiology
radiocapitellar line
radiocarcinogenesis

radiocarpal
r. angle
r. dislocation
radiocephalic
radiocephalpelvimetry
radiocesium
radiochemical impurity
radiocholangiography
radiocholecystography
radiochromic dosimetry medium
radiocineangiocardiography
radiocineangiography
radiocolloid
radiocontrast-associated
radiocurability
radiodense lesion
radiodensity area
radioenzyme
radiofibrinogen uptake scan
radiofrequency (RF)
r. absorption
r. coil
r. field
r. pulse
r. radiation
r. shield
r. spatial distribution
artifact
r. spin echo
r. transmitter-receiver coil
radiogammetry
radiograph
cephalometric r.
decubitus r.
double-contrast r.
dual-energy r. (DER)
internal oblique r.
lateral r.
lateral decubitus r.
lateral oblique r.
lateral skull r.
maxillary sinus r.
mortise r.
oblique r.
panoramic r.
plain r.
scout r.
spot r.
submentovertex r.
supine r.
Towne projection r.
Trendelenburg r.
tunnel r.

radiographer
radiographic
r. criteria
r. parallel line shadow
r. pelvimetry
radiographically
radiography
advanced multiple-beam
equalization r.
air-gap r.
bedside r.
computed r.
dental r.
digital r.
digital video
gastrointestinal r.
dual-energy r.
mobile r.
mucosal relief r.
musculoskeletal r.
plain r.
plain abdominal r. (PAR)
portable r.
scanning equalization r.
sectional r.
serial r.
slit r.
spot film r.
video digital
gastrointestinal r.
radioimmunoassay
Nichols r.
radioimmunoconjugate
radioimmunodetection
radioimmunodiagnosis
radioimmunoelectrophoresis
radioimmunoglobulin
r. scintigraphy (RIS)
r. therapy (RIT)
radioimmunoguided surgery (RIGS)
radioimmunoimaging
radioimmunolocalization
radioimmunoprecipitation
radioimmunoscintigraphy
radioimmunotherapy
radioinduced sarcoma
radioiodide

radioiodination
radioiodine uptake
radioiron
radioisotope
r. camera
carrier-free r.
r. scan
r. scanner
transplutonium r.
radiolabeled
r. antibody
r. antigen
r. thyroxine
radiolabeling
radioligand
r. assay
radiology
cardiovascular r.
chest r.
forensic r.
interventional r.
pediatric r.
skeletal r.
r. telephone access system
(RTAS)
radiolucency
relative r.
radiolucent
r. crescent line
r. crescent sign
r. defect
r. joint spaces
r. linear filling defect
r. operating room table
extension
r. stone
radiolysis
radiomutation
radionuclide
r. angiocardiography
r. angiography
r. cisternography
r. esophagram
r. generator
r. imaging
r. impurity
r. scan

NOTES

467

radionuclide *(continued)*
  r. scanning
  r. scintigraphy
  r. study
  r. venography
  r. ventriculography
radiopaque
  r. drain
  r. foreign body
  r. marker
radiopharmaceutical
  r. chemistry
  r. therapy
radiophosphate
radiopotentiation
radiopraxis
radioprotector
radioreceptor assay
radioresistance
radioresponsiveness
radiosensitivity
radiosensitization
radiosensitizer
radiosurgery
  stereotactic r.
radiotherapy
  abdominal strip r.
  continuous hyperfractionated
    accelerated r. (CHAR)
  high-dose r.
  iceberg r.
  interstitial r.
  intraoperative r. (IORT)
  intraoperative electron
    beam r. (IORT)
  involved-field r.
  r. localization
  locoregional field r.
  mantle r.
  stereotactic r.
  target r.
  teletherapy r.
radiotracer
radioulnar joint
radium (Ra)
radium-226 (^{226}Ra)
  intracavitary r.
radius
  thrombocytopenia, absent r.
    (TAR)
radix, pl. radices
radixin protein
radix-two algorithm

RadNet
radon (Rn)
  r. progeny
  r. seed implantation
radon-222 (^{222}Rn)
RadStat
raf-1 **proto-oncogene**
RAG-1 gene
RAG-2 gene
ragocyte
RAI
  radioactive iodide
  radioactive iodine
  RAI uptake
Rai
  R. classification
  R. staging system
railroad
  r. track appearance
  r. track ductus arteriosus
  r. track sign
Raindrop nebulizer
Rainier
  hemoglobin R.
raiser
  stress r.
Raji
  R. cell
  R. cell assay
rale
  Velcro r.'s
RAM
  reduced-acquisition matrix
rami (*pl. of* ramus)
Ramon flocculation
ramping
Ramsay Hunt syndrome
ram's horn sign
ramus, pl. rami
  r. intermedius artery
  mandibular r.
  pubic r., pl. pubic rami
Randall forceps
random
  r. high-dose chemotherapy
  r. motion
  r. noise
  r. walk
randomization
range
  dynamic r.
  emission r.

frequency r.
reference r.
ranine tumor
rank
Spearman r.
Ranke complex
Ransom scale
ranula
plunging r.
RAO
right anterior oblique
rapamycin
rapeseed oil
rapid
r. acquisition with
relaxation enhancement
r. dissolution formula
(RDF)
r. film changer
r. imaging
r. plasma reagin (RPR)
r. scan fluoroscopy
r. scan technique
r. tumor lysis syndrome
Rappaport
R. classification
R. classification of
lymphoma
RARα
RARα oncogene
RARα proto-oncogene
rare-earth screen
rarefaction
RAS
Rokitansky-Aschoff sinuses
ras
ras oncogene
ras proto-oncogene
rash
butterfly r.
exanthematous drug r.
morbilliform r.
papular r.
Rasheed sarcoma virus
Rashkind
R. ductus occluder device
R. procedure

Rasmussen aneurysm
Rastelli procedure
RAST inhibition assay
RAT
rotating aspiration
thromboembolectomy
rate
aldosterone secretion r.
(ASR)
count r.
digital sampling r.
dipole-dipole relaxation r.
disintegration r.
five-year cure r.
flow r.
glomerular filtration r.
(GFR)
high-dose r. (HDR)
incidence r.
lipid fraction relaxation r.
low-dose r. (LDR)
maximal midexpiratory
flow r.
morbidity r.
mortality r.
oxygen extraction r.
perinatal mortality r.
prevalence r.
relapse r.
relaxation r.
Rourke-Ernstein
sedimentation r.
sampling r.
slew r.
Solomon-Bloembergen theory
of dipole-dipole
relaxation r.
specific absorption r.
ratemeter
Rathke
R. cleft cyst
R. pouch
R. pouch tumor
ratio
A/B r.
apnea/bradycardia r. (A/B
ratio)

NOTES

ratio *(continued)*
    bicaudate r.
    cardiothoracic r.
    C/N r.
    contrast r.
    contrast-to-noise r. (C/N ratio)
    conversion r.
    cost-to-benefit r.
    diastolic velocity r.
    false negative r.
    false positive r.
    grid r.
    gyromagnetic r.
    magnetogyric r.
    myeloid/erythroid r.
    nuclear/cytoplasmic r.
    nurse-patient r.
    oxygen enhancement r.
    power r.
    proportional r.
    risk-benefit r.
    scatter r.
    S/D r.
    sensitizer enhancement r.
    signal intensity r.
    signal-to-noise r. (SNR, S/N ratio)
    stroke count r.
    stroke volume r.
    systolic/diastolic r. (S/D ratio)
    systolic velocity r.
    target-to-nontarget r.
rat tail deformity
Rauscher
    R. leukemia
    R. leukemia virus
ray
    gamma r.
    roentgen r.
    r. sum
    r. tracing
Raybar 75
Rayleigh scatter
Raynaud phenomenon
Rayvist
Razi cannula introducer
razoxane
***Rb1* oncogene**
RBE
    radiobiologic equivalent
    relative biologic effectiveness

r-beta-ser interferon
***Rb* gene**
RC50KL
    Pall filter R.
RD1 antigen
RDF
    rapid dissolution formula
RDS
    respiratory distress syndrome
    respiratory distress syndrome of newborn
^{188}Re
    rhenium-188
^{186}Re
    rhenium-186
Reach to Recovery
reaction
    adverse drug r. (ADR)
    allergic r.
    alloxan-Schiff r.
    anaphylactic r.
    anaphylactoid r.
    Arthus r.
    Bareggi r.
    brick skin r.
    cellular periosteal r.
    choriodecidual r.
    citrate r.
    complex periosteal r.
    contrast r.
    Dale r.
    decidual r.
    donor-cleavage r.
    dystonic r.
    Eisenmenger r.
    extrapyramidal r.
    fluffy periosteal r.
    giant cell r.
    glactose oxidase-Schiff r.
    hair-on-end periosteal r.
    high-energy phosphate r.
    host r.
    hypersensitivity r.
    Jarisch-Herxheimer r.
    Jones-Mote r.
    lamellar periosteal r.
    lepra r.
    leucoerythroblastic r.
    mucocutaneous r.
    Neufeld r.
    nonspecific r.
    onion skin periosteal r.
    periodic acid-Schiff r.

periosteal r.
phosphate r.
pleural r.
polymerase chain r.
Prussian blue r.
quantitative competitive
    polymerase chain r. (QC-
    PCR)
quantitative polymerase
    chain r. (Q-PCR)
quellung r.
Schultz r.
shell type of periosteal r.
Shwartzman r.
spleen immune r.
sunburst periosteal r.
symmetric periosteal r.
vagovagal r.
vasovagal r.
Watson-Ehrlich r.
wheal-and-flare r.
reactivation tuberculosis
reactive
r. cyst
r. follicular hyperplasia
r. hyperemia
r. hyperplasia
r. interface
r. lymphadenopathy
r. lymphoid hyperplasia
r. lymphoid lesion
r. proliferating
    angioendotheliomatosis
r. remodeling
r. spinal cyst
reactivity
cross r.
reactor
breeder r.
fast-breeder r.
readout
r. delay
r. gradient
reagent
cross-linking r.
F r.
Reptilase r.

Schiff r.
shift r.
Sickledex r.
tandem conjugate r.
reagin
rapid plasma r. (RPR)
reaginic antibody
real
r. image
r. reconstruction
real-time
r.-t. acquisition and velocity
    evaluation
r.-t. color Doppler imaging
r.-t. echo-planar image
r.-t. imaging
r.-t. sector scanning
transcranial r.-t. color-flow
    Doppler sonography
r.-t. ultrasonography
rearrangement
chromosome r.
gene r.
r. of genes
immunoglobulin gene r.
lymphocyte gene r.
rebound
r. sign
Rebuck skin window technique
recall phenomenon
recanalization
laser r.
r. technique
receiver
r. bandwidth
r. coil
r.'s curve
r. dead time
r. operating characteristic
r. operating characteristic
    curve
receptor
adrenergic r.
β-adrenergic r.
androgen r.

NOTES

receptor *(continued)*
anti-epidermal growth
factor r. (anti-EGFR)
antigen r.
asialoglycoprotein r.
atrial natriuretic factor r.
autocrine motility factor r.
benzodiazepine r.
r. blockade
C3 r.
cardiac r.
CD4 r.
complement r.
dopamine r.
dopamine D1 r.
dopamine D2 r.
dopaminergic r.
epidermal growth factor r.
(EGFR)
E rosette r.
estrogen r.
Fc r.
growth factor r.
histamine H1 r.
HIV r.
homing r.
hormone r.
Imubind uPAG ELISA kit
urokinase r.
interleukin-2 r.
laminin r.
mouse erythrocyte r.
mu r.
muscarinic r.
opiate r.
opioid r.
overexpressed r.
progesterone r.
progestin r.
retinoic acid r.
retinoid X r.
RGD recognition r.
serotonin r.
serum soluble r.
sigma r.
r. status
T-cell r. (TCR)
T-lymphocyte r.
transferrin r.
upregulation of the r.
urokinase r.
vesamicol r.
receptor-negative patient

recess
azygoesophageal r.
cerebellopontine r.
lacrimal r.
lateral r.
pharyngeal r.
piriform r.
rectouterine r.
rectovesical r.
sphenoethmoidal r.
subscapularis r.
superior azygoesophageal r.
Twining r.
recessive
autosomal r.
r. gene
recipient
allotransplant r.
renal allograft r.
r. twin
reciprocal gene
Recklinghausen tumor
reclining position
recognition
pattern r.
recoil
elastic r.
recombinant
r. alpha interferon
r. alpha-26 interferon
r. deoxyribonucleic
technology
r. DNA
r. fusion protein
r. G-CSF
r. hematopoietic growth
factor
r. human colony-stimulating
factor
r. human erythropoietin
r. human granulocyte
colony-stimulating factor
(rhG-CSF)
r. human granulocyte-
macrophage colony-
stimulating factor (rGM-
CSF, rhGM-CSF)
r. human granulocyte-
stimulating factor
r. human growth factor
r. human interleukin (rhIL)
r. human interleukin-3
r. human macrophage

colony-stimulating factor
(rhM-CSF)
r. interferon-α
interferon alfa-2a, r.
interferon alfa-2b, r.
r. interferon alpha (rIFN-A)
r. interferon-α-2b
r. interferon gamma (rIFN-
gamma)
r. interleukin-2 (rIL-2)
interleukin-1-alpha, r.
human
interleukin-2, liposome-
encapsulated r.
r. N-glycanase enzyme
r. N-glycanase glycerol-free
enzyme
r. platelet factor-4 (rPF4)
recombinase
lymphocyte r.
Recombinate
reconstitution
hematologic r.
immune r.
immunologic r.
reconstruction
analytic r.
r. artifact
breast r.
constrained r.
coronal r.
image r.
iterative r.
magnitude r.
nipple-areolar r.
one-sided image r.
phase-preserving r.
real r.
sagittal r.
three-dimensional r.
r. view
reconstructive imaging
recording
segmental limb pressure r.
Recovery
Reach to R.

recovery
fluid attenuated inversion r.
(FLAIR)
hematopoietic r.
inversion r. (IR)
saturation r. (SR)
selective saturation r.
short tau inversion r.
(STIR)
short TI inversion r.
(STIR)
silver r.
stem cell r.
recreational
r. drug
r. sex
recruitment factor
rectal
r. cancer
r. carcinoma
r. endosonography
r. fascia
r. fisting
r. intussusception
r. narrowing
r. opioid
r. penetration
r. sheath hematoma
r. tear
r. tip
rectangular
r. field of view
r. phalanges
rectifier
r. sub-block
r. tube
rectilinear scanner
rectitis
rectocele
rectogenital septum
rectosigmoid
r. cancer
r. irradiation tolerance
r. junction

NOTES

rectouterine
    r. fossa
    r. pouch
    r. recess
rectovaginal
    r. fistula
    r. pouch
    r. septum
rectovesical
    r. pouch
    r. recess
rectum
    benign lymphoma of r.
    r. irradiation tolerance
rectus
    r. abdominis
    r. abdominis
      musculocutaneous flap
    r. abdominis myocutaneous
      flap
    r. femoris
    r. muscle
    r. sheath
recurrence
    local r.
    pelvic r.
recurrent
    r. artery of Heubner
    r. cancer
    r. carcinoma
    r. digital fibroma
    r. fleeting lung infiltrates
    r. hyperparathyroidism
    r. laryngeal nerve
    r. lateral patellar
      subluxation
    r. lymphoma
    r. multifocal osteomyelitis
    r. pneumonia
    r. pyogenic cholangitis
    r. pyogenic hepatitis
    r. sialadenitis
    r. vermian oligoastrocytoma
red
    r. blood cell
    r. blood cell antigen
    r. blood cell scintigraphy
    r. cell antigen
    r. cell aplasia
    r. cell ghost
    r. cell index
    r. cell volume
    r. marrow

    r. pulp
    Texas R.
redistribution image
red-man syndrome
red-out
redox change
reduced-acquisition
    r.-a. matrix (RAM)
    r.-a. matrix FAST
reductase
    dihydrofolate r. (DHFR)
reduction
    fracture r.
    gradient moment r. (GMR)
    hydrostatic r.
    limb r.
    r. mammoplasty
    r. mammoplasty tissue
    pneumatic r.
    postural r.
redundancy
    phase-angle display r.
Reed cell
Reed-Sternberg (R-S)
    R.-S. cell
reference
    chemical shift r.
    frame of r.
    r. phantom
    r. range
    rotating frame of r.
    r. wave
referred pain
reflection
    r. coefficient
    mirror-image r.
    peritoneal r.
    specular r.
reflector
    diffuse r.
    specular r.
reflex
    genitourinary r.
    r. ileus
    r. sympathetic dystrophy
    r. test of adductors
refluoromyelography
reflux
    r. of barium
    duodenogastroesophageal r.
    embolic r.
    r. esophagitis
    gastroesophageal r.

GE r.
r. nephropathy
piston-like r.
vaginal r.
velopalatine r.
vesicoureteral r.
refocused
multiplanar gradient r.
reformat
reformation
DentaScan multiplanar r.
multiplanar r.'s
refraction
refractoriness
platelet r.
refractory
r. anemia
r. anemia with excess blast
r. anemia with excess blasts
in transition
r. anemia with ring
sideroblasts
r. asthma
r. tumor
Refsum disease
Regan isoenzyme
regenerating nodule
regenerative
r. polyp
regimen
circadian r.
Cooper r.
first generation r.
hybrid r.
intensification r.
intermediate-dose salvage r.
Livingstone-Wheeler r.
Maertel r.
Melacine r.
platinum-based r.
second generation r.
standard r.
third generation r.
region
abnormally contracting r.'s
axillary r.
breakpoint cluster r.

complementary
determining r.
constant r.
epigastric r.
framework r.
hinge r.
homogenously staining r.
hypervariable r.
hypothenar r.
r. of interest (ROI)
interfollicular r.
intertrochanteric r.
nuclear organizing r.
nucleolar organizing r.
occipitoparietal r.
pineal r.
pituitary r.
r.'s of protection
switch r.
variable r.
regional
r. anesthesia
r. anesthetic
r. cerebral blood flow
r. chemotherapy
r. enteritis
r. granulomatous
lymphadenitis
r. ileitis
r. lymph nodes cannot be
addressed (NX)
r. melanoma
r. migratory osteoporosis
r. neurolytic block
r. spread
r. tumor confinement
r. vascular perfusion
r. wall motion
Registrars
National Association of
Tumor R. (NATR)
registry
Herbst r.
hospital-based r.
Kiel Pediatric Tumor R.
population-based r.
Reglan

NOTES

regressing atypical histiocytosis
regression
    caudal r.
    Cox r.
    estrogen rebound r.
    spontaneous r.
regulation
    gene r.
regurgitant
    r. fraction
    r. jet
regurgitation
    aortic r.
    mitral r.
    tricuspid r.
rehabilitation
Reid base line
Reilly body
reimbursement system
reinduction chemotherapy
Reinhardt syndrome
Reinke
    R. crystal
    crystalloid of R.
Reiter syndrome
Reitman-Fränkel test
rejection
    graft r.
    hyperacute r.
    marrow graft r.
rel
    rel oncogene
    rel proto-oncogene
relapse
    bone marrow r.
    intraabdominal r.
    r. rate
    solitary r.
    testicular r.
relapse-free survival (RFS)
relapsing polychondritis
relationship
    doctor-patient r.
    dose-response r.
    pharmacodynamic-
      pharmacokinetic r.
    pharmacokinetic-
      pharmacodynamic r.
    Reynolds r.
    survival r.
    tumor cell-host bone r.

relative
    r. biologic effectiveness
      (RBE)
    r. conversion factor
    r. curative resection
    r. error
    r. noncurative resection
    r. radiolucency
    r. risk
    r. value scale
relaxation
    isovolumetric r.
    longitudinal r.
    molecular weight
      dependence of r.
    paramagnetic shift r.
    r. probe
    proton r.
    r. rate
    r. rate frequency
      dependence
    sinusoidal r.
    spin-lattice r.
    spin-spin r.
    T2 r.
    r. technique
    r. time
    transverse r. (TR)
relaxivity
    longitudinal r. (R1)
    transverse r. (R2)
relaxometry
release
    carpal tunnel r.
    catecholamine r.
    slow r. (SR)
releasing factor
remasking
remedy
    herbal r.
    plant r.
remission
    complete r. (CR)
    r. induction
remission-induction chemotherapy
remnant
    cystic duct r.
    gastric r.
    omphalomesenteric r.
    thyroglossal duct r.

remodeling
> neural foramen r.
> reactive r.

remote afterloading brachytherapy (RAB)

removable sheath helical extractor

removal
> one-session r.
> RNA r.

remyelinization

renal
> r. abscess
> r. adenocarcinoma
> r. agenesis
> r. allograft
> r. allograft-mediated hypertension
> r. allograft recipient
> r. amyloidosis
> r. angiography
> r. angiomyolipoma
> r. angioplasty
> r. arteriography
> r. artery
> r. artery aneurysm
> r. artery disease
> r. artery stenosis
> r. atrophy
> r. axis
> r. calcification
> r. calculus
> r. cancer
> r. carbuncle
> r. carcinoma
> r. carcinosarcoma
> r. cell carcinoma
> r. clearance
> r. cortex
> r. cortical adenoma
> r. cortical carcinoma
> r. cortical necrosis
> r. cortical nephrocalcinosis
> r. cyst
> r. cyst ablation
> r. cystic disease
> r. dialysis
> r. dilator

> r. disease
> r. duplication
> r. dysfunction
> r. dysgenesis
> r. dysplasia
> r. echo
> r. ectopia
> r. embolization
> r. failure
> r. fascia
> r. function
> r. fungal infection
> r. fungus ball
> r. hamartoma
> r. hilar vessel
> r. infarction
> r. infusion therapy
> r. insufficiency
> r. length measurement
> r. lymphoma
> r. malrotation
> r. mass
> r. medulla
> r. medullary pyramid
> r. obstruction
> r. osteodystrophy
> r. papillary necrosis
> r. paraneoplastic syndrome
> r. parenchyma
> r. parenchymal malakoplakia
> r. pelvis
> r. pelvis carcinoma
> polycystic r. disease
> r. and psoas shadows
> r. pyramid
> r. scintigraphy
> r. sinus complex
> r. sinus fat
> r. sinus lipomatosis
> r. stone
> r. transplant
> r. tubular acidosis
> r. tubular dysgenesis
> r. tubular ectasia
> r. tubular necrosis
> r. tumor

NOTES

renal *(continued)*
   r. vein
   r. vein thrombosis
rendering
   surface r.
Rendu-Osler-Weber disease
renin
   renin vein r.'s
   r. vein assay
reninoma
Renografin-60
Renografin-76
Reno-M-30
Reno-M-60
Reno-M drip
Renotec
renovascular
   r. cause for hypertension
   r. disease
   r. hypertension
Renovist
   R. II
Renovue
reocclusion
reordering
   data r.
   r. of phase encoding
reoxygenation
repair
   anterior posterior r.
   AP r.
   diaphragmatic crural r.
   Fontan r.
   Harrington-Allison r.
   myelomeningocele r.
   potentially lethal x-ray
    damage r.
   sublethal x-ray damage r.
   vesicovaginal r.
repair-competent
   cell r.-c.
reparative giant cell granuloma
repeat
   long terminal r.
repens
   erythema gyratum r.
reperfusion device
repetition time
repetitive pulse sequence
rephased transverse magnetization
rephasing
   echo r.
   even-echo r.

   gradient r.
   r. gradient
   gradient moment r. (GMR)
replacement
   prosthetic r.
replenisher
   Prosorba column platelet r.
Replete
replicate
replication
   DNA r.
   viral r.
replicon
repolarization
   cellular r.
report
   Walton r.
reporter gene
Reporting
   American Joint Committee
    for Cancer Staging and
    End Results R.
repository
repressed gene
repressor gene
reproductive tract embryology
reprogramming therapy
Reptilase reagent
repulsive force
rescue
   autologous bone marrow r.
    (ABMR)
   bone marrow r.
   flinic acid r.
   host r.
   leucovorin r.
   r. technique
Research
   American Association for
    Cancer R. (AACR)
   American Foundation for
    AIDS R. (AmFAR)
   Institute for Cancer R.
    (ICR)
resectability
resectable colorectal cancer
resection
   abdominoperineal r.
   abdominosacral r.
   absolute curative r.
   absolute noncurative r.
   atrial septal r. (ASR)
   coloanal r.

en bloc r.
hepatic r.
low anterior r.
pulmonary r.
relative curative r.
relative noncurative r.
rim r.
subtotal gastric r.
surgical r.
transurethral r.
UICC-RO r.
    International Union
    Against Cancer-RO
    resection
wedge r.
resective surgery
reserve
brain perfusion r.
neutrophil r.
reservoir
ICV r.
Ommaya r.
subcutaneous r.
residual
acetabular r. dysplasia
r. disease
r. ductal tissue
r. magnetization
r. paralysis
postvoid r.
r. volume
resilience
immunoglobulin r.
resistance
acquired drug r.
alkylation r.
r. to antibody
complement r.
cytokinetic r.
drug r.
drug-induced drug r.
end organ r.
inherent drug r.
kinetic r.
r. mechanism
multidrug r. (MDR)
multiple drug r.

resistive
r. index
r. magnet
resistivity
conductor r.
resistor
Starling r.
resolution
anisotropic r.
axial r.
azimuthal r.
energy r.
image spatial r.
intrinsic energy r.
isotropic r.
lateral r.
spatial r.
resolving
r. ischemic neurologic
    defect
r. power
resonance
electron paramagnetic r.
electron spin r. (ESR)
fast scan magnetic r.
r. frequency
localized magnetic r. (LMR)
magnetic r. (MR)
mobile magnetic r.
nuclear magnetic r. (NMR)
r. phenomenon
proton magnetic r.
spin-echo magnetic r.
    imaging
topical magnetic r. (TMR)
T1-weighted magnetic r.
resonant frequency
resonator
Faraday shielded r.
resorcinol spray
resorption
bony r.
periosteal r.
subarticular bone r.
subchondral r.
subperiosteal r.
resorptive atelectasis

NOTES

479

resource
respiration
  ventilator-assisted r.
respirator lung
respiratory
  r. burst
  r. burst product
  r. compensation
  r. cycle
  r. distress syndrome (RDS)
  r. distress syndrome of
    newborn (RDS)
  r. failure
  r. gating
  r. motion
  r. ordered phase encoding
  r. sorted phase encoding
  r. syncytial virus (RSV)
  r. syncytial virus infection
  r. system
  r. tract
  r. tract infection
Respirguard nebulizer
response
  anamnestic r.
  antibody r.
  anti-idiotypic
    immunoglobulin r.
  autoimmune r.
  clinical partial r. (CPR)
  complete r. (CR)
  deconditioned exercise r.
  detector r.
  dose r.
  frequency-following r.
  host r.
  immune r.
  inflammatory r.
  r. modifier
  radiation r.
  serotonergic-induced
    emetic r.
  T-helper cell r.
  TH₁ T-helper cell r.
  TH₂ T-helper cell r.
rest
  adrenal r.
  cortical r.
  r. magnetization
  pelvic r.
restaging
restenosis
  postangioplasty r.

resting energy expenditure
restoration
  r. of normal anatomic
    alignment
  physical r.
Restore hydrocolloid dressing
restraining
  physical r.
restricted diffusion
restriction
  antigen r.
  r. enzyme
  r. fragment length
    polymorphism
  lineage r.
restrictive
  r. cardiomyopathy
  r. lung disease
  r. pulmonary emphysema
restructuring
  cognitive r.
result
  surveillance-epidemiology-
    end r.'s (SEER)
resuscitation
retained
  r. barium
  r. foreign body
  r. gastric antrum
retardation
  growth r.
  intrauterine growth r.
    (IUGR)
rete
  r. mirabile
  r. ridge
retention
  r. cyst
  fluid r.
  r. polyp
reticular
  r. formation
  r. type
reticularis
  zona r.
reticulation
  coarse r.
  diffuse fine r.
  lung r.'s
reticulin
  r. deposition
  r. stain

reticulocyte
    r. count
reticulocytopenia
reticulocytosis
reticuloendothelial
    r. cell
    r. cell origin tumor
    r. imaging
    r. system
    r. tumor
reticuloendotheliosis
    leukemic r.
reticulogranular pulmonary density
reticulohistiocytic
reticulohistiocytoma
reticulohistiocytosis
reticuloid
    actinic r.
reticulonodular pattern
reticulosis
    histiocytic medullary r.
    malignant r.
    midline malignant r.
    pagetoid r.
    polymorphic r.
reticulum
    r. cell
    r. cell sarcoma
reticulum cell sarcoma
Retin-A
retinaculum, pl. retinacula
    extensor r.
    flexor r.
    peroneal r.
retinal
    r. angiomatosis
    r. anlage tumor
    r. detachment
retinalis
    lipemia r.
retinitis
retinoblastoma
    r. gene
    trilateral r.
retinocerebellar angiomatosis
retinochoroiditis

retinoic
    r. acid
    r. acid receptor
retinoid
    r. X receptor
retinol
retinopathy
    r. of prematurity
retinyl palmitate
ret **proto-oncogene**
retractile
    r. mesenteritis
    r. testis
retraction
    mediastinal r.
    nipple r.
    qualitative clot r.
retrieval
    oocyte r.
retroaortic renal vein
retrobulbar mass
retrocardiac
    r. area
    r. mass
retrocaval ureter
retrocecal appendix
retrocerebellar arachnoid cyst
retrochiasmal optic tract
retrocochlear hearing loss
Retro-Conray
retrocrural
    r. node
    r. space
retrodiskal temporomandibular joint
  pad inflammation
retroesophageal arch
retrofection
retroflexed
retrogastric space
retrogene
retrograde
    r. aortography
    r. cannulation
    r. endoscopic approach
    endoscopic r. cannulation
    r. jejunoduodenogastric
      intussusception

NOTES

retrograde *(continued)*
 r. nephrostomy puncture
 r. pyelography
 r. transurethral prostatic urethroplasty
 r. ureteral pseudodiverticulum
 r. urethrography (RUG)
retrolental fibroplasia
retrolisthesis
retromandibular
retromolar trigone cancer
retroperitoneal
 r. adenopathy
 r. calcification
 r. cyst
 r. drain
 r. fat stripe displacement
 r. fibrosis
 r. hematoma
 r. hemorrhage
 r. infection
 r. leiomyosarcoma
 r. liposarcoma
 r. lymphadenectomy
 r. lymphadenopathy
 r. lymphangioma
 r. lymph node dissection
 r. lymphoma
 r. viscera
retroperitoneum
retropharyngeal
 r. abscess
 r. hemorrhage
 r. lymph node
 r. narrowing
 r. soft tissue
retroplacental hematoma
retropneumoperitoneum
retropubic vesiculoprostatectomy
retropulsion
 r. of posterior fragment
retrospective gating
retrosternal
 r. air space
 r. area
 r. mass
 r. space
retrotracheal
 r. adenoma
 r. goiter
retroversion
retrovesical space

Retrovir
retroviral seroconversion syndrome
retrovirus
 C-type r.
 human T-lymphotropic r. (HTLV)
Rett syndrome
return
 anomalous pulmonary venous r.
 partial anomalous pulmonary venous r.
 pulmonary venous r.
 total anomalous pulmonary venous r.
Retzius
 R. foramen
 space of R.
rev
 r. gene
 r. protein
revascularization
 cerebral r.
 r. procedure
reverberation
 r. artifact
reversal
 gradient r.
reverse
 r. augmentation
 r. Barton fracture
 r. Colles fracture
 r. 3 configuration
 r. dose effect
 r. figure-3 sign
 r. genetics
 r. Hill-Sachs lesion
 r. Monteggia fracture
 r. mutation system
 r. transcriptase
 r. transcriptase inhibitor
 r. transcriptase polymerase
reversed-three sign
reversed vein graft
reverse-S sign
reversible
 r. ischemic neurologic deficit (RIND)
 r. myocardial ischemia
 r. perfusion defect
RevM10
 gene construct RevM10
rewinder

Rex protein
Reye syndrome
Reynolds
    R. number
    R. relationship
RF
    radiofrequency
    RF spoiling
RFS
    relapse-free survival
RF-spoiled FAST
RG 12915
RG 83894
RGD recognition receptor
r-GM-colony-stimulating factor
rGM-CSF
    recombinant human granulocyte-
    macrophage colony-stimulating
    factor
rgpl 60
RG 12915 serotonin antagonist
Rh
    Rhesus
    R. agglutinin
    R. antibody
    R. blood group
    R. factor
    R. factor antigen
    Gamulin R.
    R. incompatibility
    R. negative
    R. positive
RhOD immune globulin
rhabdoid tumor
rhabdomyoblast
rhabdomyoma
rhabdomyosarcoma (RMS)
    embryonal r.
    extremity r.
    genitourinary r.
    ocular r.
    orbital r.
    parameningeal r.
    paratesticular r.
    pleomorphic r.
    truncal r.
rhabdosarcoma

rhagiocrine cell
rHb1.1 recombinant hemoglobin
Rheinberg microscope
rhenium
    r. isotope
rhenium-186 (^{186}Re)
    r. etidronate
rhenium-188 (^{188}Re)
rheology of blood
rheolytic
    r. catheter
    r. thrombectomy catheter
Rhese
    R. projection
    R. view
Rhesus (Rh)
    R. factor
rheumatic
    r. disease
    r. heart disease
rheumatica
    polymyalgia r.
rheumatism
    hydroxyapatite r.
rheumatoid
    r. arthritis
    r. factor
    r. lung
    r. nodule
Rheumatrex
rhG-CSF
    recombinant human granulocyte
    colony-stimulating factor
rhGM-CSF
    recombinant human granulocyte-
    macrophage colony-stimulating
    factor
rhIL
    recombinant human interleukin
rhinitis gangrenosa progressiva
rhinocerebral mucormycosis
rhinoplasty
rhinorrhea
rhinoscleroma
rhinovirus
rhizomelia

NOTES

rhizomelic
 r. chondrodysplasia punctata
 r. dwarfism
 r. dysplasia
rhizotomy
 cranial nerve r.
Rhizoxin
rhMCAF
 human macrophage-monocyte
 chemotactic and activating
 factor
rhM-CSF
 recombinant human macrophage
 colony-stimulating factor
rhodamine
 r. analog
 r. platinum
rhodium filter
Rhodococcus
 R. equi
rhombencephalitis
rhombencephalon
rhombencephalosynapsis
rhomboid
 r. fossa
 r. ligament
 r. major
 r. of Michaelis
 r. minor
rhombotin-2/Ttg-1
 rhombotin-2/Ttg-1 oncogene
 rhombotin-2/Ttg-1 proto-
 oncogene
rhombotin/Ttg-1
 rhombotin/Ttg-1 oncogene
 rhombotin/Ttg-1 proto-
 oncogene
rhombotin/Ttg-2 **oncogene**
rhoton suction
rhythm
 biophysical r.
 circadian r.
 sinus r.
rhythmic paradoxical eruption
rib
 cervical r.
 dense r.
 r. detail
 double-exposed r.
 r. fracture
 jail-bar r.
 r. notching
 ribbon r.

 r. shadowing
 short r.
 wide r.
ribavirin
rib-bearing vertebrae
Ribbert thrombosis
ribbing disease
ribbon rib
ribonuclease (RNase)
ribonucleic acid (RNA)
ribonucleotide
 total adenine r.
riboside
 methylmercaptopurine r.
ribosome
 cellular r.
ribosome-lamella complex
ribozyme
rice-like muscle calcification
Richter
 R. syndrome
 R. syndrome-like
 transformation
 R. transformation
ricin
 r. A chain
 anti-B4 blocked r.
 B4 blocked r.
 N901 blocked r.
ricin-blocked antibody
rickets
 familial
 hypophosphatemic r.
 gastroenterogenous r.
 hypophosphatemic r.
 hypophosphatemic vitamin
 D refractory r.
 oncogenic r.
 vitamin D-dependent r.
 vitamin D-resistant r.
rickettsial infection
rider's bone
ridge
 alveolar r.
 petrous r.
 rete r.
 sphenoid r.
 transverse r.
Ridoura
Riedel
 R. lobe
 R. struma
 R. thyroiditis

Rieder
>R. cell
>R. cell leukemia

Rifabutin
rifabutin
rifampin
rifamycin
rIFN-A
>recombinant interferon alpha

rIFN-gamma
>recombinant interferon gamma

Rift Valley fever
right
>r. anterior oblique (RAO)
>r. anterior oblique view
>r. coronary artery
>r. heart
>r. lateral decubitus film
>r. lung
>r. posterior oblique (RPO)
>r. ventricle
>r. ventricular infarction
>r. ventricular outflow tract
>r. ventriculography

right-sidedness
>bilateral r.-s.

right-side-down position
right-to-left shunt
rigid
>r. bronchoscope
>r. endofluoroscopy
>r. forceps
>r. nephroscope

rigidity
>clasp-knife r.

rigidus
>hallux r.

Rigler
>R. sign
>R. triad

RIGS
>radioimmunoguided surgery

rIL-2
>recombinant interleukin-2

Riley-Day syndrome
Riley-Smith syndrome

rim
>dorsal r.
>r. resection
>r. sign
>stromal r.
>volar r.

Rimadyl
rimantadine
rim-enhancing lesion
rimming
>anal r.

RIND
>reversible ischemic neurologic
>deficit

Rindfleisch cell
ring
>A-r.
>r. apophysis
>B-r.
>r. badge
>R. biliary drainage catheter
>R. catheter
>R. drainage catheter needle
>r. epiphysis
>esophageal r.
>femoral r.
>r. fracture
>hemosiderin r.
>r. hydroxylation
>isometric contractile force r.
>Kayser-Fleischer r.
>r. lesion
>periureteric venous r.
>Schatzki r.
>r. sign
>tracheal r.
>vascular r.
>Waldeyer r.
>Wimberger r.

ring-disrupting fracture
Ringer lactate
ringing
>edge r.

Ring-MacLean sump
ring-shaped form
Riolan artery

NOTES

RIS
radioimmunoglobulin scintigraphy
Riseborough-Radin classification of intercondylar fracture
rise time
risk
cancer r.
r. factor
radiation r.
relative r.
suicidal r.
Weibull plot of adult T-cell leukemia/lymphoma r.
risk-benefit ratio
risk-directed therapy
Risser sign
ristocetin
r. cofactor test
r. von Willebrand cofactor
RIT
radioimmunoglobulin therapy
ritodrine
Rivinus ducts
RMS
rhabdomyosarcoma
rMu
r. GM-CSF
r. IL-6
r. IL-7
r. IL-1B
Rn
radon
²²²Rn
radon-222
RNA
ribonucleic acid
antisense RNA
RNA content
messenger RNA (mRNA)
RNA removal
RNA transcription
RNA tumor virus
RNase
ribonuclease
Rnase tumor marker
road mapping
Robertson
giant limb of R.
robertsonian translocation
Robert syndrome
Robinow syndrome

robotics
Robson
R. stage I-IV renal cell cancer
R. staging
R. system
ROC curve
Rochalimaea
R. *henselae*
R. *quintana*
rocker-bottom foot
rocket
r. immunoelectrophoresis
r. wire
Rockwood classification of clavicular fracture
rod
aerobic gram-negative r.
Auer r.'s
r. cell
Gram-negative r.
Harrington r.
intramedullary r.
Isolar r.
Luque r.
medullary r.
rodent facies
roentgen (R)
r. ray
roentgenographic
r. evaluation
r. finding
roentgenography
abdominal r.
Roferon
Roferon-A (*var. of* interferon alfa-2a)
Roger
maladie de R.
rogletimide
ROI
region of interest
Rokitansky-Aschoff sinuses (RAS)
Rokitansky nodule
Rokus view
rolandic artery
Rolando
fissure of R.
R. fracture
Rolland
American R.
Rollet stroma

rolling
r. hiatal hernia
r. membrane
Rolloscope II
Romer test
roof
acetabular r.
root
aortic r.
r. compression
r. end granuloma
lumbar nerve r.
r. mean square
roquinimex
Rosai-Dorfman disease
rosary
r. bead configuration
r. bead pattern
rachitic r.
Rosch modification
Rosen guidewire
Rosenmüller
fossa of R.
Rosenthal
R. aspiration needle
basal vein of R.
R. fiber
R. syndrome
rosette
r. cell
E r.
EA r.
Flexner-Wintersteiner r.
Homer Wright r.
Horner-Wright r.
malarial r.
sheep erythrocyte r.
Rose-Waaler test
ros **proto-oncogene**
Ross body
rostral
rostrocaudal extent signal
 abnormality
Rotablator thrombectomy system
Rotachrom heparin
Rotalex culture
rotamase activity

rotary
r. scoliosis
r. subluxation
rotating
r. anode
r. anode tube
r. aspiration
thromboembolectomy
(RAT)
r. frame imaging
r. frame of reference
rotating-frame
r.-f. experiment
r.-f. zeugmatography
rotation
anisotropic r.
organoaxial r.
short-T2 in anisotropic r.
r. therapy
rotational
r. burst fracture
r. contact lithotripsy
r. correlation time
r. dislocation
r. fracture
r. frequency
r. malalignment
r. motion
r. thrombectomy
rotator
r. cuff
r. cuff arthropathy
r. cuff muscle
r. cuff tear
rotavirus
Rotex
R. biopsy instrument
R. needle
Roth spot
Rotor syndrome
rotoscoliosis
rotoscoliotic deformity
rotundum
foramen r.
Rouget cell
round
r. atelectasis

NOTES

round *(continued)*
    r. back deformity
    r. cell sarcoma
    r. cell tumor
    r. ligament
    r. pneumonia
Rourke-Ernstein sedimentation rate
Rous
    R. sarcoma
    R. sarcoma virus
    R. tumor
route
    intrathecal r.
Roux-en-Y procedure
row
    first carpal r.
Rowasa enema
Roxanol
Roxicodone
roxithromycin
Royal Free disease
rPF4
    recombinant platelet factor-4
RPO
    right posterior oblique
RPR
    rapid plasma reagin
RPR-rapid plasma reagin
R ras oncogene
R-S
    Reed-Sternberg
RSV
    respiratory syncytial virus
RT
    radiation therapy
RTAS
    radiology telephone access
      system
RU 486
    mifepristone
^{82}Ru
    rubidium-82
Rubacell II culture
rubber
    r. drain
    silicone r.
rubella
    r. virus
Rubex
rubidazone
rubidium-82 (^{82}Ru)
rubidomycin
    r. hydrochloride

Rubner test
rubrospinal tract
Rudick red flags
rudimentary pronephron
ruffle
RUG
    retrograde urethrography
ruga, pl. **rugae**
rugae
    gastric r.
rugal
    r. fold
    r. pattern
rugger
    r. jersey appearance
    r. jersey vertebra
rugger-jersey spine
rule
    Hoerr r.
    Lossen r.
    modified Simpson r.
    r. of 2's
    r. of 3's
    r. of 10's
    van't Hoff r.
    Weigert-Meyer r.
ruler
    endocatheter r.
    Plexiglas radiographic r.
Rumpel-Leede test
Runeberg anemia
runoff
    epidural r.
runon transcription assay
runt disease
rupture
    amnion r.
    aortic r.
    diaphragmatic r.
    esophageal r.
    hemidiaphragm r.
    hernia r.
    intramural esophageal r.
    intraperitoneal r.
    papillary muscle r.
    splenic r.
    testicular r.
    traumatic aortic r.
    urinary bladder r.
ruptured
    r. aneurysm
    r. hollow viscus

r. spleen
r. ulcer
Rush intramedullary nail
Russell
R. body
R. classification system for soft-tissue sarcoma
R. Viper Venom (RVV)
R. viper venom clotting time
Rutledge classification of extended hysterectomy
Rutner
R. balloon dilatation helical stone extractor set

R. biopsy needle
R. cannula
R. nephroscopy adapter
R. stone basket
R-verapamil
RVV
Russell Viper Venom
RWJ 21757
RX400
Apogee RX400
Ryan White CARE Act
Rye
R. classification
R. classification of Hodgkin disease

NOTES

S 10036
S1 nuclease protection
SA
    sinoatrial node
      SA node
saber-shin
      s.-s. appearance
      s.-s. deformity
Sabin-Feldman dye test
Sabin vaccine
sabot
      coeur en s.
Sabourad plate
sac
      alveolar s.
      amniotic s.
      caudal s.
      double decidual s.
      empty gestational s.
      gestational s.
      hernial s.
      lacrimal s.
      lesser s.
      pericardial s.
      primary yolk s.
      primitive yolk s.
      pseudogestational s.
      secondary yolk s.
      thecal s.
      yolk s.
saccular
      s. aneurysm
      s. bronchiectasis
Sacks catheter
Sacks-Malecot catheter
sacral
      s. agenesis
      s. ala
      s. aneurysm
      s. bone tumor
      s. chordoma
      s. foramen
      s. fracture
      s. meningocele
      s. nerve
      s. osteomyelitis
      s. plexus
      s. promontory
sacralization

sacrococcygeal
      s. myxopapillary
        ependymoma
      s. teratoma
      s. tumor
sacroiliac
      s. fracture
      s. joint
sacrotuberous
      s. ligament
sacrum
      chordoma of s.
saddle
      s. block anesthesia
      s. coil
      s. embolus
      s. lesion
      s. nose deformity
saddlebag sign
saddle-shaped uterine fundus
S-adenosylhomocysteine (AdoHcy)
      S.-a. hydrolase (AdoHcyase)
***S*-adenosylmethionine (AdoMet)**
sadism
      anal s.
Saemisch ulcer
SafeTrak epidural catheter adapter
safety
      s. J wire
      s. wire introduction
Saf-T-coil
sagittal
      s. and coronal
        reconstruction view
      s. image
      s. plane
      s. porta hepatis
      s. reconstruction
      s. section
      s. sinus
      s. suture
      s. thrombosis
      s. view
Sahli method
SAIDS
    simian AIDS
sail-like tricuspid valve
sail sign
saimiri
      Herpesvirus s.

Sakellarides classification of calcaneal fractures
Salagen
Saldino-Noonan syndrome
Salem sump tube
salicylate
    choline s.
    sodium s.
saline
    s. cathartic
    D5 1/2 normal s.
    s. implant
salinity
Salisbury common cold virus
saliva
    s. blot test
    s. substitute
Salivart
salivary
    s. gland
    s. gland cancer
    s. gland carcinoma
    s. gland dysfunction
    s. gland infection
    s. gland lymphoepithelioma
Salk
    S. HIV Immunogen
    S. vaccine
S-allyl L cysteine
Salmon-Durie staging function
Salmonella enteritidis
salmonella meningitis
salmonellosis
salmon patch
salpingitis
    s. isthmica nodosa
salpingography
    selective s.
salpingo-oophorectomy
    bilateral s.-o. (BSO)
    total abdominal
      hysterectomy and
      bilateral s.-o. (TAHBSO)
    unilateral s.-o. (USO)
salpingopharyngeus
Salpix
Salter
    S. I-IV fracture
Salter-Harris
    S.-H. classification
    S.-H. classification of
      epiphyseal fractures
    S.-H. fracture

salt-losing nephritis
salts
    Earle s.
salvage
    autologous red cell s.
    s. chemotherapy
    s. therapy
Salzman test
samarium-153
sample
    blood s.
    s. chamber
    decalcified bone marrow s.
    fingerstick blood s.
    s. handling
    s. size
    standard s.
    s. transport
sampler
    Endopap endometrial s.
sampling
    asymmetric data s.
    blood s.
    chorionic villus s. (CVS)
    data s.
    fetal tissue s.
    Gibbs s.
    s. interval
    nodal s.
    nonlinear s.
    paraaortic node s.
    percutaneous fetal tissue s.
    percutaneous umbilical
      blood s. (PUBS)
    s. rate
    s. theorem
    s. time
    tissue s.
    transabdominal chorionic
      villus s.
    transcervical chorionic
      villus s.
    s. window
sanctuary site
sand
    hydatid s.
    s. tumor
Sandhoff disease
sandlike lucency
Sandoglobulin
Sandostatin (SSTN)
sandwich
    s. appearance

s. assay
s. configuration
s. sign
s. system
s. vertebrae
Sanfilippo syndrome
sanguineous
San Joaquin Valley fever
Santorini duct
Santyl ointment
SaO$_2$
    arterial oxygen saturation
SAPA
    spatial average-pulse average
    SAPA intensity
saphenous vein
sapphire tip probe
saquinavir
sarcoid
    Boeck s.
sarcoidal granuloma
sarcoidosis
    acinar s.
    alveolar s.
    osteosclerosis vertebral s.
sarcolysin
L-sarcolysin
sarcoma
    Abernethy s.
    African Kaposi s.
    alveolar soft part s.
    ameloblastic s.
    angiolithic s.
    bone s.
    botryoid s.
    s. botryoides
    cervical s.
    embryonal s.
    endometrial s.
    endometrial stromal s.
     (EES)
    epithelioid s.
    European Kaposi s.
    Ewing s.
    fascicular s.
    follicular dendritic s.
    giant cell s.

granulocytic s.
hemangioendothelial s.
hepatic anaplastic s.
immunoblastic s.
interdigitating dendritic
 cell s.
Jensen s.
Kaposi s. (KS)
Kupffer cell s.
leukocytic s.
lymphatic s.
mast cell s.
Mediterranean Kaposi s.
 (MEKS)
medullary s.
meningeal s.
mesodermal s.
mixed mesodermal s.
mixed müllerian s.
mixed ovarian
 mesodermal s.
monocytic s.
muscle s.
myelogenic s.
myeloid s.
non-rhabdo soft tissue s.
obesity in endometrial s.
orbital granulocytic s.
osteogenic s.
parosteal s.
periosteal s.
postirradiation s.
radioinduced s.
reticulum cell s.
round cell s.
Rous s.
Russell classification system
 for soft-tissue s.
sclerotic osteogenic s.
soft tissue s.
spindle cell s.
Sternberg s.
synovial s.
telangiectatic osteogenic s.
tendosynovial s.
undifferentiated s.
uterine s.

NOTES

sarcoma *(continued)*
    uterine mixed müllerian s.
    vascular s.
Sarcomastigophora
sarcomatodes
    lipoma s.
sarcomatoid
    s. carcinoma
    s. malignant mesothelioma
sarcomatosis
    diffuse s.
    plasmacytic s.
    sclerosing osteogenic s.
sarcomatosum
    lipoma s.
    myxoma s.
sarcomatous
sarcomere
sargramostim
sartorius
Sartorius breast pump
SATA
    spatial average-temporal average
    SATA intensity
satellite lesion
Sat pad
satumomab pentetide
saturation
    arterial oxygen s. (SaO_2)
    partial s.
    progressive s.
    progressive spin s.
    s. pulse
    s. recovery (SR)
    selective s.
    s. transfer
    transferrin s.
Sauvage filamentous velour graft
Savary-Gilliard dilator
Saver
    Haemonetics Cell S.
saw
    s. tooth sign
    s. tooth ureter
SBA
    soybean agglutinin
SBE
    self-breast examination
⁴⁷Sc
    scandium-47
scalar
    s. coupling
    s. effect

scalded skin syndrome
scale
    Adolescent and Pediatric
    Pain Tool S.
    Billingham s.
    digital gray s.
    Flint Colon Injury S.
    Glasgow Coma S.
    gray s.
    Hospital for Sick Children
    pain s.
    Internal-External Locus of
    Control S.
    Karnofsky rating s.
    Lung Cancer Symptom S.
    Miller Behavioral Style S.
    Ransom s.
    relative value s.
    Total Mood Disturbance S.
    Zubrod Performance S.
scalene node biopsy
scalenus
    s. anterior
    s. anterior muscle
    s. anticus syndrome
    s. medius
    s. tunnel syndrome
scalloping
    posterior s.
scalp
    s. hypothermia
    pilar tumor of s.
    s. tourniquet
    s. vein needle
scan
    Becton Dickinson FAC s.
    blood pool s.
    bone s.
    Cardiolite heart imaging s.
    computed tomography s.
    s. converter
    coronal s.
    CT s.
    elbow coronal s.
    EMI s.
    s. equalization
    flow portion of bone s.
    gallium s.
    gastric emptying s.
    hepatobiliary s.
    HIDA s.
    iodine-131 whole-body s.
    labeled leukocyte s.

left ventricular gated blood
pool s.
liver s.
liver-lung s.
longitudinal s.
methydiphosphonate bone s.
MUGA s.
   multiple gaited acquisition
   scan
multiple gaited
   acquisition s. (MUGA
   scan)
octreotide s.
OncoScint s.
pentretreotide s.
perfusion lung s.
PET s.
s. plane
radiofibrinogen uptake s.
radioisotope s.
radionuclide s.
sector s.
stimulation s.
strip s.
suppression s.
survey s.
thallium single-photon
   emission computed
   tomography s., thallium
   SPECT s.
transaxial s.
ventilation lung s.
scandium-47 (^{47}Sc)
scannable tumor
scanner
biplane sector s.
duplex s.
Imatron C-1000 UFCT s.
mechanical sector s.
phased array s.
radioisotope s.
rectilinear s.
whole-body s.
scanning
adiabatic fast s.
body s.
diffusion-weighted s.

s. equalization radiography
external s.
gallium s.
helical s.
IDA s.
parasternal s.
paravertebral s.
point s.
radionuclide s.
real-time sector s.
sector s.
spiral s.
spiral CT s.
suprasternal s.
whole-body s.
xenon CT s.
scanogram
scaphocephaly
scaphoid
s. abdomen
s. fracture
scapholunate
s. dislocation
s. dissociation
scapula
swallowtail malformation
   of s.
winged s.
scapulae
incisura s.
scapulothoracic joint
scar
s. cancer
s. carcinoma
epidural s.
radial s.
s. tissue
scarification of BCG
scarlet fever
scarring
fibrotic s.
parietal pleural s.
postinflammatory s.
SCAT
sheep cell agglutination test
scatter
Compton s.

NOTES

scatter *(continued)*
    s. correction
    s. degradation factor
    forward angle light s.
    s. radiation
    s. ratio
    Rayleigh s.
    side s.
scatterer depth
scattering
    Compton s.
scavenger
    s. cell
scavenging system
SCC
    squamous cell carcinoma
    SCC tumor marker
Schaedler blood agar
Schalfijew test
Schatzki ring
Schaumann lymphogranuloma
schedule
    s. dependency
    s. dependency concept
Scheffe F test
Scheie syndrome
scheme
    decay s.
    Fibonacci search s.
    gradient s.
    Kauffmann-White s.
schenckii
    Sporotrichum s.
Scheuermann
    S. disease
    S. nodule
Schick test
Schiff
    S. base
    S. reagent
    S. stain
Schilder disease
Schiller test
Schilling
    S. test
    S. type of monocytic leukemia
Schimmelbusch disease
schistocyte
schistosome granuloma
schistosomiasis
schizencephaly
Schlesinger solution

Schmid-like
    S.-l. metaphyseal chondrodysplasia
Schmorl node
schneiderian carcinoma
Schneider infusion wire
Schonander film changer
Schönlein disease
Schridde cancer hairs
Schuco nebulizer
Schuffner dot
Schultz reaction
Schumacher criteria
Schumm test
Schwachman-Diamond syndrome
schwannian lineage
schwannoma
    acoustic s.
    geniculate ganglion s.
    jugular foramen s.
Schwann tumor
Schwarten Microglide LP balloon
SCI
    spinal cord injury
sciatic
sciatica
SCID
    severe combined immunodeficiency
    severe combined immunodeficiency disease
    autosomal recessive SCID
    variant SCID
    X-linked SCID
scimitar
    s. syndrome
    s. vein
scintigraphic
    s. angiography
    s. evidence
scintigraphy
    adrenal s.
    blood pool s.
    bone s.
    bone marrow s.
    brain s.
    cardiac s.
    gallium s.
    indium-111 antimyosin s.
    In-pentetreotide s.
    long segmental diaphyseal uptake bone s.
    parathyroid s.

radioimmunoglobulin s. (RIS)
radionuclide s.
red blood cell s.
renal s.
sulfur colloid s.
^{99m}Tc-DMSA s.
transit s.
scintillation camera
scirrhous
s. carcinoma
SCIWORA
spinal cord injury without radiographic abnormality
Sclavo serum
SCLC
small cell lung cancer
sclerocystic ovary
scleroderma
diffuse s.
sclerodermoid graft-versus-host disease
scleroma
scleromyxedema
sclerosed temporal bone
sclerosing
s. adenitis
s. adenosis
s. agent
s. cholangitis
s. duct hyperplasia
s. endophthalmitis
s. lesion
s. mediastinitis
s. mesenteritis
nodular s.
s. osteogenic sarcomatosis
s. osteomyelitis of Garré
s. panencephalitis
primary s.
sclerosis, pl. scleroses
bone s.
diffuse s.
endplate s.
focal s.
hippocampal s.
marginal s.

mesial temporal s.
Mönckeberg s.
multifocal subperitoneal s.
multiple s.
nodular s.
percutaneous transhepatic s.
progressive systemic s.
temporal bone s.
tuberous s.
sclerostenosis
sclerotherapy
variceal s.
sclerotic
s. bone island
s. calvarial patch
s. lesion
s. osteogenic sarcoma
scoliosis
rotary s.
scopolamine
Scopulatiopsis
scorbutic anemia
score (*See also* scale)
functional independent measurement s.
Gleason s.
Karnofsky performance s.
scoring
biophysical profile s. (BPS)
fetal biophysical profile s.
scottie, scotty
s. dog appearance
s. dog fracture
s. dog sign
scout
s. film
s. radiograph
screen
s. craze artifact
intensifying s.
leukemia s.
lymphoma s.
rare-earth s.
two-hybrid yeast s.
screen-film contact
screening
genetic s.

NOTES

screening *(continued)*
    s. mammography
    SUDS HIV-l s.
    urine mutagenicity s.
screw
    interference s.
    lag s.
Scribner shunt
Scriptene
scrofula
scrofulaceum
    Mycobacterium s.
scrotal
    s. abscess
    s. area
    s. calcification
    s. fibroma
    s. hematocele
    s. histiocytoma
scrotum
Scully tumor
scurvy
scutum
SD
    stable disease
    SD antigen
S/D ratio
    systolic/diastolic ratio
SDZ ILE-964
^{75}Se
    selenium-75
sea
    s. algae extract
    s. urchin granuloma
    s. water drowning
sea-blue histiocyte
seagull
    s. joint
    s. sign
seam
    osteoid s.
sea proto-oncogene
seatbelt fracture
Seattle
    hemoglobin S.
sea urchin granuloma
sebaceous
    s. adenoma
    s. carcinoma
    s. cyst
    s. gland calcification
sebaceum
    adenoma s.

seborrheic
    s. dermatitis
    s. keratosis
secobarbital-hydroxyzine
second
    s. echelon lymph node
    s. generation regimen
    s. trimester gestational
    dating
secondary
    s. amyloidosis
    s. axillary adenopathy
    s. axillary lymphadenopathy
    s. calcification
    s. cancer
    s. carcinoma
    s. collimation
    s. drowning
    s. fracture
    s. hyperparathyroidism
    s. hypothyroidism
    s. malignancy
    s. radiation
    s. retroperitoneal organ
    s. sclerosing cholangitis
    s. sign
    s. skin thickening
    s. yolk sac
second-degree heart block
second-echo image
second-look operation
second-order compensation
secreted protein, acidic and rich
  in cysteine
secretin
    s. provocation
secretion
    adrenocortical s.
    mineralocorticoid s.
    sinonasal s.
secretory
    s. adenocarcinoma
    s. carcinoma
    s. component
    s. disease
    s. immunoglobulin
section
    axial s.
    cross s.
    cryostat s.
    fresh-frozen tissue s.
    frozen tissue s.
    midfrontal plane coronal s.

paraffin tissue s.
plastic s.
sagittal s.
tissue s.
sectional radiography
sector
s. scan
s. scanning
s. transducer
secular equilibrium
secundum
ostium s.
septum s.
sedation
sedative
sedimentation
sucrose gradient s.
sedimented calcium
Sedlachek program
seed
gold s.
seen on-end
SEER
surveillance-epidemiology-end
results
segment
A 1 s.
A 2 s.
aganglionic s.
atretic s.
blind s.
bronchopulmonary s.
constant s.
diversity s.
intercalated s.
joining s.
pseudogene s.
s. substitution
variable s.
segmental
s. artery
s. atelectasis
s. biliary obstruction
s. bronchus
s. limb pressure recording
s. neurofibromatosis
s. pneumonia

segmentation
s. anomaly
segmentectomy
Segond fracture
Segre chart
Segura basket
Seidelin body
Seinsheimer classification of
femoral fractures
seizure
partial complex s.
Seldinger
S. needle
S. technique
selection
s. bias
coil s.
delay time s.
gradient s.
guidance system s.
positive s.
site s.
slice s.
selective
s. arterial magnetic
resonance angiography
chemical shift s. (CHESS)
s. excitation
s. excitation projection
reconstruction imaging
s. injection
s. irradiation
s. laser sintering
s. pulse
s. reduction of pregnancy
s. salpingography
s. saturation
s. saturation recovery
s. venous magnetic
resonance angiography
selectivity
spatial s.
selenium
s. deficiency
s. plate
selenium-75 (^{75}Se)

NOTES

self-antigen
self-breast examination (SBE)
self-care
 s.-c. concept
 s.-c. deficit
self-esteem
self-expandable
 s.-e. intravascular stent
 s.-e. metallic stent
 s.-e. stent
self-expanding
 s.-e. endovascular prosthesis
 s.-e. metallic biliary stent
 s.-e. stainless steel stent
self-help group
self-renewal
sella
 dorsum s.
 s. turcica
sellae
 diaphragma s.
Seller stain
Selrodo nebulizer
semicircular canal
semi-invasive aspergillosis
semiliquid feces
semilobar holoprosencephaly
semilunar
 s. fold
 s. notch
semilunaris
 hiatus s.
semimembranosus
 s. bursa
 s. tendon
seminal
 s. tract
 s. vesicle
 s. vesicle cyst
seminiferous tubular damage
seminoma
 extragonadal s. (EGS)
 testicular s.
semiopaque
semiovate
 cerebrum s.
semirigid dilator
semisolid fecal material
semitendinosus tendon
semiupright
 s. position
 s. view
Semple vaccine

semustine
Sendai virus
Senear-Usher syndrome
senescence
 premature placental s.
senescent change
senile
 s. change
 s. fibroma
senile fibroma
Senning procedure
sensitive
 s. plane
 s. plane projection
  reconstruction imaging
 s. point
 s. volume
sensitivity
 s. analysis
 contrast s.
 culture and s.
 spectral s.
sensitization
 HLA s.
 protracted exposure s.
sensitizer
 cell s.
 s. enhancement ratio
 hypoxic s.
 hypoxic cell s.
 radiation s.
sensitizing gradient
sensitometry
Sensorcaine
sensory
 s. nucleus
 s. strip
sentinel
 s. clot
 s. fracture
 S. II
 s. loop
 s. loop sign
 s. node
SEP
 separation of ghosts
separation
 acromioclavicular joint s.
 chorioamniotic s.
 fat/water signal s.
 frequency s.
 s. of ghosts (SEP)
 meniscotibial s.

meniscocapsular s.
shoulder s.
sepsis
biliary s.
postoperative s.
septa
fibrous s.
septal
s. cartilage plate
s. defect
s. hypertrophy
interventricular s. defect
s. line
s. notch
Septata intestinalis
septate
s. hypertrophy
s. uterus
septation
gallbladder s.
septic
s. arthritis
s. diskitis
s. pulmonary embolism
s. sacroiliitis
s. shock
septicemia
bacterial s.
septic sacroiliitis
septooptic dysplasia
septostomy
atrial s.
balloon atrial s. (BAS)
Septra DS
septum
atrial s.
s. cavum vergae
femoral s.
interatrial s.
interlobular s.
interventricular s.
Körner s.
median s.
nasal s.
s. pellucidum
placental s.
s. primum

rectogenital s.
rectovaginal s.
s. secundum
subarachnoid s.
s. transversum defect
ventricular s.
septus
uterus s.
sequela, pl. sequelae
s. to recent trauma
sequelae
pulmonary s.
sequence
amino acid s.
amnion rupture s.
Carr-Purcell s. (CP sequence)
Carr-Purcell-Meiboom-Gill s.
(CPMG sequence)
CPMG s.
diffusion-sensitive s.
double inversion recovery s.
early amnion rupture s.
FAST pulse s.
FISP pulse s.
FLAIR pulse s.
FLASH pulse s.
gene s.
gradient-echo s.
GRASS pulse s.
heptamer/nonamer s.
hypervariable s.
inversion recovery s.
inversion recovery spin-
echo s. (IRSE sequence)
IRSE s.
missing pulse steady-state
free precession s.
multiplanar gradient
refocused s.
oblique sagittal s.
PRIME pulse s.
s. pulse
pulse s.
repetitive pulse s.
Shine-Dalgamo s.
short repetition time s.
simulated-echo s.

NOTES

sequence *(continued)*
- single-echo versus multiple-echo s.
- spin-echo s.
- spin-echo pulse s.
- STIR s.
- Szumowski s.
- s. time
- twin-reversed arterial perfusion s.
- velocity-encoded s.

sequencing
- DNA s.
- gene s.
- kinetic-based s.

sequential
- s. chemotherapy
- s. circulator
- s. determinant
- s. filming
- s. first-pass imaging
- s. line imaging
- s. plane imaging
- s. point imaging
- s. postremission chemotherapy (sPC)
- s. transplant

sequestered
- s. antigen
- s. disk

sequestration
- bronchopulmonary s.
- disk s.
- extralobar s.
- extrapulmonary s.
- intralobar s.
- pulmonary s.

sequestrum
- button s.

sequoiosis
sera (*pl. of* serum)
Serax
serial
- s. film changer
- s. radiography

sericite pneumoconiosis
series
- gastrointestinal s.
- Hoffmeister s.
- metabolic bone s.
- small bowel s.
- upper gastrointestinal s.
- upper GI s.

serine
- s. esterase
- s. kinase
- s. protease inhibitor
- s. proteinase

SER-IV
- supination-external rotation IV
- SER-IV fracture

seroconversion
seroconverted
serodefined
- s. antigen

serological window
serologic marker
seroma
- postoperative s.

seronegative
- s. AIDS

seropositive
seroprevalence
seroreverter
serosal invasion
serotonergic-induced emetic response
serotonin
- s. antagonist
- s. flush
- s. receptor

serous
- s. adenocarcinoma
- s. carcinoma
- s. cyst
- s. cystadenocarcinoma
- s. cystadenoma
- s. effusion
- s. ovarian tumor

serpentine aneurysm
serpiginosum
- angioma s.

serpiginous
serpin
serrated appearance
Serratia
- *S. liquefaciens*
- *S. marcescens*
- *S. proteamaculans*

serratus
- s. anterior
- s. anterior muscle

Sertoli
- S. cell
- S. cell tumor

Sertoli-Leydig cell tumor
serum, pl. **sera**
    anticrotalus s.
    antimouse lymphocyte s.
    s. bilirubin concentration
    s. chemistry
    s. creatinine
    despeciated s.
    s. glutamate pyruvate
      transaminase (SGPT)
    s. glutamic-oxaloacetic
      transaminase (SGOT)
    s. hepatitis antigen
    immune s. (IS)
    s. methylmalonic acid
    s. parathyroid hormone
    s. phenytoin level
    Sclavo s.
    s. sickness syndrome
    s. soluble receptor
    s. thyroglobulin
    s. tissue polypeptide antigen
    (S-TPA)
    s. TPA
    s. tumor marker
    Yersin s.
Servelle vein
service
    bereavement s.'s
    emotional support s.'s
Servox amplifier
sesamoid
    s. bone
    s. injury
sessile
    s. lesion
    s. polyp
sestamibi
    technetium-99m s.
    s. technetium-99m
set
    Amplatz dilator s.
    Boren-McKinney retriever s.
    Cope suture s.
    Curry intravascular
    retriever s.

    Dotter intravascular
    retrieval s.
    Greene biopsy s.
    Hawkins inside-out
    nephrostomy s.
    LifePort infusion s.
    MegaFlo infusion s.
    Myelo-Nate s.
    Rutner balloon dilatation
    helical stone extractor s.
    Soluset IV s.
    van Sonnenberg modified
    coaxial biopsy s.
Sever disease
severe
    s. combined
    immunodeficiency (SCID)
    s. combined
    immunodeficiency disease
    (SCID)
    s. combined
    immunodeficiency
    syndrome
SEW
    slice excitation wave
sex
    s. assignment
    casual s.
    communal s.
    s. cord stromal tumor
    high-risk s.
    s. hormone
    illicit s.
    recreational s.
    s. steroid
sex-conditioned gene
sex-linked
    s.-l. gene
    s.-l. hypogammaglobulinemia
    s.-l. lymphoproliferative
    syndrome
sex-reversal gene
sextuplet pregnancy
sexual
    s. activity
    s. arousal
    s. differentiation disorder

NOTES

sexual *(continued)*
    s. function
    s. problem
sexually-transmitted disease (STD)
Sézary
    S. cell
    S. lymphoma cell
    S. syndrome
SFA
    superficial femoral artery
SGO
    Society of Gynecologic Oncology
SGOT
    serum glutamic-oxaloacetic
      transaminase
SGPT
    serum glutamate pyruvate
      transaminase
shading
    image s.
shadow
    acoustic s.
    s. box
    cardiac s.
    cardiothymic s.
    cardiovascular s.
    s. cell
    concatenation of s.'s
    double-arc s.
    hilar s.
    hilar s.'s
    nipple s.
    overlying bowel s.'s
    psoas s.
    radiographic parallel line s.
    renal and psoas s.'s
    soft tissue s.
    summation of s.'s
    wall-echo s. (WES)
shadowing
    acoustical s.
    rib s.
Shaffer-Hartmann method
shaft
    femoral s.
    s. flange
    s. fracture
shaggy heart border
Shagreen rough skin patch
shallow
    s. inspiration
    s. inspiratory effort
SH antigen

shape
    line s.
    peak s.
    pulse s.
shaped pulse
shaper
    beam s.
shared epitope
shark
    s. cartilage
    s. powder
Sharpey fibers
Shaver disease
shear
    s. fracture
    s. interface
shearing
    s. force
    s. injury
sheath
    arterial s.
    axillary s.
    bicipital tendon s.
    carotid s.
    Check-Flo s.
    Colapinto s.
    femoral s.
    giant cell tumor of
      tendon s.
    introducer s.
    nerve root s.
    peel-away s.
    periarteriolar lymphoid s.
    synovial s.
    Teflon s.
    tendon s.
    working s.
sheathed needle
shedding
    viral s.
Sheehan syndrome
sheep
    s. cell agglutination test
      (SCAT)
    s. erythrocyte rosette
sheet
    beta-pleated s.
    s. sign
sheetlike growth pattern
shelf
    Blumer s.
shell
    K s.

s. nephrogram
s. type of periosteal
reaction
s. vial technique
shell-of-bone appearance
shelving edge
Shenton line
Shepherd fracture
shepherd's
s. crook catheter
s. crook configuration
s. crook deformity
shield
active s.
Dalkon s.
Faraday s.
lead s.
passive s.
radiofrequency s.
shielding
s. of the abdomen and
pelvis
lung s.
magnetic s.
passive s.
surface s.
shift
chemical s.
colloid s.
distal s.
fluorescent s.
mediastinal s.
midline s.
motion-induced phase s.
phase s.
s. probe
s. reagent
square s.
Shigella
S. *flexneri*
S. *sonnei*
shigellosis
shiitake mushroom
shim
s. coil
shimming
active s.

localized s.
passive s.
Shine-Dalgamo sequence
shin splints
Shirner test
Shirodkar cerclage
shish
s. kebab esophagus
s. kebab pattern
Shmoo sign
shock
s. block
cardiac s.
septic s.
s. wave pressure
shocklike syndrome
shock-wave lithotripsy
Shohl solution
Shone syndrome
Shope
S. fibroma
S. fibroma virus
short
s. bowel syndrome
s. esophagus type hiatal
hernia
s. inversion recovery
imaging (STIR)
s. limb dysplasia
s. oblique fracture
s. repetition time sequence
s. rib
s. rib-polydactyly syndrome
s. tau inversion recovery
(STIR)
s. TI inversion recovery
(STIR)
shortening
T1 s.
T2 s.
short-increment sensitivity index
short-range isotope
short-T2 in anisotropic rotation
shot
fast low-angle s. (FLASH)
pocket s.
shotty node

NOTES

505

shoulder
  curvilinear threshold s. (Dq)
  s. dislocation
  frozen s.
  s. girdle
  s. impingement
  s. impingement syndrome
  s. joint
  s. labral-capsular complex
  s. pad sign
  s. separation
shoulder-hand syndrome
shower
  golden s.'s
shrapnel
Shrapnell membrane
shrinkage
  tumor s.
shrinking field
shrunken bladder
shunt
  aorticopulmonary window s.
  arteriovenous s.
  Blalock-Taussig s.
  cerebral s.
  Cimino dialysis s.
  Denver ascites s.
  Denver peritoneovenous s.
  distal splenorenal s.
  end-to-side portacaval s.
  E-PTFE s.
  s. fraction
  Glenn s.
  s. infection
  intracardiac s.
  intrahepatic portacaval s.
  intrahepatic portosystemic
    venous s.
  jejunoileal s.
  left-to-right s.
  LeVeen s.
  s. to the lung
  mesoatrial s.
  mesocaval s.
  partial s.
  polytetrafluoroethylene s.
  portacaval s.
  portohepatic venous s.
  portosystemic s.
  Pott s.
  pulmonary arteriovenous s.
  right-to-left s.
  Scribner s.

  splenocaval s.
  splenorenal s.
  surgical portosystemic s.
  systemic s.
  systemic-pulmonic s.
  transjugular intrahepatic
    portosystemic s.
  Trueta s.
  s. tubing
  s. valve
  venous s.
  ventricular s.
  ventriculoatrial s.
  ventriculoperitoneal s.
  vesicoamniotic s.
  Warren s.
  Waterston-Cooley s.
shunting
  arterioportal venous s.
  blood s.
  peritoneovenous s.
  pleuroperitoneal s.
  s. of tracer to the bone
    marrow
shuntography
shuttle protein
Shwartzman reaction
Shy-Drager syndrome
SI
  International System of Units
  SI variant of HIV
S/I
  superior/inferior
SIADH
  syndrome of inappropriate
    secretion of antidiuretic
    hormone
sialadenitis
  acute suppurative s.
  autoimmune s.
  recurrent s.
sialectasis
sialic
  s. acid
  s. acid tumor marker
sialoadenitis
  myoepithelial s.
sialoglycoprotein
sialography
  parotid gland s.
  submaxillary s.
sialolithiasis
sialometaplasia

sialometry
sialophorin
sialosis
sialyl
    s. Lewis necroinflammation-
        associated carbohydrate
        antigen
    s. Lex antigen
    s. Tn antigen (STN)
Sia test
SIBC
    synchronous ipsilateral breast
    cancer
siboroxime
    technetium-99m s.
sicca
    keratoconjunctivitis s.
    s. symptom
    s. syndrome
sickle
    s. cell
    s. cell anemia
    s. cell crisis
    s. cell disease
    s. cell trait
Sickledex reagent
sickle-Thal disease
sickling
sickness
    decompression s.
side
    s. chain
    s. lobe artifact
    s. scatter
Sideris buttoned double-disk device
sideroblast
    refractory anemia with
      ring s.'s
sideroblastic
    s. anemia
siderosis
siderotica
    granulomatosis s.
siderotic nodule
sideswipe fracture
side-to-side anastomosis
sidewinder catheter

Siemens Lithostar lithotripter
sievert
sigma
    s. filter
    s. receptor
sigmoid
    s. colon
    s. diverticulum
    s. mesocolon
    s. notch
    s. sinus
    s. volvulus
sigmoidoscopy
sign
    1-2-3 s.
    air-crescent s.
    apical cap s.
    asterisk s.
    banana s.
    barber pole s.
    bare-area s.
    B6 bronchus s.
    beak s.
    Bergman s.
    bird-of-prey s.
    bladder-within-bladder s.
    bowler hat s.
    bronchus s.
    s. of the burnuous
    s. of the burnuous
      appearance
    calcification s.
    calcium s.
    s. of the camalote
    Carman meniscal s.
    caterpillar s.
    catheter-coiling s.
    celery stalk s.
    cervix s.
    chicken roosting s.
    cobra head s.
    coffee s.
    coffee bean s.
    Coke bottle s.
    collapsing cord s.
    colon cutoff s.
    comet s.

NOTES

sign *(continued)*
comet tail s.
comma s.
cord s.
crescent s.
crow-foot s.
cutoff s.
delta s.
diamond s.
diaphragm s.
differential density s.
dimple s.
displaced crus s.
dog-ear s.
double-arc shadow s.
double-ball s.
double-barrel shotgun s.
double-bleb s.
double-bubble s.
double-decidual s.
double-duct s.
double-line s.
double-target s.
double-track s.
doughnut s.
draping s.
drooping lily s.
empty delta s.
empty triangle s.
fallen fragment s.
fallen lung s.
fat pad s.
fawn tail s.
figure-3 s.
figure-8 s.
fissure s.
flag s.
Fleischner s.
floppy thumb s.
football s.
Frostberg-3 s.
Frostberg inverted-3 s.
Gage s.
garland s.
geyser s.
Gibson s.
gloved-finger s.
goblet s.
Grey Turner s.
halo s.
hatchet s.
Hellmer s.
hepatic angle s.

hilar comma s.
hilar waterfall s.
Homans s.
Hoover s.
indistinct liver s.
inferior triangle s.
infundibulum s.
intradecidual s.
inverted-V s.
Kernig s.
Kirklin s.
kissing cousin s.
knuckle s.
Kussmaul s.
lemon s.
Leser-Trélat s.
lily-pad s.
localizing s.
melting s.
meniscus s.
Mercedes-Benz s.
metacarpal s.
Mexican hat s.
moon s.
moulage s.
mouse bed s.
mucosal stripe s.
Murphy s.
mushroom s.
mustache s.
naked-facet s.
Napoleon hat s.
notch s.
nubbin s.
pad s.
parallel channel s.
Parke corner s.
pearl-and-string s.
pleural tail s.
Poppel s.
posterior drawer s.
pronator fat pad s.
pseudokidney s.
pseudotumor s.
radiolucent crescent s.
railroad track s.
ram's horn s.
rebound s.
reversed-three s.
reverse figure-3 s.
reverse-S s.
Rigler s.
rim s.

ring s.
Risser s.
saddlebag s.
sail s.
sandwich s.
saw tooth s.
scottie dog s.
seagull s.
secondary s.
sentinel loop s.
sheet s.
Shmoo s.
shoulder pad s.
signet ring s.
silhouette s.
Spalding s.
spring onion s.
squeeze s.
steeple s.
Steinberg s.
stellate s.
stretch s.
string s.
string-and-double-track s.
string-of-beads s.
stripe s.
superior triangle s.
Swiss cheese s.
tail s.
target s.
telltale triangle s.
Terry Thomas s.
Tinel s.
transverse stripe s.
triple-bubble s.
triple-track s.
trolley-track s.
trough s.
trumpet s.
urachal s.
vacuum s.
wall s.
waterfall right hilum s.
water lily s.
wave s.
Westermark s.
whirl s.

Wimberger s.
wooden shoe s.
Yergason s.
signal
    s. attenuation
    s. average
    composite s.
    s. depth
    Doppler s.
    s. drop-out artifact
    gamma s.
    high-intensity s.
    s. intensity
    s. intensity ratio
    s. joint
    s. loss
    nuclear s.
    proton magnetic
        resonance s.
    s. transducer
    s. transduction
    s. void
signal-to-noise
    s.-t.-n. calculation
    s.-t.-n. ratio (SNR, S/N
        ratio)
signature
    gut s.
signet-ring
    s.-r. cell
    s.-r. cell carcinoma
signet ring sign
significance
    atypical cell of
        undetermined s.
    s. level
    monoclonal gammopathy of
        undetermined s.
significant
    hemodynamically s.
sign-of-the-burnuous appearance
Silastic
    S. catheter
    S. double-J stent
    S. hemodialysis catheter
    S. microsphere

NOTES

Silastic *(continued)*
    S. stent
    S. tube
silent gene
silhouette
    cardiac s.
    cardiovascular s.
    heart s.
    s. sign
    s. sign of Felson
silhouetted out
silicate pneumoconiosis
silicon
    s. diode array
    s. granuloma
silicone
    s. fluid
    s. implant
    s. implant leakage
    s. injection
    s. microsphere
    s. rubber
silicon granuloma
silicoproteinosis
silicosis
    complicated s.
    simple s.
silicotic material
silicotuberculosis
silk
    s. suture
    s. tuft
sillimanite pneumoconiosis
silo-filler's
    s.-f. disease
    s.-f. lung
silver
    s. fork deformity
    Gomori methenamine s.
    Grocott methenamine s.
    s. halide film
    s. recovery
    s. stain
simiae
    Herpesvirus s.
simian
    s. AIDS (SAIDS)
    s. crease
    s. foamy virus
    s. immunodeficiency virus
    (SIV)
simian-human immunodeficiency
  virus

Simmond disease
Simmons catheter
Simon
    S. filter
    S. focus
    S. septic factor
Simon-Nitinol inferior vena cava
  filter
Simonsen phenomenon
SIM/Plant
Simplastin Excel
Simplastin L
simple
    s. achlorhydric anemia
    s. bone cyst
    s. capillary lymphangioma
    s. cortical cyst
    s. cyst
    s. silicosis
simplex
    carcinoma s.
    herpes s. (HS)
Simpson
    S. atherectomy
    S. atherectomy device
    S. atherocath
    S. directional atherectomy
    catheter
simulated-echo
    s.-e. artifact
    s.-e. sequence
simulation
    Monte Carlo s.
simulator
    Nucletron s.
simultaneous volume imaging
sincalide
Sinding-Larsen-Johansson disease
Sinemet
Sinequan
sine wave
single
    s. chemotherapy
    s. outlet of heart
    s. photon absorptiometry
    s. photon emission
    computed tomography
    (SPECT)
    s. photon emission
    tomography (SPET)
    s. umbilical artery
    s. ventricle

single-agent
   s.-a. chemotherapy
   s.-a. high-dose chemotherapy
single-day infuser
single-donor
   s.-d. apheresis
   s.-d. blood component
   s.-d. platelets
single-echo
   s.-e. diffusion imaging
   s.-e. versus multiple-echo
     sequence
single-fraction total body
  irradiation
single, nonbarbed Gianturco stent
single-shot imaging technique
single-slice
   s.-s. gradient-echo image
   s.-s. modified KEW direct
     Fournier imaging
single-stick method
single-use diagnostic system
  (SUDS)
sink
   s. effect
   quantum s.
sinoatrial
   s. node (SA)
Sinografin
sinonasal
   s. carcinoma
   s. cavity
   s. lesion
   s. lymphoma
   s. psammomatoid ossifying
     fibroma
   s. secretion
   s. tumor
sinovaginal bulb
sintering
   selective laser s.
sinus
   branchial s.
   bronchial s.
   s. cavity
   dermal s. tract
   dilated intercavernous s.

   dural s.
   endodermal s.
   ethmoid s.
   frontal s.
   s. histiocyte
   s. histiocytosis
   s. hyperplasia
   hypoechoic renal s.
   intercavernous s.
   s. lateralis
   maxillary s.
   s. of Morgagni
   occipital s.
   paranasal s.
   s. pattern
   s. pericranii
   petrosal s.
   piriform s.
   pyriform s.
   s. rhythm
   Rokitansky-Aschoff s.'s
    (RAS)
   sagittal s.
   sigmoid s.
   sphenoid s.
   sphenoparietal s.
   s. thrombosis
   s. tract
   transverse s.
   s. of Valsalva aneurysm
   s. venosus
   s. venosus atrial septal
    defect
sinusitis
   bacterial s.
   s. cerebritis
   paranasal s.
sinusoid
sinusoidal
   s. histiocyte
   s. lesion
   s. relaxation
   s. waveform
sinuum
   confluens s.
siphon
   carotid s.

NOTES

Sipple syndrome
Sips plot
sirenomelia
sirenomyelia
sister
    s. chromatid exchange
    S. Mary Joseph node
site
    angulation at the fracture s.
    antibody reaction s.
    antigen binding s.
    binding s.
    bleeding s.
    carcinoma of uncertain
     primary s. (CUPS)
    Chi s.
    donor s.
    extranodal s.
    fracture s.
    lectin-binding s.
    sanctuary s.
    s. selection
    splice s.
    unknown primary s.
site-specific
    s.-s. surgery
    s.-s. treatment
situ
    adenocarcinoma in s.
    carcinoma in s. (CIS)
    ductal carcinoma in s.
    (DCIS)
    in s.
    lobular carcinoma in s.
    malignant melanoma in s.
situs
    s. ambiguus
    atrial s.
    s. indeterminatus
    s. inversus
    s. solitus
    s. viscus inversus
sitz marker
SIV
    simian immunodeficiency virus
sixth
    s. disease
    s. nucleus
size
    borderline heart s.
    cell s.
    focal spot s.
    sample s.

    uterine s.
    voxel s.
    x-ray beam s.
Sjögren syndrome
SK
    Sloan-Kettering
    streptokinase
skeletal
    s. biopsy
    s. dysplasia
    s. hyperostosis
    s. lesion
    s. lymphoma
    s. metastasis
    s. neoplasm
    s. radiology
    s. survey
    s. system
skeleton
    appendicular s.
    axial s.
    laryngeal s.
SK & F 104864
    topotecan
skier's
    s. fracture
    s. thumb
Skillern fracture
skimming of magnetic field
skin
    s. biopsy
    s. cahedrin
    s. calcification
    s. cancer
    s. collimation
    s. depth
    s. disorder
    s. effect
    s. fold
    s. fold artifact
    granulomatous slack s.
    s. lesion
    s. lesion artifact
    mixed tumor of s.
    peau d'orange s.
    s. pore
    s. reactive factor
    s. staple
    talc on the s.
    s. thickening
skinning vulvectomy
skinny needle

skin-specific histocompatibility
  antigen
Skiodan
    S. Acacia
skip
    s. area
    s. lesion
    s. metastasis
Skipper-Schabel model
ski proto-oncogene
SKSD
    streptokinase-streptodornase
skull
    abnormally thin s.
    s. base
    s. base tumor
    cloverleaf s.
    cotton-wool s.
    s. fracture
    geographic s.
    inner table of the s.
    lacunar s.
    outer table of the s.
    thin s.
SKY pain control system
slab
slack-skin syndrome
slanting
    tibiotalar s.
SLAP
    superior labral anteroposterior
    superior labrum, anterior-to-
      posterior
    SLAP injury
    SLAP lesion
slash defect
SLE
    systemic lupus erythematosus
sleep apnea
sleeve
    Eichelter s.
    s. fracture
    s. lobectomy
    nerve root s.
    thoracic root s.
slew rate

slice
    s. excitation wave (SEW)
    s. interference
    nonplanar s.
    oblique s.
    s. point MRS
    s. profile artifact
    s. selection
    s. thickness
slice-of-sausage pattern
slice-selective excitation
slide
    poly-L-lysine s.
slider crank theory
sliding hiatal hernia
slim disease
sling
    pulmonary s.
slip
    diaphragmatic s.
    muscular s.
slipped
    s. capital femoral
    s. capital femoral epiphysis
    s. epiphysis
slip-ring gantry system
slit radiography
Sloan-Kettering (SK)
slope
    PSA s.
Slo-Phyllin
slot-blot
    s.-b. hybridization analysis
    s.-b. technique
slow
    s. exchange soft tissue
    s. hemoglobin
    s. release (SR)
SL technique
    spin-lock imaging technique
sludge
    s. ball
    gallbladder s.
    tumefactive s.
    tumefactive biliary s.
sludged blood

NOTES

sludge-like intraluminal echo
sludging of retinal vein
Sly syndrome
SM 5887
SMA
    smooth muscle actin
    superior mesenteric artery
small
    s. bone enteroscopy
    s. bore needle
    s. bowel
    s. bowel atresia
    s. bowel cancer
    s. bowel diverticulum
    s. bowel enema
    s. bowel enteroscopy
    s. bowel fold
    s. bowel follow-through
    examination
    s. bowel hemorrhage
    s. bowel obstruction
    s. bowel series
    s. bowel transit
    s. bowel tumor
    s. bowel ulcer
    s. caliber needle
    s. cell carcinoma
    s. cell lung cancer (SCLC)
    s. cell osteosarcoma
    s. cell undifferentiated
    carcinoma
    s. cleaved cell lymphoma
    s. intestine
    s. intestine cancer
    s. lymphocyte
    s. lymphocytic lymphoma
    s. lymphoid cell
    proliferation
    s. non-cleaved cell
    lymphoma
small-for-gestational-age fetus
smallpox
Sm antigen
smart
    s. laser
    s. laser catheter tip
    s. laser system
smear
    blood s.
    buffy coat s.
    cytospin s.
    Pap s.

    Papanicolaou s.
    Tzanck s.
smegma
S-method of dose calculation
SMF
    streptozotocin, mitomycin,
    5- fluorouracil
Smith
    S. fracture
    S. Malecot/ureteral stent
    S. Universal ureteral stent
Smith-Lemli-Opitz syndrome
Smith-Petersen
    S.-P. nail
    S.-P. pin
smokeless tobacco
smoking
    s. cessation
    cigarette s.
    passive s.
smoldering
    s. multiple myeloma
smooth
    s. border
    s. muscle
    s. muscle actin (SMA)
    s. muscle cell
    s. muscle tumor
smooth-bordered
smoothed curve fit
smudge cell
smudged papilla
Smythe syndrome
snake's head appearance
snare
    angiographic two-wire s.
    diathermic s.
    loop s.
    Nitinol goose-neck s.
    s. technique
sniff test
SNM
    Society of Nuclear Medicine
snowflake pattern
snowman
    s. abnormality
    s. heart configuration
snowplow effect
SNR
    signal-to-noise ratio
S/N ratio
    signal-to-noise ratio

snuffbox
anatomic s.
Snyder classification
soap
Bactoshield antibacterial s.
s. bubble appearance
calcium s.
Spectrum 2000
antibacterial s.
Soave procedure
social
s. environment
s. factor
s. support
Society
American Cancer S. (ACS)
American Roentgen Ray S.
S. of Gynecologic Oncology
(SGO)
S. of Magnetic Resonance
in Medicine
S. of Nuclear Medicine
(SNM)
Oncology Nursing S. (ONS)
Southeastern
Neuroradiological S.
S. of Surgical Oncology
(SSO)
Western
Neuroradiological S.
World Federation of
Neuroradiological S.
socioeconomic status
sodium
acyclovir s.
brequinar s.
chromotope s.
estramustine phosphate s.
s. heparin
s. imaging
s. iodide crystal
s. iodide iodine-131
ioxaglate s.
ipodate s.
liothyronine s.
meclofenamate s.
s. metrizoate

pertechnetate s.
s. phosphate
s. salicylate
technetium-99m s.
technetium-99m
pertechnetate s.
s. tetradecyl sulfate
s. thiosulfate
warfarin s.
sodium-23 (^{23}Na)
sodium-24 (^{24}Na)
sodium-2-mercaptoethane sulfonate
sodium iodide I 125
sodium iodide I 131
sodium phosphate P 32
Sof-Care
soft
s. infiltrate
s. palate
s. palate cancer
s. papilloma
s. pigment stone
s. pulse
s. tissue
s. tissue abscess
s. tissue calcification
s. tissue chondroma
s. tissue ossification
s. tissue sarcoma
s. tissue shadow
s. tissue structure
s. tissue swelling
s. tissue window
softener
stool s.
soft-tissue necrosis
software
solar radiation
**Solcotrans drainage/reinfusion
system**
sole laser therapy
solenoid
s. surface coil
soleus
solid
s. cell nest
s. organ transplant

NOTES

solid *(continued)*
    s. phase extraction
    s. tumor
    S. Tumor Autologous
      Marrow Transplant
      Program (STAMP)
solid-state detector
solitary
    s. bone cyst
    s. dilated duct
    s. gallstone
    s. myeloma
    s. osteochondroma
    s. plasmacytoma
    s. pulmonary mass
    s. pulmonary nodule
    s. relapse
    s. tumor
solitus
    situs s.
solium
    Taenia s.
Solomon-Bloembergen
    S.-B. equations
    S.-B. theory of dipole-dipole
      relaxation rate
Solu-Biloptin
soluble antigen excess
Solu-Cortef
Solu-Medrol
Soluset IV set
solute
solution
    aqueous s.
    Bouin s.
    Chloresium s.
    Drabkin s.
    Elliot B s.
    Fonio s.
    Gowers s.
    Hanks balanced salt s.
    Hayem s.
    hypertonic s.
    lactated Ringer s.
    Lugol s.
    Monsel s.
    phosphotope oral s.
    Schlesinger s.
    Shohl s.
    St. Thomas cardioplegic s.
    Xylocaine viscous s.
    Zenker s.
    zinc sulfate s.

Solutrast
solvent
    s. suppression
    s. water TI frequency
      dependence
Somacin formula
somatic
    s. hypermutation
    s. mutation
    s. mutation theory of
      cancer
somatosensory-evoked potential
somatostatin
    s. analog
somatostatinoma
somatotrophic adenoma
somatuline
    s. sulindac
somnolence
Somogyi unit
sonication
sonic thrombolysis
sonnei
    Shigella s.
sonogram
    dual transverse linear-
      array s.
    transabdominal s.
sonographic
    s. assessment
    s. guidance
sonography
    abdominal s.
    breast s.
    color-flow Doppler s.
    compression s.
    Doppler s.
    duplex s.
    endoluminal s.
    endoscopic s.
    endovaginal s.
    fatty meal s.
    intraoperative s. (IOS)
    obstetric s.
    pelvic s.
    penile s.
    thoracic s.
    transabdominal color
      Doppler s.
    transcranial real-time color-
      flow Doppler s.
    transrectal s.
    transvaginal s.

transvaginal hysterosalpingo-
contrast s.
sonologist
sonolucent
s. donut
s. halo
**Sorbie classification of calcaneal
fracture**
sorivudine
sorter
cell s.
fluorescence-activated cell s.
sorting
cell s.
Sos wire
Sotos syndrome
Sotradecol
sound
bowel s.'s
heart s.'s
pericardial knock s.
s. wave
**Southeastern Neuroradiological
Society**
Southern
S. blot
S. blot analysis
S. blot hybridization
S. blot technique
S. blot test
S. transfer analysis
soybean
s. agglutinin (SBA)
s. lectin T-lymphocyte-
depleted marrow graft
SpA
staphylococcal protein A
space
abdominal s.
acromioclavicular s.
anterior clear s.
arachnoid s.
buccal s.
coracoclavicular s.
disk s.
epidural s.
infraglottic s.

inframesocolic s.
intercostal s.
joint s.
κ s.
leptomeningeal s.
paralaryngeal s.
parapharyngeal s.
pararenal s.
peridental s.
perihepatic s.
perirenal s.
peritoneal s.
perivascular s.
pleural s.
popliteal s.
portal s.
posterior cervical s.
potassium s.
predental s.
preepiglottic s.
premasseteric s.
presacral s.
Prussak s.
retrocrural s.
retrogastric s.
retrosternal s.
retrosternal air s.
retrovesical s.
s. of Retzius
s. of Retzius abscess
subarachnoid s.
subdural s.
subhepatic s.
subphrenic s.
subpulmonic pleural s.
supracolic s.
suprahepatic s.
supratentorial s.
Traube semilunar s.
vascular s.
Virchow-Robin s.
widened retrogastric s.
κ space
space-occupying
s.-o. lesion
s.-o. process

NOTES

spade-like
> s.-l. appearance
> s.-l. hand

Spalding sign
SPARC glycoprotein
sparfloxacin
spark gap generator
Sparks mandrel graft
SPARS
> spatially-resolved spectroscopy

spasm
> arterial s.
> hemifacial s.

spastic
> s. colitis
> s. urinary bladder

spatial
> s. average-pulse average (SAPA)
> s. average-pulse average intensity
> s. average-temporal average (SATA)
> s. average-temporal average intensity
> s. encoding
> s. frequency
> s. localization procedure
> s. misregistration artifact
> s. modulation of magnetization
> s. offset image artifact
> s. peak-temporal average (SPTA)
> s. peak-temporal average intensity
> s. presaturation
> s. resolution
> s. selectivity

spatially-resolved spectroscopy (SPARS)
sPC
> sequential postremission chemotherapy

SPDP
> *N*-succinamidylproprionate

SPE
> sucrose polyester

Spearman rank
Spears laser balloon
special probe
species
> paramagnetic iron s.

therapeutic s.
toxic s.

species-specific
> s.-s. antigen
> s.-s. immunity

specific
> s. absorption rate
> s. cytoplasmic granule
> s. esterase stain
> s. immunotherapy
> s. macrophage-arming factor
> s. modulation

specificity
Specifid
specimen
> catheterized barbotage s.
> gross s.

SPECT
> single photon emission computed tomography
> dual-isotope SPECT
> SPECT imaging

spectra (*pl. of* spectrum)
spectral
> s. broadening
> s. distribution
> s. emission
> s. line
> s. pattern
> s. quality
> s. sensitivity
> s. width
> s. window

spectrin
spectrofluorometry
spectrometer
spectrophotometry
> atomic absorption s. (AAS)

spectroscopist
spectroscopy
> carbon-13 s.
> circular dichroism s.
> depth-resolved surface coil s. (DRESS)
> diffusion s.
> electrospray ionization mass s.
> flame emission s. (FES)
> fluorine-19 s.
> image-selected in vivo s.
> magnetic resonance s. (MRS)
> ^{31}P s.

phosphorus-31 s.
point-resolved s.
proton s.
proton nuclear magnetic
  resonance s.
spatially-resolved s. (SPARS)
surface-coil rotating-frame s.
spectrum, pl. **spectra**
  S. 2000 antibacterial soap
  S. DG-P pediatric cradle
  electromagnetic s.
  energy spectra
  frequency s.
  proton nuclear magnetic
    resonance s.
  ultraviolet s.
  Wiener s.
SPECTurn chair
specular
  s. reflection
  s. reflector
speech area
speed
  film s.
spell
  episodic s.'s
Spence
  tail of S.
Spengler fragment
spent phase
sperm
  s. count
  s. granuloma
spermatic
  s. artery
  s. cord
  s. vein
  s. venography
spermatocele
spermatogenesis
spermatotoxicity
SPET
  single photon emission
  tomography
SPGR
  spoiled GRASS

S-phase
  S-p. analysis
  S-p. fraction
  S-p. fractionation
sphenoethmoidal recess
sphenoid
  s. angle
  s. bone
  s. ridge
  s. ridge meningioma
  s. sinus
  s. sinus metastasis
sphenoidale
  planum s.
  pneumatosis s.
sphenoparietal
  s. sinus
  s. sulcus
sphere
  collagen s.
  gelatin s.
  s. organelle
spherical structure
spherocytosis
  hereditary s.
spheroid
sphincter
  anal s.
  external s.
  external urethral s.
  lower esophageal s.
  s. of Oddi
  s. pupillae
  pyloric s.
sphincterotome
sphincterotomy
sphincter-saving surgery
spiculated lesion
spicule
  bone s.
spider
  s. angioma
  s. cancer
  stainless steel s.
spiderlike pelvocaliceal system
Spiderlon

NOTES

spigelian
    s. fascia
    s. hernia
    s. lobe
Spigos protocol
spike
    monoclonal s.
    s. staple
spill
    ileal s.
    peritoneal s.
spin
    coupled s.
    s. density
    s. density weighted
    s. dephasing
    s. diffusion
    s. echo
    electron s.
    s. exchange
    s. flip
    high s.
    nuclear s.
    s. number
    s. quantum number
    s. tagging
    uncoupled s.
    s. vector
spina
    s. bifida
    s. bifida aperta
    s. bifida occulta
    s. ventosa
spinal
    s. accessory lymph node
    s. artery
    s. axis tumor
    s. block
    s. canal
    s. column stabilization
    s. concussion
    s. cord
    s. cord cleft
    s. cord compression
    s. cord infarct
    s. cord injury (SCI)
    s. cord injury without
      radiographic abnormality
      (SCIWORA)
    s. cord tumor
    s. dermal sinus tract
    s. diastematomyelia

    s. dural arteriovenous fistula
    s. dysraphism
    s. epidural abscess
    s. epidural angiolipoma
    s. epidural lymphoma
    s. fracture
    s. fusion
    s. growth
    s. infection
    s. inflammation
    s. meningioma
    s. muscular atrophy
    s. needle
    s. nerve
    s. osteochondrosis
    s. puncture
    s. stenosis
    s. vascular malformation
spindle
    s. cell
    s. cell carcinoma
    s. cell sarcoma
    s. cell sarcoma of vagina
    s. inhibitor
    muscle s.
    ureteral s.
spine
    bamboo s.
    caroticojugular s.
    cervical s.
    dens view of cervical s.
    dorsal s.
    fetal s.
    iliac s.
    ischial s.
    lumbar s.
    lumbosacral s.
    microcystic lumbar s.
    midthoracic s.
    nasal s.
    rugger-jersey s.
    thoracic s.
spin-echo
    s.-e. imaging
    s.-e. magnetic resonance
      imaging
    s.-e. pulse sequence
    s.-e. sequence
    s.-e. using repeated gradient
      echoes
    s.-e. versus

spin-lattice
    s.-l. relaxation
    s.-l. relaxation time
spin-lock imaging technique (SL technique)
spinnbarkeit
spinocerebellar tract
spinothalamic tract
spinous
    s. process
    s. process fracture
spin-phase
    s.-p. graph
    s.-p. phenomenon
spin-spin
    s.-s. coupling
    s.-s. relaxation
spin-warp imaging
spiral
    s. computed tomography
    s. CT
    s. CT scanning
    s. fracture
    s. oblique fracture
    s. scanning
    s. volumetric CT
spiramycin
spiritual pain
spirochetal meningoencephalitis
spirogermanium
spirohydantoin
    s. mustard
spiromustine
spironolactone
spiroplatin
Spitzer quality of life index
Spitz nevus
spitzoid malignant melanoma
splanchnic
    s. aneurysm
    s. blood
    s. nerve block
    s. vasculature
    s. venous system
splaying
spleen
    accessory s.

    s. colony assay
    ectopic s.
    s. immune reaction
    s. lesion
    ruptured s.
    wandering s.
splenectomy
splenic
    s. abscess
    s. angle
    s. arteriography
    s. artery
    s. artery pseudoaneurysm
    s. B-cell lymphoma
    s. bleeding
    s. calcification
    s. cyst
    s. embolization
    s. flexure
    s. flexure cancer
    s. hemangioma
    s. infarction
    s. lesion
    s. leukemia
    s. rupture
    s. torsion
    s. trauma
    s. vein
    s. vein thrombosis
    s. vessel
splenium
    s. of corpus callosum
splenocaval
    s. collateral
    s. shunt
splenoma
splenomegaly
splenomyelomalacia
splenoportal junction
splenorenal
    s. collateral
    s. ligament
    s. shunt
splenosis
    thoracic s.
splenunculus, pl. splenunculi
splice site

NOTES

splicing
> gene s.

splint
> shin s.'s

splinting

Spli-Prest
> S.-P. buffer
> S.-P. latex
> S.-P. negative control
> S.-P. plate
> S.-P. positive control

split
> s. cord
> s. cord syndrome
> s. cranium
> s. fracture
> s. image artifact
> s. notochord syndrome
> s. spinal cord

split-course technique

split-heel fracture

splitting fracture

Spli-Tube

spoiled
> s. gradient-echo imaging
> s. gradient-recalled
>   acquisition
> s. GRASS (SPGR)

spoiler
> s. gradient
> s. gradient patterns
> s. pulse

spoiling
> RF s.
> surface s.

spoke wheel pattern

spondylitic deformity

spondylitis
> ankylosing s.
> cryptococcal s.
> tuberculous s.

spondyloarthritis,
> pl. **spondyloarthritides**

spondyloepiphyseal dysplasia

spondylolisthesis

spondylolysis

spondylosis
> cervical spine s.
> s. deformans

sponge
> Collostat s.
> gelatin s.
> s. kidney

> medullary s.
> surgical s.

spongiform
> s. degeneration
> s. leukoencephalopathy

spongioblastoma

spongiosis

spongiosum
> corpus s.

spontanea
> dactylolysis s.

spontaneous
> s. abortion
> s. drainage
> s. fracture
> s. osteonecrosis
> s. pneumomediastinum
> s. pneumothorax
> s. regression
> s. renal hemorrhage

sporadic Burkitt lymphoma

Sporanox

sporotrichosis

Sporotrichum schenckii

spot
> blind s.
> café-au-lait s.'s
> coast of California café-au-
>   lait s.'s
> coast of Maine café au
>   lait s.'s
> cold s.
> s. compression
> s. compression magnification
>   mammography
> s. compression view
> cotton-wool s.
> cotton-wool s.
> s. film
> s. film radiography
> focal s.
> hot s.
> s. magnification
> s. radiograph
> Roth s.
> thermal hot s.

sprain fracture

spray
> Moi-Stir oral s.
> pulse fashion pulse s.
> resorcinol s.

spread
> s. Bragg peak

distant s.
halstedian concept of
   tumor s.
intraocular s.
lymphatic s.
pattern of s.
perineural tumor s.
regional s.
Sprengel deformity
springhook wire
spring onion sign
sprinter's fracture
S100 protein
Sprotte needle
sprue
   celiac s.
   nontropical s.
   tropical s.
SP-303T
SPTA
   spatial peak-temporal average
   SPTA intensity
spur
   bone s.
   bronchial s.
   calcaneal s.
   s. cell
   s. cell anemia
   Pelkan s
   plantar s.
spurious polycythemia
spurring
   marginal s.
   osteophytic s.
sputum
   induced s.
   s. study
squamocolumnar junction
squamosal suture
squamous
   s. carcinoma
   s. cell
   s. cell carcinoma (SCC)
   s. cell papilloma
   s. intraepithelial lesion
   s. metaplasia

   s. metaplasia white
     epithelium
   s. odontogenic tumor
square
   root mean s.
   s. shift
   s. wave
squared-off heart
squared patella
squeeze sign
SR
   saturation recovery
   slow release
   Oramorph S.
SR-2508
SR-4233
SR-1 antigen
***src* proto-oncogene**
SS-A antigen
SS-B antigen
S-sign of Golden
SSO
   Society of Surgical Oncology
SSTN
   Sandostatin
St.
   S. Anne-Mayo grading
     system
   S. John Wort
   S. Jude Children's Research
     Hospital
   S. Jude valve
   S. Thomas cardioplegic
     solution
^{89}St
   strontium-89
ST-1 immunotoxin
stab cell
stability
   s. of fracture
stabilization
   spinal column s.
stabilizer
   Kwik Board IV and arterial
     line s.
stable
   s. cavitation

NOTES

stable *(continued)*
  s. disease (SD)
  s. free radical
  s. xenon CT
Stachrom
  S. antiplasmin
  S. AT III
  S. dermatan sulfate
  S. heparin
  S. heparin cofactor II
  S. PA
  S. PAI
  S. PAI-3
  S. plasminogen
  S. Prekallikrein
  S. VII
  S. VIII:C
Stachrom protein C
Stachrom X
stack
  Golgi s.
stacked-coin appearance
Staclot protein
  S. p. C
  S. p. S
Stadol
staff cell
STAG
  striped tag myocardial tagging
    system
stage
  cell cycle s.
  Chang s.
  proliferative s.
  tumor s.
staghorn calculus
staging
  Ann Arbor classification of
    Hodgkin disease s.
  Black nuclear s.
  Breslow s.
  clinical s.
  Haaginsen s.
  Jewett-Strong-Marshall s.
  s. laparotomy
  League of Nations s.
  M. D. Anderson cancer s.
  multiple myeloma s.
  neoplasm s.
  physiologic s.
  Robson s.
  surgical-pathologic s.
  s. system

  Whitmore-Jewett prostate
    cancer s.
stagnant blood
stain
  acid-fast s.
  acid-Schiff s.
  calcofluor white s.
  carbolfuchsin s.
  chlorazol-fast pink s.
  chloroacetate esterase-
    butyrate esterase s.
  chromogranin s.
  Diff-Quik s.
  eosin s.
  fluorescent auramine-
    rhodamine s.
  Giemsa s.
  Gomori methenamine
    silver s.
  Gram s.
  Hansel s.
  Heidenhain iron
    hematoxylin s.
  hematoxylin and eosin s.
  immunocytochemical s.
  immunoperoxidase s.
  iron s.
  Kinyoun s.
  leukocyte acid
    phosphatase s.
  low-molecular keratin s.
  Masson trichrome s.
  mucicarmine s.
  myeloperoxidase s.
  nonspecific esterase s.
  PAS s.
  periodic acid-Schiff s.
  Perls s.
  port wine s.
  reticulin s.
  Schiff s.
  Seller s.
  silver s.
  specific esterase s.
  Sudan Black B s.
  toluidine blue s.
  TRAP s.
  trichrome s.
  Warthin-Starry s.
  Weigert iron hematoxylin s.
  Wilder reticulin s.
  Wright s.

Wright-Giemsa s.
Ziehl-Neelsen s.
staining
abnormal s.
bone marrow s.
Diff-Quik s.
immunohistologic s.
nonspecific s.
periodic acid s.
stainless
s. steel coil
s. steel microsphere
s. steel spider
stairstep fracture
stalactite phenomenon
Stamey suprapubic Malecot catheter
Stammer method
STAMP
Solid Tumor Autologous Marrow Transplant Program
STAMP therapy
standard
s. deviation
Greulich and Pyle bone age s.
s. regimen
s. sample
s. therapy
standardized care policy
standing wave
Stanford-type aortic dissection
stapedes (*pl. of* stapes)
stapedial
s. artery
s. otosclerosis
stapedius
stapes, pl. **stapedes**
staphylococcal
s. folliculitis
s. pneumonia
s. protein A (SpA)
s. scalded skin syndrome
Staphylococcus
s. albus

s. aureus
s. epidermidis
staphyloma
staple
metallic s.
skin s.
spike s.
stone s.
star
s. artifact
s. effect
starch
hydroxyethyl s.
s. microsphere
Starling
S. hypothesis
S. resistor
Starr-Edwards valve
starry sky pattern
stasis
chronic venous s.
s. edema
state
contrast-enhanced fast-acquisition steady s. (CE-FAST)
emotional s.
s. equilibrium
fast adiabatic trajectory in steady s. (FATS)
fetal behavioral s.
gradient-refocused acquisition in the steady s. (GRASS)
ground s.
high output s.
immune s.
immunodeficiency s.
neoplastic s.
oxidation s.
Profile of Mood S.'s
steady-s.
State-Trait Anxiety Inventory
static
s. coupling

NOTES

static *(continued)*
 s. gray scale ultrasound
  equipment
 s. magnetic field
station
 lymph node s.
stationary zero-order motion
Statistic
 Wilcoxan S.
statistical
 s. noise
 s. term
status
 cardiac s.
 nutritional s.
 performance s.
 ploidy s.
 receptor s.
 socioeconomic s.
 WHO performance s.
Stauffer syndrome
stave cell
stavudine
STD
 sexually-transmitted disease
SteadFAS
steady-state
 s.-s. free precession
 s.-s. gradient-echo imaging
steal
 pelvic s.
 subclavian s.
 s. syndrome
Stealth catheter balloon
STEAM
 stimulated-echo acquisition
  mode
steatosis
 hepatic s.
steel
 s. coil
 S. factor
steeple sign
steering
 beam s.
Steinberg sign
Stein-Leventhal syndrome
Steinstrasse **calculi**
**Stejskal and Tanner pulsed-
gradient spin-echo technique**
stellate
 s. border breast lesion
 s. cell necrosis

s. confluence
s. fracture
s. lesion
s. mass
s. sign
s. tear
stem
s. cell
s. cell autograft
s. cell concentrator
s. cell factor
s. cell gene therapy
s. cell infusion
s. cell leukemia
s. cell mobilization
s. cell pool
s. cell product
s. cell proliferation
s. cell recovery
s. cell transplant
stem-loop structure
stenogyria
stenosis, pl. stenoses
acquired spinal s.
ampullary s.
anastomotic s.
aortic s.
aqueductal s.
arterial s.
branch pulmonary artery s.
bronchial s.
canal s.
carotid s.
carotid artery s.
circumferential venous s.
congenital esophageal s.
foraminal s.
graft s.
hepatic artery s.
high-grade proximal s.
hourglass s.
hypertrophic pyloric s.
hypertrophic subaortic s.
idiopathic hypertrophic
 subaortic s.
ileal s.
iliac artery s.
infundibular s.
infundibular pulmonary s.
lateral recess s.
lumbar spine s.
membranous s.
mitral s.

mitral valve s.
osteal s.
papillary s.
pelvic venous s.
peripheral pulmonary
  artery s.
pulmonary valve s.
pulmonic s.
pyloric s.
renal artery s.
spinal s.
string-sign s.
subaortic s.
subglottic s.
subinfundibular
  pulmonary s.
subsonic s.
subvalvular s.
subvalvular aortic s.
subvalvular pulmonary s.
supravalvular s.
supravalvular aortic s.
supravalvular pulmonary s.
tracheal s.
tunnel subaortic s.
valvular s.
valvular aortic s.
stenotic
  s. esophagogastric
    anastomosis
  s. lesion
Stensen
  S. duct
  S. gland
Stenson foramen
stent
  Amplatz double-J s.
  Amplatz tapered
    pyeloureteral s.
  balloon-expandable s.
  balloon-expandable
    tantalum s.
  biliary s.
  Carey-Coons s.
  C-Flex s.
  C-Flex double-J s.
  s. construction

Cook s.
Cordis balloon
  expandable s.
double-barbed Gianturco s.
double-helix prostatic s.
double-J s.
double-J ureteral s.
double Malecot prostatic s.
double-pigtail s.
s. evaluation
Fabian prostatic s.
Gianturco s.
Gianturco-Rösch s.
Gianturco-Roubin balloon
  expandable s.
Gianturco self-expanding
  metallic s.
Gianturco self-expanding
  Z s.
Gianturco zigzag s.
Gibbons ureteral s.
looped Silastic Universal s.
Maass double-helix s.
Malecot s.
Medinvent s.
Medinvent vascular s.
Medtronic-Wiktor s.
Miller s.
nephroureteral s.
Nitinol s.
Palmaz balloon
  expandable s.
Palmaz-Schatz biliary s.
Percuflex antegrade s.
polyethylene double-pigtail s.
polyethylene ureteral s.
prostatic s.
Rabkin Nitinol coil s.
self-expandable s.
self-expandable
  intravascular s.
self-expandable metallic s.
self-expanding metallic
  biliary s.
self-expanding stainless
  steel s.
Silastic s.

NOTES

stent *(continued)*
    Silastic double-J s.
    single, nonbarbed
      Gianturco s.
    Smith Malecot/ureteral s.
    Smith Universal ureteral s.
    "stenting the s."
    Strecker intravascular
      flexible tantalum s.
    tandem s.
    Teflon s.
    ureteral s.
    urethral metallic s.
    urinary s.
    vascular s.
stent-graft
    covered s.-g.
Stenver view
stepladder appearance
step wedge
stercoral
    s. ulcer
    s. ulceration
stercoralis
    Strongyloides s.
stereography
stereoroentgenogram
stereoscopic view
stereotactic
    s. automated technique
    s. biopsy
    s. percutaneous needle
      biopsy
    s. radiosurgery
    s. radiotherapy
    s. surgery
    s. technique
stereotaxic localization frame
stereotaxis
stereotaxy
sterile pyuria
sterilization
Steripaque-BR
Steripaque-V
sternal
    s. abscess
    s. angle
    s. clip
    s. notch
    s. suture
Sternberger antibody sandwich
    technique
Sternberg sarcoma

Sterneedle test
sternochondral junction
sternoclavicular joint
sternocleidomastoid muscle
sternohyoid muscle
sternomanubrial joint
sternothyroid muscle
sternotomy
    median s.
    s. wire
sternum
    tie s.
steroid
    s. injection
    s. myopathy
    sex s.
    s. therapy
steroidal hormone
steroid-induced ulcer
steroidogenesis
steroid-refractory ITP
sterone
    dehydrotest s.
sterotactic brachytherapy
stertorous breathing
Stevens-Johnson syndrome
Stewart-Treves syndrome
Stickler disease
Stieda fracture
stiffener
    Dotter s.
    wire s.
stillbirth
Still disease
Stilphostrol
Stimate
stimulated
    s. echo
    s. echo artifact
stimulated-echo
    s.-e. acquisition mode
      (STEAM)
    s.-e. artifact
stimulation
    dorsal column s.
    electric s.
    high-voltage pulsed
      galvanic s. (HVPGS)
    s. scan
    TRH s.
stimulator
    long-acting thyroid s.
      (LATS)

transcutaneous electrical nerve s. (TENS)
sting
catfish s.
stipple cell
stippled
s. appearance
s. calcification
s. epiphysis
stippling
basophilic s.
STIR
short inversion recovery imaging
short tau inversion recovery
short TI inversion recovery
STIR image
STIR sequence
STIR technique
STN
sialyl Tn antigen
Stockholm technique for radium therapy
stocking
antiembolism s.'s
stoma
gastroenterostomy s.
Wang pleural s.
stomach
s. adenocarcinoma
body of the s.
s. bubble
s. cancer metastasis
cascade s.
s. cell
greater curvature of the s.
intrathoracic s.
J-shaped s.
leatherbottle s.
lesser curvature of the s.
s. narrowing
stomal
s. ulcer
s. ulceration
stomatitis
aphthous s.
mycotic s.

necrotizing s.
Vincent s.
stomatotoxicity
stone
s. basket
biliary s.
cholesterol s.
common bile duct s.
cystic duct s.
cystine s.
extrahepatic s.
fecal s.
gallbladder s.
intrahepatic s.
kidney s.
multiple s.'s
nonopaque s.
opaque s.
pigment s.
pituitary s.
radiolucent s.
renal s.
soft pigment s.
s. staple
ureteral s.
urinary s.
urinary bladder s.
stool
currant jelly s.
guaiac positive s.
melenic s.
occult blood in s.
s. softener
s. swabbing
stop
Waterhouse s.
storage
long-term s.
magnetic tape s.
storiform neurofibroma
storiform-pleomorphic pattern
Storm Von Leeuwen chamber
Stortz thoracoscope
S-TPA
serum tissue polypeptide antigen
straddle fracture

NOTES

straight
  s. back syndrome
  s. line recovery period
strand
  rabbit ears s.'s
strandy infiltrate
strangulated obstruction
S-transferase
  glutathione S.-t.
strap muscle
stratified squamous epithelium of portio vaginalis
strawberry gallbladder
straw-colored fluid
streak
  bunch-of-flowers s.'s
  candle-wax-dripping s.'s
  primitive s.
streaky density
streamer
Strecker intravascular flexible tantalum stent
strength
  field s.
streptavadin-biotin-peroxidase complex technique
streptavidin
streptococcal pneumonia
Streptococcus
  S. bovis
  S. faecalis
  S. mitis
  S. pneumoniae
  S. pyogenes
  S. viridans
streptococcus
  Bargen s.
streptokinase (SK)
  s. infusion
  s. resistance test
  s. therapy
streptokinase-streptodornase (SKSD)
streptolysin
Streptomyces
  S. antibioticus
  S. verticillus
streptomycin
streptozocin
streptozotocin (STZ)
streptozotocin, mitomycin, 5-fluorouracil (SMF)

stress
  s. endpoint
  endpoint of s.
  s. fracture
  hoop s.
  s. incontinence
  s. injury
  s. raiser
  s. reaction in exenteration
  s. test
  s. thallium image
  s. ulcer
  s. view
stress-induced ischemia
stress-strain curve
stretchability
  mucus s.
stretch sign
striated
  s. muscle
  s. nephrogram
striate vein
striations across image
striatum
  corpus s.
stricture
  anastomotic s.
  antral s.
  biliary s.
  choledochojejunostomy s.
  colonic s.
  common bile duct s.
  congenital urethral s.
  duodenal s.
  enteric s.
  esophageal s.
  gastroesophageal junction s.
  lye s.
  Makar s.
  pyloric s.
  ureteral s.
  urethral s.
stridor
  inspiratory s.
  laryngeal s.
string-and-double-track sign
string-of-beads
  s.-o.-b. appearance
  s.-o.-b. sign
string-of-pearls appearance
string sign
string-sign stenosis

strip
 Chiron s.
 s. scan
 sensory s.
stripe
 central high-signal
  intensity s.
 paratracheal tissue s.
 pleural s.
 psoas s.
 s. sign
 tracheal s.
 tracheal wall s.
striped tag myocardial tagging system (STAG)
stripping program
stroke
 cardiogenic s.
 s. count image
 s. count ratio
 embolic s.
 thrombotic s.
 s. volume
 s. volume ratio
stroke-like syndrome of aphasia
stroma
 bone marrow s.
 cartilage s.
 cervical s.
 collagen s.
 gonadal s.
 osteoid s.
 Rollet s.
stromal
 s. carcinoid of ovary
 s. cell
 s. cell tumor
 s. elements
 s. fibroblast
 s. rim
 s. tetranectin
 s. tumor
stromelysin
stromelysin-3
Strongyloides stercoralis
strongyloidiasis, strongyloidosis

strontium
 s. isotope
strontium-89 (^{89}St)
 s. chloride
structural
 s. anomaly
 s. gene
structure
 cervical s.
 collagenous s.
 cyclobutane dicarboxylation
  ring s.
 cystic s.
 glandular s.
 helix-loop-helix s.
 midline cystic s.
 müllerian s.
 musculoaponeurotic s.
 osseous s.
 ossification of
  cartilaginous s.
 peritubular vascular s.
 prominent ductal vascular s.
 soft tissue s.
 spherical s.
 stem-loop s.
 test tube s.
 tuboreticular s.
 vascular s.
structured
 s. noise
 s. water
struma
 s. ovarii
 Riedel s.
strut
 bone s.
 s. fracture
Stryker
 S. frame
 S. notch view
Stuart
 S. factor
 S. index
Stuart-Prower factor
stuck twin
study, pl. studies

NOTES

study *(continued)*
    animal s.
    barium s.
    bone length s.
    case-control s.
    cerebral perfusion s.
    Childhood Cancer
      Survivor S. (CCSS)
    cohort s.
    correlational s.
    correlative Doppler s.
    DNA hybridization s.
    double blind s.
    double-contrast barium s.
    DPTA CSF flow s.
    efficacy s.
    epidemiological s.
    gated blood pool s.
    gene rearrangement s.
    imaging s.
    intervention s.
    laboratory s.
    molecular s.
    molecular hybridization s.
    Multicenter AIDS Cohort S.
      (MACS)
    phantom s.
    postirradiation s.
    preclinical s.
    PVB s.
    radiobiologic s.
    radionuclide s.
    sputum s.
    thymidine suicide s.
    urodynamic s.
stump
    s. cancer
    cervical s.
Sturge-Weber
    S.-W. disease
    S.-W. syndrome
Sturge-Weber-Dimitri syndrome
stutzeri
    Pseudomonas s.
style
    coping s.
    life s.
styloglossus muscle
stylohyoid muscle
styloidium
    os s.
styloid process

stylomastoid
    s. foramen
stylopharyngeus
styptic
    Binelli s.
Stypven time test
STZ
    streptozotocin
subacromial
    s. bursa
    s. bursitis
subacute
    s. granulomatous
    s. necrotizing myelopathy
    s. sclerosing panencephalitis
    s. thyroiditis
subadditivity
subaortic stenosis
subarachnoid
    s. cistern
    s. cyst
    s. cysticercosis
    s. hemorrhage
    s. injection
    s. nerve block
    s. septum
    s. space
subarticular
    s. bone resorption
    s. pseudocyst
subastrocytic tumor
subblock
    rectifier s.
subcapital
    s. fracture
subcapsular
    s. hematoma
    s. hepatic necrosis
    s. renal hematoma
subcardinal vein
subcarinal
    s. angle
    s. lymph node
subchondral
    s. cyst
    s. osteosclerosis
    s. resorption
subchorial hemorrhage
subchorionic
    s. fibrin deposition
    s. hematoma
    s. hemorrhage

subclavian
s. apheresis
s. apheresis catheter
s. artery
s. catheter
s. central venous catheter insertion
s. line
s. steal
s. steal syndrome
s. thrombosis
s. vein
s. vein access catheter
s. vein occlusion
s. vein thrombosis
s. vessel
s. vessel thrombosis
subclavicular
subclavius
subclone
subcortical
s. arteriosclerotic encephalopathy
s. atherosclerotic encephalopathy
s. encephalopathy
subcostal plane
subcutaneous
s. arterial bypass graft
s. edema
s. emphysema
s. fat
s. implanted injection port
s. infusion
s. injection of contrast artifact
s. mastectomy
s. nodule
s. reservoir
s. sacrococcygeal myxopapillary ependymoma
s. tissue
s. tumor
subdeltoid
s. bursa
s. bursal effusion
s. fat plane obliteration

subdiaphragmatic abscess
subdivision
histologic s.
subdural
s. effusion
s. empyema
s. hematoma
s. hemorrhage
s. interhemispheric hematoma
s. needle
s. space
subendometrial halo
subependymal
s. cyst
s. germinolysis
s. giant cell
s. giant cell astrocytoma
s. hemorrhage
s. oligodendroglioma
s. vein
subependymoma
suberosis
subfascial hematoma
subgaleal hematoma
subglottic
s. hemangioma
s. inverted V
s. narrowing
s. stenosis
subhepatic
s. abscess
s. space
subinfundibular pulmonary stenosis
subintimal filling
sublethal
s. gene
s. x-ray damage repair
subleukemic leukemia
sublingual gland
subluxation
atlantoaxial s.
recurrent lateral patellar s.
rotary s.
submandibular
s. duct

NOTES

submandibular *(continued)*
   s. ganglion
   s. gland
submaxillary
   s. gland
   s. sialography
   s. view
submembranous placental
  hematoma
submental vertex projection
submentovertex
   s. radiograph
   s. view
submentovertical projection
submicron
   s. magnetic particle
   s. magnetic principle
submucosal
   s. circular fold
   s. fold
suboptimal
   s. examination
   s. surgery
subpectoral implant
subperiosteal
   s. cortical abrasion
   s. cortical defect
   s. desmoid
   s. fracture
   s. hematoma
   s. hemorrhage
   s. infection
   s. resorption
subphrenic
   s. abscess
   s. fluid
   s. space
subpopulation
subpulmonic
   s. effusion
   s. pleural space
subscapulans tendon tear
subscapular
   s. bursa
   s. notch syndrome
subscapularis
   s. recess
   s. tendon
subsecond FLASH imaging
subsegmental
   s. atelectasis
   s. perfusion defect

subseptus
   uterus s.
subset
   organ-restricted lymphoid s.
   T-lymphocyte s.
subsonic stenosis
substance
   brain s.
   diamagnetic s.
   thyrotropic s.
substantia nigra
substernal thyroid gland
substitute
   blood s.
   saliva s.
substituted benzamide
substitution
   creeping s.
   segment s.
substrate
   Brown s.
subsulfate
   ferric s.
subtalar
   s. joint
   s. view
subthalamus
subtotal gastric resection
subtraction
   s. cloning
   digital s.
   dual-energy s.
   s. image
   s. imaging
   s. technique
subtrochanteric fracture
subungual melanoma
subunit
subvalvular
   s. aortic stenosis
   s. pulmonary stenosis
   s. stenosis
succedaneum
   caput s.
succenturiate lobe
succimer
   technetium-99m s.
succinate
   hydrocortisone sodium s.
   methylprednisolone
    sodium s.
succinic acid ester carboxorolone

sucralfate
  gadolinium s.
sucrose
  s. gradient sedimentation
  s. polyester (SPE)
suction
  s. catheter
  s. curettage
  s. device
  s. drainage
  rhoton s.
Sudan Black B stain
Sudeck
  S. atrophy
  S. dystrophy
sudotox
  alvircept s.
SUDS
  single-use diagnostic system
    SUDS HIV-1
    SUDS HIV-1 screening
sufentanil
sugar
  blood s.
  s. tumor
suicidal risk
suicide gene
suit
  anti-G s.
  antishock s.
  hot-water circulating s.
  MAST s.
sulcal
  s. enhancement
  s. enlargement
sulcus, pl. **sulci**
  callosal s.
  central s.
  cerebral s.
  cingulate s.
  costophrenic s.
  hippocampal s.
  lateral s.
  pulmonary s.
  sphenoparietal s.
  superior pulmonary s.
sulfadiazine

sulfamerazine
sulfamethazine
sulfamethoxazole
sulfate
  barium s.
  bleomycin s.
  chondroitin s.
  curdlan s. (CRDS)
  dehydroepiandrosterone s.
    (DHEAS)
  dextran s.
  hydrazine s.
  manganese s.
  morphine s. (MS)
  phenylzine s.
  piperazine estrone s.
  quinine s.
  sodium tetradecyl s.
  Stachrom dermatan s.
  vinblastine s.
  vincristine s.
sulfatide
sulfhydryl
  s. group
sulfinpyrazone
sulfonamide
sulfonate
  methylene dimethane s.
    (MDMS)
  sodium-2-mercaptoethane s.
sulfoxide
  dimethyl s. (DMSO)
sulfoximine
  buthionine s. (BSO)
  L-buthionine s.
sulfur
  s. colloid
  s. colloid scintigraphy
  s. dioxide
  s. granules
sulindac
  somatuline s.
sum
  field-echo s.
  ray s.
Sumacal

NOTES

summation
  s. shadow artifact
  s. of shadows
sump
  s. drain
  Ring-MacLean s.
  van Sonnenberg s.
sunburst
  s. appearance
  s. nephrogram
  s. pattern
  s. periosteal reaction
sunlight
sunrise view
superantigen
superbound water
superconducting magnet
superconductor
  niobium/titanium s.
superfamily
  immunoglobulin s.
superfecundation
superfemale syndrome
superficial
  s. angioma
  s. femoral artery (SFA)
  s. lymphadenopathy
  s. radiation
  s. spreading carcinoma
  s. spreading melanoma
  s. temporal artery
  s. temporal artery to
    posterior cerebral artery
    bypass
  s. thrombophlebitis
superficialis
  flexor s.
Superflab
superimposition artifact
superinfection
superior
  s. azygoesophageal recess
  s. cervical ganglion
  s. colliculus
  s. labral anteroposterior
    (SLAP)
  s. labral anteroposterior
    injury
  s. labrum, anterior-to-
    posterior (SLAP)
  s. longitudinal fasciculus
  s. mesenteric
  s. mesenteric artery (SMA)

  s. mesenteric artery
    syndrome
  s. mesenteric vein
  s. oblique
  s. occipitofrontal fasciculus
  s. ophthalmic vein
  s. ophthalmic vein
    thrombosis
  s. orbital fissure
  s. pulmonary sulcus
  s. pulmonary sulcus tumor
  s. sagittal sinus thrombosis
  s. sulcus tumor
  s. triangle sign
  s. vena cava
  s. vena cava filter
  s. vena cava obstruction
  s. vena cava syndrome
superior/inferior (S/I)
superiosus
  levator palpebrae s.
supernatant
supernormal artery
supernumerary kidney
superolateral displacement
superoxide dismutase
superparamagnetic
  s. agent iron oxide
  s. contrast agent
  s. microsphere
superparamagnetism
Superscan
super-still guide wire
supervoltage radiation
supination
supination-adduction fracture
supination-eversion fracture
**supination-external rotation IV
  (SER-IV)**
**supination-external rotation IV
  fracture**
supinator
supine
  s. bicycle stress
    echocardiography
  s. oblique approach
  s. position
  s. radiograph
supplement
  Ensure nutritional s.
  enteral nutritional s.
supply
  arterial s.

blood s.
three-phase voltage s.
tumor blood s.
vascular s.

support
autologous bone marrow s. (ABMS)
blood component s.
home nutritional s.
income s.
nutritional s.
psychological s.
social s.

supportive care

suppression
bone marrow s.
Chopper fat s.
drug-induced bone marrow s.
fat s.
HPA s.
immune s.
immunologic s.
light chain isotype s.
s. scan
solvent s.

suppressor
s. gene
immune s. (IS)
s. T-cell
tumor s.

suppurative
s. ascending cholangitis
s. pancreatitis
s. pyelonephritis
s. thyroiditis

supraanal fascia
supracardinal vein
supracervical hysterectomy
supraclavicular
s. fossa
s. lymph node
s. node involvement

supraclavicular fossa
supraclinoid
s. carotid aneurysm
s. portion

supracolic space
supracondylar
s. humeral fracture
s. Y-shaped fracture

supracristal ventricular septal defect
supradditivity
supraglottic
s. carcinoma
s. laryngectomy
s. narrowing

suprahepatic
s. hypertension
s. space

suprahyoid
suprailiac aortic mesenteric graft
supramesocolic compartment
supraorbital
s. artery
s. foramen

suprapancreatic obstruction
suprapatellar bursa
suprarenal aortic aneurysm
suprascapular notch syndrome
suprasellar
s. lesion
s. low-density lesion
s. mass
s. meningioma
s. subarachnoid cistern

supraspinatus tendon
suprasternal scanning
supratentorial
s. astrocytoma
s. flow compensation
s. glioma
s. neoplasm
s. space
s. tumor

supratrochlear
s. artery
s. node

supratubercular ridge of Meyer
supravalvular
s. aortic stenosis
s. pulmonary stenosis
s. stenosis

NOTES

supraventricular
  s. level
  s. tachyarrhythmia (SVT)
  s. tachycardia
  s. venous echo
supraventricularis
  crista s.
Suprefact
SUR
  suramin
suramin (SUR)
SureCath port access catheter
Sure-Cut needle
surface
  s. antigen
  articular s.
  cell s.
  s. coil
  s. coils in rotating-frame
    experiment
  s. configuration
  s. epithelium
  s. epithelium vascular
    channel
  s. immunoglobulin
  s. irradiation
  s. membrane
  s. membrane antigen
  s. membrane
    immunoglobulin
  s. osteosarcoma
  palmar s.
  plantar s.
  s. projection
  s. rendering
  s. shielding
  s. spoiling
surface-coil
  s.-c. NMR
  s.-c. rotating-frame
    spectroscopy
surface-projection rendering image
surfactant
  synthetic s.
surgery
  bypass s.
  coronary artery bypass s.
  cytoreductive s.
  debulking s.
  endoscopic sinus s.
  functional endoscopic
    sinus s. (FESS)
  inadequate s.

  limb-sparing s.
  local s.
  Mohs micrographic s.
  palliative s.
  radical s.
  radioimmunoguided s.
    (RIGS)
  resective s.
  site-specific s.
  sphincter-saving s.
  stereotactic s.
  suboptimal s.
  transsphincteric s.
  video-assisted
    thoracoscopic s. (VATS)
surgical
  s. cholecystectomy
  s. cholecystostomy
  s. clip
  s. emergency
  s. endarterectomy
  s. excision biopsy
  s. neurangiographic
    technique
  s. oncology
  s. pathology
  s. portosystemic shunt
  s. resection
  s. sponge
surgical-pathologic staging
surgical-radiologic
  minicholecystostomy
surrogate marker
surveillance
  immune s.
  immunologic s.
surveillance-epidemiology-end results
  (SEER)
survey
  s. film
  s. scan
  skeletal s.
  Third National Cancer S.
survival
  actuarial s.
  cell s.
  s. curve
  disease-free s.
  failure-free s.
  s. function
  life table s.
  progression-free s. (PFS)
  relapse-free s. (RFS)

s. relationship
s. trend
survivor
long-term s.
Survivorship
National Coalition for
Cancer S. (NCCS)
susceptibility
s. artifact
s. effect
genetic s.
s. imaging
magnetic s.
s. mapping
suspended inspiration
suspension
barium s.
cell s.
cellular s.
chromic phosphate P 32
colloidal s.
colloidal s.
fast exchange-cellular s.
fresh cell s.
Megace oral s.
monocellular s.
suspicion
high index of s.
Sustacal
S. HC
S. liquid
sustentaculum
s. lienis
s. tali
sutural
s. calcification
s. diastasis
s. marking
suture
coronal s.
cranial s.
lambdoid s.
lambdoidal s.
s. line
s. line cancer
metallic s.
metopic s.

palatine s.
silk s.
squamosal s.
sternal s.
wide s.
zygomaticofrontal s.
zygomaticotemporal s.
SV40 virus
Svedberg unit
SVT
supraventricular
tachyarrhythmia
swabbing
stool s.
throat s.
swabstick
Moi-Stir s.
swallow
barium s.
Gastrografin s.
Hypaque s.
swallowing
fetal s.
**swallowtail malformation of
scapula**
swamp-static artifact
Swan-Ganz catheter
swan-neck deformity
sweat
s. duct adenoma
s. gland carcinoma
night s.'s
sweep
duodenal s.
widened duodenal s.
Sweet syndrome
swelling
soft tissue s.
Swenson pull-through procedure
swept gain
swimmer's view
swimming pool granuloma
swinging heart
swish and swallow mouthwash
Swiss
S. Alps appearance
S. cheese air bronchogram

NOTES

Swiss *(continued)*
- S. cheese hyperplasia
- S. cheese nephrogram
- S. cheese sign
- S. mouse leukemia virus
- S. roll technique

Swiss-type agammaglobulinemia

switch
- genetic s.
- lineage s.
- s. region

switched B-gradient technique

switching
- gene s.

swollen hemisphere

Swyer-James-Macleod syndrome

Swyer syndrome

Sydenham chorea

Syed template

sylvian
- s. aqueduct
- s. cistern
- s. fissure
- s. point
- s. triangle

Sylvius
- aqueduct of S.
- fissure of S.

symmetric
- s. echo
- s. hypertrophy
- s. periosteal reaction

sympathectomy

sympathetic
- s. block
- s. dystrophy

sympathomimetic amine

symphysis pubis

symptom
- B-s.'s
- mediator-related s.
- menopausal s.
- objective s.'s
- sicca s.
- vasomotor s.

synapsin Ia protein

synaptic vesicle

synaptophysin

synchronous
- s. carcinoma
- s. colorectal cancer
- s. ipsilateral breast cancer (SIBC)

synchrotron

syncope

syncytial variant

syncytiotrophoblast
- s. cell

syndactyly

syndesmophyte
- bridging s.

syndesmosis, pl. **syndesmoses**

syndrome
- acquired immunodeficiency s. (AIDS)
- acute respiratory distress s. (ARDS)
- acute retroviral s.
- Adam s.
- Adams-Stokes s.
- Addison s.
- adenomatous polyposis s.
- adrenal feminizing s.
- adrenal virilizing s.
- adrenogenital s.
- adult respiratory distress s. (ARDS)
- afferent loop s.
- Albright s.
- Aldrich s.
- Alport s.
- AMBRI s.
- aminopterin s.
- amniotic band s.
- analgesic s.
- angioosteohypertrophy s.
- anomalous innominate artery compression s.
- anterior spinal artery s.
- antiphospholipid s.
- apallic s.
- Apert s.
- Arnold-Chiari s.
- Asherman s.
- asplenia s.
- ataxia-hemiparesis s.
- autoimmune polyendocrine-candidiasis s.
- Bafverstedt s.
- Bannayan s.
- bare lymphocyte s.
- Barlow s.
- Bartter s.
- basal cell nevus s.
- battered baby s.

battered child s.
Bearn-Kunkel-Slater s.
Beckwith-Wiedemann s.
Behçet s.
Bernard-Soullier s.
Berry s.
bile plug s.
biliary obstruction s.
Birt-Hogg-Dube s.
blind loop s.
blind pouch s.
Bloom s.
blueberry muffin s.
blue digit s.
blue-rubber-bleb-nevus s.
blue toe s.
Blum s.
body cast s.
Boerhaave s.
Bonnevie-Ullrich s.
Brown-Sequard s.
Buckley s.
Budd-Chiari s.
Butler-Albright s.
Caffey-Kempe s.
cancer, anorexia, cachexia s. (CACS)
Caner-Decker s.
capillary leak s.
Caplan s,
carcinoid s.
cardiomelic s.
cardiosplenic s.
Carney s.
carotid cavernous s.
carpal tunnel s.
Carpenter s.
cast s.
cauda equina s.
caudal regression s.
cavernous sinus s.
cellular immunity deficiency s. (CIDS)
cerebral s.
cerebrohepatorenal s.
cervical disk s.
cervical pain s.

cervical rib s.
Chédiak-Higashi s.
Chilaiditi s.
chronic brain s.
chronic fatigue and immune dysfunction s. (CFIDS)
chronic pain s.
chronic pluripotential immunoproliferative s.
chronic venous statis s.
Churg-Strauss s.
cleft face s.
cleft lip and palate s.
Clough and Richter s.
coarctation s.
Cockayne s.
Conn s.
Cornelia De Lange s.
CREST s.
cri-du-chat s.
Cronkhite-Canada s.
Crow-Fukase s.
crush s.
Cruveilhier-von Baumgarten s.
Cushing s.
Dandy-Walker s.
defibrination s.
de Morsier s.
DeToni-Debré-Fanconi s.
DiFerrante s.
DiGeorge s.
distress s.
disuse s.
Down s.
Dresbach s.
Dressler s.
dumping s.
Duncan s.
Dyke-Davidoff-Masson s.
dysarthria s.
dysgenetic s.
dysmotile cilia s.
dysmyelopoietic s.
Eagle-Barrett s.
Eaton-Lambert s.
ectopic ACTH s.

NOTES

syndrome *(continued)*
  Ehlers-Danlos s.
  Eisenmenger s.
  Ellis-van Creveld s.
  EMG s.
  empty sella s.
  encephalotrigeminal s.
  eosinophilia myalgia s.
  Epstein-Barr virus-associated
    lymphoproliferative s.
  Escobar s.
  Evans s.
  failed back surgery s.
  failing ovary s.
  Fallot s.
  familial atypical multiple
    mole melanoma s.
    (FAMMM)
  familial dysplastic nevus s.
    (FDNS)
  familial polyposis s.
  Fanconi s.
  Felton s.
  Felty s.
  feminizing testes s.
  fetal cardiosplenic s.
  Fiessinger-Leroy s.
  Fiessinger-Leroy-Reiter s.
  Fitz-Hugh and Curtis s.
  floppy valve s.
  focal cerebral s.
  Foster-Kennedy s.
  functional bowel s.
  Gardner s.
  Garland s.
  gastrointestinal s.
  gay bowel s.
  gay lymph node s.
  gender dysphoria s.
  Gignotti-Crosti s.
  Glanzmann s.
  Goltz s.
  Good s.
  Goodpasture s.
  Gorham s.
  Gorham-Stout s.
  Gorlin s.
  Gorlin-Pindborg s.
  Gradenigo s.
  granulomatous slack skin s.
  gray platelet s.
  Grisel s.
  Guillain-Barré s.

Hakim s.
Halbrecht s.
Hamman-Rich s.
hand-foot s.
Heerfordt s.
HELLP s.
hemichorea-hemiballismus s.
hemisensory s.
hemolytic uremic s.
hemophagocytic s.
Hermansky-Pudlak s.
HIV wasting s.
Holt-Oram s.
Horner s.
Hunter s.
Hurler s.
Hutchinson s.
hyperabduction s.
hypereosinophilic s.
hyperviscosity s.
hypogenetic lung s.
hypoperistalsis s.
hypoplastic heart s.
hypoplastic left heart s.
hypoplastic right heart s.
Imerslund s.
Imerslund-Graesbeck s.
immotile cilia s.
immunodeficiency s.
impingement s.
s. of inappropriate secretion
  of antidiuretic hormone
  (SIADH)
infantile choriocarcinoma s.
infratentorial s.
innominate artery
  compression s.
intestinal
  pseudoobstruction s.
intrauterine parabiotic s.
irritable bowel s.
isolated tethered cord s.
Ivemark s.
Jaffe-Campanacci s.
Jeune s.
Job s.
jugular foramen s.
Kallman s.
Karroo s.
Kartagener s.
Kasabach-Merritt s.
Kast s.
Kawasaki s.

Ketron-Goodman s.
Kimmelstiel-Wilson s.
kinky-hair s.
Kleffner-Landau s.
Klinefelter s.
Klippel-Feil s.
Klippel-Trenaunay s.
Klippel-Trenaunay-Weber s.
Klippel-Trenaunay-Weber-
  Rubashov s.
Kostmann s.
Laurence-Moon-Biedl s.
lazy leukocyte s.
left heart s.
left parietal s.
Leriche s.
Leri-Layani-Weill s.
Lesch-Nyhan s.
Li-Fraumeni cancer s.
Lightwood s.
Löffler s.
Löfgren s.
Louis-Bar s.
low back s.
Lucey-Driscoll s.
Lutembacher s.
Lyell s.
lymphadenopathy s.
lymphoproliferative s.
Lynch s.
Macleod s.
Maffucci s.
malabsorption s.
male Turner s.
malignant carcinoid s.
Malin s.
Mallory-Weiss s.
Marfan s.
Maroteaux-Lamy s.
Mayer-Rokitansky-Küster-
  Hauser s.
Mazabraud s.
McCune-Albright s.
McKusick-Kaufman s.
Meckel s.
Meckel-Gruber s.
meconium aspiration s.

meconium plug s.
megacystis-microcolon-
  intestinal hypoperistalsis s.
Meigs s.
Meigs-Salmon s.
Melnick-Needles s.
Mendelson s.
Menkes s.
mermaid s.
metastatic carcinoid s.
middle fossa s.
Mikity-Wilson s.
Mikulicz s.
milk-alkali s.
milkman's s.
Miller-Duker s.
Milwaukee shoulder s.
Mirizzi s.
monosomy 7 s.
monosomy 5q-s.
Morgagni s.
Morquio s.
Mosse s.
Mounier-Kuhn s.
mucosal neuroma s.
mucous plug s.
multiple basal cell
  neuromas s.
multiple endocrine
  neoplasia s.
multiple hamartoma s.
murine-acquired
  immunodeficiency s.
  (MAIDS)
myasthenic s.
mycosis fungoides/Sézary s.
myelodysplastic s. (MDS)
myeloproliferative s.
myofascial pain
  dysfunction s.
nail-patella s.
Nelson s.
nephrotic s.
neurocutaneous s.
neurologic paraneoplastic s.
Nezelof s.
Nievergelt s.

NOTES

syndrome *(continued)*
    Noonan s.
    nuchal cyst s.
    Ogilvie s.
    Omenn s.
    opsomyoclonus s.
    orbital apex s.
    orofacial-digital s.
    Osler s.
    ovarian hyperstimulation s.
    (OHS)
    ovarian remnant s.
    ovarian vein s.
    palmoplantar
    erythrodysesthesia s.
    Papillon-Lefevre s.
    parabiotic s.
    paraneoplastic s.
    parent-infant traumatic
    stress s.
    Parinaud s.
    Parkes-Weber s.
    Paterson-Brown-Kelly s.
    Paterson-Kelly s.
    Pena Shokeir s.
    Pendred s.
    Pepper s.
    pericardiotomy s.
    Peutz-Jeghers s
    Pfeiffer s.
    phenytoin-induced
    pseudolymphoma s.
    Pierre Robin s.
    Plummer-Vinson s.
    pluripotential
    immunoproliferative s.
    POEMS s.
    Poland s.
    polyglandular autoimmune s.
    (PGA)
    polyposis s.
    polysplenia s.
    Pompe s.
    pontine s.
    postcardiac injury s. (PCIS)
    postcholecystectomy s.
    postembolization s.
    postmaturity s.
    postmyocardial infarction s.
    postpericardiotomy s.
    postphlebitic syndrome
    postpolio s.
    postrubella s.

    Potter s.
    primary antiphospholipid
    antibody s. (PAPS)
    proteus s.
    proximal loop s.
    prune belly s.
    pseudo-blind loop s.
    pseudo-Kaposi s.
    pseudolymphoma s.
    pulmonary venolobar s.
    Purtillo s.
    5q s.
    Ramsay Hunt s.
    rapid tumor lysis s.
    red-man s.
    Reinhardt s.
    Reiter s.
    renal paraneoplastic s.
    respiratory distress s. (RDS)
    retroviral seroconversion s.
    Rett s.
    Reye s.
    Richter s.
    Riley-Day s.
    Riley-Smith s.
    Robert s.
    Robinow s.
    Rosenthal s.
    Rotor s.
    Saldino-Noonan s.
    Sanfilippo s.
    scalded skin s.
    scalenus anticus s.
    scalenus tunnel s.
    Scheie s.
    Schwachman-Diamond s.
    scimitar s.
    Senear-Usher s.
    serum sickness s.
    severe combined
    immunodeficiency s.
    sex-linked
    lymphoproliferative s.
    Sézary s.
    Sheehan s.
    shocklike s.
    Shone s.
    short bowel s.
    short rib-polydactyly s.
    shoulder-hand s.
    shoulder impingement s.
    Shy-Drager s.
    sicca s.

Sipple s.
Sjögren s.
slack-skin s.
Sly s.
Smith-Lemli-Opitz s.
Smythe s.
Sotos s.
split cord s.
split notochord s.
staphylococcal scalded
 skin s.
Stauffer s.
steal s.
Stein-Leventhal s.
Stevens-Johnson s.
Stewart-Treves s.
straight back s.
Sturge-Weber s.
Sturge-Weber-Dimitri s.
subclavian steal s.
subscapular notch s.
superfemale s.
superior mesenteric artery s.
superior vena cava s.
suprascapular notch s.
Sweet s.
Swyer s.
Swyer-James-Macleod s.
systemic s.
Takatsuki s,
TAR s.
Teitze s.
thoracic inlet s.
thoracic outlet s.
thrombocytopenia, absent
 radius s.
Tietze s.
Tolosa-Hunt s.
Toni-Debre-Fabry-Fanconi s.
TORCH s.
toxic-oil s.
toxic shock s.
transfusion s.
trash-foot s.
Treacher Collins s.
Trinquoste s.
tumor lysis s.

Turcot s.
Turner s.
twiddler's s.
twin-twin transfusion s.
ugly foot s.
ulnar tunnel s.
upper limb-cardiac s.
urethral s.
VACTERL s.
van Buchem s.
vanishing bone s.
vascular leak s.
vasodepressor s.
vasovagal s.
venolobar s.
Verner-Morrison s.
von Hippel-Lindau s.
Waardenburg s.
Wallenburg s.
wasting s.
Waterhouse-Friderichsen s.
WDHA s.
Weill-Marchesani s.
Weingarten s.
Weismann-Netter s.
Werner s.
white clot s.
Williams s.
Williams-Campbell s.
Wilson-Mikity s.
Wiskott-Aldrich s.
Wolf-Parkinson-White s.
Woringer-Kolopp s.
Wyburn-Mason s.
X-linked
 lymphoproliferative s.
XLP s.
XXY s.
Yunis-Varon s.
Zellweger s.
Zieve s.
Zollinger-Ellison s.
synechia vulvae
synergism
 therapeutic s.
synergy
 therapeutic s.

NOTES

syngeneic
- s. bone marrow transplant
- s. tissue

syngraft

synostosis
- craniofacial s.
- lambdoid s.
- metatarsal s.

synovectomy

synovial
- s. bursa
- s. chondromatosis
- s. cyst
- s. joint
- s. membrane
- s. osteochondromatosis
- s. pannus
- s. sarcoma
- s. sheath
- s. tissue

synovioma

synovitis
- intraarticular localized nodular s.
- pigmented villonodular s.
- purulent s.
- toxic s.
- transient s.
- s. tumor

syntenic gene

synthase
- thymidylate s.

synthesis
- heme s.
- IgA s.
- s. phase
- prostaglandin s.

synthesizer
- frequency s.

synthetase
- fatty acyl-Co-A s.
- folylpolyglutamate s.
- glutamylcysteine s.

synthetic
- s. surfactant
- s. vascular bypass graft

syphilis
- congenital s.
- tertiary s.

syphilitic aortitis

syringe
- electric s.
- tuberculin s.

syringes (*pl. of* syrinx)

syringobulbia

syringocarcinoma

syringohydromyelia

syringohydromyelic cavity

syringoma
- chondroid s.

syringomyelia
- cervical s.

syrinx, pl. syringes

system
- AEGIS sonography management s.
- air filtration s.
- Ann Arbor staging s. I-IV
- anterolateral s.
- antibody-based detection s.
- aortoiliac inflow s.
- Arizona Cancer Center multiple myeloma staging s.
- Astler-Coller staging s.
- Aviva mammography s.
- Bard rotary atherectomy s. (BRAS)
- Bethesda s.
- bifid collecting s.
- biliary s.
- Boden-Gibb staging s.
- Dorrmunn classification s.
- Breslow microstaging s.
- bursa-dependent s.
- CADD-TPN ambulatory infusion s.
- Cancer Rehabilitation Evaluation S. (CARES)
- carbon dioxide laser s.
- cardiovascular s.
- carrier-mediated transport s.
- cartesian coordinate s.
- central nervous s. (CNS)
- ChemoBloc vial venting s.
- Clark classification s.
- coagulation s.
- collecting s.
- collimating s.
- condenser discharge s.
- Cope retention s.
- Cope single-stick biliary drainage s.
- CrystalEYES video s.
- data s.
- detection s.

digestive s.
dye laser s.
Edwards hypothetical double
  aortic arch s.
effaced collecting s.
electrostatic imaging s.
endocrine s.
Enneking staging s.
Excimer laser s.
extrapyramidal s.
femoropopliteal outflow s.
fetal musculoskeletal s.
fibrinolytic s.
fiducial alignment s.
FIGO staging s.
folate polyglutamylation s.
Fränkel classification s.
free radical scavenging s.
Gleason tumor grading s.
gradient s.
guided coaxial balloon
  catheter s.
Helios laser s.
Helix multihead nuclear
  imaging s.
hematopoietic s.
hepatic venous s.
host vector s.
image recording s.
imaging center
  information s.
immune s.
immunoregulatory effector s.
implantable drug delivery s.
information s.
Intra-Op autotransfusion s.
Jass grading s.
Kagan staging s.
Kernohan histologic
  grading s.
laser s.
Leukotrap RC s.
Leukotrap red cell
  storage s.
light collection s.
lymphatic s.
Magnes biomagnetometer s.

mammillary s.
M. D. Anderson grading s.
Medilase angioscope-laser
  delivery s.
Mini-Balloon s.
model s.
multileaf collimating s.
musculoskeletal s.
nervous s.
Neurostat Mark II
  cryoanalgesia s.
ONCOCIN information s.
OPAL knowledge-entry s.
optical s.
Pageblot s.
particulate air filtration s.
PDQ information s.
pelvocalyceal s.
peripheral nervous s.
photoelectric s.
picture archival
  communication s. (PACS)
portal venous s.
primary central nervous s.
protein C anticoagulant s.
purple mutation s.
pyelocalyceal s.
pyramidal s.
Q-prep s
radiology telephone access s.
  (RTAS)
Rai staging s.
reimbursement s.
respiratory s.
reticuloendothelial s.
reverse mutation s.
Robson s.
Rotablator thrombectomy s.
sandwich s.
scavenging s.
single-use diagnostic s.
  (SUDS)
skeletal s.
SKY pain control s.
slip-ring gantry s.
smart laser s.

NOTES

system *(continued)*
 Solcotrans
  drainage/reinfusion s.
 spiderlike pelvocaliceal s.
 splanchnic venous s.
 staging s.
 St. Anne-Mayo grading s.
 striped tag myocardial
  tagging s. (STAG)
 television s.
 tibioperoneal runoff s.
 trumpet-like pelvocaliceal s.
 Uni-frame patient
  immobilization s.
 Urocyte diagnostic
  cytometry s.
 Vac-Lok patient
  immobilization s.
 vertebrobasilar s.
 VEST s.
 widened collecting s.
 XERG s.
systematic
 s. noise
 s. relaxation effect

systemic
 s. lupus erythematosus
  (SLE)
 s. lymphoma
 s. lymphoproliferative
  disorder
 s. nodular panniculitis
 s. polyclonal immunoblastic
  proliferation
 s. radioimmunoglobulin
  therapy
 s. shunt
 s. syndrome
 s. therapy
systemic-pulmonic shunt
systole
systolic
 s. anterior movement
 s. function
 s. velocity ratio
systolic/diastolic ratio (S/D ratio)
Szumowski sequence

T
    T antigen
    T-cell
    T-lymphocyte
T1
    T1 relaxation time
    T1 shortening
T2
    T2 relaxation
    T2 shortening
T3
    triiodothyronine
    T3 uptake
T4
    thyroxine
    T4 count
    T4 helper cell
    T4 uptake
    WHO classification for
        transitional cell carcinoma
        of the urinarybladder:
        stages Ta through T4
T$_d$
    diffusion time
T11 antigen
t(14,18) chromosomal translocation
T-2 protocol
Ta
    tantalum
^{182}Ta
    tantalum-182
^{178}Ta
    tantalum-178
TAA
    tumor-associated antigen
Tabar pattern
tabes dorsalis
table
    Hadlock t.
Tac antigen
TACE
    transcatheter arterial
        chemoembolization
Tace
tachyarrhythmia
    supraventricular t. (SVT)
tachycardia
    paroxysmal auricular t.
        (PAT)

    paroxysmal
        supraventricular t.
    supraventricular t.
    ventricular t.
tachykinin
tachyphylaxis
tachypnea
    transient t.
tacrolimus
TAD 9/HAM combination
Taenia solium
TAG
    tumor-associated glycoprotein
TAG-72
    tumor-associated glycoprotein-72
tagging
    bolus t.
    myocardial t.
    spin t.
TAHBSO
    total abdominal hysterectomy
    and bilateral salpingo-
    oophorectomy
taheebo tea
tail
    axillary t.
    comet t.
    Dacron t.
    dural t.
    t. sign
    t. of Spence
    wool t.
tailored
    t. excitation
    t. pulse
Takatsuki syndrome
Takayasu arteritis
tal-1
    tal-1 oncogene
    tal-1 proto-oncogene
tal-1/SIL **fusion gene**
talar
    t. avulsion fracture
    t. dome cyst
    t. fracture
    t. neck fracture
    t. osteochondral fracture
talc
    t. on the skin
    t. pneumoconiosis

talcosis
tali (*var. of* talus)
    sustentaculum t.
talin protein
talipes equinovarus
tallysomycin
talocalcaneal, talocalcanean
    t. angle
    t. articulation
talocalcaneonavicular
    t. joint
talofibular
    t. ligament
    t. ligament injury
talonavicular
    t. joint
tal **oncogene**
talus, tali
    vertical t.
Talwin
TAM
    tamoxifen
Tamm-Horsfall proteinuria
tam-o-shanter appearance
tamoxifen (TAM)
    t. citrate
tampon
    vaginal t.
tamponade
    balloon t.
    cardiac t.
    t. needle tract
tan-1
    tan-1 oncogene
    tan-1 proto-oncogene
tandem
    t. conjugate reagent
    t. construction
    t. double dose
    t. stent
    t. technique
    t. transplant
tangential view
tangent screen testing
tanned red cell
tannic acid fixative
tantalum (Ta)
    t. bronchography
    t. mesh
    t. powder
tantalum-178 (^{178}Ta)
tantalum-182 (^{182}Ta)

tape
    clonidine transdermal t.
    Dermiform hypo-allergenic
      knitted t.
    genetic masking t.
    Johnson & Johnson
      waterproof t.
    Micropore t.
tapered fingers
tapered-tip dilator
tapeworm
Taq polymerase
TAR
    thrombocytopenia, absent radius
      TAR syndrome
TARAP assay
tarda
    osteogenesis imperfecta t.
    porphyria cutanea t.
target
    antigenic t.
    assay t.
    t. cell
    t. erythrocyte
    intracellular t.
    molybdenum t.
    t. organ
    t. radiotherapy
    t. sign
    tungsten t.
targeted imaging for fetal anomalies
targeting
    t. agent
    magnetite in tumor t.
target-to-nontarget ratio
Tarlov cyst
tarsal
    t. joint
    transverse t. joint
    t. tunnel
tarsoepiphyseal aclasis
tart cell
tartrate
    butorphanol t.
    thorium t.
tartrate-resistant
    t.-r. acid phosphatase
Tasmar
taste abnormality
TAT
    thrombin-antithrombin III
    complex

tat
- t. gene
- t. inhibitor
- t. protein
- T. protein of HIV

TATA
- tumor-associated transplantation antigen
- TATA box

tattoo
Taub test
tauromustine (TCNU)
Taussig-Bing
- T.-B. disease
- T.-B. heart

tax
- t. gene

Taxol
Taxotere
Tax protein
TB
- tuberculosis
  - covitary TB

TBI
- total body irradiation
- tracheobronchial injury

Tc
- technetium

^{99m}Tc
- technetium-99m
  - ^{99m}Tc macroaggregated albumin

TCC
- transitional cell carcinoma

^{99m}Tc-DMSA scintigraphy
^{99m}Tc-DTPA
T-cell
- T.-c. acute lymphoblastic leukemia
- cytolytic T.-c.
- T.-c. disorder
- T.-c. function test
- T.-c. growth factor
- T.-c. lineage antigen
- T.-c. lymphoblastic lymphoma
- T.-c. lymphoma
- T.-c. lymphoma variant
- T.-c. malignancy
- T.-c. neoplasm
- T.-c. phenotype
- T.-c. prolymphocytic leukemia
- T.-c. pseudoclonality
- T.-c. receptor (TCR)
- T.-c. replacement factor

T-cell-mediated immunity
T-cell-rich
- T.-c.-r. B cell
- T.-c.-r. B-cell lymphoma

TcHIDA
^{99m}Tc-HMPAO
- ^{99m}Tc-H. cerebral perfusion SPECT imaging
- ^{99m}Tc-H. SPECT imaging

***tcl-1* oncogene**
***tcl-2* oncogene**
***tcl-3* oncogene**
***tcl-4* oncogene**
TCNU
- tauromustine

T-condylar fracture
tcPO$_1$
- transcutaneous oxygen pressure measurement

TCR
- T-cell receptor

T-cytotoxic cell
TdT
- terminal deoxynucleotidyl transferase

TDTH cell
TE
- thromboembolic
  - TE fistula

tea
- herbal t.
- taheebo t.

teacup fracture

NOTES

team
interdisciplinary t.
transplant t.
tear
anulus fibrosus t.
bucket-handle t.
esophageal t.
flap t.
intimal t.
Mallory-Weiss esophageal t.
parrot's beak t.
parrot's beak labral t.
quadriceps tendon t.
rectal t.
rotator cuff t.
stellate t.
subscapulans tendon t.
tibial tendon t.
traumatic aortic t.
teardrop
t. appearance
t. fracture
teat
pyloric t.
teboroxime
technetium-99m t.
TEC
transluminal extraction catheter
TEC-2100 positioning laser
Technegas
Techneplex
Technescan MAG3
technetium (Tc)
t. pertechnate
t. stannous pyrophosphate
t. sulfur colloid
technetium-99m (^{99m}Tc)
t. albumin
t. albumin colloid
t. antibody labeling
t. bicisate
t. colloid
t. dimercaptosuccinic acid
t. disofenin
t. etidronate
t. ferpentetate
t. furifosmin
t. glucepate
t. HIDA
t. iron-ascorbate-DTPA
t. lidofenin
t. macroaggregated albumin
(MAA)

t. medronate
t. mertiatide
t. oxidronate
t. pertechnetate
t. pertechnetate sodium
t. PIPIDA
t. pyrophosphate
sestamibi t.
t. sestamibi
t. siboroxime
t. sodium
t. succimer
t. sulfur colloid
t. teboroxime
t. tetrofosmin
technetium-tagged
t.-t. Cardiolite
t.-t. red blood cell
technetium-thallium subtraction imaging
technical
t. charge
t. factor
technique
afterloading t.
air-gap t.
alkaline phosphatase-antialkaline phosphatase t.
APAAP t.
assay t.
avidin-biotin binding t.
avidin-biotin-peroxidase-antiperoxidase t.
balloon catheter t.
basket fragmentation t.
basketing t.
biotin-streptavidin peroxidase conjugate t.
boost t.
bougienage t.
Braasch bulb t.
cardiovascular imaging t.
catheter-securing t.
cognitive t.
composite addition t.
Cope t.
DEFT t.
Deisting prostatic dilation t.
dephase-rephase magnitude subtraction t.
depth pulse t.
Dixon t.
DNA microinjection t.

double-freeze t.
double-stick t.
driven equilibrium Fourier
transform t.
dynamic bolus tracking t.
Eklund t.
electron arc t.
endofluoroscopic t.
endovascular t.
enzyme-multiplied
immunoassay t. (EMIT)
FLAK t.
flow cytometry t.
fluorescent antibody t.
fluoroscopic t.
fluoroscopic pushing t.
flushing t.
Fourier-acquired steady-
state t. (FAST)
Fourier imaging t.
Fraunfelder t.
FRODO t.
graded compression
sonography t.
gradient-echo t.
grasping t.
grid t.
guidewire exchange t.
half-Fourier
transformation t.
Hawkins t.
Hawkins inside-out
nephrostomy t.
Hawkins single-stick t.
high-kV t.
high-resolution bone
algorithm t.
hybridization-subtraction t.
hybridoma t.
hybrid subtraction t.
immersion t.
immune monitoring t.
immunoadsorption t.
immunofluorescence t.
inside-out t.
interleaved phase contrast t.
jugular t.

kissing-balloon t.
large-core t.
Laurell t.
localization t.
magnetization transfer t.
MAST t.
mathematical modeling t.
Menghini biopsy t.
molecular t.
molecular genetic t.
monitoring t.
Mose t.
motion artifact
suppression t. (MAST)
MPGR t.
MP-RAGE t.
neuroablative t.
no-touch t.
Oakley-Fulthorpe t.
Overhauser t.
partial Fourier t.
perfusion measurement t.
presaturation t.
projection-reconstruction t.
pseudobiopsy t.
PSSE t.
pulsed-gradient spin-echo t.
rapid scan t.
Rebuck skin window t.
recanalization t.
relaxation t.
rescue t.
Seldinger t.
shell vial t.
single-shot imaging t.
SL t.
slot-blot t.
snare t.
Southern blot t.
spin-lock imaging t. (SL
technique)
split-course t.
Stejskal and Tanner pulsed-
gradient spin-echo t.
stereotactic t.
stereotactic automated t.

NOTES

553

technique *(continued)*
    Sternberger antibody
      sandwich t.
    STIR t.
    streptavadin-biotin-peroxidase
      complex t.
    subtraction t.
    surgical neurangiographic t.
    Swiss roll t.
    switched B-gradient t.
    tandem t.
    time-of-flight t.
    tissue-sparing t.
    trocar t.
    trocar-cannula t.
    two-needle t.
    two-step t.
    venous access t.
    water-suppression t.
    whole blood lysis t.
technology
    acoustic response t. (ART)
    antisense t.
    bull's-eye t.
    recombinant
      deoxyribonucleic t.
tectal beaking
tectospinal tract
tectum
TEE probe
teeth
    carious t.
    floating t.
TEF
    tracheoesophageal fistula
Teflon
    T. catheter
    T. dilator
    T. sheath
    T. stent
Teflon-coated needle
teflonized J-wire
Tegaderm
    T. dressing
    T. TFD
tegafur
tegmentum of brainstem
tegmen tympani
Tegtmeyer catheter
TEGwire
    T. angioplasty catheter
    T. balloon
Teichmann crystal

Teitze syndrome
tela choroidea
telangiectasia, teleangiectasia
    ataxia t.
    hemorrhagic t.
    hereditary hemorrhagic t.
    pulmonary t.
telangiectasis, pl. telangiectases
    capillary t.
    hereditary hemorrhagic t.
telangiectatic
    t. angioma
    t. cancer
    t. fibroma
    t. osteogenic
    t. osteogenic sarcoma
telangiectaticum
    granuloma t.
teleangiectasia *(var. of*
  telangiectasia)
Telebrix
telecobalt therapy
TeleMax
telemeric DNA
telencephalic
    t. malformation
    t. ventriculofugal artery
telencephalon
TelePACS
Telepaque
telephone handle bone
teleradiology
teletherapy
    t. radiotherapy
television system
$t_{1/2}$**elim**
    elimination half-life
telltale triangle sign
telogen
    t. effluvium
telomerase
telomere
telosome
temafloxacin
temozolomide
temperature
    t. distribution measurement
    Neel t.
template
    Syed t.
temporal
    t. artery
    t. average intensity

t. bone
t. bone fracture
t. bone sclerosis
t. bone tumor
t. filter
t. fossa
t. granulomatous arteritis
t. horn
t. instability artifact
t. lobe
t. lobe epilepsy
t. meningioma
t. peak
t. peak intensity
t. process
t. space infection
temporalis muscle
temporary diverting colostomy
temporomandibular joint (TMJ)
temporooccipital artery
temporoparietooccipital junction
TEN
total enteral nutrition
Vivonex TEN
Tenckhoff catheter
tendineae
chordae t.
tendinitis
calcific t.
tendinopathy
tendinosis
tendo calcaneus
tendon
Achilles t.
anterior tibial t.
biceps t.
biceps brachii t.
extensor t.
flexor t.
gracilis t.
iliopsoas t.
infrapatellar t.
infraspinatus t.
patellar t.
peroneal brevis t.
peroneal longus t.
popliteal t.

posterior tibial t.
quadriceps t.
semimembranosus t.
t. sheath
subscapularis t.
supraspinatus t.
tendonitis
tendosynovial sarcoma
tenesmus
teniposide (VM-26)
tennis elbow
tenography
tenonavicular
tenosynovial osteochondromatosis
tenosynovitis
de Quervain t.
TENS
transcutaneous electrical nerve
stimulator
tensile injury
Tensilon
tensin protein
tension
t. cyst
t. endothorax
t. fracture
t. pneumothorax
tensor
t. fascia femoris
t. tympani
t. veli palatini
t. veli palatini muscle
tenth-value layer
tentorial
t. meningioma
t. traversal
tentorium cerebelli
tenuin protein
teratoblastoma of ovary
teratocarcinoma
t. of ovary
pineal t.
teratogen
teratogenesis
teratogenic effect
teratogenicity
t. of contrast agent

NOTES

teratoid tumor
teratoma
    cystic t.
    embryonal t.
    immature t.
    immature ovarian t.
    malignant t.
    malignant ovarian t.
    mature cystic t.
    mature ovarian t.
    ovarian cystic t.
    ovarian embryonal t.
    pineal t.
    sacrococcygeal t.
terazosin
terbutaline
terconazole
teres
    ligamentum t.
    t. major
    t. minor
Teridax
terlipressin
term
    hierarchy of t.'s
    statistical t.
terminal
    t. care
    t. deoxynucleotidyl
      transferase (TdT)
    t. duct lobular unit
    t. ileitis
    t. ileum
    t. progression
    t. tufts
    t. ureterectasis
terminale
    filum t.
terminalis
    ventriculus t.
terminally ill patient
terminator
    conditional chain t.
    DNA chain t.
    obligate chain t.
teroxirone
Terry-Mayo needle
Terry Thomas sign
tertiary
    t. collimation
    t. hypothyroidism
    t. syphilis
    t. wave

tertius
    peroneus t.
Terumo guidewire
Teslac
TESPA
    triethylenethiophosphoramide
test
    Achilles tendon reflex t.
    acid t.
    Allen t.
    Ames t.
    anergy t.
    Barlow t.
    beta-hCG t.
    biceps brachii tendon
      reflex t.
    bilirubin t.
    blood t.
    blood urea nitrogen t.
    blot t.
    brachioradialis tendon
      reflex t.
    B/T Blue Gene
      Rearrangement t.
    CA 15-2 RIA t.
    Casoni skin t.
    chi squared t.
    Cochran-Mantel-Haensel t.
    CombiBlot t.
    conglutinating complement
      absorption t. (CCAT)
    contraction stress t.
    Coombs t.
    Cortrosyn stimulating t.
    creatinine t.
    Davidsohn t.
    D-Di t.
    Dick t.
    dipyridamole/thallium
      stress t.
    Dunnet t.
    dye reduction spot t.
    Envacor t.
    Enzymune t.
    EPIblot HIV-1 t.
    EPIblot HIV Western
      blot t.
    Farr t.
    Fisher exact t.
    Fouchet t.
    FS t.
    GeneAmp PCR t.
    germ tube t.

Graham-Cole t.
Hammarsten t.
Hanger t.
Heaf t.
Hemoccult t.
Henry t.
Herp-Check antibody t.
Hicks-Pitney thromboplastin
  generation t.
Hinton t.
HIVAGEN t.
HIV phenotype t.
Hoppe-Seyler t.
immunobead-binding
  assay t.
immunoblot t.
indirect fluorescent
  antibody t.
induced sputum t.
t. injection
Integra PBS Pageblot t.
internal carotid balloon t.
iron-binding capacity t.
Kitzmiller t.
Kleihauer t.
Kobert t.
Kolmer t.
Kowarsky t.
Kveim t.
La Bross spot t.
Ladendorff t.
Leclercq t.
Linsman water t.
liver function t. (LFT)
Luria-Delbruck fluctuation t.
Machado t.
Machado-Guerreiro t.
Mann-Whitney U t.
Mantel-Cox t.
Mecholyl t.
Middlebrook-Dubos
  hemagglutination t.
Moloney t.
Molulsky dye reduction t.
Mono-Diff t.
Monospot t.
Müller t.

Nippe t.
Noguchi t.
nonstress t. (NST)
Northern blot t.
one-tail t.
OraQuick t.
OraSure t.
Ortolani t.
osmotic fragility t.
p24 antigen t.
Papanicolaou t.
paper
  radioimmunosorbent t.
  (PRIST)
Paul-Bunnell-Davidsohn t.
pelvic steal t.
perchlorate washout t.
platelet suspension
  immunofluorescence t.
  (PSIFT)
Pohl t.
postcoital t.
PPD t.
predictive value of t.
predictive value of
  negative t.
predictive value of
  positive t.
pregnancy t.
pulmonary function t.
Purdue Pegboard T.
quadriceps femoris tendon
  reflex t.
quanti-Pirquet t.
Quick t.
RA latex fixation t.
Reitman-Fränkel t.
ristocetin cofactor t.
Romer t.
Rose-Waaler t.
Rubner t.
Rumpel-Leede t.
Sabin-Feldman dye t.
saliva blot t.
Salzman t.
Schalfijew t.
Scheffe F t.

NOTES

test *(continued)*
    Schick t.
    Schiller t.
    Schilling t.
    Schumm t.
    sheep cell agglutination t.
      (SCAT)
    Shirner t.
    Sia t.
    sniff t.
    Southern blot t.
    Sterneedle t.
    streptokinase resistance t.
    stress t.
    Stypven time t.
    Taub t.
    T-cell function t.
    Thrombo-Wellco t.
    tine t.
    Triboulet t.
    tuberculin skin t.
    t. tube structure
    Tuttle t.
    two-tail t.
    ultrastructural platelet
      peroxidase t.
    ureteral perfusion t.
    van den Bergh t.
    Vironostika ELISA AIDS t.
    Voges-Proskauer t.
    Vollmer t.
    von Zeynek and Mencki t.
    Waaler-Rose t.
    Wassermann t.
    water-siphon t.
    Weichbrodt t.
    Weil-Felix t.
    Western blot t.
    Wetzel t.
    Whitaker t.
    Widal-Felix t.
    Widmark t.
    Wilcoxon rank-sum t.
    Williamson blood t.
    Winn t.
    Wishart t.
    Zaleski t.
Testamone
testes (*pl. of* testis)
Testex
testicle
    undescended t.

testicular
    t. abscess
    t. artery
    t. artery avulsion
    t. biopsy
    t. cancer
    t. cyst
    t. ectopia
    t. feminization
    t. infarct
    t. ischemia
    t. leukemia
    t. metastasis
    t. posttraumatic edema
    t. relapse
    t. rupture
    t. seminoma
    t. torsion
    t. trauma
    t. tubular adenoma
    t. tumor
    t. vein
testing
    fecal occult blood t.
    guaiac t.
    hypothesis t.
    lung function t.
    occult blood t.
    perimetry t.
    prenatal t.
    provocative t.
    radiation sensitivity t.
    tangent screen t.
    toxicology t.
    visual acuity t.
testis, pl. **testes**
    t. cancer
    t. dysfunction
    t. dysplasia
    ectopia t.
    t. fracture
    interstitial cell tumor of t.
    maldescended t.
    malpositioned t.
    mediastinum t.
    occult primary tumor of t.
    retractile t.
testolactone
Testone LA 100, 200
testosterone
    t. enanthate
    t. propionate
Testred

Testrin
Tesuloid
tetanus
    t. antigen
    t. immune globulin
tetany
tethered
    t. cord
    t. spinal cord
tetraazacyclododecanetetraacetic
    t. acid (DOTA)
    t. tetramethylene
      phosphonate (DOTP)
tetrabromophenolphthalein
tetracycline
tetradentate thioiminato
tetradiploid tumor
δ-9-tetrahydrocannabinol (THC)
tetrahydrouridine (THU)
tetraiodophenolphthalein
tetralogy
    t. of Fallot
    pink t.
tetrameric antibody complex
tetranectin
    plasma t.
    stromal t.
tetraphenylborate
tetraphocomelia
tetraplatin
tetraploid tumor
tetrazolium
    nitroblue t.
tetrazolium-based colorimetric assay
tetrofosmin
    technetium-99m t.
texaphyrins
Texas Red
texture
    echo t.
T1-FAST
TFD
    thin-film dressing
      Bioclusive TFD
      Op-Site TFD
      Tegaderm TFD
      Uniflex TFD

TG
    thioguanine
β-TG
    Asserachrom β-TG
6-TG
    6-thioguanine
T-gamma
    T.-g. lymphoma
    T.-g. lymphoproliferative
      disorder
    T.-g. proliferative disease
TGF-alpha
    transforming growth factor-alpha
    4
thalamic
    t. plane
    t. vein
thalamoperforating artery
thalamostriate vein
thalamus
thalassemia
    alpha chain t.
    t. intermedia
    t. major
thalidomide
thallium
    t. imaging
    t. myocardial scan with
      SPECT imaging
    t. single photon emission
      computed tomography scan
    t. SPECT scan
thallium-201
    t. chloride
    dipyridamole t.
thanatophoric
    t. dwarfism
    t. dysplasia
Thaw protocol
Thayer-Doisy unit
Thayer-Martin culture medium
THC
    delta-9-tetrahydrocannabinol
    δ-9-tetrahydrocannabinol
THE
    transhiatal esophagectomy

NOTES

theca
    t. cell tumor
thecal sac
theca-lutein cyst
thecoma
    t. of ovary
Theiler virus
thelarche
    premature t.
T-helper cell response
thenylidene
Theobald Smith phenomenon
theophylline
theorem
    Nyquist t.
    Nyquist sampling t.
    sampling t.
theory
    Anderson-Carr-Randall t.
    BPP t.
    clonal deletion t.
    clonal selection t.
    crystal field t. (CFT)
    decision t.
    Ehrlich side chain t.
    Fisher-Race t.
    Fourier optical t.
    Frerich t.
    lattice t.
    Metchnikoff cellular
        immunity t.
    natural selection t.
    network t.
    slider crank t.
    unitarian t.
    Wood-Fildes t.
theraccine
TheraCys
therapeutic
    t. approach
    t. drug monitoring
    t. embolism
    t. embolization
    t. index
    t. microsphere
    t. species
    t. synergism
    t. synergy
therapy
    ablation t.
    adjuvant t.
    androgen deprivation t.
    antibiotic t.

antifungal t.
antimycotic t.
antineoplastic t.
antiplatelet t.
antiretroviral t.
antiviral t.
biologic t.
blood component t.
boron neutron-capture t.
Cancell t.
cesium t.
chemoendocrine t.
chemoradiation t.
combined modality t.
compartmental
    radioimmunoglobulin t.
concomitant t.
contact dissolution t.
cyclosporine t.
cytoreductive t.
dietary t.
directly observed t. (DOT)
electroconvulsive t.
electron t.
empiric t.
endocrine t.
endourological t.
estrogen replacement t.
experimental t.
extended field irradiation t.
external x-ray t.
ex vivo gene t.
fast neutron radiation t.
fibrinolytic t.
Fletcher-Suit system for
    radium t.
fluoride t.
fractionated radiation t.
Functional Assessment of
    Cancer T. (FACT)
gastrointestinal complication
    of radiation t.
gene t.
gene replacement t.
gold t.
HDR intracavitary
    radiation t.
hematoporphyrin t.
hepatic arterial t.
high-dose t.
hormonal t.
hormonal ablative t.

hormone t.
hyperthermia t.
ImmTher t.
immunoaugmentative t.
immunosuppressive t.
innovative t.
instillational t.
interlesional t.
internal radiation t.
interstitial t.
intraarterial t.
intracavitary t.
intralesional t.
intrathecal t.
intravenous ozone t.
intraventricular t.
invasive t.
isolation perfusion t.
laser t.
LDR intracavitary
  radiation t.
Manchester system for
  radium t.
medical t.
megavitamin t.
monoclonal antibody t.
multimodality t.
multiple agent t. (MAT)
myoablative t.
neoadjuvant t.
neodymium·YAG laser t.
neutron rupture t.
nutritional t.
occlusion t.
ocular radiation t. (ORT)
oxygen t.
palliative t.
parenteral t.
Paris method for radium t.
particle beam radiation t.
PEIT t.
percutaneous ethanol
  injection t. (PEIT)
percutaneous microwave
  coagulation t.
percutaneous transcatheter t.
perfusion t.

photodynamic t.
postmenopausal estrogen t.
postradiation t.
primary healing after
  radiation t.
prophylactic t.
pyretic t.
radiation t. (RT, XRT)
radioimmunoglobulin t.
  (RIT)
radiopharmaceutical t.
renal infusion t.
reprogramming t.
risk-directed t.
rotation t.
salvage t.
sole laser t.
STAMP t.
standard t.
stem cell gene t.
steroid t.
Stockholm technique for
  radium t.
streptokinase t.
systemic t.
systemic
  radioimmunoglobulin t.
telecobalt t.
thrombolytic t.
timed sequential t.
total D t.
t-PA t.
trimodality t.
triple t.
triple intrathecal t. (TIT)
ventilator t.
warfarin t.
whole-brain radiation t.
  (WBRT)
wide-field radiation t.
wide-range radiation t.
xenogenic cell t.
x-ray t.
thermal
  t. balloon
  t. bioeffect
  t. effect

NOTES

thermal *(continued)*
    t. equilibrium
    t. hot spot
    t. noise
    t. occlusion
    t. shape memory
Thermex
    Direx T.
thermochemotherapy
    intraperitoneal t.
thermography
thermoluminescent dosimeter
thermometer
    First Temp Genius
    tympanic t.
    Thermoscan Pro-1 instant t.
thermometry
thermonic emission
thermoregulatory mechanism
**Thermoscan Pro-1 instant
  thermometer**
thesaurosis
thickened
    t. fold
    t. irregular endometrium
thickening
    antral mucosal t.
    apical pleural t.
    bladder wall t.
    capsular t.
    diffuse t.
    focal gallbladder wall t.
    heel pad t.
    ligamentum flavum t.
    mucosal t.
    mural t.
    nuchal t.
    nuchal skin t.
    peau d'orange skin t.
    postbiopsy skin t.
    postlumpectomy skin t.
    secondary skin t.
    skin t.
thickness
    bladder wall t.
    endometrial t.
    slice t.
thiethylperazine maleate
thin-film dressing (TFD)
thinning
    cortical t.
thin-section axial image
thin skull

thioflavin T
thioguanine (TG)
6-thioguanine (6-TG)
**6-thioguanine, procarbazine,
  CCNU, hydroxyurea (TPCH)**
**6-thioguanine, procarbazine,
  dibromodulcitol, CCNU
  (lomustine), vincristine (TPDCV)**
**6-thioguanine, rubidomycin, ara-C,
  prednisone (TRAP)**
**6-thioguanine, rubidomycin, ara-C,
  methotrexate, prednisolone,
  cyclophosphamide, Oncovin,
  L-asparaginase (TRAMPCOL)**
thioiminato
    tetradentate t.
thiol
    t. augmentation
    t. modification
thiopental
Thioplex
6-thiopurine
thiosemicarbazone
    copper pyruvaldehyde t.
thiosulfate
    sodium t.
thiotepa
thiourea linkage
Third
third
    t. generation regimen
    T. National Cancer Survey
    t. trimester gestational
      dating
    t. ventricular
      hemangioblastoma
third-degree heart block
Thixokon
Thoma-Zeiss counting cell
**Thompson-Epstein classification of
  femoral fractures**
Thora-Cath catheter
thoracentesis
    misplaced t.
thoraces (*pl. of* thorax)
thoracic
    t. adenopathy
    t. angiography
    t. aorta
    t. aorta aneurysm
    t. circumference
    t. crush
    t. cyst

t. deformity
t. disk
t. disk herniation
t. duct
t. duct cyst
t. dysplasia
t. inlet
t. inlet soft tissue
t. inlet syndrome
t. outlet
t. outlet syndrome
t. pulsion diverticulum
t. root sleeve
t. root sleeve diverticulum
t. sonography
t. spinal cord
t. spinal neoplasm
t. spine
t. spine fracture
t. splenosis
transaxial t. inlet
t. vascular embolization
t. vent
t. vertebra
thoracoabdominal gradient
thoracoacromial artery
thoracolumbar
t. fascia
t. spine fracture
thoracoomphalopagus
thoracopagus
thoracoscope
Stortz t.
thoracotomy
thorax, pl. thoraces
bony t.
Thorazine
Thoreau filter
thorium
t. compound
t. dioxide
t. tartrate
Thornwaldt cyst
Thorotrast
thorotrast
thread-and-streaks vascular channels

threatened abortion
three-dimensional (3D)
t.-d. fast low-angle shot imaging
t.-d. Fourier imaging (3DFr)
t.-d. Fourier transform (3DFT)
t.-d. imaging
t.-d. neuroimaging
t.-d. projection reconstruction imaging
t.-d. reconstruction
three-dimensional-FATS method
three-level Haar wavelet decomposition
three-part fracture
three-phase voltage supply
threonine kinase
threshold
t. of Firooznia
ultrasound t.
throat swabbing
Thrombate III
thrombectomy
chemical t.
mechanical t.
rotational t.
thrombi (*pl. of* thrombus)
thrombin
thrombin-antithrombin III complex (TAT)
Thrombin-Prest
thromboangiitis obliterans
thromboanoic acid
thrombocyte
thrombocythemia
essential t.
thrombocytic leukemia
thrombocytopenia
idiopathic t.
thrombocytopenia,
t. absent radius (TAR)
t. absent radius syndrome
thrombocytosis
paraneoplastic t.

NOTES

thromboembolectomy
    percutaneous aspiration t.
    (PAT)
    rotating aspiration t. (RAT)
thromboembolic (TE)
    t. disease
    t. pulmonary arterial
    hypertension
thromboembolism
    pulmonary t.
thrombogenic coil
β-thromboglobulin
thrombolysis
    sonic t.
thrombolytic
    t. therapy
    t. time
thrombomodulin
thrombopenic anemia
thrombophlebitis
    superficial t.
thromboplastin
thrombopoiesis
thrombopoietin
thrombosed giant vertebral artery aneurysm
thrombosis
    aortic t.
    ascending medullary vein t.
    atrial t.
    axillosubclavian vein t.
    calf vein t.
    catheter-induced subclavian
    vein t.
    coronary t.
    cortical vein t.
    deep vein t. (DVT)
    deep venous t. (DVT)
    dural sinus t.
    ileofemoral t.
    iliofemoral t.
    intervillous t.
    jugular vein t.
    pelvic vein t.
    portal vein t.
    portosplenic t.
    renal vein t.
    Ribbert t.
    sagittal t.
    sinus t.
    splenic vein t.
    subclavian t.
    subclavian vein t.

    subclavian vessel t.
    superior ophthalmic vein t.
    superior sagittal sinus t.
    venous t.
    venous sinus t.
thrombospondin
    Asserachrom t.
thrombotherapy
thrombotic
    t. endocarditis
    t. microangiopathy
    t. obstruction
    t. obstructions
    t. occlusion
    t. stroke
Thrombo-Wellco test
thromboxane
Thrombozyme
thrombus, pl. thrombi
    anechoic t.
    ball t.
    bland t.
    coral t.
    t. extension
    iliocaval t.
    intraluminal t.
    mural t.
    tumor t.
through-and-through
    t.-a.-t. fracture
    t.-a.-t. guidewire
through transfer imaging
through-transmission
thrower's fracture
thrush
    oral t.
TH₁ T-helper cell response
TH₂ T-helper cell response
THU
    tetrahydrouridine
thumb
    fingerized hypoplastic t.
    gamekeeper's t.
    hitchhiker's t.
    hypoplastic t.
    skier's t.
    triphalangeal t.
thumbprinting appearance of the colon
Thy 1 antigen
thymectomy
thymic
    t. agenesis

t. cyst
t. enlargement
t. hyperplasia
t. interdigitating dendritic
   cell
t. leukemia
t. lymphocyte
t. lymphocyte antigen
t. mass
t. neoplasm
thymic-dependent deficiency
thymidine
t. suicide study
tritiated t. (TT)
thymidylate
t. complex
t. synthase
t. synthase expression
thymine dimer
thymocyte
thymolipoma
thymoma
invasive t.
thymopentin
thymosin
thymotaxin
thymus
t. gland
t. nurse cell
thymus-dependent
t.-d. antigen
t.-d. cell
thymus-independent antigen
thymus-replacing factor
thyroarytenoid
thyroglobulin
serum t.
thyroglossal
t. duct cyst
t. duct remnant
thyroid
t. abscess
t. acropachy
t. adenoma
Bavarian t.
t. calcification
t. cancer

t. carcinoma
t. cartilage
t. cyst
t. cystadenoma
t. disease
follicular adenocarcinoma
   of t.
t. function
t. gland
t. hormone
t. hyperplasia
lingual t.
t. lymphoma
t. needle biopsy
t. nodule
t. nodule ablation
occult carcinoma of the t.
t. orbitopathy
thyroidectomy
thyroiditis
acute suppurative t.
chronic lymphocytic t.
de Quervain t.
Hashimoto t.
lymphocytic t.
painless t.
Riedel t.
subacute t.
suppurative t.
thyroid-stimulating hormone (TSH)
thyrotropic substance
thyrotropin
thyrotropin-producing adenoma
thyrotropin-releasing
t.-r. factor
t.-r. hormone (TRH)
thyroxin-binding globulin
thyroxine (T4)
labeled t.
radiolabeled t.
TI
inversion time
tricuspid incompetence
tricuspid insufficiency
TI-23
^{201}**TI**
tian hau fen

NOTES

tiazofurin
TIBC
    total iron-binding capacity
tibia
    proximal t.
    t. vara
tibial
    t. artery
    t. bending fracture
    t. condyle fracture
    t. diaphyseal fracture
    t. fracture
    t. open fracture
    t. plafond
    t. plafond fracture
    t. plateau
    t. plateau fracture
    t. shaft fracture
    t. tendon tear
    t. triplane fracture
    t. tuberosity
    t. tuberosity fracture
    t. vein
tibialis
    t. anterior
    t. posterior
tibiofibular joint
tibioperoneal
    t. runoff system
    t. trunk angioplasty
tibiotalar
    t. joint
    t. slanting
ticarillin
Tice
    T. BCG
tidal volume
tie-on needle
tie sternum
Tietze
    T. cyclic reduction assay
    T. syndrome
Tilden method
Tillaux-Chaput fracture
Tillaux fracture
Tillaux-Kleiger fracture
till birth and death model
tilorone
tilt
    base-ring t.
    lunate t.
time
    acquisition t.

activated partial
    thromboplastin t. (APTT)
t. activity function
background equivalent
    radiation t.
bleeding t.
carcinoembryonic antigen
    doubling t. (CEA-DT)
cell generation t.
cerebral circulation t.
circulation t.
clot lysis t.
clot retraction t.
concentration times t. (C x
    T)
t. constant
correlation t.
cycle t.
Dale-Laidlaw clotting t.
dead t.
decay t.
delay t.
diffusion t. (T_d)
t. domain
doubling t.
Duke bleeding t.
dwell t.
echo t.
effective transverse
    relation t.
efficient relaxation t.
euglobulin lysis t.
t. of flight
t. gain compensation
hematologic recovery t.
image acquisition t.
image reconstruction t.
interpulse t.
inversion t. (TI)
Ivy bleeding t.
Lee-White clotting t.
longitudinal recovery t.
longitudinal relaxation t.
mean transit t.
median survival t. (MST)
partial thromboplastin t.
    (PTT)
t. points
0 t. points
prothrombin t. (PT)
proton spin-lattice
    relaxation t.
pulse repetition t.

receiver dead t.
relaxation t.
repetition t.
rise t.
rotational correlation t.
Russell viper venom
  clotting t.
sampling t.
sequence t.
spin-lattice relaxation t.
thrombolytic t.
transit t.
transverse relaxation t.
T1 relaxation t.
t. trend
tumor doubling t.
t. without symptoms or
  toxicity (Q-TWiST)
time-compensated gain
timed-sequential therapy
time-gain compensation
Timentin
time-of-flight
  t.-o.-f. angiography
  t.-o.-f. effect
  t.-o.-f. flow measurement
  t.-o.-f. signal loss
  t.-o.-f. technique
time-to-treatment
  t.-t.-t. bias
  t.-t.-t. failure (TTF)
time-varied gain
time-varying magnetic field
time-velocity measurement
timing
  gradient t.
  t. parameters
Tinel sign
tine test
tip
  t. angle
  catheter t.
  Cope-Saddekni catheter t.
  t. deflector
  t. dispersion characteristic
  rectal t.

smart laser catheter t.
waiter's t. palsy
tirapazamine
Tiselius apparatus
tissue
  t. adhesive
  adipose t.
  anisotropic t.
  t. bank
  t. blocking
  bronchial-associated
    lymphoid t.
  t. characterization
  t. conductivity
  connective t.
  denuded connective t.
  ectopic t.
  fast exchange-soft t.
  fatty t.
  fatty prostatic t.
  fetal lymphoid t.
  fibrofatty breast t.
  fibrous connective t.
  freeze-dried paraffin-
    embedded t.
  gastrointestinal-associated
    lymphoid t.
  glandular t.
  gut-associated lymphoid t.
  histiocytic t.
  t. immunity
  t. imprint
  intralobular connective t.
  isotropic t.
  lymphoid t.
  mammary t.
  mesothelial t.
  microscopically normal t.
  mucosa-associated
    lymphoid t.
  neural t.
  normal t.
  t. oxygenation
  paravaginal soft t.
  perilobular connective t.
  t. plasminogen activator

NOTES

tissue *(continued)*
    t. polypeptide antigen (TPA)
    preepiglottic soft t.
    prevertebral soft t.
    reduction mammoplasty t.
    residual ductal t.
    retropharyngeal soft t.
    t. sampling
    scar t.
    t. section
    slow exchange soft t.
    soft t.
    subcutaneous t.
    syngeneic t.
    synovial t.
    thoracic inlet soft t.
    t. tolerance to radiation
    vascular t.
    t. water content
    t. weighting factor
    xenogeneic t.
tissue-sparing technique
tissue-specific antigen
TIT
    triple intrathecal therapy
titanium
    t. compound
    t. Greenfield vena cava filter
titer
    antigen t.
    ASO t.
    CEA t
    hemagglutination t.
titration
    Dean and Webb t.
Tl-201
    Cardiolite Tl-201
TLA
    translumbar aortography
    TLA needle
TLI
    total lymphoid radiation
    tritiated thymidine labeling index
T-lymphocyte
    T.-l. activation
    T.-l. binding
    T.-l. differentiation
    T.-l. homing
    T.-l. receptor
    T.-l. receptor gene
    T.-l. subset
TMJ
    temporomandibular joint
TMR
    topical magnetic resonance
TMTX
    trimetrexate
TNF
    tumor necrosis factor
TNM
    tumor node metastasis
    TNM classification
TNP-470
tobacco
    t. mosaic virus
    smokeless t.
tobramycin
Tocantins bone marrow biopsy needle
tocolysis
tocopherol
    alpha t.
toddler's fracture
togavirus
tolazoline
    t. hydrochloride
tolerance
    antigen t.
    drug t.
    Fletcher rule of irradiation t.
    immunologic t.
    irradiation t.
    rectosigmoid irradiation t.
    rectum irradiation t.
Tolosa-Hunt syndrome
toluene
toluidine
    t. blue
    t. blue stain
tomato tumor
tomography
    computed t. (CT)
    computerized axial t. (CAT)
    conventional t.
    dynamic computed t.
    emission computed t. (ECT)
    expiratory computed t.
    flow mode ultrafast computed t.
    helical computed t.

high-resolution computed t. (HRCT)
limited-slice computed t.
linear t.
nuclear magnetic resonance t.
positron emission t. (PET)
quantitative computed t.
single photon emission t. (SPET)
single photon emission computed t. (SPECT)
single photon emission computed t. (SPECT)
spiral computed t.
trispiral t.
ultrafast computed t.
xenon-enhanced computed t.
x-ray computed t.
Tomosar
tomosynthesis
Tomudex
tone
    fetal t.
    vascular t.
tongs
    Crutchfield t.
tongue
    t. cancer
    t. disorder
    t. fasciculation
    t. fracture
Toni-Debre-Fabry-Fanconi syndrome
Tonnesen catheter
tonsil
    t. cancer
    cerebellar t.'s
    lingual t.'s
tonsillar
    t. area cancer
toothbrush
    biotene t.
tooth mass
toothpaste
    biotene t.
    t. shadows mucous plug

tophaceous gout
tophus, pl. tophi
topical
    t. anesthetic
    t. effect
    t. magnetic resonance (TMR)
    t. photochemotherapy
topogram
Topo II
topoisomerase
    t. II (Topo II)
    t. I inhibitor
    t. inhibitor
topoisomerase I
topoisomerase II (Topo II)
topotecan (SK & F 104864, TPT)
TOR
    toremifene
Toradol
TORCH
    toxoplasmosis, rubella, cytomegalovirus, herpes virus
    TORCH group
    TORCH syndrome
torcula
torcular-lambdoid inversion
Torecan
toremifene (TOR)
Tornwaldt cyst
torpedoes
    Gelfoam t.
torque
    t. attenuating diameter wire
    t. control guidewire
torreus
    Aspergillus t.
torsion
    acute testicular t.
    extravaginal testicular t.
    gallbladder t.
    intravaginal t.
    missed testicular t.
    ovarian t.
    splenic t.
    testicular t.

NOTES

torsional
    t. attenuating diameter guidewire
    t. fracture
torticollis
tortuosity
tortuous
    t. aortic arch
tortuous aortic arch
toruloma
Torulopsis
    T. flabrata
torulosis
torus
    t. fracture
    t. mandibularis
    t. tibarius
    t. tubarius
total
    t. abdominal hysterectomy
    t. abdominal hysterectomy and bilateral salpingo-oophorectomy (TAHBSO)
    t. adenine deoxyribonucleotide
    t. adenine ribonucleotide
    t. anomalous pulmonary venous return
    t. body irradiation (TBI)
    t. B therapy
    t. dose over time concept
    t. enteral nutrition (TEN)
    t. exenteration
    t. glossectomy
    t. image noise
    t. iron-binding capacity (TIBC)
    t. lung capacity
    t. lymphoid radiation (TLI)
    t. mastectomy
    T. Mood Disturbance Scale
    t. nodal irradiation
    t. parenteral nutrition (TPN)
totally-implantable catheter
Touraine-Solente-Gole disease
tourniquet
    scalp t.
Touton giant cell
towering cerebellum
Towne
    T. projection radiograph
    T. view

toxic
    t. epidermal necrolysis
    t. megacolon
    t. nodular goiter
    t. shock syndrome
    t. species
    t. synovitis
toxicity
    bismuth t.
    bone marrow t.
    cardiac t.
    chemotherapy-induced pulmonary t.
    cyclosporine t.
    dermatologic t.
    dose-limiting t. (DLT)
    drug t.
    endocrine t.
    epithelial t.
    extramedullary t.
    gastrointestinal t.
    genitourinary t.
    gonadal t.
    hematologic t.
    mucosal t.
    myocardial t.
    nonmyelosuppressive t.
    ocular t.
    organ t.
    pulmonary t.
    radiation-induced pulmonary t.
    time without symptoms or t. (Q-TWiST)
    vascular t.
toxic-oil syndrome
toxicology testing
toxin
    bacterial t.
    Coley t.
    two-chain t.
Toxocara
    T. canis
    T. canis endophthalmitis
toxocariasis
Toxoplasma
    T. gondii
toxoplasma IgG antibody
toxoplasmosis
    t. lymphadenopathy
    ocular t.
    t., rubella, cytomegalovirus, herpes virus (TORCH)

TP-40
TPA
    tissue polypeptide antigen
      serum TPA
      TPA tumor marker
t-PA therapy
TPCH
    6-thioguanine, procarbazine,
      CCNU, hydroxyurea
TPDCV
    6-thioguanine, procarbazine,
      dibromodulcitol, CCNU
      (lomustine), vincristine
TP intensity
TPN
    total parenteral nutrition
TPT
    topotecan
TR
    transverse relaxation
      TR image
TRA
    trans-retinoic acid
trabecular carcinoma
trabeculated
    t. bone
    t. bone lesion
tracer
    carbon dioxide t.
    deposition of t.
    t. principle
    radioactive t.
    uptake of t.
trachea
    carrot-shaped t.
    intrathoracic t.
    lunate-shaped t.
    napkin-ring t.
tracheal
    t. bifurcation angle
    t. caliber
    t. diverticulosis
    t. fracture
    t. lumen
    t. ring
    t. stenosis

    t. stripe
    t. wall stripe
tracheobiliary fistula
tracheobronchial
    t. hypersensitivity
    t. injury (TBI)
    t. papillomatosis
tracheobronchoesophageal fistula
tracheobronchomalacia
tracheobronchomegaly
tracheobronchopathia
  osteochondroplastica
tracheocele
tracheoesophageal fistula (TEF)
tracheomalacia
tracheopathia osteochondroplastica
tracheostomy
    t. tube
trachomatis
    Chlamydia t.
tracing
    ray t.
track
    needle t.
    t. of pin
Tracker-18 Unibody catheter
Tracker coaxial infusion catheter
tracking
    bolus t.
    lymphatic t.
    magnetic bolus t.
tract
    abnormal fetal urogenital t.
    alimentary t.
    association t.
    biliary t.
    bronchial t.
    corticobulbar t.
    corticospinal t.
    dermal sinus t.
    t. dilation
    fetal urogenital t.
    fistulous t.
    gastrointestinal t.
    genitourinary t.
    iliotibial t.
    internodal t.'s

NOTES

tract *(continued)*
    lateral lemniscus t.
    lateral spinothalamic t.
    left ventricular outflow t.
    olfactory t.
    pulmonary outflow t.
    pyramidal t.
    respiratory t.
    retrochiasmal optic t.
    right ventricular outflow t.
    rubrospinal t.
    seminal t.
    sinus t.
    spinal dermal sinus t.
    spinocerebellar t.
    spinothalamic t.
    tamponade needle t.
    tectospinal t.
    tree-barking urinary t.
    UGI t.
    upper aerodigestive t.
    upper gastrointestinal t.
    urinary t.
    urogenital t.
    uveal t.
    ventricular outflow t.
    vestibulospinal t.
traction
    breast t.
    t. diverticulum
    t. fracture
Trac-Wright catheter
TRAIDS
    transfusion-related AIDS
train
    Carr-Purcell-Meiboom-Gill
      echo t.
    echo t.
trait
    Lepore t.
    sickle cell t.
tram
    t. line
    t. track cortical calcification
TRAMPCOL
    6-thioguanine, rubidomycin, ara-C, methotrexate, prednisolone, cyclophosphamide, Oncovin, L-asparaginase
trampoline fracture
tranexamic acid
transabdominal
    t. chorionic villus sampling

    t. color Doppler sonography
    t. sonogram
transacting
transactivation
transaminase
    serum glutamate pyruvate t. (SGPT)
    serum glutamic-oxaloacetic t. (SGOT)
transarterial platinum coil embolization
transaxial
    t. plane
    t. scan
    t. scan plane
    t. thoracic inlet
transaxillary needle
transbronchial biopsy
transcaphoid fracture
transcapitate fracture
transcatheter
    t. arterial chemoembolization (TACE)
    t. closure
    t. embolization
    t. occlusion
    t. splenic embolization
    t. therapeutic infarction
transceiver
transcerebral medullary vein
transcervical
    t. chorionic villus sampling
    t. femoral fracture
transchondral fracture
transcondylar fracture
transcranial
    t. Doppler
    t. real-time color Doppler imaging
    t. real-time color-flow Doppler sonography
transcript
    leukemia t.
transcriptase
    reverse t.
transcription
    t. factor
    gene t.
    RNA t.
transcriptional mutation
transcubital approach

transcutaneous
    t. electrical nerve stimulator (TENS)
    t. oxygen pressure measurement ($tcPO_2$)
transdermal medication patch
transducer
    Acuson linear array t.
    ART t.
    t. beam pattern
    biopsy t.
    end-viewing t.
    high-frequency t.
    high-resolution t.
    linear array t.
    phased array t.
    piezoelectric t.
    puncture t.
    sector t.
    signal t.
    ultrasound t.
transduction
    signal t.
transduodenal endosonography
transection, transsection
    aortic t.
    traumatic aortic t.
transepiphyseal fracture
transesophageal echocardiography
transfection
    DNA t.
    gene t.
transfemoral
    t. venous catheterization
transfemoral venous catheterization
transfer
    t. characteristic
    embryo t.
    t. factor
    Fourier t.
    gamete interfallopian t. (GIFT)
    gene t.
    t. imaging
    immunity t.
    inversion t.
    linear energy t. (LET)

    magnetization t.
    placental t.
    saturation t.
    in vivo gene t.
transferase
    adenine phosphoribosyl t.
    alkyl t.
    deoxynucleotidyl t.
    glutathione t.
    terminal deoxynucleotidyl t. (TdT)
transferrin
    t. receptor
    t. saturation
transform
    discrete Fourier t. (DFT)
    driven equilibrium Fourier t. (DEFT)
    fast Fourier t.
    Fourier t.
    inverse Fourier t. (IFT)
    three-dimensional Fourier t. (3DFT)
    two-dimensional Fourier t. (2DFT)
    wavelet t.
transformation
    blastic t.
    cavernous t.
    t. constant
    Fourier t.
    photo t.
    plasmacytoid t.
    prolymphocytic t.
    prolymphocytoid t.
    Richter t.
    Richter syndrome-like t.
    vascular t.
    t. zone
transforming
    t. gene
    t. growth factor-α
    t. growth factor
    t. growth factor-β
    t. growth factor-alpha 4 (TGF-alpha)
    t. principle

NOTES

transfused blood
transfusion
    blood t.
    cellular blood product t.
    erythrocyte t.
    fetomaternal t.
    granulocyte t.
    leukocyte t.
    matched lymphocyte t.
    monovular twin t.
    platelet t.
    t. syndrome
    white blood cell t.
transfusion-acquired HIV
transfusion-related AIDS
  (TRAIDS)
transgastric endosonography
transgene
transgenic mouse
transgluteal approach
transhamate fracture
transhepatic
    t. biliary disease
    t. catheter
    t. cholangiography
    t. drainage
    t. protogram
transhiatal esophagectomy (THE)
translent
    t. acantholytic dermatosis
    t. cavitation
    t. chyle leak
    t. equilibrium
    t. hemispheric attack
    t. hiatal hernia
    t. ischemic attack
    t. myeloproliferative disease
    t. osteoporosis of hip
    t. pleural effusion
    t. respiratory distress of
    newborn
    t. synovitis
    t. synovitis of hip
    t. tachypnea
    t. tachypnea of newborn
    (TTN)
transiliac fracture
transit
    delayed small bowel t.
    t. scintigraphy
    small bowel t.
    t. time

    tubular t.
    t. volume
transition
    cell phase t.
    t. electron
    isometric t.
    t. metal
    refractory anemia with
    excess blasts in t.
    t. zone
transitional
    t. cell cancer
    t. cell carcinoma (TCC)
    t. cell neoplasm
    t. cell papilloma
    t. vertebra
transjugular
    t. intrahepatic portosystemic
    shunt
    t. venography
translation
    nick t.
translational
    t. diffusion
    t. motion
translocation
    chromosomal t.
    chromosome t.
    robertsonian t.
    t(14,18) chromosomal t.
translumbar
    t. access
    t. aortography (TLA)
    t. aortography needle
transluminal
    t. angioplasty
    t. endarterectomy catheter
    t. extraction catheter (TEC)
transmissible venereal tumor
transmission
    airborne t.
transmitter coil
transmural invasion
transonic
transpapillary placement
transperineal implant
transphosphorylation
transplant
    allogeneic bone marrow t.
    (ABMT)
    allogeneic peripheral cell t.
    autologous bone marrow t.
    (ABMT)

bone marrow t. (BMT)
cardiac t.
double t.
heart t.
hepatic t.
HLA-identical sibling t.
human-leukocyte-antigen-
  identical t.
kidney t.
liver t.
lung t.
MUD t.
organ t.
pancreatic t.
peripheral blood stem
  cell t.
peripheral stem cell t.
renal t.
sequential t.
solid organ t.
stem cell t.
syngeneic bone marrow t.
tandem t.
t. team
twin t.
twin donor t.
transplantation
  t. antigen
  autologous blood stem
    cell t.
  bone marrow t
  t. immunology
transplatin
transplutonium radioisotope
transport
  sample t.
transposed adnexa
transposition
  t. complex
  congenitally corrected t.
  t. of great arteries
  t. of great vessels
  t. of ovary
transposon
transrectal
  t. biopsy

t. sonography
t. ultrasonography
trans-retinoic acid (TRA)
transsacral fracture
transscaphoid
  t. dislocation fracture
  t. perilunate dislocation
transsection (*var. of* transection)
transseptal catheterization
transsexual
transsphincteric surgery
transstenotic gradient
transthoracic
  t. esophagectomy
  t. needle biopsy
  t. percutaneous fine-needle
    aspiration biopsy
transtriquetral fracture
transtubercular plane
transudative pleural effusion
transurethral
  t. balloon dilatation
  t. incision of the prostate
    (TUIP)
  t. resection
  t. resection of bladder
    (TURB)
  t. resection of bladder
    tumor
  t. resection of prostate
    (TURP)
  t. resection of prostate
    ulceration
transvaginal
  t. approach
  t. cone
  t. fallopian tube
    catheterization
  t. hysterosalpingo-contrast
    sonography
  t. implant
  t. sonography
  t. ultrasonography
transversalis fascia
transversarium
  foramen t.

NOTES

transverse
  t. acoustic wave
  t. colon
  t. colon carcinoma
  t. comminuted fracture
  t. diameter between ischia
  t. fracture
  t. lines of Park
  t. lucent metaphyseal lines
  t. magnetization
  t. mesocolon
  t. myelitis
  t. plane
  t. process
  t. processes
  t. process fracture
  t. relaxation (TR)
  t. relaxation time
  t. relaxivity (R2)
  t. ridge
  t. section imaging
  t. sinus
  t. stripe sign
  t. tarsal joint
  t. view
transversely oriented endplate compression fracture
transverse/neutral view
transversus abdominis muscle
transvesical oocyte retrieval
transvestite
TRAP
  6-thioguanine, rubidomycin, ara-C, prednisone
  TRAP positive
  TRAP stain
trap
  t. door fragment
  promoter t.
trapeziometacarpal joint
trapezium, pl. trapezia
  t. fracture
trapezius
trapezoid ligament
trapping
  air t.
  t. defect
trash-foot syndrome
Traube semilunar space
trauma
  abdominal t.
  birth t.
  cardiothoracic t.

  nonaccidental t.
  pelvic vascular t.
  sequela to recent t.
  splenic t.
  testicular t.
  vascular t.
traumatic
  t. aortic disruption
  t. aortic injury
  t. aortic rupture
  t. aortic tear
  t. aortic transection
  t. bone cyst
  t. diaphragmatic hernia
  t. fat necrosis
  t. lipid cyst
  t. lung cyst
  t. meningocele
  t. pneumatocele
  t. pneumomediastinum
  t. pneumothorax
  t. rupture of the diaphragm (TRD)
Travase ointment
Travenol
  T. biopsy needle
  T. Infusor pump
traversal
  tentorial t.
trazodone
TRD
  traumatic rupture of the diaphragm
  iatrogenic TRD
  penetrating TRD
Treacher Collins syndrome
treatment
  Allen t.
  allocation of t.
  conservative t.
  curative t.
  experimental t.
  ex vivo marrow t.
  ferromagnetic microembolization t.
  hyperthermia t.
  hypothermia t.
  indomethacin t.
  P32 intraperitoneal t.
  site-specific t.
treatment-related secondary cancer
tree
  t. artifact

biliary t.
bronchial t.
decision t.
tree-barking urinary tract
tree-in-winter appearance
trefoil appearance
Treitz
ligament of T.
trend
survival t.
time t.
Trendelenburg radiograph
Trental
Trentin hematopoietic-inductive
microenvironment model
trephine biopsy
Treponema pallidum
treponematosis
tretinoin
Trevor disease
TRH
thyrotropin-releasing hormone
TRH stimulation
triad
Bergquist t.
Carney t.
Charcot t.
Hutchinson t.
Kartagener t.
Phemister t.
portal t.
Rigler t.
wall-echo shadow t.
WES t.
Whipple t.
trial
clinical t.
crossover t.
triamenedithiol
triamine
triangle
anal t.
Codman t.
femoral t.
Garland t.
Kager t.
t. of Laimer

sylvian t.
urogenital t.
triangular ligament
triangulation method
triatriatum
cor t.
triazinate (TZT)
triazofurin
tribavirin
Triboulet test
triceps brachii
trichinosis
trichloracetic acid
trichobezoar
Trichomonas
trichomoniasis
trichosanthin
Trichosporon
trichrome stain
trichuriasis
triciribine phosphate
tricuspid
t. atresia
t. incompetence (TI)
t. insufficiency (TI)
t. regurgitation
t. valve
tricyclic nucleotide
trident hand
triethylenethiophosphoramide
(TESPA)
trifluoperazine
trifurcation
popliteal artery t.
trigeminal
t. nerve
t. neuroma
trigger
EKG t.
t. point injection
triggering
triglycerides
medium chain t.
trigonocephaly
trigonum
os t.

NOTES

triiodobenzoic acid
triiodothyronine (T3)
trilateral retinoblastoma
trilineage
    t. engraftment
    t. hematopoiesis
Trilisate
trilogy of Fallot
trilostane
trimalleolar
    t. ankle fracture
    t. fracture
trimalleolar fracture
trimeric protein
trimester
trimethoprim
trimethoprim-sulfamethoxazole
trimethylanilinium
trimetrexate (TMTX)
    t. gluconate
    t. gluconurate
trimodality therapy
Trinquoste syndrome
Triosil
tripartite duodenal carcinoma
tripelennamine hydrochloride
triphalangeal thumb
triphasic
triphosphate
    adenosine t. (ATP)
    deoxyadenosine t. (dATP)
    guanosine t. (GTP)
    nucleoside t. (NTP)
5'-triphosphate
    ara C 5'-t. (ara-CTP)
triplane fracture
triple
    t. intrathecal therapy (TIT)
    t. therapy
triple-bubble sign
triple-head camera
triple-lumen catheter
triple-peak configuration
triplet gestation
triple-track sign
triploidy
tripod fracture
Tripter
    Direx T.
triquetral
    t. bone
    t. fracture
triquetropisiform articulation

triquetrum
trisalicylate
    choline magnesium t.
trisomic fetus
trisomy
trisomy 13-15
trisomy 16-18
trisomy 18
trisomy 21
trispiral tomography
tritiated
    t. thymidine (TT)
    t. thymidine labeling index
        (TLI)
triton tumor
trk proto-oncogene
trocar
    t. catheter
    t. drainage method
    t. needle
    t. technique
trocar-cannula technique
trochanter
    greater t.
    lesser t.
trochanteric
troche
    Mycelex t.
trochlea, pl. trochleae
trochlear
    t. nerve
    t. nerve neoplasm
    t. notch
troland
trolley-track sign
Trombostat
tromethamine
    ketorolac t.
Tronzo classification of
  intertrochanteric fractures
tropane
    methyl-2-carbomethoxy-3-
      phenyl t.
trophic fracture
trophoblast
trophoblastic
    t. disease
    t. tumor
tropica
    Leishmania t.
tropical
    t. eosinophilia
    t. hemobilia

t. macrocytic anemia
t. pancreatitis
t. spastic paraparesis
t. sprue
tropicalis
 Candida t.
tropicum
 granuloma t.
tropisetron
tropism
tropolone
tropomyosin
trough
 t. drug measurement
 t. line
 t. sign
Trousseau-Lallemand body
Tru-Cut
 T.-C. biopsy needle
 T.-C. liver biopsy needle
 T.-C. needle biopsy
true
 t. aneurysm
 t. conjugate measurement
 t. histiocytic lymphoma
 t. knot
 t. porencephaly
 t. ventricular aneurysm
Trueta shunt
Trümmerfeld zone
trumpet-like pelvocaliceal system
trumpet sign
truncal rhabdomyosarcoma
truncation
 t. artifact
 t. band artifact
 t. phenomenon
truncus arteriosus
trunk
 brachiocephalic t.
 pulmonary t.
Trypanosoma cruzi
trypanosomiasis
trypsinization
TSH
 thyroid-stimulating hormone
T-shaped uterus

TSH-displacing antibody
TSPP
TSTA
 tumor-specific transplantation
 antigen
TT
 tritiated thymidine
T1-T4
TTF
 time-to-treatment failure
TTN
 transient tachypnea of newborn
TTPA
T-tube cholangiography
tubal
 t. mass
 t. obstruction
 t. occlusion
 t. pregnancy
tubarius
 torus t.
tube
 Argyle feeding t.
 Blakemore-Sengstaken t.
 Cantor t.
 Carlen endotracheal t.
 cathode ray t. (CRT)
 Celestin t.
 chest t.
 Contigen t.
 Crookes-Hittorf t.
 Dennis t.
 Dobbhoff feeding t.
 endotracheal t.
 enteral feeding t.
 ET t.
 eustachian t.
 fallopian t.'s
 feeding t.
 field emission t.
 Frederick-Miller t.
 gastrointestinal t.
 gastrostomy t.
 Hemagard collection t.
 Herring t.
 Hymlek portable chest t.
 intestinal t.

NOTES

tube *(continued)*
Levin t.
mediastinal t.
MIC t.
Miller-Abbott t.
Minnesota t.
molybdenum target t.
nasogastric t.
nasojejunal feeding t.
neural t.
Newvicon camera t.
NG t.
percutaneous endoscopic
gastrostomy t., PEG t.
Plumicon camera t.
rectifier t.
rotating anode t.
Salem sump t.
Silastic t.
T-t.
tracheostomy t.
uterine t.
Vidicon camera t.
Wintrobe t.
Xomed endotracheal t.
tubercidin
tuber cinereum
tubercle
intercondylar t.
jugular t.
t. of Morgagni
tuberculin
new t.
t. skin test
t. syringe
t. unit
tuberculoma
tuberculosis (TB)
anorectal t.
atypical t.
cavitary t.
endobronchial t.
exudative t.
fibroproductive t.
miliary t.
miliary pulmonary t.
multidrug-resistant t. (MDR-
TB)
Mycobacterium t.
postprimary pulmonary t.
primary pulmonary t.
progressive primary t.

pulmonary t.
reactivation t.
tuberculous
t. arthritis
t. cystitis
t. effusion
t. mediastinal adenopathy
t. peritonitis
t. spondylitis
tuberculum sellae meningioma
tuberosity
ischial t.
tibial t.
tuberous sclerosis
tubing
dialysis t.
polyethylene t.
shunt t.
tublin protein
tubogram
tuboovarian abscess
tuboreticular structure
tubular
t. adenoma
t. bronchiectasis
t. carcinoma
t. dysgenesis
t. fertility index
t. function
t. gas pattern
t. hypoplasia
t. necrosis
renal t. dysgenesis
t. transit
t. wire mesh
tubulovillous adenoma
tuft
t. fracture
penciling of terminal t.'s
silk t.
terminal t.'s
ungual t.
TUIP
transurethral incision of the
prostate
tularemia
tulip bulb aorta
tumbling
macromolecular t.
tumefactive
t. biliary sludge
t. sludge

tumor

abdominal wall desmoid t.
t. ablation
acinic cell t.
acoustic nerve sheath t.
acute splenic t.
adenoid t.
adenomatoid t.
adenomatoid odontogenic t.
adipose t.
adrenal t.
adrenocortical rest cell t.
ameloblastic adenomatoid t.
amyloid t.
aneuploid t.
aneuploid NBX t.
t. aneuploidy
t. angiogenesis
t. angiogenesis factor
t. angiogenic factor
angiomatoid t.
t. antigen
t. antigenicity
aortic body t.
apudoma t.
Askin t.
autochthonous t.
t. autocrine mobility factor
Azzopardi t.
B cell t.
Bednar t.
benign t.
benign lymphoepithelial
  parotid t.
benign ovarian t.
Berkson-Gage method t.
t. biology
bipotential precursor cell t.
bladder t.
blood t.
t. blood supply
t. blush
bone t.
bone-forming t.
brain t.
Brenner t.
bronchial carcinoid t.

Brooke t.
brown t.
t. burden
burned-out t.
Buschke-Löwenstein t.
carcinoid t.
cardiac t.
carotid body t.
cartilage-containing giant
  cell t.
cartilage-forming t.
cartilaginous t.
t. cell
cell t.
t. cell-host bone relationship
cellular t.
central nervous system t.
central neuroepithelial cell
  origin t.
cerebellopontine angle t.
cervical t.
chemoreceptor t.
chemoresistant t.
chromaffin t.
Codman t.
collision t.
congenital cardiac t.
connective t.
connective tissue t.
cutaneous t.
cutaneous Merkel cell t.
debulking of t.
deep t.
t. defect
t. d'emblee mycosis
  fungoides
t.-derived activated cells
dermal duct t.
dermoid t.
desmoid t.
t. doubling time
drug resistant t.
ductectatic mucinous t.
dumbbell t.
eighth nerve t.
t. embolism
embryonal t.

NOTES

tumor *(continued)*
  embryonic t.
  endocrine t.
  endodermal sinus t.
  endometrioid t.
  epidermoid t.
  epithelial t.
  Erdheim t.
  t. erosion
  esophageal t.
  Ewing t.
  extrahepatic primary
    malignant t.
  extratesticular t.
  fatty t.
  fecal t.
  feminizing adrenal t.
  fibroid t.
  fungating t.
  ganglion cell t.
  G cell t.
  germ cell t.
  gestational trophoblastic t.
  giant cell t.
  Glazunov t.
  glial brain t.
  glomus t.
  glomus body t.
  glomus caroticum t.
  glomus jugulare t.
  Godwin t.
  granular cell t.
  granulosa cell t.
  granulosa-stromal cell t.
  Grawitz t.
  t. growth
  Gubler t.
  gynecologic t.
  haarscheibe t.
  hepatic t.
  heterologous t.
  hilar t.
  histoid t.
  homologous t.
  human t.
  Hürthle cell t.
  hylic t.
  hyperdiploid t.
  hypodiploid t.
  hypopharyngeal t.
  t. hypoxia
  t. immunology
  t. immunotherapy

  t. implant
  inflammatory
    myofibroblastic t.
  infratentorial t.
  innocent t.
  INSS stage 1 t.
  interstitial cell t.
  intestinal carcinoid t.
  intracranial t.
  intramural t.
  intraorbital granular cell t.
  intraventricular t.
  islet cell t.
  juxtaglomerular t.
  Keasby t.
  Klatskin t.
  Koenen t.
  Krukenberg t.
  Landschutz t.
  leiomyomatous t.
  Leydig cell t.
  Lindau t.
  lipogenic t.
  Lugano classification for
    testicular t.
  lung t.
  lymphoepithelial t.
  lymphoepithelial parotid t.
  t. lysis syndrome
  malignant t.
  malignant mixed t.
  malignant mixed
    müllerian t.
  malignant ovarian t.
  malignant small round
    cell t.
  t. marker
  t. mass
  mediastinal germ cell t.
  melanotic
    neuroectodermal t.
  meningeal cell t.
  Merkel cell t.
  mesenchymal t.
  mesenchymal sex cord
    stromal t.
  mesonephroid t.
  metastatic t.
  metastatic lymph node t.
  Middeldorph t.
  mixed t.
  mixed germ cell t.
  mixed mesodermal t.

mucinous t.
mucoepidermoid t.
müllerian t.
multifocal brain t.
multiploid t.
musculoskeletal t.
myofibroblastic t.
t. necrosis factor (TNF)
t. necrosis factor-α
t. necrosis factor-alpha
t. necrosis factor-β-
lymphotoxin
Nelson t.
t. neovasculature
nerve cell t.
nerve sheath t.
neural t.
neuroectodermal t.
neuroendocrine t.
neuroepithelial t.
neurogenic t.
neuroglial t.
neuronal cell origin t.
t. node metastasis (TNM)
nonencapsulated sclerosing t.
nonepithelial t.
nonsclerosing t.
nonseminomatous t.
nonseminomatous germ
cell t.
odontogenic t.
oil t.
oncocytic hepatocellular t.
optic complex t.
oral cavity t.
organoid t.
osteocartilaginous t.
osteoclastoma giant cell t.
ovarian t.
ovarian carcinoid t.
ovarian granulosa-stromal
cell t.
ovarian granulosa-theca
cell t.
ovarian hilar cell t.
t. oxygenation

Page grade (2/2, 3/3) for
breast t.
Pancoast t.
pancreatic islet cell t.
papillary t.
paracardiac t.
paraffin t.
parasellar dermoid t.
paratesticular t.
parathyroid t.
parotid t.
pearl t.
pearly t.
pediatric solid t.
Pepper t.
percutaneous ethanol
ablation of t.
peripheral
neuroectodermal t.
peritoneum desmoid t.
permeative
neuroectodermal t.
phantom t.
phyllodes t.
Pindborg t.
pineal t.
pineal germ cell t.
pineal gland t.
pineal parenchymal t.
pineal region t.
pituitary t.
t. ploidy
t. plop
pontine angle t.
posterior fossa t.
Pott puffy t.
precursor cell t.
pregnancy t.
primary implanted t.
primitive neuroectodermal t.
primitive neuroepithelial t.
t. progression
pulmonary t.
radiation-induced peripheral
nerve t.
ranine t.
Rathke pouch t.

NOTES

tumor *(continued)*
    t. receptor protein negative
    Recklinghausen t.
    refractory t.
    renal t.
    reticuloendothelial t.
    reticuloendothelial cell
      origin t.
    retinal anlage t.
    rhabdoid t.
    round cell t.
    Rous t.
    sacral bone t.
    sacrococcygeal t.
    sand t.
    scannable t.
    Schwann t.
    Scully t.
    serous ovarian t.
    Sertoli cell t.
    Sertoli-Leydig cell t.
    sex cord stromal t.
    t. shrinkage
    sinonasal t.
    skull base t.
    small bowel t.
    smooth muscle t.
    solid t.
    solitary t.
    spinal axis t.
    spinal cord t.
    squamous odontogenic t.
    t. stage
    stromal t.
    stromal cell t.
    subastrocytic t.
    subcutaneous t.
    sugar t.
    superior pulmonary sulcus t.
    superior sulcus t.
    t. suppressor
    t. suppressor gene
    supratentorial t.
    synovitis t.
    temporal bone t.
    teratoid t.
    testicular t.
    tetradiploid t.
    tetraploid t.
    theca cell t.
    t. thrombus
    tomato t.
    transmissible venereal t.
    transurethral resection of
      bladder t.
    triton t.
    trophoblastic t.
    turban t.
    ulcerative t.
    urethral t.
    uroepithelial t.
    t. vaccine
    vaginal t.
    vanishing t.
    vascular t.
    t. vascularity
    villous t.
    t. virus
    t. volume
    von Hippel t.
    Warthin t.
    well-differentiated polycystic
      Wilms t.
    Wilms t.
    Yaba t.
    yolk sac t.
    Zollinger-Ellison t.
tumoral calcinosis
tumor-associated
    t.-a. antigen (TAA)
    t.-a. glycoprotein (TAG)
    t.-a. glycoprotein-72
      (TAG-72)
    t.-a. glycoprotein-72 antigen
    t.-a. transplantation antigen
      (TATA)
tumor-cell product
tumoricidal
    t. effect
    t. potential
tumorigenesis
tumorigenicity
tumorigenic mechanism
tumor-infiltrating lymphocyte
tumor-like bone condition
tumor-limiting factor
tumor-specific
    t.-s. antigen
    t.-s. transplantation antigen
      (TSTA)
tumor-targeting ability
tungstate
    antimonium t. (HPA-23)
    calcium t.

tungsten
    t. carbide pneumoconiosis
    t. target
tungsten-188 (^{188}W)
tunica
    t. adventitia
    t. albuginea
    t. albuginea cyst
    t. intima
    t. media
    t. vaginalis
tunnel
    carpal t.
    t. radiograph
    t. subaortic stenosis
    tarsal t.
Tuohy aortography needle
Tuohy-Borst
    T.-B. adapter
    T.-B. introducer
TURB
    transurethral resection of
    bladder
turban tumor
turbinate
    nasal t.
    paradoxical middle t.
turboFLASH
turbulence
turbulent flow
turcica
    sella t.
Turcot syndrome
Turk cell
Turkel needle
Turner
    T. needle
    T. syndrome
TURP
    transurethral resection of
    prostate
turricephaly
Tuttle test
T1-weighted
    T.-w. FAST
    T.-w. image
    T.-w. magnetic resonance

    T.-w. spin echo
    T.-w. spin-echo examination
T2-weighted
    T.-w. image
    T.-w. spin-echo examination
twiddler's syndrome
twin
    conjoined t.'s
    dichorionic t.
    dichorionic-diamniotic t.
    discordant t.
    dizygotic t.
    t. donor
    donor t.
    t. donor transplant
    t. ectopic pregnancy
    fraternal t.
    identical t.
    monochorionic t.
    monochorionic-
    monoamniotic t.
    monozygotic t.
    perfused t.
    t. pregnancy
    pump t.
    recipient t.
    stuck t.
    t. transplant
twin-beam CT
twining
    T. line
    T. recess
twin-peaked pulse
twin-reversed arterial perfusion
    sequence
twin-twin transfusion syndrome
twist
    myocardial t.
twister pulse
TwoCal HN
two-chain toxin
two-dimensional (2D)
    t.-d. Fourier imaging (2DFr)
    t.-d. Fourier transform
    (2DFT)
    t.-d. Fourier transformation
    imaging

NOTES

two-dimensional *(continued)*
    t.-d. imaging
    t.-d. immunoelectrophoresis
    t.-d. mapping
two-dye method
two-hit hypothesis
two-hybrid yeast screen
two-needle technique
two-part fracture
Tworek bone marrow-aspirating
    needle
Twort-d'Herelle phenomenon
two-step
    t.-s. procedure
    t.-s. technique
two-tail test
tylectomy
tylosis
Tylox
tympani
    chorda t.
    tegmen t.
tympanic
    t. cavity
    t. membrane
    t. plexus
tympanicum
    glomus t.
tympanosclerosis
type
    centrocyte-like t.

    diffuse fibrosis t.
    hand-mirror cell t.
    L&H t.
    lymphomatous t.
    mixed cellularity t.
    nonconvoluted t.
    pleomorphic t.
    reticular t.
typhlitis
typhoid
typing
    Mostofi histologic t.
    primed lymphocyte t.
tyropanoate
tyropanoic acid
tyrosinase
tyrosine
    t. hydroxylase
    t. kinase
    t. phenolic group
    t. phosphorylation
    t. protein kinase
tyrosinemia
Tzanck smear
T-zone lymphoma
TZT
    triazinate
Tzu
    Ya Yan T.

UBCR probe
UC
    undifferentiated carcinoma
U-cell lymphoma
U-87201E
U-87291E
UGI
    upper gastrointestinal
        UGI tract
ugly foot syndrome
UICC
    International Union Against
      Cancer
    Union Internationale Contre le
      Cancer
UICC-RO resection
UK
    urokinase
ulcer, ulceration
    antral u.
    aphthous u.
    atherosclerotic u.
    benign gastric u.
    Buruli u.
    channel pyloric u.
    collar button u.
    colonic u.
    Curling u.
    u. disease
    duodenal u.
    duodenal u. disease
    esophageal u.
    frontier u.
    gastric u.
    giant duodenal u.
    kissing u.'s
    malignant gastric u.
    oral u.
    penetrating aortic u.
    peptic u.
    peptic u. disease
    perforated u.
    postbulbar u.
    prepyloric u.
    ruptured u.
    Saemisch u.
    small bowel u.
    stercoral u.
    steroid-induced u.

    stomal u.
    stress u.
ulcerans
    Mycobacterium u.
Ulcerase
ulcerating granuloma of pudenda
ulceration (*var. of* ulcer)
    marginal u.
    mucosal u.
    postbulbar u.
    stercoral u.
    stomal u.
    transurethral resection of
      prostate u.
ulcerative
    u. colitis
    u. jejunitis
    u. tumor
***Ulex europaeus* I lectin**
Ullmann line
ulna, pl. **ulnae**
ulnar
    u. artery
    u. fracture
    u. tunnel syndrome
    u. variance
ulnaris
    extensor carpi u.
U-loop nephrostomy catheter
ultrafast computed tomography
ultrafiltration
ultrasmall-shafted balloon
ultrasonic
    u. atherolysis
    u. attenuation
    u. lithotripsy
    u. lithotripter cannula
    u. nebulizer
ultrasonographically-guided injection
ultrasonography, ultrasound (US)
    B-mode u.
    carotid duplex u.
    compression u.
    continuous-wave Doppler u.
    CW Doppler u.
    Doppler u.
    duplex u.
    endorectal u.
    endoscopic u.
    endovaginal u.

ultrasonography *(continued)*
    gray scale u.
    intraductal u.
    intraoperative u.
    intravascular u.
    obstetric u.
    periorbital directional
      Doppler u.
    real-time u.
    transrectal u.
    transvaginal u.
ultrasound-guided
    u.-g. biopsy
    u.-g. needle aspiration
    u.-g. nephrostomy puncture
ultrastructural platelet peroxidase
  test
ultrastructure
ultrathin balloon
ultraviolet
    u. detector
    u. radiation
    u. spectrum
umbilical
    u. artery
    u. cord
    u. cord cyst
    u. cord edema
    u. cord hematoma
    u. hernia
    u. mass
    u. vein
    u. vein varix
umbilicovesical fascia
umbilicus
Umbradil
umbrella filter
uncinate
    u. process
    u. process fracture
    u. process mass
uncoupled spin
uncovertebral joint
undertreatment
undescended testicle
undifferentiated
    u. carcinoma (UC)
    u. carcinoma of ovary
    u. cell adenoma
    u. sarcoma
undisplaced fracture
undiversion
    urinary u.

Undritz anomaly
unequal pulmonary blood flow
unexplained fever
ungual
    u. fibroma
    u. tuft
unicaliceal kidney
unicameral bone cyst
unicollis
    bicornuate u.
unicondylar fracture
unicornis
    uterus u.
unicornuate uterus
Uniflex
    U. dressing
    U. TFD
uniformity
    differential u.
    extrinsic field u.
    field u.
    integral u.
    intrinsic field u.
Uni-frame patient immobilization
  system
unilateral
    u. diaphragmatic elevation
    u. hydrocephalus
    u. hyperlucent lung
    u. intrafacetal dislocation
    u. large smooth kidney
    u. lobar emphysema
    u. lung perfusion
    u. pleural effusion
    u. pulmonary agenesis
    u. pulmonary edema
    u. salpingo-oophorectomy
      (USO)
    u. small kidney
unilocular cystic lesion
unimalleolar fracture
Unimist
union
    fibrous u.
    U. Internationale Contre le
      Cancer (UICC)
    osseous u.
unipapillary kidney
unit
    adapted standard
      mammography u.
    Ansbacher u.
    Bessey-Lowrey u.

Bethesda u.
blast colony-forming u.
burst-forming u.
central processing u. (CPU)
colony-forming u. (CFU)
erythroid burst-forming u.
fibrinogen equivalent u.
granulocyte colony-
 forming u. (G-CFU)
granulocyte-macrophage
 colony-forming u. (CFU-
 GM)
gray u.
Hounsfield u. (HU)
kallikrein-inhibiting u.
King-Armstrong u.
Lf u.
Mammotest u.
megakaryocyte colony-
 forming u.
murine colony-forming u.
osteomeatal u.
pressor u.
Somogyi u.
Svedberg u.
terminal duct lobular u.
Thayer-Doisy u.
tuberculin u.
unitarian theory
unit-culture
 colony-forming u.-c, (CFU-
 C)
unit-eosinophil
 colony-forming u.-e.
 (CFU$_{EOS}$)
unit-erythroid
 burst-forming u.-e. (BFU-E)
unit-fibroblast
 colony-forming u.-f. (CFU-F)
UniTone
univariant analysis
univentricular heart
Universal
 U. basket
 U. handle
universalis
 calcinosis u.

unknown
 u. primary
 u. primary site
unmasking
 antigen u.
unrelated
 u. bone marrow donor
 u. donor (URD)
unresectable colorectal cancer
unresponsiveness
 immunologic u.
unsaturated fat
unsharp masking
unsharpness
 u. of the costophrenic
 angles
 motion u.
unstable
 u. angina
 u. fracture
ununited fracture
unused colon
unusual interstitial pneumonitis
uphill varices
UPJ
 ureteropelvic junction
upper
 u. aerodigestive tract
 u. gastrointestinal (UGI)
 u. gastrointestinal endoscopy
 u. gastrointestinal series
 u. gastrointestinal tract
 u. GI series
 u. limb-cardiac syndrome
 u. motor neuron
upregulate
upregulation of the receptor
upright position
UPSC
 uterine papillary serous
 carcinoma
uptake
 amine precursor u.
 antimyosin u.
 increased isotope u.
 isotope u.
 radioiodine u.

NOTES

uptake *(continued)*
 RAI u.
 T3 u.
 T4 u.
 u. of tracer
UR-2 sarcoma virus
urachal
 u. abnormality
 u. carcinoma
 u. cyst
 u. sign
urachus
uracil
 u. mustard
uranium mining
urate nephropathy
URD
 unrelated donor
urea
urealyticum
 Ureaplasma u.
Ureaplasma urealyticum
uremia
uremic medullary cystic disease
ureter
 beaded u.
 bifid u.
 circumcaval u.
 corkscrew u.
 extravesical intrasphincteric
 ectopic u.
 hockey-stick appearance of
 the u.'s
 pipestem u.
 retrocaval u.
 saw tooth u.
ureteral
 u. calculus
 u. carcinoma
 u. fistula
 u. jet
 u. obstruction
 u. occlusion
 u. perforation
 u. perfusion test
 u. peristalsis
 u. spindle
 u. stent
 u. stone
 u. stricture
ureterectasis
 terminal u.
ureteric calculus

ureteritis cystica
ureterocele
 ectopic u.
 orthotopic u.
 pyoureter ectopic u.
ureterolysis
ureteroneocystostomy
ureteropelvic
 u. junction (UPJ)
 u. junction obstruction
ureteroperitoneal fistula
ureteropyelostomy
ureterostomy
ureteroureteral anastomosis
ureterovaginal fistula
ureterovesical
 u. junction
 u. junction obstruction
urethra
 penile u.
 prostatic u.
 prostatic portion of the u.
urethral
 u. diverticulum
 u. metallic stent
 u. stricture
 u. syndrome
 u. tumor
 u. valve
urethritis
urethrography
 retrograde u. (RUG)
urethroplasty
 prostatic u.
 retrograde transurethral
 prostatic u.
urethroscopy
urethrotomy
 internal u.
uric
 u. acid
 u. acid calculus
 u. acid nephropathy
uridine
urinary
 u. bladder
 u. bladder diverticulum
 u. bladder rupture
 u. bladder stone
 u. bladder wall calcification
 u. calculus
 u. conduit
 u. diversion

u. diverticulum
u. excretion
u. extravasation
u. fistula
u. obstruction
u. stent
u. stone
u. tract
u. tract anomaly
u. tract infection
u. undiversion
urine
u. leak
u. mutagenicity screening
urinoma
Urocyte diagnostic cytometry system
urodynamic study
uroepithelial
u. malignancy
u. tumor
Urogastrone
urogenital
u. embryology
u. malignancy
u. tract
u. triangle
Urografin
urogram
intravenous u. (IVU)
urographic density
urography
excretory u. (EU)
intravenous u.
urokinase (UK)
u. receptor
urokinase-type plasminogen activator
urolithiasis
urologic emergency
Uromiro
Uropac
uropathy
chronic obstructive u.
obstructive u.
uropod
uroporphyrinogen

urosepsis
urothelial
urothelium
Urovision
ursodeoxycholic acid
ursodiol
urticaria
u. pattern
u. pigmentosa
US
ultrasonography
ultrasound
Imagent US
USO
unilateral salpingo-oophorectomy
Ussing equation
usual
u. interstitial pneumonia
u. interstitial pneumonia of Liebow
u. interstitial pneumonitis
uteri (*pl. of* uterus)
uteric fold
uterine
u. agenesis
u. angiosarcoma
u. anomaly
u. aplasia
u. artery
u. artery waveform
u. bleeding
u. cancer
u. carcinosarcoma
u. cervical cancer
u. cervix
u. chondrosarcoma
u. contraction
u. corpus lymphoma
u. fibroid
u. hypoplasia
u. isthmus
u. leiomyoma
u. leiomyosarcoma
u. mass
u. mixed müllerian sarcoma
u. myoma

NOTES

uterine *(continued)*
> u. papillary serous
> carcinoma (UPSC)
> u. sarcoma
> u. sarcoma metastasis
> u. size
> u. tube

utero
> fetal death in u.

uteroplacental
> u. circulation
> u. insufficiency

uterosacral ligament
uterovesical
> u. fossa
> u. junction
> u. pouch

uterus, pl. **uteri**
> adenocarcinoma of u.
> anteflexed u.
> anteverted u.
> u. arcuatus
> u. bicornis
> bicornuate u.
> body of the u.
> corpus u.
> u. didelphys
> liposarcoma of u.
> müllerian sarcoma of u.
> septate u.
> u. septus
> u. subseptus
> T-shaped u.
> u. unicornis
> unicornuate u.

utricle cyst
U-tube
uveal
> u. melanoma
> u. tract

UV irradiation

V2 loop
V3 loop
VAB
  vinblastine, actinomycin D,
    bleomycin
VAB-6
  vinblastine, actinomycin D,
    bleomycin, cisplatin,
    cyclophosphamide
Vabra aspirator
VAC
  vincristine, actinomycin D,
    cyclophosphamide
  vincristine, Adriamycin,
    cisplatin
    pulse VAC
      vincristine, actinomycin D,
        cyclophosphamide
VACA
  vincristine, actinomycin A
    (dactinomycin),
    cyclophosphamide, Adriamycin
vaccination
  phase II autologous v.
vaccine
  B7 transfected melanoma
    cell v.
  combined immunotherapy
    with levamisole and
    bacillus Calmette-Guérin v.
  duck embryo v.
  GD2T herpes v.
  HIV v.
  killed v.
  killed virus v.
  live virus v.
  measles v.
  melanoma cell lysate v.
  melanoma whole-cell v.
    (MCV)
  meningococcal v.
  methanol extraction residue
    of bacillus Calmette-
    Guérin v.
  Pasteur Institute bacillus
    Calmette-Guérin v.
  pneumococcal v.
  polysaccharide v.
  Sabin v.
  Salk v.

  Semple v.
  tumor v.
  varicella-zoster virus v.
  Vaxsyn HIV-1 v.
vaccinia
  v. melanoma oncolysate
    (VMO)
  v. virus
Vac-Lok patient immobilization
  system
VACTERL
  vertebral, anal, cardiac, tracheal,
    esophageal, renal, limb
    VACTERL syndrome
vacuo
  hydrocephalus ex v.
vacuole
  pinocytotic v.
vacuolization
  cytoplasmic v.
Vacutainer needle
vacuum
  v. disk phenomenon
  v. extraction
  v. phenomenon
  v. sign
VAD
  vascular access dressing
  vincristine, Adriamycin,
    dexamethasone
    Covaderm plus VAD
vagale
  glomus v.
vagi (*pl. of* vagus)
vagina
  intraepithelial neoplasia
    of v.
  in situ carcinoma of v.
  spindle cell sarcoma of v.
vaginal
  v. agenesis
  v. bleeding
  v. candle
  v. carcinoma
  v. condom
  v. discharge
  v. endosonography
  v. fornix
  v. hysterectomy

vaginal *(continued)*
    v. intraepithelial neoplasm
      (VAIN)
    v. reflux
    v. tampon
    v. tumor
vaginalis
    Gardnerella v.
    portio v.
    processus v.
    stratified squamous
      epithelium of portio v.
    tunica v.
vaginectomy
vaginoperineoplasty
vaginosis
    bacterial v.
vagotomy
vagovagal reaction
vagus, pl. **vagi**
VAIN
    vaginal intraepithelial neoplasm
valaciclovir
valence bond
Valergen
valga
    coxa v.
valgum
    genu v.
valgus
    v. deformity
    hallux v.
valgus-external rotation injury
validation
    histopathologic v.
Valium
Vallbracht slow rotational
    recanalizing wire
vallecula, pl. **valleculae**
vallecular narrowing
valproate
valproic acid
Valsalva maneuver
Valtrex
value
    Astrup blood gas v.
    negative predictive v.
    P-v.
    positive predictive v.
    S-v.
valve
    aortic v.
    atrioventricular v.

    attenuation v.
    Björk-Shiley heart v.
    Carpentier-Edwards v.
    v. cinefluoroscopy
    congenital absence of
      pulmonary v.
    v. cusps
    Ebstein malformation of
      tricuspid v.
    flail mitral v.
    floppy mitral v.
    hammock-like posterior
      bowing of mitral v.
    heart v.
    Heimlich v.
    v. of Heister
    incompetent ileocecal v.
    Ionescu-Shiley v.
    v. leaflet
    v. leaflet calcification
    Lillehei-Kaster v.
    miniaturized mitral v.
    mitral v.
    posterior urethral v.
    prosthetic v.
    pulmonary v.
    sail-like tricuspid v.
    shunt v.
    Starr-Edwards v.
    St. Jude v.
    tricuspid v.
    urethral v.
    v. vegetation
    v. wrapping
valve-ended catheter
valvoplasty (*var. of* valvuloplasty)
valvula, pl. **valvulae**
    valvulae conniventes
valvular
    aortic v. disease
    v. aortic stenosis
    v. heart disease
    v. stenosis
valvuloplasty, valvoplasty
    balloon dilation v. (BDV)
VAM
    vinblastine, Adriamycin,
      mitomycin C
VAMP
    vincristine, Adriamycin,
      methylprednisolone
van
    V. Andel tapered catheter

v. Buchem syndrome
v. den Bergh test
v. Sonnenberg modified
coaxial biopsy set
v. Sonnenberg sump
vancomycin
vanillylmandelic acid (VMA)
vanishing
v. bone syndrome
v. tumor
van't Hoff rule
VAPA
vincristine, Adriamycin
(doxorubicin), prednisone,
ara-C
VAPEC-B
Vaquez-Osler disease
vara
Blount tibia v.
coxa v.
tibia v.
variable
v. region
v. segment
variance
Kruskal-Wallis
nonparametric analysis
of v.
ulnar v.
variant
anatomical v.
blastic v.
Dandy-Walker v.
erythrodermatous v.
fibroblastic v.
fibrolamellar v.
fibrosarcoma v.
hyaline-vascular v.
Japanese v.
L-phase v.
lymphohistiocytic v.
macrophage v.
normal v.
paraimmunoblastic v.
plasmacytoid v.
prolymphocytoid v.
v. SCID

syncytial v.
T-cell lymphoma v.
variation
circadian v.
coefficient of v.
developmental v.
ethnic v.
geographic v.
variceal
v. bleeding
v. sclerotherapy
varicella
v. macule
v. papule
varicella-zoster
v.-z. immune globulin
(VZIG)
v.-z. infection
v.-z. pneumonia
v.-z. virus
v.-z. virus infection
v.-z. virus vaccine
varices (*pl. of* varix)
varicocele
Varicocid
varicoid
v. carcinoma
v. esophageal cancer
varicose bronchiectasis
variocele
varioliform erosion
VariTone
varix, pl. varices
colonic v.
downhill varices
duodenal varices
esophageal varices
orbital v.
pulmonary v.
umbilical vein v.
uphill varices
varum
genu v.
varus
v. deformity
hallux v.

NOTES

vasa
  v. previa
  v. vasorum
vascular
  v. abnormality
  v. access
  v. access device
  v. access dressing (VAD)
  v. anomaly
  v. assessment
  v. bypass graft
  v. calcification
  v. cast
  v. channel
  collagen v. disease (CVD)
  v. compartment
  v. complication
  v. disease
  v. disorder
  v. ectasia
  v. embolotherapy
  v. fibrous polyp
  v. graft
  v. insufficiency
  intracranial v. abnormality
  v. invasion
  v. leak syndrome
  v. leiomyoma
  v. malformation
  mesenteric v. insufficiency
  v. necrosis
  v. pedicle
  v. perforation
  v. ring
  v. sarcoma
  v. space
  v. stent
  v. structure
  v. supply
  v. tissue
  v. tone
  v. toxicity
  v. transformation
  v. trauma
  v. tumor
vascularity
  overcirculation v.
  pulmonary v.
  tumor v.
vascularization
vasculature
  cerebral v.

  extracranial v.
  extracranial cerebral v.
  peripheral v.
  pulmonary v.
  splanchnic v.
vasculitis
  bacterial v.
  leukocytoclastic v.
  Pneumocystis-related v.
vasculosus
  nevus v.
vas deferens
Vasiodone
vasoactive intestinal peptide (VIP)
Vaso-Cath catheter
vasodepressor syndrome
vasodilating agent
vasodilator
  v. administration
vasogenic
  v. edema
  v. impotence
vasomotor symptom
vasoocculsive crisis
vasopressin (VP)
  arginine v.
  desamino-D-arginine v.
  v. infusion
vasoreactivity
  cerebral v.
vasorum
  vasa v.
vasospasm
Vasotec
vasovagal
  v. reaction
  v. syndrome
vastus
  v. intermedius
  v. lateralis
  v. medialis
VATER
  vertebral, anal, tracheal,
  esophageal, renal
  VATER association
  VATER complex
Vater
  ampulla of V.
  papilla of V.
VATH
  vinblastine, Adriamycin,
  thiotepa, Halotestin

VATS
  video-assisted thoracoscopic
  surgery
vault
   cranial v.
Vaxsyn HIV-1 vaccine
VBAP
  vincristine, BCNU, Adriamycin,
   prednisone
VBC
  vinblastine, bleomycin, cisplatin
VBL
  vinblastine
VC
  vincristine
VCA
  viral capsid antigen
VCAP
  vincristine, cyclophosphamide,
   Adriamycin, prednisone
V-2 carcinoma
VCMP
  vincristine, cyclophosphamide,
   melphalan, prednisone
VCR
  vincristine
VCUG, VCU
  vesicoureterogram
  voiding cystourethrogram
VDBCC
  vincristine, dactinomycin,
   bleomycin, cisplatin,
   cyclophosphamide
VDD
  vincristine, doxorubicin,
   dexamethasone
VDP
  vinblastine, dacarbazine,
   Platinol
VDRL
  Venereal Disease Research
   Laboratories
VDS
  vindesine
vector
   v. genome

macroscopic
  magnetization v.
 v. profile
 spin v.
Veegam
Veenema-Gusberg prostatic biopsy
  needle
vegetation
   valve v.
veiled cell
veiling glare
vein
   accessory hepatic v.
   adrenal v.
   antecubital v.
   axillary v.
   azygos v.
   basilic v.
   basivertebral v.
   brachial v.
   bridging v.
   cardinal v.
   caudate v.
   cavernous transfer of
    portal v.
   cephalic v.
   cerebral v.
   circumaortic left renal v.
   circumaortic renal v
   condylar emissary v.
   cortical v.
   dilated collateral v.
   dorsal penile v.
   epigastric v.
   esophageal v.
   femoral v.
   v. of Galen
   v. of Galen aneurysm
   v. of Galen malformation
   gastric v.
   greater saphenous v.
   hemiazygous v.
   hemispheric v.
   hepatic v.
   ileofemoral v.
   iliac v.
   inferior mesenteric v.

NOTES

vein *(continued)*
    innominate v.
    internal jugular v.
    jugular v.
    mastoid emissary v.
    mediastinal v.
    mesencephalic v.
    mesenteric v.
    ophthalmic v.
    orbital varix ophthalmic v.
    ovarian v.
    parathyroid v.
    paraumbilical v.
    penile v.
    perforating v.
    pericallosal v.
    perithyroid v.
    peroneal v.
    petrosal v.
    pontomesencephalic v.
    popliteal v.
    portal v.
    portal v. system
    posterior cardinal v.
    pulmonary v.
    quadrigeminal v.
    renal v.
    retroaortic renal v.
    saphenous v.
    scimitar v.
    Servelle v.
    sludging of retinal v.
    spermatic v.
    splenic v.
    striate v.
    subcardinal v.
    subclavian v.
    subependymal v.
    superior mesenteric v.
    superior ophthalmic v.
    supracardinal v.
    testicular v.
    thalamic v.
    thalamostriate v.
    tibial v.
    transcerebral medullary v.
    umbilical v.
    v. valve wrapping
velamentous
    v. insertion
    v. insertion of cord
Velban
Velcro rales

Veldona
velocity
    acoustic v.
    angular v.
    blood v.
    blood flow v.
    carotid v.
    encoding v.
    flow v.
    v. gradient
    high v.
    v. imaging
    v. mapping
    peak v.
    v. profile
    PSA v.
velocity-compensating gradient pulse
velocity-density imaging
velocity-encoded
    v.-e. cine MR imaging
    v.-e. sequence
velocity-evaluation phantom
velopalatine reflux
Velsar
vena, pl. **venae**
    v. cava
    v. cava anomaly
    v. cava filter
    venae comitantes
venacavagram
venacavography
    inferior v.
venacavotony
venae (*pl. of* vena)
Vena Tech dual vena cava filter
Venereal
    V. Disease Research
      Laboratories (VDRL)
venereal lymphogranuloma
venereum
    granuloma v.
    lymphogranuloma v.
    papilloma v.
venipuncture
venoablation
    percutaneous v.
venobiliary fistula
Venoglobulin
Venoglobulin-S
venography
    antegrade v.
    digital free hepatic v.

gonadal v.
hepatic v.
magnetic resonance v.
portal v.
radionuclide v.
spermatic v.
transjugular v.
wedged hepatic v.
venolobar syndrome
Venom
Russell Viper V. (RVV)
venoocclusive disease (VOD)
venospasm
venosus
ductus v.
sinus v.
venotomy
venous
v. access
v. access device
v. access device-related
bacteremia
v. access technique
v. angioma
v. blood
v. calcifications
v. catheter
v. collateral
collateral v. channel
v. congestion
v. distention
v. drainage
v. fistulogram
v. hum
v. hypertension
v. infarction
v. interposition graft
v. lake
v. malformation
v. obstruction
v. occlusion
v. oozing
periureteric v. ring
portohepatic v. shunt
v. shunt
v. sinus thrombosis
v. thrombosis

v. thrombosis embolism
transfemoral v.
catheterization
v. waveform
vent
thoracic v.
ventilation
v. agent
v. defect
v. lung scan
mechanical v.
ventilation-perfusion (V/Q)
v.-p. imaging
v.-p. inequality
v.-p. mismatch
ventilator-assisted respiration
ventilator therapy
ventosa
spina v.
ventral
v. epidural abscess
v. epidural fat
v. hernia
ventricle
CAD right v.
cerebral v.
colloid cyst of third v.
common atrium, aortic
atresia, double-outlet
right v,
double-inlet single v.
double-outlet right v.
high-riding third v.
hourglass v.
ipsilateral lateral v.
lateral v.
left v.
right v.
single v.
ventricular
v. aneurysm
v. dilation
v. endomyocardial biopsy
v. enlargement
v. function
v. myocardium
v. obstruction

NOTES

ventricular *(continued)*
    v. outflow tract
    v. septal defect
    v. septum
    v. shunt
    v. tachycardia
    v. view
ventriculitis
ventriculoatrial shunt
ventriculofugal artery
ventriculogram
    iohexol CT v.
ventriculography
    cerebral v.
    cine left v.
    left v.
    radionuclide v.
    right v.
ventriculomegaly
ventriculoperitoneal shunt
ventriculus terminalis
Venturi effect
venule
    high endothelial v.
VEPA
    vinblastine, etoposide,
    prednisone, Adriamycin
VePesid
    etoposide
    VP-16
vera
    polycythemia v.
    polycythemia rubra v.
verapamil
Vercyte
Veress needle
vergae
    cavum v.
    septum cavum v.
Verifuse
    V. ambulatory infusion pump
vermian
    v. agenesis
    v. pseudotumor
vermicularis
    Enterobacter v.
vermiform appendix
Verner-Morrison syndrome
vernis
verruciformis
    epidermodysplasia v.
verrucosus
    nevus v.

verrucous
    v. carcinoma
    v. nevus
Versed
versus
    spin-echo v.
vertebra, pl. vertebrae
    accordion v.
    anterior scalloping of
    vertebrae
    block v.
    bone-within-bone v.
    bullet-shaped v.
    cervical v.
    coin-on-edge v.
    corduroy v.
    coronal cleft v.
    fishtail v.
    fused vertebrae
    ghost v.
    hamburger vertebrae
    honeycomb v.
    H-shape vertebrae
    ivory v.
    limbus v.
    Lincoln log v.
    lumbar v.
    non-rib-bearing
    vertebrae
    picture frame v.
    v. plana
    rib-bearing vertebrae
    rugger jersey v.
    sandwich vertebrae
    thoracic v.
    transitional v.
    vertebra plana fracture
    wedge-shaped v.
vertebral
    v., anal, cardiac, tracheal,
    esophageal, renal, limb
    (VACTERL)
    v., anal, tracheal,
    esophageal, renal (VATER)
    v. angiography
    v. arch ligament ossification
    v. artery
    v. body
    v. body fracture
    v. border abnormality
    v. canal
    v. column
    v. compression fracture

v. endplate abnormality
v. foramen
v. hemangioma
v. hyperostosis
v. lamina
osteosclerosis v. sarcoidosis
v. wedge compression
fracture
vertebrobasilar
v. artery
v. insufficiency
v. occlusion
v. system
vertical
v. partial laryngectomy
v. sheer fracture
v. talus
verticillus
Streptomyces v.
vertigo
very late antigen
vesamicol receptor
vesical
v. fascia
vesicancy
vesicant
vesicle
brain region v.
lipid-containing v.
seminal v.
synaptic v.
vesicoamniotic shunt
vesicosacral ligament
vesicoureteral reflux
vesicoureterogram (VCUG, VCU)
vesicovaginal
v. fistula
v. repair
vesiculoprostatectomy
retropubic v.
vessel
abdominal great v.
axillary v.
blood v.
brachiocephalic v.
cerebral blood v.
collateral v.

complexes of v.'s
corkscrew v.
v. dilator
femoropopliteal v.
great v.'s
hairpin v.
hilar v.
iliac v.
lenticulostriate v.
mesenteric v.
native v.
penile v.
peripheral v.
portosystemic collateral v.
puff-of-smoke v.'s
pulmonary v.
renal hilar v.
splenic v.
subclavian v.
transposition of great v.'s
vestigial v.
vestibular aqueduct
vestibule
esophageal v.
vestibulocochlear
vestibulospinal tract
vestigial vessel
VEST system
veto
v. activity
v. cell
V factor
VH
Bebulin VH
VHL
von Hippel-Lindau disease
Vi
V. antigen
vibrio
El Tor v.
NAG v.
Vibrio cholerae
vicarious excretion of contrast material
VI cranial nerve palsy
vidarabine

NOTES

video
    v. digital gastrointestinal
      radiography
    v. display camera
    v. fluoroscopy
    v. imaging
    v. signal generator
video-assisted thoracoscopic surgery
  (VATS)
videodensitometry
videofluoroscopy
Videx
    Zerit with V.
vidian
    v. artery
    v. canal
Vidicon camera tube
view
    air contrast v.
    Alexander v.
    amputated-foot v.
    apical lordotic v.
    axial v.
    axillary v.
    base v.
    v. box
    Broden v.
    Caldwell v.
    Carter Rowe v.
    cephalic tilt v.
    cerebellar v.
    Chamberlain-Towne v.
    classic carpal tunnel v.
    Cleopatra v.
    closed-mouth v.
    cone-down v., coned-
      down v.
    coronal v.
    coronal reconstruction v.
    craniocaudal v.
    cross-table v.
    cross-table lateral v.
    decubitus v.
    Eklund v.
    exaggerated craniocaudal v.
    expiratory v.
    extended field of v.
    extension v.
    external rotation v.
    field of v. (FOV)
    Fleckinger v.
    flexion v.
    flexion and extension v.'s

    Fuchs odontoid v.
    full-column v.
    Garth v.
    Grashey v.
    half axial v.
    Hampton v.
    Heinig v.
    Hughston v.
    infrapatellar v.
    inspiratory v.
    v. insufficiency artifact
    internal rotation v.
    Judet v.
    lateral decubitus v.
    lateral extension v.
    lateral flexion v.
    lateral oblique v.
    lateromedial oblique v.
    Law v.
    left anterior oblique v.
    long axis v.
    lordotic v.
    magnification v.
    Mayer v.
    medial oblique v.
    mediolateral v.
    Merchant v.
    mortise v.
    Mukherjee-Sivaya v.
    navicular v.
    oblique v.
    open-mouth v.
    Panorex v.
    parallax v.
    plumbline v.
    portable v.
    posterooblique v.
    postreduction v.
    reconstruction v.
    rectangular field of v.
    Rhese v.
    right anterior oblique v.
    Rokus v.
    sagittal v.
    sagittal and coronal
      reconstruction v.
    semiupright v.
    spot compression v.
    Stenver v.
    stereoscopic v.
    stress v.
    Stryker notch v.
    submaxillary v.

submentovertex v.
subtalar v.
sunrise v.
swimmer's v.
tangential v.
Towne v.
transverse v.
transverse/neutral v.
ventricular v.
Waters v.
weightbearing v.
West Point v.
Zanca v.
Viewing Wand
vif **protein**
VIG
 vinblastine, ifosfamide, gallium
 nitrate
Vigilon
 V. gel dressing
vignetting
 cone of v.
VII
 Stachrom VII
VII:Ag
 factor VII antigen
 Asserachrom VII:Ag
VIII
 clotting factor VIII
 VIII nerve complex
 VIII nerve herpetic neuritis
 VIII nerve neuritis
VIII:C
 Stachrom VIII:C
VIIIR
 factor VIIIR
 von Willebrand factor
villi (*pl. of* villus)
villotubular adenoma
villous
 v. adenoma
 v. carcinoma
 v. lymphocyte
 v. papilloma
 v. polyp
 v. tumor
villus, pl. villi

arachnoid villi
chorionic v.
vilona
vimentin
Vim-Silverman needle
vinblastine (VBL)
 v. amide desacetyl
 L-phenylalanine mustard, v.
 (PAVe)
 v. sulfate
vinblastine, actinomycin D,
 bleomycin (VAB)
vinblastine, actinomycin D,
 bleomycin, cisplatin,
 cyclophosphamide (VAB-6)
vinblastine, Adriamycin, mitomycin
 C (VAM)
vinblastine, Adriamycin, thiotepa,
 Halotestin (VATH)
vinblastine, bleomycin, cisplatin
 (VBC)
vinblastine, dacarbazine, Platinol
 (VDP)
vinblastine, etoposide, prednisone,
 Adriamycin (VEPA)
vinblastine, ifosfamide, Platinol
 (VIP)
vinca alkaloid
vincaleukoblastine
vinca-related neuropathy
Vincasar
Vincent stomatitis
vincristine (VC, VCR)
 v. sulfate
vincristine, actinomycin A
 (dactinomycin), cyclophosphamide,
 Adriamycin (VACA)
vincristine, actinomycin D,
 cyclophosphamide (pulse VAC,
 VAC)
vincristine, Adriamycin, cisplatin
 (VAC)
vincristine, Adriamycin,
 dexamethasone (VAD)
vincristine, Adriamycin
 (doxorubicin), prednisone, ara-C
 (VAPA)

NOTES

vincristine, Adriamycin,
   methylprednisolone (VAMP)
vincristine, BCNU, Adriamycin,
   prednisone (VBAP)
vincristine, carmustine,
   cyclophosphamide, melphalan,
   prednisone (M2)
vincristine, cyclophosphamide,
   Adriamycin, prednisone (VCAP)
vincristine, cyclophosphamide,
   melphalan, prednisone (VCMP)
vincristine, dactinomycin,
   bleomycin, cisplatin,
   cyclophosphamide (VDBCC)
vincristine, doxorubicin,
   dexamethasone (VDD)
vincristine, melphalan,
   cyclophosphamide, prednisone
   (VMCP)
vincristine, prednisone,
   cyclophosphamide, ara-C (VPCA)
vinculin protein
vindesine (VDS)
vindolin
vinorelbine
violet
   gentian v.
VIP
   vasoactive intestinal peptide
   vinblastine, ifosfamide, Platinol
   VP-16, ifosfamide, Platinol
vipoma
viral
   v. budding
   v. capsid antigen (VCA)
   v. envelope protein
   v. hepatitis
   v. infection
   v. load
   v. oncogene
   v. pneumonia
   v. replication
   v. shedding
   v. spasmodic laryngitis
Virchow
   V. cell
   V. metastasis
   V. node
Virchow-Robin
   V.-R. space
   V.-R. space dilatation
viremia
Virend

viridans
   Streptococcus v.
virilization
virion
   intranuclear v.
virology
Vironostika ELISA AIDS test
virucidal
virulent
virus
   Abelson murine leukemia v.
   adenoassociated v.
   apeu v.
   avian E26 v.
   avian leukosis-sarcoma v.
   avian sarcoma v.
   Balb/C sarcoma v.
   bovine leukemia v.
   Brunhilde v.
   Butzler Campylobacter v.
   Bwamba v.
   CA v.
   Cache valley v.
   California v.
   Catu v.
   Chenuda v.
   Coe v.
   Colorado tick fever v.
   croup-associated v.
   dengue v.
   Ebola v.
   Ebola-Marburg v.
   ECBO v.
   ECHO v.
   ECMO v.
   Epstein-Barr v. (EBV)
   feline ataxia v.
   feline leukemia v.
   feline leukemia-sarcoma v.
   fluorescent treponemal
      antibody v. (FTA-ABS)
   Friend v.
   Friend leukemia v.
   Gardner-Rasheed sarcoma v.
   Germistan v.
   gibbon ape
      lymphosarcoma v.
   Graffi v.
   Gross leukemia v.
   Guama v.
   Guaroa v.
   Hardy-Zuckerman 2 feline
      sarcoma v.

Harvey sarcoma v.
hepatitis A v.
hepatitis B v.
hepatitis C v. (HCV)
hepatitis delta v.
hepatitis E v.
herpes v., herpesvirus
herpes simplex v. (HSV)
horizontal transmission
of v.
human immunodeficiency v.
(HIV)
human immunodeficiency v.
1 (HIV-1)
human immunodeficiency v.
2 (HIV-2)
human T-cell leukemia v.
(HTLV)
human T-cell leukemia v.
type 1-5, human T-
lymphotropic virus
human T-cell
lymphotropic v. (HTLV)
Ilheus v.
infectious papilloma v.
influenza v.
Itaqui v.
Japanese B encephalitis v.
JC v.
Jeryl Lynn mumps v.
Junin v.
Kemerova v.
killed v.
Kirsten sarcoma v.
Kumba v.
Langat v.
Lansing v.
Lassa fever v.
Latino v.
Leon v.
Lepore v.
lipid-coated v.
Lucke v.
Lunyo v.
lymphadenopathy-
associated v.

lymphogranuloma
venereum v.
Machupo v.
Makonde v.
Marburg v.
Marituba v.
masked v.
Mason-Pfizer monkey v.
Mayaro v.
McDonough sarcoma v.
McKrae herpes simplex v.
Mengo v.
Mossuril v.
mouse leukemia v.
mouse mammary tumor v.
mouse parotid tumor v.
mumps v.
murine sarcoma v.
Murray Valley
encephalitis v.
Ntaya v.
parainfluenza v.
Parodi-Irgens sarcoma v.
Powassan v.
rabbit fibroma v.
Rasheed sarcoma v.
Rauscher leukemia v.
respiratory syncytial v.
(RSV)
RNA tumor v.
Rous sarcoma v.
rubella v.
Salisbury common cold v.
Sendai v.
Shope fibroma v.
simian foamy v.
simian-human
immunodeficiency v.
simian immunodeficiency v.
(SIV)
SV40 v.
Swiss mouse leukemia v.
Theiler v.
tobacco mosaic v.
tumor v.
UR-2 sarcoma v.
vaccinia v.

NOTES

virus *(continued)*
    varicella-zoster v.
    Wesselsbron v.
    Willowbrook v.
    Yale SK v.
    Yamaguchi sarcoma v.
virus-2
    herpes v.-2
viscera
visceral
    v. artery
    v. calcification
    v. heterotaxy
    v. larva migrans
    v. lesion
    v. peritoneum
    v. pleura
viscosity coefficient
viscous lidocaine
viscus
    perforated hollow v.
    ruptured hollow v.
Vistaril
visual acuity testing
visualization
    needle v.
vital capacity
vitamin
    v. A deficiency
    v. B_{12} deficiency
    v. D-dependent rickets
    v. D-resistant rickets
vitelline duct
vitiligo
    v. autoantibody
vitreous
    persistent hyperplastic
      primary v.
vitritis
vitro
    in v.
vivo
    ex v.
    in v.
Vivonex TEN
VM-26
    teniposide
VMA
    vanillylmandelic acid
VMCP
    vincristine, melphalan,
      cyclophosphamide, prednisone

VMO
    vaccinia melanoma oncolysate
vocal
    v. cord
    v. cord cancer
    v. cord paralysis
vocational issue
VOD
    venoocclusive disease
Voges-Proskauer test
Vogt cephalosyndactyly
void
    flow v.
    signal v.
voiding cystourethrogram (VCUG, VCU)
Vokes chemotherapy protocol
volar
    v. angulation
    v. intercalated segment
    instability
    v. rim
Volkmann
    V. contracture
    V. fracture
Vollmer test
volt
    electron v. (eV)
    kiloelectron v. (kev, keV)
volume
    amniotic fluid v.
    aortic flow v.
    v. averaging
    break-even v.
    caudate v.
    cerebellar v.
    cerebral blood v.
    cerebrospinal fluid v.
    closing v.
    v. coil
    Coulter v.
    erythrocyte v.
    fetal aortic flow v.
    forced expiratory v.
    heart v.
    v. imaging
    v. loss
    lung v.
    mean corpuscular v. (MCV)
    organ v.
    patient v.
    ping-pong v.

quantitative amniotic
fluid v.
red cell v.
residual v.
sensitive v.
stroke v.
tidal v.
transit v.
tumor v.
voxel v.
volume-selective excitation
volumetry
CT-aided v.
volvulus
cecal v.
colonic v.
gastric v.
mesenteroaxial v.
midgut v.
organoaxial v.
sigmoid v.
vomer
vomiting
anticipatory v.
delayed v.
projectile v.
Von
V. Jaksch anemia
von
v. Brunn cell nests
v. Gierke disease
v. Hippel-Lindau disease
(VHL)
v. Hippel-Lindau syndrome
v. Hippel tumor
v. Meyenburg complex
v. Recklinghausen disease
v. Recklinghausen
neurofibromatosis
v. Willebrand disease
v. Willebrand factor (factor
VIIIR, vWF)
v. Zeynek and Mencki test
von Hippel-Lindau syndrome
von Hippel tumor
vorozole

**Vostal classification of radial
fractures**
voxel
v. size
v. volume
voxel-gradient rendering image
VP
vasopressin
VP-16 (VePesid)
etoposide
vpa gene
VPCA
vincristine, prednisone,
cyclophosphamide, ara-C
VP-16, ifosfamide, Platinol (VIP)
vpr
v. gene
v. protein
vpu gene
vpx gene
V/Q
ventilation-perfusion
V/Q inequality
V-sign of Naclerio
vulva, pl. vulvae
bowenoid papulosis of v.
epidermoid carcinoma of v.
intraepithelial neoplasia
of v.
nevus of v.
preinvasive disease of
cervix, vagina, and v.
synechia vulvae
vulvar
v. adenoid cystic
adenocarcinoma
v. biopsy
v. carcinoma
v. intraepithelial neoplasia
v. intraepithelial neoplasm
v. malignancy
v. melanoma
v. pruritus
vulvectomy
radical v.
skinning v.
vulvovaginal carcinoma

NOTES

Vumon
vWF
   von Willebrand factor
     Assera vWF
     Assera-Plate vWF

VZIG
   varicella-zoster immune globulin

[188]W
    tungsten-188
Waaler-Rose test
Waardenburg syndrome
Wackenheim line
wagon wheel fracture
Wagstaffe fracture
waiter's tip palsy
Waldenström macroglobulinemia
Waldeyer
    W. fossa
    W. ring
    W. ring lesion
    W. ring lymphoma
Waldhausen procedure
Walinsky catheter
walk
    random w.
Walker
    W. carcinoma
    W. carcinosarcoma
walking
    chromosome w.
walking-stick appearance
wall
    anterolateral abdominal w.
    arterial w.
    bowel w.
    w. calcification
    chest w.
    fetal abdominal w.
    w. filter
    gallbladder w.
    lateral pharyngeal w.
    myocardial w.
    orbital w.
    pelvic w.
    w. sign
wall-echo
    w.-e. shadow (WES)
    w.-e. shadow triad
Wallenburg syndrome
wallerian degeneration
Wallner interstitial prostate
    implanter
Wallstent
    W. biliary endoprosthesis
Walter Reed classification for
    HIV infection
Walther fracture

Waltman loop
Walton report
Wand
    Viewing W.
wandering
    w. cell
    w. spleen
Wang pleural stoma
WAP
    whole abdominopelvic
    irradiation
Warburg apparatus
warfarin
    w. sodium
    w. therapy
warmer
    blood w.
warm-reactive antibody
Warren shunt
wart
    genital w.
Warthin
    W. cell
    W. tumor
Warthin-Finkeldy giant cell
Warthin-Starry stain
washed red cells
washing
    endometrial jet w.
washin phase
washout phase
Wassermann test
wastage
    pregnancy w.
wasting
    AIDS w.
    w. syndrome
water
    w. bottle heart configuration
    bound w.
    bulk w.
    w. cancer
    w. density area
    w. density line
    free w.
    hydration w.
    hydration layer w.
    ion-bound w.
    irrotationally bound w.
    w. lily sign

water *(continued)*
    oxygen-free w.
    polar-bound w.
    structured w.
    superbound w.
waterfall
    w. appearance
    w. right hilum sign
water-hammer
    w.-h. pulse
    w.-h. pulse waveform
Waterhouse
    W. stop
    W. transpubic procedure
Waterhouse-Friderichsen syndrome
Waters
    W. projection
    W. view
watershed
    w. areas
    w. infarct
    w. mechanism
water-siphon test
water-soluble contrast media
Waterston-Cooley shunt
water-suppression technique
watery diarrhea, hypokalemia, achlorhydria (WDHA)
Watson-Ehrlich reaction
Watson-Jones classification of tibial tubercle avulsion fractures
wave
    acoustic w.
    circular polarization w.
    continuous w. (CW)
    electromagnetic w.
    extracorporeal shock w.
    longitudinal acoustic w.
    peristaltic w.
    pulsed w.
    R-w.
    reference w.
    w. sign
    sine w.
    slice excitation w. (SEW)
    sound w.
    square w.
    standing w.
    tertiary w.
    transverse acoustic w.
waveform
    arterial w.
    Doppler w.

    flow velocity w.
    pulsed Doppler w.'s
    sinusoidal w.
    uterine artery w.
    venous w.
    water-hammer pulse w.
wavelength
wavelet
    w. encoding
    w. transform
wavelet-encoded magnetic resonance imaging
waves
wax phantom
WBC count
WBRT
    whole-brain radiation therapy
WDHA
    watery diarrhea, hypokalemia, achlorhydria
    WDHA syndrome
web
    antral w.
    esophageal w.
webbed neck
Weber-Christian disease
weblike appearance
Webster strain mouse
wedge
    w. compression fracture
    w. fracture
    w. resection
    step w.
wedged hepatic venography
wedge-shaped vertebra
Wegener granulomatosis
Wegner line
Weibel-Palade body
Weibull plot of adult T-cell leukemia/lymphoma risk
Weichbrodt test
Weigert iron hematoxylin stain
Weigert-Meyer rule
weight
    w. estimation and assessment
    fetal w.
    w. loss
    molecular w.
weightbearing view
weighted
    N(H) w.
    spin density w.

T1-w.
T2-w.
weighting
Weil-Felix test
Weill-Marchesani syndrome
Weingarten syndrome
Weismann-Netter syndrome
Weitbrecht foramen
Welcker method
well-circumscribed
    w.-c. carcinoma
    w.-c. lesion
Well-Cogen
well counter
Wellcovorin
well-defined mass
well-differentiated
    w.-d. lymphocytic
    w.-d. polycystic Wilms
      tumor
Wellferon (*var. of* interferon alfa-n1)
Werdnig-Hoffmann disease
Werlhof disease
Werner syndrome
Wernicke area
WES
    wall-echo shadow
    WES triad
Wesselsbron virus
Westcott needle
Westergren method
Westermark sign
Western
    W. blot
    W. blot analysis
    W. blot test
    W. Neuroradiological
      Society
"western boot" in open fracture
the western yew, Taxus blevifolia
West Point view
wet lung disease
wetting
Wetzel test

Wharton
    W. duct
    W. gland
wheal-and-flare reaction
wheat germ agglutinin
wheelchair artifact
whiplash
Whipple
    W. disease
    W. operation
    W. procedure
    W. triad
whirl sign
Whitaker test
white
    w. blood cell
    w. blood cell contamination
    w. blood cell count
    w. blood cell depletion
    w. blood cell engraftment
    w. blood cell function
    w. blood cell transfusion
    w. cell
    w. clot syndrome
    w. epithelium
    w. matter
    w. matter disease
    w. matter shearing injury
    w. noise
    w. pulp
white-out
whitlow
    herpes w.
Whitmore-Jewett prostate cancer
  staging
WHO
    World Health Organization
    WHO classification for
      transitional cell carcinoma
      of the urinarybladder:
      stages Ta through T4
    WHO performance status
    WHO toxicity assessment
whole
    w. abdominopelvic
      irradiation (WAP)

NOTES

whole *(continued)*
  w. blood
  w. blood lysis technique
whole-body
  w.-b. hyperthermia
  w.-b. irradiation
  w.-b. scanner
  w.-b. scanning
**whole-brain radiation therapy
  (WBRT)**
whole-pelvis irradiation
whole-volume coil
Wholey
  W. reperfusion atherolytic
  wire
  W. steerable guidewire
whorling
  cellular w.
Wiberg
  CE angle of W.
  center-edge angle of W.
Wickham-Miller nephroscope
Widal-Felix test
wide
  w. rib
  w. suture
wide-field radiation therapy
wide-latitude film
widened
  w. anterior meningeal index
  w. collecting system
  w. duodenal sweep
  w. retrogastric space
widening
  infundibulum w.
  mediastinal w.
wide-range radiation therapy
Widmark test
width
  line w.
  prevertebral w.
  spectral w.
  window w.
Wiener spectrum
Wilcoxan Statistic
Wilcoxon rank-sum test
Wilder reticulin stain
wild-type
  w.-t. cell
  w.-t. gene
**Wilkins classification of radial
  fractures**

Williams
  W. copulating pouch
  operation
  W. syndrome
Williams-Campbell syndrome
Williamson blood test
Willis
  circle of W.
Willowbrook virus
willow fracture
Will Rogers phenomenon
Wills factor
Willson torque wire
Wilms tumor
Wilson
  W. disease
  W. fracture
Wilson-Mikity syndrome
Wimberger
  W. ring
  W. sign
wimp mutation
Winckel disease
window
  acquisition w.
  aortic w.
  aorticopulmonary w., aortic-
  pulmonic w.
  Brewster w.
  W. center
  data acquisition w.
  w. efficiency
  energy w.
  lung w.
  mediastinal w.
  oval w.
  w. period
  sampling w.
  serological w.
  soft tissue w.
  spectral w.
  w. width
window-period phenomenon
windsock appearance
wineglass
  w. appearance
  w. pelvis
wing
  greater sphenoid w.
winged scapula
Winn test
**Winquist-Hansen classification of
  femoral fractures**

Winslow
    foramen of W.
Wintrobe
    W. index
    W. and Landsberg method
    W. tube
wire
    Amplatz w.
    Amplatz stiffening w.
    atherolytic reperfusion w.
    Bentson w.
    coat-hanger w.
    Cragg w.
    Dasher guide w.
    eel w.
    floppy-tip w.
    gold-198 w.
    guide w.
    iridium w.
    Katzen infusion w.
    Lunderquist w.
    Lunderquist-Ring torque
      control w.
    Nitinol hydrophilic-
      coated w.
    pacemaker w.
    rocket w.
    safety J w.
    Schneider infusion w
    Sos w.
    springhook w.
    sternotomy w.
    w. stiffener
    super-still guide w.
    torque attenuating
      diameter w.
    Vallbracht slow rotational
      recanalizing w.
    Wholey reperfusion
      atherolytic w.
    Willson torque w.
    Zeitler pulsating w.
Wirsung duct
Wishart test
Wiskott-Aldrich syndrome
within-view motion

Wolfe
    W. breast carcinoma
      classification
    W. classification of breast
      carcinoma
wolffian
    w. duct
    w. duct carcinoma
Wolff law
Wolf-Parkinson-White syndrome
Wolf Piezolith 2200 lithotripter
Wolman disease
woman
    postmenopausal w.
wooden shoe sign
Wood-Fildes theory
wool
    w. coil
    w. tail
Woringer-Kolopp syndrome
working
    w. formulation of non-
      Hodgkin lymphoma
    w. sheath
workstation
    Pegasys w.
World
    W. Federation of
      Neuroradiological Societies
    W. Health Organization
      (WHO)
    W. Health Organization
      classification
wormian bone
wormy appearance
Wort
    St. John W.
wound
    w. breakdown
    gunshot w. (GSW)
WR-2721
    ethiofos
wrap
    no frequency w.
wraparound
    w. artifact
    w. ghost artifact

NOTES

wrapping
    valve w.
    vein valve w.
wrestler's herpes
Wright-Giemsa
    W.-G. evaluation
    W.-G. stain
Wright stain
wrinkle artifact

Wrisberg ligament
wrist
    w. dislocation
    w. joint
Wroblewski method
Wucheria bancrofti
Wu-Kabat plot
Wyburn-Mason syndrome

X

X chromosome
X factor
X gradient

X:Ag
factor X antigen
Asserachrom X:Ag

Xanax
xanthemia
xanthine
xanthinuria
xanthoastrocytoma
pleomorphic x.
xanthogranuloma
juvenile x.
necrobiotic x.
xanthogranulomatous
x. pyelonephritis
xanthoma
xanthomatosis
familial x.
xanthomatous pseudotumor
Xanthomonas maltophilia
xanthosarcoma
^{133}**Xe**
xenon-133
^{127}**Xe**
xenon 127
xenobiotic
xenogeneic
x. antigen
x. tissue
xenogenesis
xenogenic cell therapy
xenograft
bovine x.
human-murine x.
porcine x.
xenon
x. CT measurement
x. CT scanning
xenon-127 (^{127}Xe)
xenon-133 (^{133}Xe)
xenon-enhanced
x.-e. computed tomography
x.-e. CT
xenopi
Mycobacterium x.

XERG system
xeroderma pigmentosum
xeromammography
xerophthalmia
xerorhinia
xerosis
xerostomia
xiphoidalgia
xiphoid process
x-line method
X-linked
X.-l. agammaglobulinemia
X.-l. Duchenne muscular dystrophy
X.-l. gene
X.-l. hyper-IgM immunodeficiency
X.-l. hypogammaglobulinemia
X.-l. lymphoproliferative syndrome
X.-l. SCID
X.-l. spastic paraparesis
XLP syndrome
xomazyme
XomaZyme-H65
Xomed endotracheal tube
x-ray
x-r. beam
x-r. beam size
chest x-r.
x-r. computed tomography
x-r. crystallography
x-r. diffraction analysis
x-r. generator
x-r. of kidneys, ureters, and bladder
x-r. mammography
x-r. therapy
XRT
radiation therapy
XXY syndrome
xylazine
xylene
Xylocaine
X. viscous solution
Xyloxylin
xyxoid

Y
  yttrium
    Y gradient
^{50}Y
  yttrium-50
^{90}Y
  yttrium-90
Yaba tumor
Yakima
    hemoglobin Y.
Yale SK virus
Yamaguchi sarcoma virus
yaws
Y-axis
Ya Yan Tzu
yeast
    budding y.
yellow fever
yellow-out
Yergason sign
Yersinia
    Y enterocolitica
    Y pestis
yersinia
    y. enterocolitis
    y. terminal ileitis
yersiniosis
Yersin serum
yes proto-oncogene
yew
        European y.
        Himalayan y.
        Pacific y.

yield
    fluorescence y.
y-interferon
YLF
    yttrium lithium fluoride
Y-linked gene
yoga
yohimbine
yoke
yolk
        y. sac
        y. sac tumor
York-Mason procedure
yo-yo peristalsis
Y-shaped acetabulum
Y-T fracture
ytterbium
ytterbium-169 DTPA
yttrium (Y)
        ferritin-labeled y.
        y. lithium fluoride (YLF)
yttrium-50 (^{50}Y)
yttrium-90 (^{90}Y)
yttrium-90-labeled
        y.-l. anti-B2
          immunoconjugate
        y.-l. antiferritin
yttrium-labeled immunoconjugate
yttrium lithium fluoride (YLF)
Yunis-Varon syndrome
Y-view

Z

Z
- Z band
- Z direction
- Z gradient
- Z line

Zacopride
Zahn line
zalcitabine
Zaleski test
Zanca view
Zanosar
zanoterone
Zavala lung biopsy needle
zearaleone
zeatin
ZEBRA
- Z. antigen
- Z. protein

zebra
- z. artifact
- z. stripe artifact
- z. stripe image

Zeitler pulsating wire
Zellweger syndrome
zeniplatin (CL286558)
Zenker
- Z. diverticulum
- Z. pouch
- Z. solution

Zen macrobiotic diet
zeolite pneumoconiosis
Zerit with Videx
zero
- z. filling
- z. line
- z. net flow
- z. phase

zeroth moment
zetacrit
zeta potential
zeugmatography
- rotating-frame z.

Zickel nail
zidovigne
zidovudine
Ziehl-Neelsen stain
Zieve syndrome
ZIG
- zoster immune globulin

Zimmerman-Brittin exchange model

Zimmerman elementary particle
zinc
- z. oxide
- z. peroxide
- z. sulfate solution

zindoxifene
zinostatin
zipper
- z. artifact
- leucine z.

zirconium granuloma
Zithromax
Z line
Zofran
Zoladex
Zollinger-Ellison
- Z.-E. syndrome
- Z.-E. tumor

zona
- z. fasciculata
- z. glomerulosa
- z. reticularis

zonal anatomy
zone
- chemoreceptor trigger z.
- focal z.
- z. focusing
- Fraunhofer z.
- Grenz z.
- junctional z.
- large loop excision of transformation z. (LLETZ)
- Looser z.
- lung z.
- mantle z.
- prostatic transition z.
- transformation z.
- transition z.
- Trümmerfeld z.

zonography
zoo-agglutinin
zooprecipitin
zooprophylaxis
zootoxin
zorubicin hydrochloride
zoster
- dermatomal z.
- herpes z.
- z. immune globulin (ZIG)

Zovirax

Z-plasty
Z-technique
Zubrod Performance Scale
Zuckerkandl
organs of Z.
Zung Depression Inventory
ZVD
zydoridine
zydoridine (ZVD)
zygomatic arch
zygomaticofacial foramen

zygomaticofrontal suture
zygomaticomaxillary fracture
zygomaticotemporal suture
zygomaxillary
zygomycete
zygomycosis
zygosity
zygote
zymosis
zymotic papilloma
zyxin protein

Appendices

Appendix 1

Radiographic Anatomy and Positioning

Anatomic Planes

A plane is a flat surface formed by making a cut (imaginary or real) through the body or a part of it. In radiography, various planes are used as points of reference that assist in localizing areas of the body to permit specific centering guidelines. The major anatomic planes used in radiographic positioning are as follows:

Longitudinal plane	Made by cutting along the long (longitudinal) axis of the body or body part. In the erect position, this plane is termed *vertical* and is perpendicular to the horizontal.
Transverse plane	Made by cutting across the body or body part crosswise (at a right angle to the long axis). If the patient is erect, this plane is termed *horizontal* (parallel to the horizon).
Midsagittal or median plane	Longitudinal plane made by cutting from front (anterior) to back (posterior) along the median line of the body and along the sagittal suture of the skull.
Sagittal plane	Longitudinal plane made by cutting from front (anterior) to back (posterior) on either side of the sagittal suture and parallel to the midsagittal or median plane.
Coronal plane	Longitudinal plane made by cutting lengthwise from side to side through the head and body (or body part) along the coronal suture of the skull or parallel to it. The coronal suture lies behind the frontal bone and extends toward the sides of the skull.
Transpyloric plane	Transverse plane made by cutting across the body from one side to the other at the level of the 9th costal cartilages. The plane is situated about halfway between the superior border of the sternum (manubrial, or sternal, notch) and the symphysis pubis (junction of the two anterior or superior portions of the pubic bones). The name of this plane reflects the fact that it should cut across the pylorus of the stomach.
Midcoronal (midaxillary) plane	Longitudinal plane made by cutting through the head and body along the coronal suture of the head and extending the cut down the body.

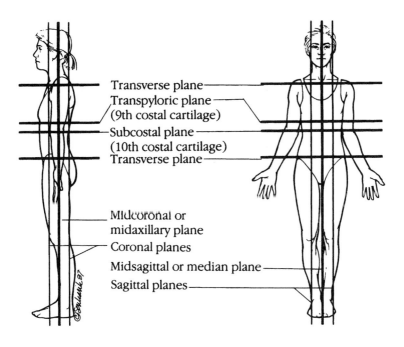

Transverse plane
Transpyloric plane
(9th costal cartilage)
Subcostal plane
(10th costal cartilage)
Transverse plane

Midcoronal or
midaxillary plane
Coronal planes
Midsagittal or median plane
Sagittal planes

Appendix 1

Anterior	In front of (toward the front of the body or a structure within it); sometimes referred to as *ventral*.
Posterior	In back of (toward the back of the body or a structure within it); sometimes referred to as *dorsal*.
Medial	Toward the midline of the body.
Lateral	Away from the midline of the body (to the side).
Proximal	Closer to the point of attachment or origin; in the extremities, closest to the trunk.
Distal	Farther from the point of attachment or origin; in the extremities, farthest from the trunk.
Cephalad, cephalic, superior	Toward the head or the upper part of a structure.
Caudad, caudal, inferior	Away from the head or the lower part of a structure (literally means ''toward the tail'').

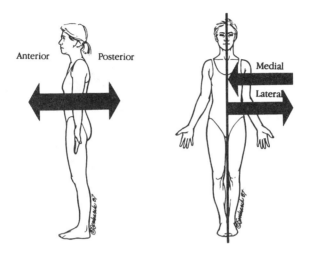

Anterior   Posterior

Medial
Lateral

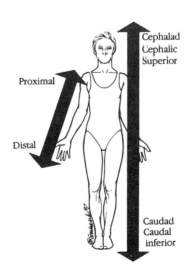

Cephalad
Cephalic
Superior

Proximal

Distal

Caudad
Caudal
inferior

Abduction	Movement of a limb or body part further from or away from the midline of the body.
Adduction	Movement of a limb or body part closer to or toward the midline of the body.
Extension	Straightening of a joint or extremity so that the angle between contiguous (adjoining) bones is increased.
Flexion	Bending of a joint or extremity so that the angle between contiguous (adjoining) bones is decreased.
Eversion	Movement of turning a body part outward (away from the midline).
Inversion	Movement of turning a body part inward (toward the midline).
Pronation	Movement of turning the body to face downward or turning the hand so that the palm is facing downward.
Supination	Movement of turning the body to face upward or turning the hand so that the palm faces upward.

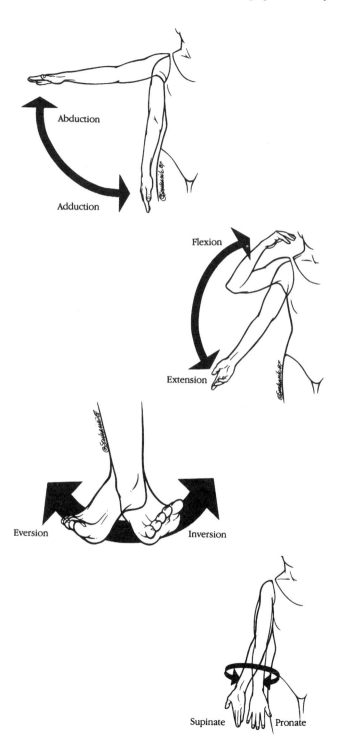

Abduction

Adduction

Flexion

Extension

Eversion

Inversion

Supinate

Pronate

Anatomic position	Position of the body when the subject is facing the front in the erect position with the arms and legs fully extended. The palms of the hands are facing forward and the feet are together. In radiography, this term is used as the reference position of the body to describe the various different positions.
Supine position	Position in which the subject is lying on the back with the face up. Sometimes referred to as the *dorsal recumbent* (lying down) or *dorsal decubitus* position, since the back (dorsal surface) of the body is dependent (nearer the table).
Prone position	Position in which the subject is lying face down on the front of the body. Sometimes referred to as the *ventral recumbent* or *ventral decubitus* position, since the front (ventral surface) of the body is dependent (nearer the table).
Lateral position	Position in which the side of the subject is next to the film. A lateral position is named by the side of the subject that is situated adjacent to the film. Sometimes referred to as an *erect lateral* if the subject is sitting or standing and a *lateral recumbent* or *lateral decubitus* if the subject is lying down.
Oblique position	Position in which the subject is neither prone nor supine, but rotated somewhere in between. In radiographic terminology, the subject is in a posterior oblique position if some part of the posterior surface of the body is closer to the film, and in an anterior oblique position if some part of the anterior surface of the body is closer to the film.
Right anterior oblique (RAO)	Patient is lying semiprone (face down) on the radiographic table or standing facing a vertical grid device with the *right* side closer to the film.

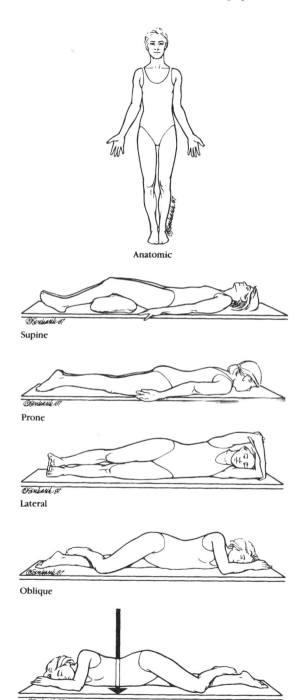

Anatomic

Supine

Prone

Lateral

Oblique

Right anterior oblique (RAO)

Left anterior oblique (LAO)	Patient is lying semiprone (face down) on the radiographic table or standing facing a vertical grid device with the *left* side closer to the film.
Right posterior oblique (RPO)	Patient is lying semisupine (face up) on the radiographic table or standing facing away from a vertical grid device with the *right* side closer to the film.
Left posterior oblique (LPO)	Patient is lying semisupine (face up) on the radiographic table or standing with the back against a vertical grid device with the *left* side closer to the film.
Decubitus position	Patient is lying down, and the central ray is horizontal (parallel to the floor).
Dorsal decubitus	Patient is lying supine (face up) on the radiographic table or on a stretcher placed next to a vertical grid device. The x-ray beam enters from one side of the patient and exits the other.
Ventral decubitus	Patient is lying prone (face down) on the radiographic table or on a stretcher placed next to a vertical grid device. The x-ray beam enters from one side of the patient and exits the other.
Lateral decubitus	Patient is lying on either side on the radiographic table or on a stretcher placed next to a vertical grid device. For a *left* lateral decubitus, the patient is lying on the *left* side with the *right* side up, while for a *right* lateral decubitus, the patient is lying on the *right* side with the *left* side up. The x-ray beam passes through the patient from front to back or back to front, depending on whether the patient is facing toward or away from the radiographic tube.

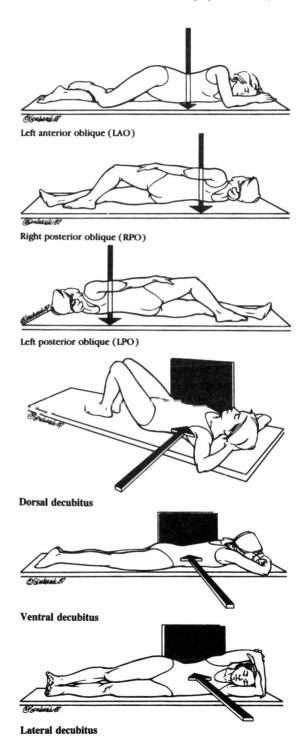

Left anterior oblique (LAO)

Right posterior oblique (RPO)

Left posterior oblique (LPO)

Dorsal decubitus

Ventral decubitus

Lateral decubitus

S ___
R ___
L ___

In radiography, the term *projection* is described by the path along which the x-rays travel from the radiographic tube through the subject to the image receptor.

Anteroposterior (AP) projection	Patient is either supine (face up) on the radiographic table (dorsal decubitus) or erect with the back against a vertical grid device. The x-ray beam enters the front (anterior) surface of the body and exits the back (posterior) surface.
Posteroanterior (PA) projection	Patient is either prone (face down) on the radiographic table (ventral decubitus) or erect facing a vertical grid device. The x-ray beam enters the back (posterior) surface of the body and exits the front (anterior) surface.
Lateral projection	Patient is lying on either side on the radiographic table (lateral decubitus) or standing with either side against a vertical grid device. The lateral projection is always named by the side of the patient that is placed next to the film.
Oblique projection	Patient is rotated into a position that does not produce either a frontal (AP or PA) or lateral projection.
Axial projection	Any projection in which there is longitudinal angulation of the central ray with respect to the long axis of the body part.
Tangential projection	Any projection in which the central ray passes between or passes by (skims) body parts to project an anatomic structure in profile and free of superimposition

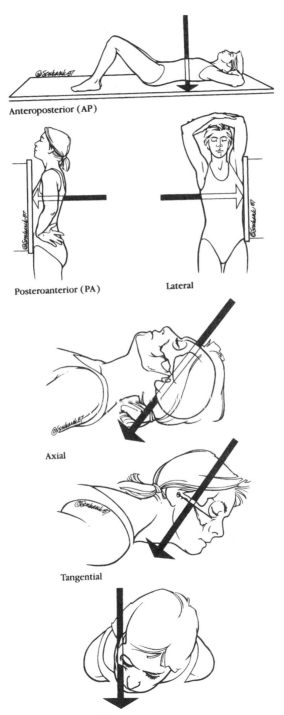

Anteroposterior (AP)

Posteroanterior (PA)   Lateral

Axial

Tangential

Tangential

From Eisenberg R. Radiographic positioning. Boston: Little, Brown and Company, 1989.

A13

Appendix 2
Contrast Media

^{99m}Tc CEA
Abrodil
acetrizoate
acetrizoic acid
adipiodone
amidotrizoic acid
Amipaque
Angioconray
Angiografin
barium sulfate
benzoic acid
Biligrafin
Biligram
Biliodyl
Bilivistan
Bilopaque
Biloptin
bismuth
Bracco
brominized oil
bunamiodyl
calcium
Cardio-Conray
Cardiografin
Cardiolite
CardioTek
CEA-Tc 99m
cerium
Cholebrine
Cholografin
Cholovue
Clysodrast
Conray
Cystografin
Cystokon
diaginol
diatrizoate
diatrizoate meglumine
diatrizoic acid
diodine

diodone
Diodrast
Dionosil
diprotrizoate
disofenin
Duografin
Duroliopaque
dysprosium
Echovist
Endobile
Endografin
Ethiodane
ethiodized oil
Ethiodol
ethyliodophenylundecyl
Feridex
gadodiamide
gadolinium
gadolinium diethlenetriamine-penta-
  acetate
gadopentetate dimeglumine
gadoteriodol
Gastrografin
Gastrozepine
Gd-DTPA
glucagon
Hexabrix
high-osmolar contrast medium
Hippuran
Hypaque
Hytrast
Intropaque
Imagent BP
Imagent GI
Imagent LN
Imagent US
indium 111
iobenzamic acid
iobutoic acid
iocarmate meglumine

iocarmic acid
iocetamate
iodamic acid
iodamide
iodatol
iodide
iodine 131 MIBG
iodipamide
iodipamide meglumine
iodipamide methylglucamine
iodized oil
iodoalphionic acid
iodohippurate
iodomethamate
iodophendylate
iodophthalein
iodopyracet
iodoxamate
iodoxamic acid
iodoxyl
ioglicate
ioglicic acid
ioglucol
ioglucomide
ioglunide
ioglycamic acid
ioglycamide
iogulamide
iohexol
iomide
iopamidol
iopanoate
iopanoic acid
iophendylate
iophenoxic acid
ioprocemic acid
iopromide
iopronic acid
iopydol
iopydone
iosefamate
iosefamic acid
ioseric acid
iosulamide

iosumetic acid
iotasul
ioteric acid
iothalamate
iothalamic acid
iotrol
iotroxamide
iotroxic acid
ioxaglate
ioxaglic acid
ioxithalamate
ioxithalamic acid
iozomic acid
ipodate
ipodic acid
IR-192
iridium
Iriditope
Isopaque
Isovue
Isovue M
Kinevac
Kontrast U
Levolist
Lipiodol
Liquipake
Macrotec
magnesium
Magnevist
manganese chloride
meglumine
meglumine diatrizoate
Metastron
methiodal
methylglucamine
metrizamide
metrizoate
metrizoic acid
Micropaque
Microtrast
Monophen
Myodil
Myoscint
Neo-Iopax

Neurolite
Niopam
Novopaque
Nyegaard
Octreoscan
Omnipaque
Omniscan
OncoRad OV103
OncoScint CR/OV
OncoScint CR103
OncoScint OV103
OncoScint PR
OncoTrac
Orabilex
Oragrafin
Oravue
Osbil
Pantopaque
Pertscan 99m
phenobutiodyl
phentetiothalein
potassium bromide
Praestholm
Priodax
Prograf
ProHance
propyliodone
radioactive iodide
Raybar 75
Rayvist
Renografin-60
Renografin-76
Reno-M-30
Reno-M-60
Reno-M-Dip
Renotec
Renovist
Renovist II
Renovue
Retro-Conray
Salpix
satumomab pentetide
sincalide
Sinografin

Skiodan
Skiodan Acacia
sodium
Solu-Biloptin
Solutrast
Steripaque-BR
Steripaque-V
tacrolimus
tantalum-178
TcHIDA
teboroxime
Techneplex
Technescan MAG3
technetium 99m, or ^{99m}Tc
technetium stannous pyrophophate
technetium-tagged Cardiolite
technetium-99m albumin
technetium-99m albumin aggregated
technetium-99m albumin colloid
technetium-99m bicisate
technetium-99m colloid
technetium-99m disofenin
technetium-99m etidronate
technetium-99m ferpentetate
technetium-99m furifosmin
technetium-99m glucepate
technetium-99m HIDA
technetium-99m iron-ascorbate-DTPA
technetium-99m lidofenin
technetium-99m macroaggregated
    albumin
technetium-99m medronate
technetium-99m mertiatide
technetium-99m oxidronate
technetium-99m penetate
technetium-99m pertechnetate sodium
technetium-99m PIPIDA
technetium-99m pyrophosphate
technetium-99m sestamibi
technetium-99m siboroxime
technetium-99m sodium
technetium-99m succimer
technetium-99m sulfur colloid
technetium-99m teboroxime
technetium-99m tetrofosmin

technetium 99m tetrofosmin
technetium stannous pyrophosphate
Telebrix
Telepaque
Teridax
Tesuloid
tetrabromophenolphthalein
tetraiodophenolphthalein
thallium 201
Thixokon
thorium dioxide
thorium tartrate

Thorotrast
triiodobenzoic acid
Triosil
TSPP
tyropanoate
tyropanoic acid
Umbradil
Urografin
Uromiro
Uropac
Urovision
Vasiodone

AIDS Laboratory Tests

This list of tests is not intended in any way to suggest patterns of physician's orders, nor is it complete. These tests may support possible clinical diagnoses or rule out other diagnostic possibilities. Each laboratory test relevant to AIDS is listed and weighted. Two symbols (**) indicate that the test is diagnostic, that is, documents the diagnosis if the expected is found. A single symbol (*) indicates a test frequently used in the diagnosis or management of the disease. The other listed tests are useful on a selective basis with consideration of clinical factors and specific aspects of the case.

Acid-Fast Stain
Acid-Fast Stain, Modified, *Nocardia* Species
Babesiosis Serological Test
Bacteremia Detection, Buffy Coat Micromethod
Beta$_2$-Microglobulin
Biopsy or Body Fluid Anaerobic Bacterial Culture
Biopsy or Body Fluid Fungus Culture
Biopsy or Body Fluid Mycobacteria Culture
Blood and Fluid Precautions, Specimen Collection
Blood Culture, Aerobic and Anaerobic
Blood Fungus Culture
Bronchial Washings Cytology
Bronchoalveolar Lavage
Bronchoalveolar Lavage Cytology
Brushings Cytology
Candida Antigen
Candidiasis Serologic Test
Cerebrospinal Fluid Cytology
Cerebrospinal Fluid Fungus Culture
Cerebrospinal Fluid Mycobacteria Culture
Chromosome Analysis, Blood or Bone Marrow
Complete Blood Count

Cryptococcal Antigen Titer, Serum or Cerebrospinal Fluid
Cryptosporidium Diagnostic Procedures, Stool
Cytomegalic Inclusion Disease Cytology
Cytomegalovirus Antibody
Cytomegalovirus Culture
Cytomegalovirus Isolation, Rapid
Darkfield Examination, Syphilis
Electron Microscopy
Estrogen Receptor Immunocytochemical Assay
Folic Acid, Serum
Hemoglobin A$_2$
Hepatitis B Surface Antigen
Herpes Cytology
Herpes Simplex Virus Antigen Detection
Herpes Simplex Virus Culture
Herpes Simplex Virus Isolation, Rapid
Histopathology
Histoplasmosis Serology
**HIV-1/HIV-2 Serology
HTLV-I/II Antibody
*Human Immunodeficiency Virus Culture
*Human Immunodeficiency Virus DNA Amplification
India Ink Preparation

Inhibitor, Lupus, Phospholipid Type
KOH Preparation
Leishmaniasis Serological Test
*Lymphocyte Subset Enumeration
Lymphocyte Transformation Test
Migration Inhibition Test
Mycobacteria by DNA Probe
Neisseria gonorrhoeae Culture
Nocardia Culture, All Sites
*p24 Antigen
Ova and Parasites, Stool
Platelet Count
Pneumocystis carinii Preparation
Pneumocystis Fluorescence
Polymerase Chain Reaction
Red Blood Cell Indices
Risks of Transfusion
Skin Biopsies
Skin Mycobacteria Culture
Skin Test, Tuberculosis
Sputum Culture

Sputum Cytology
Sputum Fungus Culture
Sputum Mycobacteria Culture
Stool Culture
Stool Fungus Culture
Stool Mycobacteria Culture
Susceptibility Testing, Fungi
Susceptibility Testing, Mycobacteria
T- and B-Lymphocyte Subset Assay
Throat Culture
Toxoplasmosis Serology
Urine Culture, Clean Catch
Urine Fungus Culture
VDRL, Serum
Viral Culture
Viral Culture, Blood
Viral Culture, Body Fluid
Viral Culture, Dermatological
   Symptoms
Viral Culture, Tissue
White Blood Count

From Quick Look drug book 1995. Baltimore: Williams & Wilkins, 1995.

Appendix 4
AIDS-Related Drugs

Currently on market:
aminosidine (Gabbromicina®)
atovaquone (Mepron®)
bovine colostrum
bovine whey protein concentrate
(Immuno-C®)
bropirimine [ABPP]
carbovir
CD4, human recombinant soluble
[rCD4] (Receptin®)
CD4, human truncated-369 AA
polypeptide (Soluble T4®)
CD4, immunoglobulin G,
recombinant human
clindamycin (Cleocin®)
co-trimoxazole (Bactrim™, Septra®,
and others)
Cryptosporidium hyperimmune
bovine colostrum IgC concentrate
Cryptosporidium parvum bovine
immunoglobulin concentrate
(Sporidin-G®)
dapsone
didanosine (Videx®)
2'-3'-dideoxyadenosine
2'-3'-dideoxycytidine
2'-3'-dideoxyinosine
dronabinol (Marinol®)
eflornithine hydrochloride
(Orinidyl®)
eooetin alfa (Epogen®, Procrit®)
filgrastim (Neupogen®)-new
indication
fluconazole (Diflucan®)
foscarnet (Foscavir®)
gentamicin liposome infection
L-glutathione (Cachexon®)
granulocyte marcophage colony-
stimulating factor [molgramostim,
GM-CSF] (Leucomax®)

HIV neutralizing antibodies
(Immupath®)
HIV protease inhibitor (Vertex®)
HPA-23
human T-lymphotropic virus
type III gp 160 antigens,
recombinant
human immunodeficiency virus (HIV-
1) immune globulin
immune globulin I.V., human
(Gamimune N®)
interferon alfa-2a (Roferon-A®)
interferon alfa-2b (Intron® A)
lactobin
megestrol acetate (Megace®)
mitoguazone
monoclonal antibody to CD4, 5a8
muramyl-tripeptide [MTP-PE]
oxandrolone (Oxandrin®,
Hepandrin®)
pentamidine isethionate (NebuPent™,
Pentam-300®)
piritrexim isethionate
poloxamer 331 (Protox®)
primaquine phosphate
rifabutin (Mycobutin™)
roquinimex (Linomide®)
SDZ MSL-109
sermorelin acetate (Geref®)
somatropin (Biotropine®,
Humatrope®, Norditropine®,
Nutrotropin®, Protropin®II,
Saizen®)
stavudine [d4T; didehydrothymidine]
(Zerit®)
sulfadiazine
trimetrexate glucuronate
(Neutrexin®)
zalcitabine (Hivid®)
zidovudine [AZT] (Retrovir®)

AIDS/ARC drugs soon to be released or in development

acemannan (Carrisyn®)
AIDS vaccine
AL-271 [AZT]
alvicept sudotox [CD4-PE40]
AR-121 (Nystatin-LF®, I.V.)
AS-101
atevirdine mesylate
azidouridine (AzdU®)
AZT-P-ddi (Scriptene®)
bropirimineK [ABPP]
CD4-IgG
curdlan sulfate [CRDS]
delavirdine mesylate
deoxynojirimycin, n-butyl [DNJ]
dextran sulfate sodium
diethyldithiocarbamate [DTC]
(Imuthiol®)
fiacitabine [FIAC]
fialuridine [FIAU]
FK-565
fluorothymidine [FLT]
hypericin (VIMRxyn®)
interferon alfa-NL (Wellferon®)
interferon beta, recombinant [r-IFN-beta] (R-Fone®)
interferon beta, recombinant human (Betaseron®)
interleukin-2 (Proleukin®)
interleukin-3
iscador
isoprinosine
lamivudine [3TC]
lentinan
methionine-enkephalin
molgramostim (Leucomax®)
nevirapine
oxothiazolidone carboxylate (Procysteine®)
poly I: poly C12U (Ampligen®)
PR-225 [redox-acyclovir]
PR-239 [redox-penicillin G]
TAT antagonist
thymopentin (Timunox®)
thymostimuline [TP-1]
trichosanthin [GLQ223; Compound Q]
tumor necorsis factor [TNF] binding protein I
tumor necorsis factor [TNF] binding protein II

From Quick Look drug book 1995. Baltimore: Williams & Wilkins, 1995.

Appendix 5
Chemotherapy Protocols

AA	ara-C, Adriamycin
AAA	adenosine-adenosine-adenosine
ABC	Adriamycin, BCNU, cyclophosphamide
ABCD	Adriamycin, bleomycin, CCNU, dacarbazine
ABCM	Adriamycin, bleomycin, cyclophosphamide, mitomycin-C
ABCX	Adriamycin, bleomycin, cisplatin, radiation therapy
ABD	Adriamycin, bleomycin, DTIC
ABDIC	Adriamycin, bleomycin, dacarbazine, CCNU, prednisone
ABDV	Adriamycin, bleomycin, DTIC, vinblastine
ABP	Adriamycin, bleomycin, prednisone
ABV	actinomycin-D, bleomycin, vincristine
ABV	Adriamycin, bleomycin, vinblastine
ABVD	Adriamycin, bleomycin, vinblastine, dacarbazine
ABVE	Adriamycin, bleomycin, vincristine, etoposide
AC	Adriamycin, carmustine
AC	Adriamycin, CCNU
AC	Adriamycin, cisplatin
AC	Adriamycin, cyclophosphamide
ACe	Adriamycin, cyclophosphamide
ACE	Adriamycin, cyclophosphamide, etoposide
ACE-II	Adriamycin, cyclophosphamide, etoposide in high-dose infusion
ACFUCY	actinomycin-D, 5-FU, cyclophosphamide
ACID	Adriamycin, cyclophosphamide, imidazole, dactinomycin
ACM	Adriamycin, cyclophosphamide, methotrexate

ACOAP	Adriamycin, cyclophosphamide, Oncovin, cytosine arabinoside, prednisone
ACOP	Adriamycin, cyclophosphamide, Oncovin, prednisone
ACOPP	Adriamycin, cyclophosphamide, Oncovin, prednisone, procarbazine
ACT-FU-Cy	actinomycin-D, 5-FU, cyclophosphamide
A+D or 7+3	ara-C, daunorubicin
ADBC	Adriamycin, DTIC, bleomycin, CCNU
ADE	ara-C, daunorubicin, etoposide
ADIC	Adriamycin, DTIC
AdOAP	Adriamycin, Oncovin, ara-C, prednisone
AdOP	Adriamycin, Oncovin, prednisone
Adria+BCNU	Adriamycin, BCNU
Adria-L-PAM	Adriamycin, melphalan
AFM	Adriamycin, 5-FU, methotrexate
AID	Adriamycin, ifosfamide, dacarbazine, mesna
AIM	L-asparaginase, ifosfamide, methotrexate
ALOMAD	Adriamycin, Leukeran, Oncovin, methotrexate, actinomycin-D, dacarbazine
Alpha-Beta	alpha tocopherol and beta carotene
ALT-RCC	autolymphocyte-based treatment for renal cell carcinoma
AMSA; m-AMSA	acridinylamine methanesulfon anisidide
anti-MY9BMT	bone marrow transplant
anti-T12	allogeneic BMT bone marrow transplant
AOPA	ara-C, Oncovin, prednisone, asparaginase
AOPE	Adriamycin, Oncovin, prednisone, etoposide
APC	AMSA, prednisone, chlorambucil
APE	Adriamycin, Platinol, etoposide
APO	Adriamycin, Platinol, Oncovin
ara-c+ADR	ara-C, Adriamycin
ara-c-HU	ara-C, hydroxyurea

ara-C+DNR+PRED+HP	cytarabine, daunorubicin, prednisolone, mercaptopurine
ara-C+6TG	cytarabine, thioguanine
A-SHAP	Adriamycin, Solu-Medrol, high-dose ara-C, Platinol
AV	Adriamycin, vincristine
AVDP	aspraginase, vincristine, daunorubicin, prednisone
AVM	Adriamycin, vinblastine, methotrexate
AVM	Adriamycin, vincristine, mitomycin-C
AVP	actinomycin-D, vincristine, procarbazine
BAC	BCNU, cytarabine, cyclophosphamide
BACO	bleomycin, Adriamycin, CCNU, Oncovin
BACOD	bleomycin, Adriamycin, cyclophosphamide, Oncovin, dexamethasone
BACON	bleomycin, Adriamycin, CCNU, Oncovin, nitrogen mustard
BACOP	bleomycin, Adriamycin, cyclophosphamide, Oncovin, prednisone
BACT	BCNU, cytarabine, cyclophosphamide, thioguanine
BACT	BCNU, ara-C, cyclophosphamide, 6-thioguanine
BACT	bleomycin, Adriamycin, cyclophosphamide, tamoxifen
BAM/BLITZ	B4 locked ricin
BAMON	bleomycin, Adriamycin, methotrexate, Oncovin, nitrogen mustard
BAP	bleomycin, Adriamycin, prednisone
BAVIP	bleomycin, Adriamycin, vinblastine, imidazole, carboxamide, prednisone
BBVP-M	BCNU, bleomycin, VePesid, prednisone, methotrexate
BCAVe	bleomycin, CCNU, Adriamycin, Velban
B-CAVe	bleomycin, CCNU, Adriamycin, vinblastine

BCD	bleomycin, cyclophosphamide, dactinomycin
BCDT	BCNU, cisplatin, dacarbazine, tamoxifen
B-CHOP	bleomycin, cyclophosphamide, hydroxydaunomycin, Oncovin, prednisone
BCMF	bleomycin, cyclophosphamide, methotrexate, fluorouracil
BCOP	BCNU, cyclophosphamide, Oncovin, prednisone
BCP	BCNU, cyclophosphamide, prednisone
BCVP	BCNU, cyclophosphamide, vinblastine, prednisone
BCVPP	BCNU, cyclophosphamide, vinblastine, procarbazine, prednisone
B-DOPA	bleomycin, dacarbazine, Oncovin, prednisone, Adriamycin
BEAC	BCNU, etoposide, ara-C, cyclophosphamide
BEAM	BCNU, etoposide, cytarabine, melphalan
BEMP	bleomycin, Eldisine, mitomycin, Platinol
BEP	bleomycin, etoposide, Platinol
BHD	BCNU, hydroxyurea, dacarbazine
BHDV	BCNU, hydroxyurea, dacarbazine, vincristine
BIP	bleomycin, ifosfamide, cisplatin
BLEO-COMF	bleomycin, cyclophosphamide, Oncovin, methotrexate, fluorouracil
BLEO-MOPP	bleomycin, nitrogen mustard, Oncovin, procarbazine, prednisone
B-MOPP	bleomycin, mechlorethamine, Oncovin, procarbazine, prednisone
BMP	BCNU, methotrexate, procarbazine
BLITZ	monoclonal antibodies
BOAP	bleomycin, Oncovin, Adriamycin, prednisone
BOLD	bleomycin, Oncovin, lomustine, dacarbazine
BOMP	bleomycin, Oncovin, Matulane, prednisolone

BOP	BCNU, Oncovin, prednisone
BOP	bleomycin, Oncovin, Platinol
BOPAM	bleomycin, Oncovin, prednisone, Adriamycin, mechlorethamine, methotrexate
BOPP	BCNU, Oncovin, procarbazine, prednisone
BT	BCNU, triazinate
BVAP	BCNU, vincristine, Adriamycin, prednisone
BVCPP	BCNU, vinblastine, cyclophosphamide, procarbazine, prednisone
BVD	BCNU, vincristine, dacarbazine
BVDS	bleomycin, Velban, doxorubicin, streptozocin
BVPP	BCNU, vincristine, procarbazine, prednisone
CABOP	cyclophosphamide, Adriamycin, bloemycin, Oncovin, prednisone
CABS	CCNU, Adriamycin, bleomycin, streptozocin
CAC	cisplatin, ara-C, caffeine
CAD	cyclophosphamide, Adriamycin, dacarbazine
CAD	cytosine arabinoside, daunorubicin
CADIC	cyclophosphamide, Adriamycin, DTIC
CADO	cyclophosphamide, doxorubicin, vincristine
CAE	cyclophosphamide, Adriamycin, etoposide
CAF	cyclophosphamide, Adriamycin, 5-FU
CAFFI	cyclophosphamide, Adriamycin, 5-FU by continuous infusion
CAFP	cyclophosphamide, Adriamycin, 5-FU, prednisone
CAFTH	cyclophosphamide, Adriamycin, 5-FU, tamoxifen, Halotestin
CAFVP	cyclophosphamide, Adriamycin, 5-FU, vincristine, prednisone
CALF	cyclophosphamide, Adriamycin, leucovorin calcium, 5-FU

CALF-E	cyclophosphamide, Adriamycin, leucovorin calcium, 5-FU, ethinyl estradiol
CAM	cyclophosphamide, Adriamycin, methotrexate
CAMB	cyclophosphamide, Adriamycin, methotrexate, bleomycin
CAMELEON	cytosine arabinoside, high-dose methotrexate, leucovorin, Oncovin
CAMEO	cyclophosphamide, Adriamycin, methotrexate, etoposide, Oncovin
CAMF	cyclophosphamide, Adriamycin, methotrexate, 5-FU
CAMF	cyclophosphamide, Adriamycin, methotrexate, folic acid
CAMLO	cytosine arabinoside, methotrexate, leucovorin, Oncovin
CAMP	cyclophosphamide, Adriamycin, methotrexate, procarbazine
CAO	cyclophosphamide, Adriamycin, Oncovin
CAP	cyclophosphamide, Adriamycin, Platinol
CAP-I	cyclophosphamide, Adriamycin, prednisone
CAP-II	cyclophosphamide, Adriamycin, high-dose Platinol
CAP-BOP	cyclophosphamide, Adriamycin, procarbazine, bleomycin, Oncovin, prednisone
CAPPr	cyclophosphamide, Adriamycin, Platinol, prednisone
CARBOPEC	carboplatin, etoposide, cyclophosphamide
CAT	cytosine arabinoside, Adriamycin, 6-thioguanine
CAT	cytosine arabinoside, thioguanine
CAV	cyclophosphamide, Adriamycin, Velban
CAV	cyclophosphamide, Adriamycin, vincristine
CAVe	CCNU, Adriamycin, Velban
CAVP	cyclophosphamide, Adriamycin, VM-26, prednisone

CAVP-I	cyclophosphamide, Adriamycin, vincristine, prednisone
CAVP-16	cyclophosphamide, Adriamycin, VP-16
CAVPM	cyclophosphamide, Adriamycin, VP-16, prednisone, methotrexate
CBPPA	cyclophosphamide, bleomycin, procarbazine, prednisone, Adriamycin
CBV	cyclophosphamide, BCNU, VP-16–213
CBV	cyclophosphamide, BCNU, VePesid
CBVD	CCNU, bleomycin, vinblastine, dexamethasone
CC	carboplatin, cyclophosphamide
CCAVV	CCNU, cyclophosphamide, Adriamycin, vincristine, VP-16
CCFE	cyclophosphamide, Adriamycin, vincristine, VP-16
CCM	cyclophosphamide, CCNU, methotrexate
CCMA	CCNU, cyclophosphamide, methotrexate, Adriamycin
CCNU-OP	CCNU, Oncovin, prednisone
CCOB	CCNU, cyclophosphamide, Oncovin, bleomycin
CCV	CCNU, cyclophosphamide, vincristine
CCV-AV	CCNU, cyclophosphamide, vincristine, plus Adriamycin, vincristine
CCVB	CCNU, cyclophosphamide, vincristine, bleomycin
CCVPP	CCNU, cyclophosphamide, Velban, procarbazine, prednisone
CCVV	cyclophosphamide, CCNU, VP-16, vincristine
CCVVP	cyclophosphamide, CCNU, VP-16, vincristine, Platinol
CD	cytarabine, daunorubicin
CDC	carboplatin, doxorubicin, cyclophosphamide
CDE	cyclophosphamide, doxorubicin, etoposide

Got a Good Word for STEDMAN'S?

Help us keep STEDMAN'S products fresh and up-to-date with new words and new ideas!

Do we need to add or revise any items? Is there a better way to organize the content?

Be specific! How can we make this STEDMAN'S product the best medical word reference possible for you? Fill in the lines below with your thoughts and recommendations. Attach a separate sheet of paper if you need to— *you* are our most important contributor and we want to know what's on *your* mind. Thanks!

(PLEASE TYPE OR PRINT CAREFULLY)

Terms you believe are incorrect:

Appears as: Suggested revision:

_____

_____

_____

New terms you would like us to add:

_____

_____

Other comments:

_____

_____

_____

All done? Great, just mail this card in today. No postage necessary, and thanks again!

Name / Title: _____

Facility / Company: _____

Address: _____

City / State / Zip: _____

Day Telephone No. (   )

Williams & Wilkins
A WAVERLY COMPANY
351 West Camden Street
Baltimore, Maryland 21201-2436

To order or to receive a catalog call toll free 1-800-527-5597.

rad/onc 2ed

#07966-2

BUSINESS REPLY MAIL

FIRST CLASS   PERMIT NO. 724   BALTIMORE, MD

POSTAGE WILL BE PAID BY ADDRESSEE

ATTN: STEDMAN'S EDITORIAL
ELECTRONIC MEDIA DIVISION
WILLIAMS & WILKINS
PO BOX 1496
BALTIMORE   MD   21298-9724

CE .... cisplatin, etoposide
CEB .... carboplatin, etoposide, bleomycin
CECA .... cisplatin, etoposide,
                                 cyclophosphamide, Adriamycin
CEF .... cyclophosphamide, epirubicin, 5-FU
CEM .... cytosine arabinoside, etoposide,
                                 methotrexate
CEP .... CCNU, etoposide, prednimustine
CEP .... cyclophosphamide, etoposide,
                                 Platinol
CEPT .... cyclophosphamide, fluorouracil,
                                 prednisone, tamoxifen
CEV .... cyclophosphamide, etoposide,
                                 vincristine
CF .... cisplatin, 5-FU
CFL .... cisplatin, 5-FU, leucovorin calcium
CFM .... cyclophosphamide, 5-FU,
                                 mitoxantrone
CFP .... cyclophosphamide, 5-FU, prednisone
CFPT .... cyclophosphamide, 5-FU,
                                 prednisone, tamoxifen
CHAD .... cyclophosphamide,
                                 hexamethylmelamine, Adriamycin,
                                 DDP
CHAMOCA .... cyclophosphamide, hydroxyurea,
                                 actinomycin-D, methotrexate,
                                 Oncovin, folinic acid, Adriamycin
CHAP .... cyclophosphamide,
                                 hexamethylmalamine, Adriamycin,
                                 cisplatin
CHAP .... cyclophosphamide, Hexalen,
                                 Adriamycin, Platinol
CHD .... cyclophosphamide,
                                 hexamethylmelamine, DDP
CHD-R .... cyclophosphamide,
                                 hexamethylmelamine, DDP,
                                 radiotherapy
CHEX-UP .... cyclophosphamide,
                                 hexamethylmelamine, 5-FU, Platinol
CHF .... cyclophosphamide,
                                 hexamethylmelamine, 5-FU
CHL+PRED .... chlorambucil, prednisone
Chl-VPP .... chlorambucil, vinblastine,
                                 procarbazine, prednisone

CHOB	cyclophosphamide, hydroxydaunomycin, Oncovin, bleomycin
CHOD	cyclophosphamide, hydroxydaunomycin, Oncovin, dexamethasone
CHOP	cyclophosphamide, hydroxydaunomycin, Oncovin, prednisone
CHOP-BLEO	cyclophosphamide, hydroxydaunomycin, Oncovin, prednisone, bleomycin
CHOPE	cyclophosphamide, Halotestin, Oncovin, prednisone, etoposide
CHOR	cyclophosphamide, hydroxydaunomycin, Oncovin, radiotherapy
CHVP	cyclophosphamide, hydroxydaunomycin, VM-26, prednisone
CIA	CCNU, isophosphamide, Adriamycin
CISCA	ciplatin, cyclophosphamide, Adriamycin
CISCAii/DViv	cisplatin, cyclophosphamide, Adriamycin, vinblastine, bleomycin
CIVPP	chlorambucil, vinblastine, procarbazine, prednisone
CMC	cyclophosphamide, methotrexate, CCNU
CMC-VAP	cyclophosphamide, methotrexate, CCNU, vincristine, Adriamycin, procarbazine
CMED	cyclophosphamide, methotrexate, etoposide, dexamethasone
CMF	cyclophosphamide, methotrexate, 5-FU
CMF-AV	cyclophosphamide, methotrexate, 5-FU, Adriamycin, vincristine
CMFAVP	cyclophosphamide, methotrexate, 5-FU, Adriamycin, vincristine, prednisone
CMF-BLEO	cyclophosphamide, methotrexate, 5-FU, bleomycin

CMF-FLU	cyclophosphamide, methotrexate, 5-FU, fluoxymesterone
CMFH	cyclophosphamide, methotrexate, 5-FU, hydroxyurea
CMFP	cyclophosphamide, methotrexate, 5-FU, prednisone
CMFpT	cyclophosphamide, methotrexate, 5-FU, low-dose prednisone, tamoxifen
CMFPTH	cyclophosphamide, methotrexate, 5-FU, prednisone, tamoxifen, Halotestin
CMFP-VA	cyclophosphamide, methotrexate, 5-FU, prednisone, vincristine, Adriamycin
CMFT	cyclophosphamide, methotrexate, 5-FU, tamoxifen
CMF-TAM	cyclophosphamide, methotrexate, 5-FU, tamoxifen
CM-5-FU	cyclophosphamide, methotrexate, 5-FU
CMFV	cyclophosphamide, methotrexate, 5-FU, vincristine,
CMFVAT	cyclophosphamide, methotrexate, 5-FU, vincristine, Adriamycin, testosterone
CMFVP	cyclophosphamide, methotrexate, 5-FU, vincristine, prednisone
CMH	cyclophosphamide, m-AMSA, hydroxyurea
C-MOPP	cyclophosphamide, mechlorethamine, Oncovin, procarbazine, prednisone
CMP	CCNU, methotrexate, procarbazine
CMPF	cyclophosphamide, methotrexate, prednisone, 5-FU
CMV	cisplatin, methotrexate, vinblastine
CNF	cyclophosphamide, Novantrone, 5-FU
CNOP	cyclophosphamide, Novantrone, Oncovin, prednisone
COAP	cyclophosphamide, Oncovin, ara-C, prednisone
COAP-BLEO	cyclophosphamide, Oncovin, ara-C, prednisone, bleomycin

COB	cisplatin, Oncovin, bleomycin
COBMAM	cyclophosphamide, Oncovin, bleomycin, methotrexate, Adriamycin, MeCCNU
COF/COM	cyclophosphamide, Oncovin, 5-FU plus cyclophosphamide, Oncovin, MeCCNU
COM	cyclophosphamide, Oncovin, MeCCNU
COM	cyclophosphamide, Oncovin, methotrexate
COM-A	cyclophosphamide, Oncovin, methotrexate, Adriamycin, ara-C
COMB	cyclophosphamide, Oncovin, MeCCNU, bleomycin
COMB	cyclophosphamide, Oncovin, methotrexate, bleomycin
COMBAP	cyclophosphamide, Oncovin, methotrexate, bleomycin, Adriamycin, prednisone
COMe	cyclophosphamide, Oncovin, methotrexate
COMET-A	cyclophosphamide, Oncovin, methotrexate, leucovorin, etoposide, ara-C
COMF	cyclophosphamide, Oncovin, methotrexate, 5-FU
COMLA	cyclophosphamide, Oncovin, methotrexate, leucovorin, ara-C
COMP	cyclophosphamide, Oncovin, methotrexate, prednisone
Cooper CMFVP	cyclophosphamide, methotrexate, 5-FU, vincristine, prednisone
COP	cyclophosphamide, Oncovin, prednisolone
COP	cyclophosphamide, Oncovin, prednisone
COPA	cyclophosphamide, Oncovin, prednisone, Adriamycin
COPAC	CCNU, Oncovin, prednisone, Adriamycin, cyclophosphamide
COP-B	cyclophosphamide, Oncovin, prednisone, bleomycin

COP-BAM	cyclophosphamide, Oncovin, prednisone, bleomycin, Adriamycin, Matulane
COP-BLAM	cyclophosphamide, Oncovin, prednisone, bleomycin, Adriamycin, Matulane
COP-BLEO	cyclophosphamide, Oncovin, prednisone, bleomycin
COPE	cyclophosphamide, Oncovin, Platinol, etoposide
COPP	CCNU, Oncovin, procarbazine, prednisone
COPP	cyclophosphamide, Oncovin, procarbazine, prednisone
CP	Cytoxan, Platinol
CPB	cyclophosphamide, Platinol, BCNU
CPC	cyclophosphamide, Platinol, carboplatin
CPOB	cyclophosphamide, prednisone, Oncovin, bleomycin
CROP	cyclophosphamide, rubidazone, Oncovin, prednisone
CROPAM	cyclophosphamide, rubidazone, Oncovin, prednisone, L-asparaginase, methotrexate
CT	cytarabine, 6-thioguanine
CTCb	cyclophosphamide, thiotepa, carboplatin
CTX-Plat	cyclophosphamide, Platinol
CV	cisplatin, VP-16
CVA	cyclophosphamide, vincristine, Adriamycin
CVA-BMP	cyclophosphamide, vincristine, Adriamycin, BCNU, methotrexate, procarbazine
CVAD	cyclophosphamide, vincristine, Adriamycin, dexamethasone
CVB	CCNU, vinblastine, bleomycin
CVD	cisplatin, vinblastine, dacarbazine
CVEB	cisplatin, Velban, etoposide, bleomycin
CVI	carboplatin, VePesid, ifosfamide, Mesnex uroprotection

CVM	cyclophosphamide, vincristine, methotrexate
CVP	cyclophosphamide, vincristine, prednisone
CVP-BLEO	cyclophosphamide, vincristine, prednisone, bleomycin
CVPP	CCNU, vinblastine, prednisone, procarbazine
CVPP	cyclophosphamide, vinblastine, procarbazine, prednisone
CVPP-CCNU	cyclophosphamide, vinblastine, procarbazine, prednisone, CCNU
CyADIC	cyclophosphamide, Adriamycin, DTIC
CyHOP	cyclophosphamide, Halotestin, Oncovin, prednisone
CYTABOM	cytarabine, bleomycin, Oncovin, mechlorethamine
CyVADACT	cyclophosphamide, vincristine, Adriamycin, dactinomycin
CyVADIC	cyclophosphamide, vincristine, Adriamycin, DTIC
CyVMAD	cyclophosphamide, vincristine, methotrexate, Adriamycin, DTIC
DAP I	dianhydrogalactitol, Adriamycin, Platinol
DAP II	dianhydrogalactitol, Adriamycin, high-dose Platinol
DAP/TMP	dapsone, trimethoprim
DAT	daunomycin, ara-C, 6-thioguanine
DATVP	daunomycin, ara-C, thioguanine, vincristine, prednisone
DAV	dibromodulcitol, Adriamycin, vincristine
DAVH	dibromodulcitol, Adriamycin, vincristine, Halotestin
DBV	dacarbazine, BCNU, vincristine
DC	daunorubicin, cytarabine
DCCMP	daunorubicin, cyclocytidine, 6-mercaptopurine, prednisone
DCMP	daunorubicin, cytarabine, 6-mercaptopurine, prednisone
DCT	daunorubicin, cytarabine, thioguanine
DCV	dacarbazine, CCNU, vincristine

DDP	diamminedichloroplatinum
DECAL	dexamethasone, etoposide, cisplatin, ara-C, L-asparaginase
DFV	DDP, 5-FU, VePesid
DHAP	dexamethasone, high-dose ara-C, Platinol
DIMOPP	dose-intensified MOPP
DMC	dactinomycin, methotrexate, cyclophosphamide
DOAP	daunorubicin, Oncovin, ara-C, prednisone
DTIC	dacarbazine
DTIC-ACTD	DTIC, actinomycin D
DVB	DDP, vindesine, bleomycin
DVP	daunorubicin, vincristine, prednisone
DVPA	daunorubicin, vincristine, prednisone, asparaginase
DVPL-ASP	daunorubicin, vincristine, prednisone, L-asparaginase
DZAPO	daunorubicin, azactidine, ara-C, prednisone, Oncovin
EAP	etoposide, Adriamycin, Platinol
EBAP	Eldisine, BCNU, Adriamycin, prednisone
ECHO	etoposide, cyclophosphamide, hydroxydaunomycin, Oncovin
EDAP	etoposide, dexamethasone, ara-C, Platinol
EFP	etoposide, 5-FU, cisplatin
ELF	etoposide, leucovorin, 5-FU
EMA-CO	etoposide, methotrexate-leucovorin, actinomycin D, cyclophosphamide, Oncovin
E-MVAC	escalated methotrexate, vinblastine, Adriamycin, cisplatin
E-MVAC	escalated methotrexate, vinblastine, Adriamycin, cyclophosphamide
EP	etoposide, Platinol
EPOCH	etoposide, prednisone, Oncovin, cyclophosphamide, Halotestin
ESHAP	etoposide, Solu-Medrol, ara-C, Platinol
EVA	etoposide, vinblastine, Adriamycin

FAC	5-FU, Adriamycin, cyclophosphamide
FAC-BCG	Ftorafur, Adriamycin, cyclophosphamide, bacille Calmette-Guerin
FAC-LEV	5-FU, Adriamycin, cyclophosphamide, levamisole
FAC-M	5-FU, Adriamycin, cyclophosphamide, methotrexate
FACP	Ftorafur, Adriamycin, cyclophosphamide, Platinol
FACS	5-FU, Adriamycin, cyclophosphamide, streptozocin
FACVP	5-FU, Adriamycin, cyclophosphamide, VP-16
FAM	5-FU, Adriamycin, mitomycin-C
FAM-C	5-FU, Adriamycin, methyl-CCNU
FAM-CF	5-FU, Adriamycin, mitomycin, citrovorum factor
FAMe	5-FU, Adriamycin, semustine
FAME	5-FU, Adriamycin, MeCCNU
FAMMe	5-FU, Adriamycin, mitomycin-C, MeCCNU
FAM-S	5-FU, Adriamycin, mitomycin-C, streptozocin
FAMTX	5-FU, Adriamycin, high-dose methotrexate
FAP	5-FU, Adriamycin, Platinol
FCAP	5-FU, cyclophosphamide, Adriamycin, Platinol
FCE	5-FU, cisplatin, etoposide
F-CL	5-FU, leucovorin calcium
FCP	5-FU, cyclophosphamide, prednisone
FDC	fluorouracil, doxorubicin, cisplatin
FEC	5-FU, epirubicin, cyclophosphamide
FED	5-FU, etoposide, DDP
FIMe	5-FU, ICRF-159, MeCCNU
FL	flutamide, leuprolide acetate
FL	flutamide, Lupron Depot
FLAC	5-FU, leucovorin calcium, Adriamycin, cyclophosphamide
FLAP	5-FU, leucovorin calcium, Adriamycin, Platinol
FLe	5-FU, levamisole
Fluosol/BCNU	fluosol-DA20, BCNU

F-MACHOP	fluorouracil, methotrexate, Adriamycin, vincristine, prednisone
FMS	5-FU, mitomycin-C, streptozocin
FMV	5-FU, methyl CCNU, vincristine
FNM	5-FU, Novantrone, methotrexate
FOAM	5-FU, Oncovin, Adriamycin, mitomycin-C
FOM	5-FU, Oncovin, mitomycin-C
FOMi	5-FU, Oncovin, mitomycin-C
FOMI	5-FU, Oncovin, mitomycin
FRACON	framycetin, colistin, nystatin
5-FU/LV	fluorouracil, leucovorin
FUM	5-FU, methotrexate
FURAM	Ftorafur, Adriamycin, mitomycin-C
FUVAC	5-FU, vinblastine, Adriamycin, cyclophosphamide
HAD	hexamethylmelamine, Adriamycin, DDP
HAM	hexamethylmelamine, Adriamycin, melphalan
HAM	hexamethylmelamine, Adriamycin, methotrexate
HAMP	hexamethylmelamine, Adriamycin, methotrexate, Platinol
HCAO	hexamethylmelamine, cyclophosphamide, Adriamycin, Oncovin
H-CAP	hexamethylmelamine, cyclophosphamide, Ariamycin, Platinol
HDPEB	high-dose PEB or Platinol, etoposide, bleomycin
HD-VAC	high-dose methotrexate plus vinblastine, Adriamycin, cisplatin
Hexa-CAF	Hexalen, cyclophosphamide, Adrucil, Folex
HiC-COM	ara-C, citrovorum factor, allopurinol, Elliot B solution, cyclophosphamide, Oncovin, methotrexate
HILDAC	high-dose ara-C
high-risk ATAC	L-asparaginase, ara-C, VP-16, anti-J2 26 monoclonal antibody, anti-CALLA hybridoma antibody

HMTX	high-dose methotrexate
HOAP-BLEO	hydroxydaunomycin, Oncovin, ara-C, prednisone, bleomycin
HOP	hydroxydaunomycin, Oncovin, prednisone
IC	idarubicin, cytarabine
ICE	ifosfamide, carboplatin, etoposide
ID	ifosfamide, mesna, doxorubicin
IMAC	ifosfamide, mesna, Adriamycin, cisplatin
IMF	Ifex, Mesnex, Folex, 5-FU
IMVP-16	ifosfamide, methotrexate, VP-16
KGC	Keflin, getamicin, carbenicillin
LAM	L-asparaginase, methotrexate
LAPOCA	L-asparaginase, prednisone, Oncovin, cytarabine, Adriamycin
LMF	Leukeran, methotrexate, 5-FU
LOMAC	leucovorin, Oncovin, methotrexate, Adriamycin, cyclophosphamide
L VAM	Lupron, Velban, Adriamycin, Mutamycin
LVVP	Leukeran, vinblastine, vincristine, prednisone
M2	vincristine, carmustine, cyclophosphamide, melphalan, prednisone
MABOP	Mustargen, Adriamycin, bleomycin, Oncovin, prednisone
MAC	methotrexate, actinomycin D, cyclophosphamide
MAC	methotrexate, Adriamycin, cyclophosphamide
MAC	mitomycin-C, Adriamycin, cyclophosphamide
MAC-III	methotrexate, actinomycin D, chlorambucil
MACC	methotrexate, Adriamycin, cyclophosphamide, CCNU

MACHO .... methotrexate, asparaginase, cyclophosphamide, hydroxydaunomycin, Oncovin

MACOP-B .... methotrexate, Adriamycin, cyclophosphamide, Oncovin, presnidone, bleomycin

MAD .... MeCCNU, Adriamycin

MADDOC .... mechlorethamine, Adriamycin, dacarbazine, DDP, Oncovin, cyclophosphamide

MAID .... mesna, Adriamycin, interleukin-3, dacarbazine

MAID .... Mesnex, Adriamycin, Ifex, dacarbazine

MAP .... melphalan, Adriamycin, prednisone

MAP .... melphalan, Adriamycin, prednisone

MAT .... multiple agent therapy

MAZE .... m-AMSA, azactidine, etoposide

M-BACOD .... moderate dose methotrexate, bleomycin, Adriamycin, cyclophosphamide, Oncovin, dexamethasone

M-BACOD .... high-dose methotrexate, bleomycin, Adriamycin, cyclophosphamide, Oncovin, dexamethasone

M-BACOS .... methotrexate, bleomycin, Adriamycin, cyclophosphamide, Oncovin, Solu-Medrol

M-BAM .... cyclophosphamide, total body irradiation, monoclonal antibodies

MBC .... methotrexate, bleomycin, cisplatin

MBD .... methotrexate, bleomycin, DDP

MC .... mitoxantrone, cytarabine

MCBP .... melphalan, cyclophosphamide, BCNU, prednisone

MCP .... melphalan, cyclophosphamide, prednisone

MCV .... methotrexate, cisplatin, vinblastine

MDLO .... metoclopramide, dexamethasone, lorazepam, ondansetron

MeCP .... methyl-CCNU, cyclophosphamide, prednisone

MECY .... methotrexate, cyclophosphamide

MeFA .... methyl-CCNU, 5-FU, Adriamycin

MF	methotrexate, 5-FU
MF	mitomycin, 5-FU
MFP	melphalan, 5-FU, Provera
MIFA	mitomycin, fluorouracil, Adriamycin
MIME	mitoguazone, ifosfamide, methotrexate, etoposide
MINE	mesna, ifosfamide, Novantrone, etoposide
mini-COAP	cyclophosphamide, Oncovin, ara-C, prednisone
MM	mercaptopurine, methotrexate
MMC	methotrexate, mercaptopurine, cyclophosphamide
MMOPP	methotrexate, mechlorethamine, Oncovin, procarbazine, prednisone
MMPT	methylprednisolone pulse therapy
MOAD	methotrexate, Oncovin, L-asparaginase, dexamethasone
MOB	Mustargen, Oncovin, bleomycin
MOB-III	mitomycin-C, Oncovin, bleomycin, cisplatin
MOCA	methotrexate, Oncovin, cyclophosphamide, Adriamycin
MOF	MeCCNU, Oncovin, 5-FU
MOF	methotrexate, Oncovin,5-FU
MOF-STREP	MeCCNU, Oncovin, 5-FU, streptozocin
MOMP	mechlorethamine, Oncovin, methotrexate, prednisone
MOP	mechlorethamine, Oncovin, prednisone
MOP	mechlorethamine, Oncovin, procarbazine
MOP	melphalan, Oncovin, methylprednisolone
MOP-BAP	mechlorethamine, Oncovin, procarbazine, bleomycin, Adriamycin, prednisone
MOPP	mechlorethamine, Oncovin, procarbazine, prednisone
MOPP	methotrexate, Oncovin, procarbazine, prednisone

MOPP-ABV .... mechlorethamine, Oncovin, procarbazine, prednisone, Adriamycin, bleomycin, vinblastine

MOPP-ABV Hybrid .... mechlorethamine, Oncovin, procarbazine, prednisone, Adriamycin, bleomycin, vinblastine, hydrocortisone

MOPP-ABVD .... mechlorethamine, Oncovin, procarbazine, prednisone, Adriamycin, bleomycin, vinblastine, dacarbazine

MOPP-BLEO .... mechlorethamine, Oncovin, procarbazine, prednisone, bleomycin

MOPr .... mechlorethamine, Oncovin, procarbazine

MP .... melphalan, prednisone

M-PFL .... methotrexate, Platinol, 5-FU, leucovorin calcium

MPL+PRED .... melphalan, prednisone

MTX+MP .... methotrexate, mercaptopurine

MTX+MP+CTX .... methotrexate, mercaptopurine, Cytoxan

MV .... mitoxantrone, VP-16

MVAC .... methotrexate, vinblastine, Adriamycin, cisplatin

MVF .... mitoxantrone, vincristine, 5-FU

MVP .... mitomycin-C, vinblastine, Platinol

MVPP .... mechlorethamine, vinblastine, procarbazine, prednisone

MVT .... mitoxantrone, VP-16, thiotepa

MVVPP .... mechlorethamine, vincristine, vinblastine, procarbazine, prednisone

NAC .... nitrogen mustard, Adriamycin, CCNU

OAP .... Oncovin, ara-C, prednisone

OAP-BLEO .... Oncovin, ara-C, prednisone, bleomycin

O-DAP .... Oncovin, dianhydrogalactitol, Adriamycin, Platinol

OMAD .... Oncovin, methotrexate, Adriamycin, dactinomycin

OPAL	Oncovin, prednisone, L-asparaginase
OPP	Oncovin, procarbazine, prednisone
OPPA	Oncovin, procarbazine, prednisone, Adriamycin
PAB-Esc-C	Platinol, Adriamycin, bleomycin, escalating doses of cyclophosphamide
PAC	Platinol, Adriamycin, cyclophosphamide
PAC-1	cisplatin, Adriamycin, cyclophosphamide
PAC-4D 5-day infusion	Platinol, Adriamycin, cyclophosphamide
PACE	Platinol, Adriamycin, cyclophosphamide, etoposide
PATCO	prednisone, ara-C, thioguanine, cyclophosphamide, Oncovin
PAVe	procarbazine, Alkeran, Velban or L-phenylalanine mustard, Vinblastine
PBV	Platinol, bleomycin, vinblastine
PCE	Platinol, cyclophosphamide, Eldesine
PCV	procarbazine, CCNU, vincristine
PEB	Platinol, etoposide, bleomycin
PEC	Platinol, etoposide, cyclophosphamide
PEP	Procytox, epipodophyllotoxin-derivative, prednisolone
PF+E	Platinol, 5-FU plus etoposide, methotrexate, leucovorin
PFL	Platinol, 5-FU, leucovorin calcium
PFM	Platinol, 5-FU, moderate-dose methotrexate
PFT	phenylalanine mustard, 5-FU, tamoxifen
PHRT	procarbazine, hydroxyurea, radiotherapy
PIA	Platinol, ifosfamide, Adriamycin
PMB	Platinol, methotrexate, bleomycin
PMF	L-phenylalanine mustard, methotrexate, 5-FU
PMFAC	prednisone, methotrexate, and FAC protocol [5-FU, Adriamycin, cyclophosphamide]

P-MVAC	Platinol, methotrexate, vinblastine, Adriamycin, carboplatin
POC	procarbazine, Oncovin, CCNU
POCA	prednisone, Oncovin, cytarabine, Adriamycin
POCC	procarbazine, Oncovin, cyclophosphamide, CCNU
POMP	prednisone, Oncovin, methotrexate, Purinethol
PRH-E	Platinol, etanidazole
PRIME	procarbazine, isophosphamide, methotrexate
ProMACE	prednisone, methotrexate, Adriamycin, cyclophosphamide, etoposide
ProMACE	prednisone, methotrexate-leucovorin, Adriamycin, cyclophosphamide, etoposide
ProMACE-CytaBOM	prednisone, methotrexate-leucovorin, Adriamycin, cyclophosphamide, etoposide, cytarabine, bleomycin, Oncovin, methotrexate
ProMACE-CytaBOM	prednisone, Adriamycin, cyclophosphamide, etoposide, cytarabine, bleomycin, Oncovin, methotrexate
ProMACE-CytaBOM	prednisone, methotrexate, doxorubicin, cyclophosphamide, etoposide, cytarabine, bleomycin, vincristine, methotrexate
ProMACE-MOPP	procarbazine, methotrexate, Adriamycin, cyclophosphamide, etoposide, Mustargen, Oncovin, procarbazine, prednisone
ProMACE-MOPP	prednisone, methotrexate, doxorubicin, cyclophosphamide, etoposide, mechlorethamine, vincristine, procarbazine, prednisone
PT	Platinol, Taxol
pulse VAC	vincristine, actinomycin D, cyclophosphamide
PUVA	psoralens, ultraviolet A
PVA	prednisone, vincristine, asparaginase

PVB .... Platinol, vinblastine, bleomycin
PVDA .... prednisone, vincristine,
                                            daunorubicin, asparaginase
PVP .... Platinol, VP-16

RIDD .... recombinant interleukin-2,
                                            dacarbazine, DDP
ROAP .... rubidazone, Oncovin, ara-C,
                                            prednisone

SAM .... streptozocin, Adriamycin, methyl-
                                            CCNU
SCAB .... streptozocin, CCNU, Adriamycin,
                                            bleomycin
SD .... streptozocin, doxorubicin
SIMAL-pilot .... ara-C, hydrocortisone, mesna,
                                            prednisone, VP-16, leucovorin
SIMAL—2nd induction/maintenance ...... prednisone, L-asparaginase,
                                            daunomycin, VM-26, methotrexate,
                                            ara-C, VP-16, leucovorin
SIMAL—BMT .... [bone marrow transplant] ara-C,
                                            methotrexate, prednisone
SK .... Sloan-Kettering procotol
SMF .... streptozocin, mitomycin-C, 5-FU
STAMP .... protocol
STEAM .... streptonigrin, thioguanine,
                                            cyclophosphamide, actinomycin,
                                            mitomycin
super-CM regimen .... cyclophosphamide, methotrexate,
                                            5-FU
SWOG CMFVP .... cyclophosphamide, methotrexate,
                                            5-FU, vincristine, prednisone

T-2 .... dactinomycin, Adriamycin,
                                            vincristine, cyclophosphamide,
                                            radiation
T-10 .... methotrexate, calcium leucovorin
                                            rescue, Adriamycin, cisplatin,
                                            bleomycin, cyclophosphamide,
                                            dactinomycin
TAD .... 6-thioguanine, ara-C, daunomycin
TC .... 6-thioguanine, cytarabine
T-CAP .... Baker Antifol, cyclophosphamide,
                                            Adriamycin, Platinol

T-CAP III	triazinate, cyclophosphamide, Adriamycin, Platinol
TEC	Thiotepa, etoposide, carboplatin
TEMP	tamoxifen, etoposide, mitoxantrone, Platinol
T-MOP	6-thioguanine, methotrexate, Oncovin, prednisone
TOAP	thioguanine, Oncovin, cytosine arabinoside
TPCH	thioguanine, procarbazine, CCNU, hydroxyurea
TPDCV	thioguanine, procarbazine, DBC, CCNU, vincristine
TRAMACOL	6-thioguanine, rubidomycin, cytarabine, methotrexate, prednisolone, cyclophosphamide, Oncovin, L-asparaginase
TRAP	thioguanine, rubidomycin, ara-C, prednisone
VA	vincristine, Adriamycin
VAAP	vincristine, asparaginase, Adriamycin, prednisone
VAB	vinblastine, actinomycin D, bleomycin
VAB1	vinblastine, actinomycin D, bleomycin
VAB2	vinblastine, actinomycin D, bleomycin, cisplatin
VAB3	vinblastine, actinomycin D, bleomycin, cisplatin, chlorambucil, cyclophosphamide
VAB4	vinblastine, actinomycin D, bleomycin, cisplatin, cyclophosphamide
VAB5	vinblastine, actinomycin D, bleomycin, cisplatin, cyclophosphamide
VAB6	cyclophosphamide, dactinomycin, vinblastine, bleomycin, cisplatin
VABCD	vinblastine, Adriamycin, bleomycin, CCNU, DTIC
VAC	vincristine, actinomycin D, cyclophosphamide

VAC	vincristine, Adriamycin, cyclophosphamide
VAC pulse	vincristine, actinomycin D, cyclophosphamide administered in a pulsed fashion
VAC standard	vincristine, Adriamycin, cyclophosphamide administered daily
VACA	vincristine, actinomycin D, cyclophosphamide, Adriamycin
VACAD	vincristine, Adriamycin, cyclophosphamide, actinomycin D, dacarbazine
VACP	VePesid, Adriamycin, cyclophosphamide, Platinol
VAD	vincristine, Adriamycin, dexamethasone
VAD/V	vincristine, Adriamycin, dexamethasone, verapamil
VAFAC	vincristine, amethopterin, 5-FU, Adriamycin, cyclophosphamide
VAI	vincristine, actinomycin D, ifosfamide
VAIE	vincristine, Adriamycin, ifosfamide, etoposide
VAM	VP-26–213, Adriamycin, methotrexate
VAMP	vincristine, Adriamycin, methotrexate, prednisone
VAMP	vincristine, amethopterin, 6-mercaptopurine, prednisone
VAP	vincristine, Adriamycin, procarbazine
VAP	vincristine, asparaginase, prednisone
VAP-II	vinblastine, actinomycin D, Platinol
VAPEC-B	vincristine, doxorubicin, prednisone, etoposide, cyclophosphamide, bleomycin
VAT	vinblastine, Adriamycin, thiotepa
VAT	vincristine, ara-A, 6-thioguanine
VATD	vincristine, ara-C, 6-thioguanine, daunorubicin
VATH	vinblastine, Adriamycin, thiotepa, Halotestin

VAV	VP-26–213, Adriamycin, vincristine
VB	vinblastine, bleomycin
VBA	vincristine, BCNU, Adriamycin
VBAP	vincristine, BCNU, Adriamycin, prednisone
VBC	VePesid, BCNU, cyclophosphamide
VBC	vinblastine, bleomycin, cisplatin
VBD	vinblastine, bleomycin, DDP
VBM	vincristine, bleomycin, methotrexate
VBMCP	vincristine, BCNU, melphalan, cyclophosphamide, prednisone
VBMF	vincristine, bleomycin, methotrexate, 5-FU
VBP	vinblastine, bleomycin, Platinol
VC	VP-16, carboplatin
VCAP	vincristine, cyclophosphamide, Adriamycin, prednisone
VCAP-I	VP-16, cyclophosphamide, Adriamycin, Platinol
VCAP-III	VP-16–213, cyclophosphamide, Adriamycin, Platinol
VCF	vincristine, cyclophosphamide, 5-FU
VCMP	vincristine, cyclophosphamide, melphalan, prednisone
VCP	vincristine, cyclophosphamide, prednisone
VCP-1	VP-16, cyclophosphamide, Platinol
VDP	vinblastine, dacarbazine, Platinol
VDP	vincristine, daunorubicin, prednisone
VelP	Velban, ifosfamide, Platinol
VEMP	vincristine, Endoxan, 6-mercaptopurine, prednisone
VIC	vinblastine, ifosfamide, CCNU
VIC	VP-16, ifosfamide, carboplatin
VIE	vincristine, ifosfamide, etoposide
VIP	VePesid, ifosfamide, Platinol
VIP-B	VP-16, ifosfamide, Platinol, bleomycin
VLP	vincristine, L-asparaginase, prednisone
VM-26PP	VM-26, procarbazine, prednisone
VMAD	vincristine, methotrexate, Adriamycin, actinomycin D

VMC	VP-16, methotrexate, citrovorum factor
VMCP	vincristine, melphalan, cyclophosphamide, prednisone
VMP	VePesid, mitoxantrone, prednimustine
VOCA	VP-16, Oncovin, cyclophosphamide, prednisone
VOCAP	VP-16–213, Oncovin, cyclophosphamide, Adriamycin, Platinol
VP	vincristine, prednisone
VP+A	vincristine, prednisone, asparaginase
VPB	vinblastine, Platinol, bleomycin
VPBCPr	vincristine, prednisone, vinblastine, chlorambucil, procarbazine
VPCA	vincristine, prednisone, cyclophosphamide, ara-C
VPCMF	vincristine, prednisone, cyclophosphamide, methotrexate, 5-FU
VP-16+DDP	etoposide, cisplatin
VP+L-Asparaginase	vincristine, prednisone, L-asparaginase,
VP-16-P	VP-16, Platinol
VPP	VePesid, Platinol
VPVCP	vincristine, prednisone, vinblastine, chlorambucil, procarbazine

Appendix 6
Cancer Classification/Grading/Staging Systems

American Joint Committee on Cancer (AJCC) (0, I–IV, IA–IIIB)
Ann Arbor staging system (I–IV)
Astler-Coller staging system (A–D, A1–D3)
Bennett classification system for lymphoma
Black nuclear staging system
Boden-Gibb staging system
Bombriski classification system for melanoma
Borrmann classification system for gastric tumors (I–IV, 1–4)
Breslow microstaging system for melanoma
Broder system
Butchart staging system (I–IV, IA, IB)
Chang staging system (T1–T4)
Child-Pugh classification system (A–C)
Children's Cancer Study Group System (CCSG) (I–IVS)
Clark microstaging system (I–V)
Clark-Breslow classification system
Dripps classification system
Dukes classification (A–D)
Dukes-Astler-Coller classification (B2–C2)
Dutch classification of cutaneous T-cell lymphoma
Eastern Cooperative Oncology Group (ECOG) scale (0–4)
Edmondson-Steiner classification system
Enneking staging system for bone (IA–IIIB)
Evans staging system for neuroblastoma (I–IV)
French/American/British (FAB) classification system for hematological
    malignancies (M0-M7, M4E, M5A, M5B)
Goldman classification system for gliomyosarcoma
Goseki grading system for gastric carcinoma
Haggitt classification system for colorectal adenocarcinoma (level 1–4)
Host performance scale (H0–H4)
International Staging System (INSS) for lung cancer (I–IIIB)
International Staging System (INSS) for neuroblastoma (1–4S)
Jass grading system for colorectal malignancies (I–IV)
Jewett classification system for prostatic carcinoma (A–D)
Jewett-Marshall scale (A–D)
Jewett-Strong scale (A1–D)
Karnofsky scale: Criteria of Performance Status (100–0)
Keil classification system for leukemia and lymphoma
Kernohan histologic grading system (1–4)
Lancefield classification system for group A–G and K streptococcus

Lauren classification system for gastric cancer

Linell-Ljungberg classification system for breast carcinoma

Lugano classification system for testicular tumors

Mattson staging system (IA, IB, II–IV)

Mayo grading system (1–3)

M. D. Anderson grading system (1–4)

Ming grading system for gastric cancer

National Cancer Institute-Veterans' Administration (NCI-VA) grading system (1–4)

Page grading system

Radiation Therapy Oncology (RTOG) classification system (stage II–IV, phase I–III, grade 1–5)

Rappaport classification system for lymphoma (also Modified Rappaport classification system) (I–IV)

Ringertz grading system for glial tumors (astrocytoma, anaplastic astrocytoma, and glioblastoma multiforme)

Robson staging system for renal cell carcinoma (I–IV)

Russell classification system for soft tissue sarcomas

Rye classification system for Hodgkin disease (0–IV)

St. Ann-Mayo grading system

TNM staging (T=extent of primary tumor, N=absence or presence and extent of regional lymph node involvement, M=absence or presence of distant metastases)

> TX, T0-T4, T1a-T1c, T4a-T4b
> TX=primary tumor cannot be assessed, T0=no evidence of primary tumor
> Tis=carcinoma in situ
> NX, N0-N3, N1a, N1b, N1bi-iv (1bi-iv refers to size of lymph node metastases)
> MX, M0, M1
> GX–G4=histopathologic grade
> LX, L0–L2=lymphatic invasion
> RX, R0–R2=residual tumor
> VX, V0–V2=venous invasion
> Prefixes under TNM:
> aTNM=classification first determined at autopsy
> cTNM=clinical classification
> (m)=multiple primary
> pTNM=pathologic classification
> r=recurrent tumors, when staged after disease-free interval
> y=classification during or following multinodal therapy

Wolfe breast carcinoma classification

World Health Organization (WHO) classification system for transitional cell carcinoma of the bladder (Ta–T4)

World Health Organization (WHO) classification system for CNS, intracranial, meningioma, astrocytic, lung, GI and liver tumors (grade 1–4)

World Health Organization (WHO) classification system for glial neoplasms (I–XII)

Whitmore-Jewett staging system (A–D)

Working Formulation Equivalent of non-Hodgkin lymphoma (I–IV)

National Cancer Institute (NCI) Comprehensive Cancer Centers

Comprehensive Cancer Center at Wake Forest University
Medical Center Boulevard
Winston-Salem, NC 27157-1082
(910) 716-4606

Dana-Farber Cancer Institute
44 Binney Street
Boston, Ma 02115
(617) 632-3476

Dartmouth-Hitchcock Medical Center
One Medical Center Drive
Lebanon, NH 03756
(603) 650-5527

Duke University Medical Center
Box 3814
Durham, NC 27710
(919) 684-3377

Fox Chase Cancer Center
7701 Burholme Avenue
Philadelphia, PA 19111
(215) 728-2570

Fred Hutchinson Cancer Research Center
1124 Columbia Street
Seattle, WA 98104
(206) 667-5000

Jonsson Comprehensive Cancer Center
University of California at Los Angeles
10920 Wilshire Boulevard, Suite 1010
Los Angeles, CA 90024-6502
(800) 825-2631

Kaplan Cancer Center
New York University Medical Center
550 First Avenue
New York, NY 10016
(212) 263-6485

Lombardi Cancer Research Center
Georgetown University Medical Center
3800 Reservoir Road, NW
Washington, DC 20007
(202)687-2192

Memorial Sloan-Kettering Cancer Center
1275 York Avenue
New York, NY 10021
(800) 525-2225

Meyer L. Prentis Comprehensive Cancer Center of Metropolitan Detroit
110 East Warren Avenue
Detroit, MI 48201
(313) 833-0710

Norris Cotton Cancer Center
Dartmouth-Hitchcock Medical Center
One Medical Center Drive
Lebanon, NH 03756
(603) 650-5527

Roswell Park Cancer Institute
Elm and Carlton Streets
Buffalo, NY 14263
(800) ROSWELL (800) 767-9355)

Ohio State University Comprehensive Cancer Center
Arther G. James Cancer Hospital
300 West 10th Avenue
Columbus, OH 43210
(800) 293-5066
(614) 293-5066

Pittsburgh Cancer Institute
Information & Referral Service
Suite 405, Iroquois Building
3600 Forbes Avenue
Pittsburgh, PA 15213
(800) 537-4063

Sylvester Comprehensive Cancer Center
University of Miami Medical School
1475 Northwest 12th Avenue
Miami, FL 33136
(305) 545-1000

The Johns Hopkins Oncology Center
601 North Caroline Street
Baltimore, MD 21287-0992
(410) 955-8964

The University of Texas M.D. Anderson
Cancer Center
1515 Holcombe Boulevard
Houston, TX 77030
(713) 792-6161

UNC Lineberger Comprehensive Cancer
Center
School of Medicine
Campus Box 7295
University of North Carolina
Chapel Hill, NC 27599-7295
(919) 966-3036

University of Alabama Comprehensive
Cancer Center
Wallace Turner Institute
1824 6th Avenue South
Birmingham, AL 35294-3300
(205) 934-5077

University of Arizona Cancer Center
Department of Hematology/Oncology
1515 North Campbell Avenue
Tucson, AZ 85724
(602) 626-6372

University of Michigan Comprehensive
Cancer Center
101 Simpson Drive
Ann Arbor, MI 48109-0752
(313) 936-9583

University of Pennsylvania Cancer
Center
Penn Tower Hotel, 6th Floor
3400 Spruce Street
Philadelphia, PA 19104
(215) 662-3914

University of Wisconsin Comprehensive
Cancer Center
600 Highland Avenue
Madison, WI 53792
(608) 263-8090

USC/Norris Comprehensive Cancer
Center
University of Southern California
1441 Eastlake Avenue
Los Angeles, CA 90033-0804
(213) 226-2370

Vermont Regional Cancer Center
University Health Center
Associates of Medicine,
Hematology/Oncology
One South Prospect Street
Burlington, VT 05401
(802) 656-4580

Yale University Comprehensive Cancer
Center
333 Cedar Street
New Haven, CT 06520
(203) 785-4095

Courtesy of National Cancer Institute's Cancer Information Service of Maryland, DC, and Northern Virginia. For more information about the National Cancer Institute, call 1-800-4-CANCER